BSAVA Manual of Canine and Feline Endocrinology

Fourth edition

Editors:

Carmel T. Mooney
MVB MPhil PhD DipECVIM-CA MRCVS

Veterinary Clinical Studies Section, School of Veterinary Medicine,
University College Dublin, Belfield, Dublin 4, Republic of Ireland

and

Mark E. Peterson
DVM DipACVIM

Director of Endocrinology and Nuclear Medicine, Animal Endocrine Clinic,
New York, NY 10025, USA

Published by:

British Small Animal Veterinary Association
Woodrow House, 1 Telford Way, Waterwells
Business Park, Quedgeley, Gloucester GL2 2AB

A Company Limited by Guarantee in England.
Registered Company No. 2837793.
Registered as a Charity.

Copyright © 2012 BSAVA
First published 1990
Second edition 1998
Third edition 2004
Fourth edition 2012

A catalogue record for this book is available from the British Library.

ISBN 978-1-905319-28-2

The publishers, editors and contributors cannot take responsibility for information provided on dosages and methods of application of drugs mentioned or referred to in this publication. Details of this kind must be verified in each case by individual users from up to date literature published by the manufacturers or suppliers of those drugs. Veterinary surgeons are reminded that in each case they must follow all appropriate national legislation and regulations (for example, in the United Kingdom, the prescribing cascade) from time to time in force.

Printed by: Replika Press Pvt. Ltd, India
Printed on ECF paper made from sustainable forests

Other titles in the BSAVA Manuals series:

For information on these and all BSAVA publications please visit our website: www.bsava.com

Contents

Contributors

Amanda K. Boag MA VetMB DipACVIM DipACVECC FHEA MRCVS
Clinical Director, Vets Now, Penguin House, Castle Riggs, Dunfermline KY11 8SG

Rosario Cerundolo DVM CertVD DipECVD MRCVS
European and RCVS Recognized Specialist in Veterinary Dermatology
Honorary Associate Professor of Veterinary Dermatology, University of Nottingham
Consultant in Dermatology, Dick White Referrals, Station Farm, London Road,
Six Mile Bottom, Suffolk CB8 0UH

Dennis J. Chew DVM DipACVIM
The Ohio State University College of Veterinary Medicine, Columbus, OH 43210, USA

David B. Church BVSc PhD MACVSc ILTM MRCVS
Professor of Small Animal Studies, Department of Veterinary Clinical Sciences,
The Royal Veterinary College, Hawkshead Lane, North Mymms, Hatfield, Hertfordshire AL9 7TA

Sylvie Daminet DMV PhD DipACVIM DipECVIM-CA
Companion Animal Clinic, University of Ghent, Salisburylane 133, 9820, Belgium

Lucy J. Davison MA VetMB PhD DSAM DipECVIM-CA
The Queen's Veterinary School Hospital, Department of Veterinary Medicine,
University of Cambridge, Madingley Road, Cambridge CB3 0ES

Steve Dodkin BSc MSc
Diagnostic Laboratories, Langford Veterinary Services, University of Bristol, Langford,
Bristol BS40 5DU

Peter A. Graham BVMS PhD CertVR DipECVCP MRCVS
Cambridge Specialist Laboratory Services, Unit 2 Sawston Park, London Road, Pampisford,
Sawston, Cambridgeshire CB22 3EE

Danièlle Gunn-Moore BSc BVM&S PhD FHEA MACVSc MRCVS
RCVS Recognized Specialist in Feline Medicine
Professor of Feline Medicine and Head of Companion Animal Sciences,
Royal (Dick) School of Veterinary Studies, Division of Veterinary Clinical Sciences,
The University of Edinburgh, Hospital for Small Animals, Easter Bush Veterinary Centre,
Roslin, Midlothian EH25 9RG

Andrea M. Harvey BVSc DSAM(Feline) DipECVIM-CA MRCVS
RCVS Recognized Specialist in Feline Medicine
International Society of Feline Medicine, Taeselbury, High Street, Tisbury, Wiltshire SP3 6LD

Michael E. Herrtage MA BVSc DVSc DVR DVD DSAM DipECVIM-CA DipECVDI MRCVS
European and RCVS Recognized Specialist in Veterinary Internal Medicine
Department of Veterinary Medicine, University of Cambridge, Madingley Road, Cambridge CB3 0ES

Peter P. Kintzer DVM DipACVIM
Bost Road Animal Hospital, Springfield, MA 01119, USA

Hans S. Kooistra DVM PhD DipECVIM-CA
Department of Clinical Sciences of Companion Animals, Faculty of Veterinary Medicine,
Utrecht University, Yalelaan 108, 3584 CM, Utrecht, The Netherlands

Carlos Melian DVM PhD
Veterinary Teaching Hospital, Faculty of Veterinary Medicine, University of Las Palmas de Gran
Canaria, Trasmontana s/n, 35416 Arucas, Las Palmas, Gran Canaria, Spain

Carmel T. Mooney MVB MPhil PhD DipECVIM-CA MRCVS
Veterinary Clinical Studies Section, School of Veterinary Medicine, University College Dublin,
Belfield, Dublin 4, Republic of Ireland

Raymond F. Nachreiner DVM PhD
Professor, Endocrine Section, Diagnostic Center for Population and Animal Health,
Michigan State University, 4125 Beaumont Road, Lansing, MI 48910-8104, USA

Rhett Nichols DVM DipACVIM
Antech Diagnostics, Lake Success, New York and Animal Endocrine Clinic,
New York, NY 10025, USA

Stijn J.M. Niessen DVM PhD DipECVIM-CA PGCVetEd FHEA MRCVS
Lecturer, Department of Veterinary Clinical Sciences, The Royal Veterinary College,
Hawkshead Lane, North Mymms, Hatfield, Hertfordshire AL9 7TA and
Research Associate, Diabetes Research Group, Newcastle Medical School,
Framlington Place, Newcastle-upon-Tyne NE2 4HH

Kostas Papasouliotis DVM PhD DipRCPath DipECVCP MRCVS
Diagnostic Laboratories, Langford Veterinary Services and School of Veterinary Sciences,
University of Bristol, Langford, Bristol BS40 5DU

Mark E. Peterson DVM DipACVIM
Director of Endocrinology and Nuclear Medicine, Animal Endocrine Clinic,
New York, NY 10025, USA

Ian K. Ramsey BVSc PhD DSAM DipECVIM-CA FHEA MRCVS
Professor, School of Veterinary Medicine, University of Glasgow, Bearsden Road,
Bearsden, Glasgow G61 1QH

Jacquie Rand BVSc(Hons) MACVS DVSc DipACVIM
Professor of Companion Animal Health and Director, Centre for Companion Animal Health,
School of Veterinary Science, The University of Queensland, St Lucia, QLD 4072, Australia

Nicki Reed BVM&S Cert VR DSAM(Feline) DipECVIM-CA MRCVS
European Veterinary Specialist in Internal Medicine
Lecturer in Companion Animal Medicine, Royal (Dick) School of Veterinary Studies,
The University of Edinburgh, Hospital for Small Animals, Easter Bush Veterinary Centre,
Roslin, Midlothian EH25 9RG

Kent R. Refsal DVM PhD
Professor, Endocrine Section, Diagnostic Center for Population and Animal Health,
Michigan State University, 4125 Beaumont Road, Lansing, MI 48910-8104, USA

Patricia A. Schenck DVM PhD
Section Chief, Endocrine Section, Diagnostic Center for Population and Animal Health,
Michigan State University, 4125 Beaumont Road, Lansing, MI 48910-8104, USA

Johan P. Schoeman BVSc MMedVet PhD DSAM DipECVIM-CA MRCVS
Professor, Small Animal Internal Medicine and Head, Department of Companion Animal Clinical
Studies, Faculty of Veterinary Science, University of Pretoria, Onderstepoort, South Africa

Robert E. Shiel MVB PhD DipECVIM-CA
Section of Small Animal Medicine, School of Veterinary and Biomedical Sciences,
Faculty of Health Sciences, Murdoch University, Murdoch, WA 6150, Australia

Barbara J. Skelly MA VetMB PhD CertSAM DipACVIM DipECVIM MRCVS
Department of Veterinary Medicine, University of Cambridge, Madingley Road,
Cambridge CB3 0ES

Annemarie M.W.Y. Voorbij DVM
Department of Clinical Sciences of Companion Animals, Faculty of Veterinary Medicine,
Utrecht University, Yalelaan 108, 3584 CM, Utrecht, The Netherlands

Foreword

The field of small animal endocrinology has expanded significantly over the last 20 years. Since publication of the third edition of the *BSAVA Manual of Canine and Feline Endocrinology* (2004) there have been further important advances in knowledge of the discipline. In particular, the diagnosis and treatment of some endocrine disorders now warrant more detailed information and discussion.

The editors, Carmel Mooney and Mark Peterson, are to be congratulated on the format and content of this fourth edition of the Manual. The impressive international author list features well known veterinarians working in the field of endocrinology, all of whom bring significant experience and a practical approach to the chapters of this Manual. The book provides an excellent resource for both practising veterinarians and veterinary students to update their knowledge. More experienced specialist readers will also find the content valuable and easy to navigate. In its 300 pages, the Manual contains illustrations, tables and algorithms to assist understanding and allow easy access to information. The first section addresses hormone assays, sample collection and the principles of interpretation of test results. Subsequent chapters on each endocrine gland are complemented by chapters on presenting complaints and their investigation.

This Manual should be on the bookshelf of every small animal clinic and veterinary hospital. The information it provides can be easily applied to the clinical diagnosis and treatment of endocrine diseases for the benefit of animal patients and their owners.

Boyd R. Jones BVSc FACVSc DipECVIM-CA MRCVS
Emeritus Professor, Small Animal Clinical Studies,
University College Dublin, Republic of Ireland
Adjunct Professor of Companion Animal Medicine,
Massey University, New Zealand

Preface

This is the fourth edition of the *BSAVA Manual of Canine and Feline Endocrinology*. In introducing the third edition in 2004, the unprecedented advances in diagnostic tests and therapies were highlighted. Surprisingly, another 6 years on the advance in these and other areas has continued unabated. For example: disorders once considered rare, such as Conn's disease, are now investigated more readily and consequently encountered more frequently; the management of diabetic cats has moved from palliation to achieving remission; and, significantly, the genetic risks associated with many disorders have been elucidated.

There has been a change in the format of the Manual to provide easier access to relevant information. The first chapter deals with the type of assays used for hormone measurement and the collection and storage of samples and how this may influence the results obtained. The second chapter represents a new and exciting venture, outlining the principles for interpreting endocrine test results and introduces the reader to assessment of test performance and how to improve our diagnostic confidence.

The following 17 chapters follow a traditional route, describing disorders associated with each major endocrine gland. Where applicable, chapters outlining feline and canine disorders are divided. The final 9 chapters provide information on solving both clinical and clinicopathological abnormalities for which endocrine disorders are a major consideration.

As Editors we have been privileged to work with an internationally renowned panel of experts in their field. Our authors emanate from most corners of the world and have shown true dedication in contributing to this work. Endocrine diseases may vary in prevalence from place to place but essentially require the same diagnostic tests and treatments, whatever their geographical location. As a consequence, treatments that may not be available worldwide are highlighted where applicable, maintaining the international appeal of the Manual.

This new edition of the *BSAVA Manual of Canine and Feline Endocrinology* has been a long time hatching but each chapter provides the reader with the most up-to-date information available. It is a valuable resource not only to those with a specific interest in small animal endocrinology but to all other general practitioners, veterinary nurses and technicians and to undergraduate veterinary students. We hope that it is a worthwhile addition to the practice library.

Carmel T. Mooney
Mark E. Peterson
December 2011

Whatever the future holds, be with the BSAVA

Membership plans to suit every stage of your veterinary career.

Members of the BSAVA receive a wide range of benefits to support them during their professional life.

- Subsidised CPD
- Postgraduate Certificates
- *BSAVA Small Animal Formulary* – print, online & Smartphone app
- *BSAVA Guide to Procedures in Small Animal Practice* – online & Smartphone app
- *BSAVA/VPIS Poisons Triage Tool* – online and **new printed booklet for members renewing for 2012**
- Congress registration discount
- Congress podcasts
- Discount on BSAVA manuals
- Subscriptions to JSAP and **companion**
- Access to exclusive online resources

Join online at **www.bsava.com** or call 01452 726700

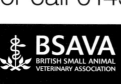 **BSAVA** BRITISH SMALL ANIMAL VETERINARY ASSOCIATION   **Follow BSAVA** www.facebook.com/thebsava www.twitter.com/thebsava

Hormone assays and collection of samples

Kent R. Refsal and Raymond F. Nachreiner

Introduction

Veterinary endocrine laboratories have recently faced challenges from the loss of commercial assay methods that were known to work well for samples from animal species. Several assays previously used in published veterinary studies, including immunoradiometric assays for endogenous adreno-corticotropic hormone (ACTH) and intact para-thyroid hormone (PTH), are no longer available. In addition, other radioiodine-based immunoassays have been discontinued in favour of automated chemiluminescence-based assay systems. There is uncertainty as to whether the performance of some of these assays, developed for humans, will be similar for samples from dogs and cats. This chapter provides an overview of assay methods currently used or available for companion animal diagnostics, and summarizes the recommended procedures for sample collection and handling.

Hormone assays

Competitive immunoassays

Principle
Competitive immunoassays involve mixing a patient sample containing an unknown concentration of endogenous hormone with a known standard quantity of labelled hormone, in the presence of an antibody specific for that hormone. The assay is based on the premise that the antibody has equal binding affinity for the endogenous unlabelled hormone and the labelled hormone. After sufficient incubation time has passed the hormone–antibody binding reaches equilibrium. The amount of labelled hormone bound to the antibody is inversely proportional to the concentration of unlabelled hormone in the sample (Figure 1.1).

A separation step is required to isolate the hormone bound to the assay antibody.

- A common technique employs tubes where the assay antibody is coated on to the inner surface of the bottom of a test tube. The antibody-bound hormone (labelled and unlabelled) is then isolated when the supernatant is poured out of the tube.

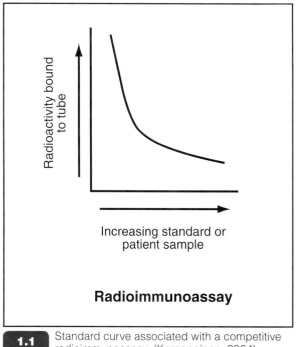

Radioimmunoassay

1.1 Standard curve associated with a competitive radioimmunoassay. (Kemppainen, 2004)

- If the assay antibody is added in solution, a common separation method employs the addition of a second antibody, raised against the IgG of the species in which the assay antibody was produced. The second antibody reagent may also contain an agent such as polyethylene glycol, to promote precipitation. After incubation and centrifugation, the large complexes of anti-hormone–anti-IgG form a pellet at the bottom of the tube. The supernatant containing the unbound hormone is poured off, taking care to leave the pellet intact.

Data obtained from assays performed on samples containing known quantities of hormone are used to plot a standard curve. Curve-fitting calculations are used to define a mathematical relation between the percentage of antibody-bound labelled hormone and the concentration of unlabelled hormone in a sample. A computer data reduction program can then be used to calculate the concentration of hormone in the patient sample.

A competitive immunoassay is well suited for hormones that are easily available or synthesized, so that there is a ready source of labelled hormone (ligand or tracer) for use in assays and for generating standard curves. This type of immunoassay has been the mainstay in veterinary diagnostics for measurement of thyroid hormones, steroid hormones, metabolites of vitamin D, and some peptide hormones such as insulin, gastrin, and insulin-like growth factor 1 (IGF-1).

Labelling options

Over the past 40 years, the radioimmunoassay (RIA) has been the most commonly used competitive immunoassay, with ^{125}I being the predominant isotope used to label hormones. A laboratory equipped with a gamma counter and data reduction programs can use RIA kits from different manufacturers or can develop in-house assays. Most commercial RIA kits are manufactured for diagnostic application in humans. In some instances, the hormone concentrations are higher than in animal species (e.g. total thyroxine (T4) and cortisol) and slight modifications of the kit protocol (e.g. extension of the incubation time for hormone and assay antibody, increased volume of standard and sample, and addition of a lower standard to the curve) are necessary to improve the performance for veterinary samples.

Disadvantages of RIA include:

- Relatively short shelf-life of the radioligand (approximately 2 months)
- Cost of disposal of radioactive waste
- Need to perform laboratory surveys to ensure against accidental contamination of personnel and the environment.

Hormones being used as ligands may also be labelled with enzymes that catalyse colour change or with compounds that produce fluorescence or chemiluminescent signals when a substrate is added to the antibody-bound fraction of hormone. These assays have the advantages of a longer shelf-life and easier disposal of waste materials. Commercially available chemiluminescent assays are developed around manufacturer-specific automated instruments, which perform all the assay steps. However, these automated systems may not be as amenable to modification of the assay procedures as RIAs.

A study comparing methods for cortisol measurement demonstrated that RIAs were better able to distinguish very low from low-normal cortisol concentrations than was a chemiluminescent immunoassay (Russell *et al.*, 2007). Comparison of commercially available RIAs, a chemiluminescent enzyme immunoassay, and an enzyme-linked immunoassay (for in-clinic use) for measurement of total T4 depicted similar performance in samples from dogs and cats (Kemppainen and Birchfield, 2006).

Immunometric assays

Principle

This type of immunoassay relies on separate antibodies that bind to different specific segments of the hormone to be measured. A capture antibody is coated on the wall of a tube, or microtitre plate, or on a bead placed in a tube. The second antibody is labelled, usually with ^{125}I or an enzyme that provides a means of detection. The samples and reagents are combined for the time necessary to achieve full binding of the hormone and antibodies. At the end of the incubation period the supernatant is decanted or aspirated to remove labelled antibody that is not bound to the hormone. A wash step is employed for maximum removal of the unbound labelled antibody. In assays using a non-isotopic detection system, the substrate is then added.

This type of assay detects hormone that is captured between both antibodies. The amount of radioiodine, colour intensity or chemiluminescent signal is directly proportional to the concentration of hormone in the standards or unknown sample (Figure 1.2). A standard curve is included in each assay run and the concentration of hormone in

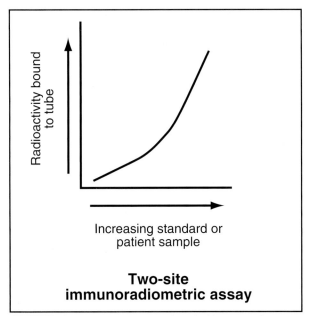

Two-site immunoradiometric assay

1.2 Standard curve associated with a two-site immunoradiometric assay. (Kemppainen, 2004)

unknown samples is determined using curve-fitting calculations. An advantage of this type of assay is the measurement of biologically active hormone without cross-reactivity of inactive fragments, which may also be bound in a competitive assay utilizing one antibody.

Applications

The first reported use of commercial immunoradiometric assays in veterinary diagnostics involved the human intact PTH (Torrance and Nachreiner, 1989) and ACTH (Randolph et al., 1998) assays. Today, the canine thyroid-stimulating hormone (TSH; thyrotropin) immunometric assay, available in both radioiodine and chemiluminescent forms, is almost universally used in veterinary laboratories (see Chapter 9). There is some evidence of cross-reactivity with feline TSH and therefore possibility of its use for diagnosing feline hyper- and hypothyroidism (see Chapters 10 and 11). An enzyme-linked immunometric assay for canine TSH has just been announced (www.oxfordlabs.com). At present, there are no published data comparing this with other available methods. There are also commercial enzyme-linked immunometric assays for insulin, which utilize different combinations of antibodies and reagents intended to optimize standard curves for dogs and cats (www.mercodia.com). Numerical results from immunometric assays may differ, depending on the specificity of the antibodies and the nature of hormone production and metabolism. An example can be seen with whole PTH and intact PTH immunoradiometric assays.

Parathyroid hormone: The intact PTH assay, which first appeared in the late 1980s, was developed around a capture antibody against the C-terminal of PTH and a detection (labelled) antibody against PTH 1–34. In the ensuing years, truncated forms of PTH (PTH 7–84) were discovered that are actively secreted by the parathyroid glands and not products of degradation (Friedman and Goodman, 2006). It was soon recognized that some of these truncated products cross-react in intact PTH assays. Eventually, antibodies against PTH 1–4 were developed for use as detection antibodies. The whole PTH assay utilizes a detection antibody against PTH 1–4 compared with the intact PTH assay that employs an antibody against PTH 1–34. Both assays utilize a capture antibody against PTH 39–84. In dogs, results from both PTH assays are positively correlated, but are higher with the intact PTH assay (Estepa *et al.*, 2003), presumably because this also measures the 7–84 PTH fragment produced by the parathyroid glands. Initially, PTH 7–84 was considered to be inactive, but there is now evidence that it may antagonize actions of PTH 1–84 (Friedman and Goodman, 2006). If production of PTH 7–84 is incrementally higher in states of secondary hyperparathyroidism, the whole PTH assay would, in theory, give the best estimate of production of the biologically active hormone, but the intact PTH assay may provide a better means of distinguishing baseline from increased parathyroid gland function. This may be of particular relevance in the cat, where normal baseline concentrations of PTH are lower than in dogs.

The majority of case reports, clinical studies and experimental studies containing intact PTH results in dogs and cats have utilized immunoradiometric (radioiodine based) assays. More recently, there have been several studies in dogs using a chemiluminescent immunometric assay to quantify intact PTH (Ham *et al.*, 2009; Cortadellas *et al.*, 2010). In the clinical study by Ham *et al.*, paired results of intact PTH assays were compared using

an immunoradiometric assay; numerically lower values were reported with the chemiluminescent assay, but there was a high correlation of results between the two assay methods. To date, use of the chemiluminescent intact PTH assay has not been reported in cats.

Assays for free thyroxine
In a competitive immunoassay for total T4, a chemical is included in the assay reagents to dissociate T4 from its binding proteins in the serum. This allows direct competition between unlabelled and labelled T4 in binding to the assay antibody. A similar straightforward approach cannot be used for estimation of free T4, as there is also binding of labelled hormone to thyroid-binding proteins in the serum. The challenge in measurement of free T4 by immunoassay is to isolate the hormone–antibody reaction from the effects of binding proteins in the serum.

Measurement of free T4 by equilibrium dialysis has been regarded as the 'gold standard' for laboratory assessment. In the commercially available kit, a dialysis membrane separates an aliquot of serum from an assay buffer solution. Over time, free T4 diffuses across the membrane. When the distribution of free T4 between the two compartments reaches equilibrium (overnight duration), an aliquot of the assay buffer is used to measure T4 concentration; this is done using a sensitive competitive assay.

In an attempt to simplify assay procedures, direct serum-free T4 assays were developed for human diagnostics. One approach involves synthesizing T4 analogues with a decreased affinity for serum-binding proteins and performing a competitive immunoassay using the analogue as the labelled hormone. Another approach is the so-called two-step assay, where serum is pipetted into a tube coated with T4 antibody. In a short, precisely timed, incubation, free T4 in the sample begins to bind to the assay antibody and the serum is poured out of the assay tube. A longer first incubation would begin to strip T4 from serum-binding proteins and invalidate the assay as a free fraction assay. The solution of labelled T4 is then added to bind to antibody not already occupied by endogenous T4 in the sample.

Results from five different commercially available free T4 analogue assays have been compared with equilibrium dialysis using samples from healthy dogs, hypothyroid dogs, and dogs with non-thyroidal illness (Schachter *et al.*, 2004). All the assays were generally good at distinguishing reference interval concentrations of free T4 in healthy dogs from low values in hypothyroid dogs. However, the analogue assays could not distinguish sick euthyroid from hypothyroid dogs as reliably as the equilibrium dialysis assay. Most veterinary clinical studies reporting free T4 results in dogs and cats have determined free T4 by equilibrium dialysis and, whilst the manufacturers have recently changed, similar results are produced. A commercial solid-phase chemiluminescent canine free T4 analogue immunoassay has been recently introduced (Immulite, Siemens Medical Solutions Diagnostics). To date, there are no peer-reviewed published reports comparing the performance of the contemporary equilibrium dialysis free T4 assay with the two-step radioimmunoassay or the analogue free T4 chemiluminescent immunoassays used by veterinary laboratories.

Liquid chromatography–mass spectrometry

At the risk of oversimplification, the liquid chromatography–mass spectrometry (LCMS) analytical technique isolates and quantifies single or multiple analytes in a sample, based on the molecular weight, structure and properties of ionization when impacted by an electron beam. Advances in sample preparation (serum or urine), instrumentation and tools for data analysis have resulted in widespread utilization of LCMS in research and clinical diagnostics. In human medicine LCMS is widely used in the assessment of disorders of steroidogenesis and offers the advantages of high sensitivity, better specificity than immunoassays and the ability to measure multiple steroids simultaneously (Shackleton, 2010). LCMS has been particularly useful in defining the site of enzyme deficiency in the many manifestations of congenital adrenal hyperplasia in humans. Human laboratories that offer testing for a wide array of corticosteroids have been used by veterinary surgeons to identify congenital adrenal hyperplasia and to define unusual patterns of steroid production by adrenal tumours (Reine et al., 1999; Knighton, 2004). If this type of testing is to be undertaken in the future, it is likely that the results will be determined using LCMS technology.

Similar techniques using high-powered liquid chromatography (HPLC) and electrochemical detection have application in the measurement of multiple catecholamines and their metabolites, and have been used for the assessment of phaeochromocytoma in dogs (Kook et al., 2010). In assessment of vitamin D status, LCMS offers advantages in its ability to detect multiple metabolites (those in nmol/l and pmol/l concentrations), and distinguish the D2 from D3 forms. In RIAs for 25-hydroxycholecalciferol (25(OH)-vitamin D; calcidiol), there is similar antibody cross-reactivity with D2 and D3 forms of this metabolite. More recently, LCMS has been used to quantify concentrations of free T4 and triiodothyronine (T3) in human serum (Gu et al., 2007).

Assay validation

Several features of assay performance must be considered when evaluating the utility of an assay for research or clinical applications. Most comments here are directed to immunoassays, but there is general relevance for LCMS methods.

Specificity

To ensure each assay is measuring what is intended, serum samples are 'spiked' with varying known quantities of other similar hormones or relevant substances. Results from the serum sample, with and without added hormone, are compared to see whether the addition of another hormone increases the measured value. Specificity data are presented as percentage cross-reactivity and are typically provided by the assay manufacturer. An example of clinical relevance is the >30% cross-reactivity of prednisolone in competitive immunoassays for cortisol. Thus, if a sample intended for measurement of cortisol is collected within 12 hours of administration of prednisolone (or perhaps longer, depending on the dose), the test result obtained will be a summation of cortisol and prednisolone cross-reacting in the assay and not an accurate reflection of the concentration of cortisol. For example, if there is 100 nmol/l of prednisolone in the circulation at the time of sampling, the result of the cortisol assay would be increased by >30 nmol/l.

Accuracy

If a known quantity of the hormone to be measured is added to a sample, it is important to know how much is detected in the assay. This endpoint is often not optimally assessed, as there may not be a source of purified hormone from the species of interest.

Parallelism

In addition to the specificity of an assay antibody, the binding of the antibody with the hormone may be influenced by other components in the sample, referred to as the 'matrix' effect. In commercial assays the standard curve usually has components of human serum and it is important to know whether dilutions of a veterinary sample will yield expected results that parallel the standard curve.

Sensitivity

An immunoassay has a finite limit of detection, based on the relative amounts of antibody used in the assay. The lower limit of detection can be assessed by different methods, including the calculated result that is two standard deviations from the mean of several total binding (0 standard) tubes. Another example is the point on the standard curve that is 10% from total binding. The upper limit of detection can be assessed by adding hormone to samples and identifying the value where measured and known amounts diverge. Expansion of the upper limit of detection can be accomplished by dilution of the sample and adjusting the result by the dilution factor.

Precision

There is the need for assurance that results are similar in repeat assays of the same sample, both within and between assay runs. Ideally, this is done with at least two samples or pools, representing values at the low, middle or high end of the range of values observed in the species. Repeatability is often expressed as the coefficient of variation of repeat assays (standard deviation/mean).

Physiological responses and clinical confirmation

Another important aspect of assay validation is whether hormone results change appropriately in response to physiological stimuli, or correlate with the clinical diagnosis by independent confirmation.

An example of an appropriate response to a physiological stimulus in dogs is in the demonstration of a decrease in PTH with infusion of calcium and a compensatory increase of PTH when ionized calcium is decreased by infusion of EDTA (Estepa *et al.*, 2003). In the authors' laboratory, identification of a high concentration of TSH with the canine immunoradiometric assay in a cat with very low concentrations of thyroid hormones, due to treatment with methimazole, provided evidence that the canine assay may be suitable for cats.

Pronounced elevations of glucagon using commercial human assays have been reported in dogs with a confirmed diagnosis of glucagonoma (Cave *et al.*, 2007; Mizuno *et al.*, 2009). The correlation of a test result with the clinical diagnosis may be the first recognition that an assay is suitable in a particular species, which would then prompt efforts to pursue the other analytical steps detailed above.

Sometimes, the challenge is to obtain samples suitable to meet the needs for assay validation. For example, if results from healthy animals are at the low end of the detection range of an assay, it may be difficult to obtain a sufficient volume of serum from clinical cases with high concentrations or situations of physiological stimulus to assess dilutional parallelism.

Optimal assessment of assay performance also includes screening for potentially interfering substances, including icterus, haemolysis and lipaemia.

Sample collection and handling

To obtain the best diagnostic information from endocrine assays, veterinary surgeons and hospital staff must be aware of factors in sample type and condition, handling, and storage that may affect the assays used by the laboratory. A general summary of sample requirements for commonly requested assays is provided in Figure 1.3. Clinicians are advised to contact the laboratory if questions arise as to specimen type, sample handling and shipment.

Analyte	Sample type	Handling considerations	Interfering factors	Comments from human assays
Adrenocorticotropic hormone	EDTA plasma	Collect blood in siliconized glass or plastic tubes. Centrifuge as soon as possible. Transfer plasma to plastic tube. Freeze for prolonged storage. Avoid repeated freeze–thaw cycles. Protease inhibitors help preservation. Must ship by overnight express. Must be cold on arrival at laboratory	Lipaemia	
Aldosterone	Serum or EDTA/heparinized plasma		None listed	EDTA yields results 15% higher. Stable for 7 days at 2–8°C
Cortisol	Serum or EDTA/heparinized plasma	Slight degradation at 72 hours at >20°C	None listed	Avoid repeated freeze–thaw cycles
1,25-Dihydroxycholecalciferol (1,25(OH)$_2$-vitamin D)	Serum or EDTA plasma		Not tested	
Gastrin	Serum only	Ship on frozen gel packs	None listed	Lipaemia/haemolysis interfere. Freeze for prolonged storage. Ship frozen
Growth hormone	EDTA plasma	Freeze for transport. Ship express in frozen gel packs		
25-Hydroxycholecalciferol (25(OH)-vitamin D)	Serum or EDTA/heparinized plasma	Stable in separated serum	Not tested	
Insulin	Serum or EDTA/heparinized plasma	Serious degradation at >4°C. Refrigerate or freeze. Ship on frozen gel packs for <72 hours. Haemolysis speeds degradation	Lipaemia, haemolysis	Serum yields approximately 9% higher
Insulin-like growth factor-1	Serum or EDTA/heparinized plasma	Quite stable during shipment	None listed	For chemiluminescent assay avoid EDTA/heparinized plasma. Avoid repeated freeze–thaw cycles
Parathyroid hormone	Serum or EDTA/heparinized plasma	Significant degradation at >20°C. Ship on frozen gel packs by overnight express. Protease inhibitors help but 4°C best	None listed	Avoid repeated freeze–thaw cycles. Stability may be enhanced in EDTA

1.3 Handling suggestions for hormones and hormone-related analytes. (continues) ▶

Analyte	Sample type	Handling considerations	Interfering factors	Comments from human assays
Parathyroid hormone-related protein	EDTA plasma	Significant degradation at >20°C. Ship on frozen gel packs by overnight express	Not tested	Centrifuge within 2 hours. Freeze if stored >4 hours
Progesterone	Serum or EDTA/ heparinized plasma	Avoid separator gel tubes. Quite stable in separated serum	Assess parallelism in direct serum assays	Avoid repeated freeze–thaw cycles
Renin	EDTA plasma	Pre-chilled blood collection tubes. Add aprotinin. Centrifuge in refrigerated centrifuge. Freeze and store in plastic tubes. Ship frozen on dry ice. Must remain frozen until assay	None listed	Avoid heparin
Testosterone	Serum or heparinized plasma	Stable at 20°C in separated serum Freeze for prolonged serum	Assess parallelism in direct serum assays	EDTA plasma approximately 10% lower
Thyroxine, total	Serum	Stable in separated serum for 7 days at room temperature. Freeze for longer storage	None listed	Avoid EDTA or citrate plasma. Avoid repeated freeze–thaw cycles
Free thyroxine, equilibrium dialysis	Serum	Stable in separated serum for 5 days at ≤20°C. More than 50% increase after 5 days at ≤37°C	Avoid severe lipaemia (false increases)	
Free thyroxine, 2-step RIA	Serum	Stable in separated serum for 5 days at ≤20°C. More than 50% increase after 5 days at ≤37°C	Not tested	Avoid EDTA or citrate plasma. Gross lipaemia interferes. Avoid sample agitation
Triiodothyronine, total	Serum	Less stable than thyroxine at 20°C	Avoid severe lipaemia	
Thyroglobulin autoantibody	Serum or blood spot	Stable at room temperature. Blood spot must remain dry	None listed	Avoid gross haemolysis/ lipaemia and hyperbilirubinaemia for chemiluminescence. Avoid freeze–thaw cycles
Thyroid-stimulating hormone	Serum	Stable at room temperature. Freeze for long storage. Stable with freeze–thaw cycles	None listed	Avoid gross haemolysis/ lipaemia for chemiluminescence
Vasopressin	EDTA plasma	Pre-chilled blood collection tubes. Add aprotinin. Centrifuge in refrigerated centrifuge. Freeze and store in plastic tubes. Ship frozen on dry ice	Not tested	Avoid platelets

1.3 (continued) Handling suggestions for hormones and hormone-related analytes.

Sample type and condition

Some hormones can be measured in either serum or plasma. However, some tests require serum only or a specific type of plasma. After collection and centrifugation, it is safest to transfer the serum or plasma into a plain tube for shipment to the laboratory. As a general rule, serum is the preferred sample for tests related to assessment of thyroid status, and is specifically required for free T4 assays. Good quality serum or plasma is typically suitable for assays of steroids.

Manufacturers of kits for the following assays typically specify EDTA plasma:

- ACTH
- Growth hormone
- Antidiuretic hormone (vasopressin)
- Parathyroid hormone-related protein
- Plasma renin activity.

Most immunoassays are resistant to interference from mild haemolysis or lipaemia. However, if there are severe changes in the sample, there is concern that altered matrix effects will alter binding of the hormone and antibody. There are occasional instances of lipaemic sera showing pronounced, and seemingly spurious, elevations of free T4 when measured by equilibrium dialysis. The result is repeatable on the original sample but typically not duplicated when a less lipaemic follow-up sample is assayed. It is suspected that this change occurs as a result of *in vitro* metabolism of triglycerides to non-esterified fatty acids, which, in turn, displace T4 from the binding proteins.

Collection tubes

Contemporary sample collection tubes are made from either plastic or glass, sealed with a vacuum, and may also contain several additional substances. The inner wall of the tube may be coated with a surfactant, to prevent adhesion of red blood cells, and there may or may not be silica as a clot activator. There is a stopper lubricant to maintain the vacuum seal and allow ease of removal. A serum tube may contain a separator gel. In one study of human samples using an automated chemiluminescent technique, T3 values differed depending on the type of sample tube used, with higher values resulting from samples placed in serum separator tubes (Bowen *et al.*, 2007). Although published data are limited, it is recognized that significant decreases of progesterone in canine serum occur from prolonged contact (e.g. overnight) with separator gel. The decrease may be of sufficient magnitude to alter prediction of the time of breeding. It is presumed that the progesterone is absorbed by the gel.

Limited studies of other hormones in the authors' laboratory have shown no difference in results from samples divided between plain tubes and those with separator gels, using RIAs or immunoradiometric assays. The comparisons were made on freshly collected samples, where the serum was removed from collection tubes immediately following centrifugation. There is a need for a systematic study comparing hormone assay results from different collection tubes in different assay systems.

References and further reading

Bowen RAR, Vu C, Remaley AT, Hortin GL and Csako G (2007) Differential effect of blood collection tubes on total free fatty acids (FFA) and total triiodothyronine (TT3) concentration: a model for studying interference from tube constituents. *Clinica Chimica Acta* **378**, 181–193

Cave TA, Evans H, Hargreaves J and Blunden AS (2007) Metabolic epidermal necrosis in a dog associated with pancreatic adenocarcinoma, hyperglucagonaemia, hyperinsulinaemia and hypoaminoacidaemia. *Journal of Small Animal Practice* **48**, 522–526

Cortadellas O, Fernandez del Palacio MJ, Talavera J and Bayon A (2010) Calcium and phosphorus homeostasis in dogs with spontaneous chronic kidney disease at different stages of severity. *Journal of Veterinary Internal Medicine* **24**, 73–79

Estepa JC, Lopez I, Felsenfeld AJ *et al.* (2003) Dynamics of secretion and metabolism of PTH during hypo- and hypercalcemia in the dog as determined by the 'intact' and 'whole' PTH assays. *Nephrology Dialysis Transplantation* **18**, 1101–1107

Friedman PA and Goodman WG (2006) PTH(1-84)/PTH(7-84): a balance of power. *American Journal of Physiology – Renal Physiology* **290**, 975–984

Gu J, Soldin OP and Soldin SJ (2007) Simultaneous quantification of free triiodothyronine and free thyroxine by isotope dilution tandem mass spectrometry. *Clinical Biochemistry* **40**, 1386–1391

Ham K, Greenfield CL, Barger A *et al.* (2009) Validation of a rapid parathyroid hormone assay and intraoperative measurement of parathyroid hormone in dogs with benign naturally occurring primary hyperparathyroidism. *Veterinary Surgery* **38**, 122–132

Kemppainen RJ (2004) Hormone assays. In: *BSAVA Manual of Canine and Feline Endocrinology, 3rd edn*, ed. CT Mooney and ME Peterson, pp. 6–10. BSAVA Publications, Gloucester

Kemppainen RJ and Birchfield JR (2006) Measurement of total thyroxine concentration in serum from dogs and cats by use of various methods. *American Journal of Veterinary Research* **67**, 259–265

Knighton EL (2004) Congenital adrenal hyperplasia secondary to 11-beta-hydroxylase deficiency in a domestic cat. *Journal of the American Veterinary Medical Association* **225**, 238–241

Kook PH, Grest P, Quante S, Boretti FS and Reusch CE (2010) Urinary catecholamines and metadrenaline to creatinine ratios in dogs with a phaeochromocytoma. *Veterinary Record* **166**, 169–174

Mizuno T, Hiraoka H, Yoshioka C et al. (2009) Superficial necrolytic dermatitis associated with extrapancreatic glucagonoma in a dog. *Veterinary Dermatology* **20**, 72–79

Randolph JF, Toomey J, Center SA *et al.* (1998) Use of the urine cortisol-to-creatinine ratio for monitoring dogs with pituitary-dependent hyperadrenocorticism during induction treatment with mitotane (o,p'-DDD). *American Journal of Veterinary Research* **59**, 258–261

Reine NJ, Hohenhaus AE, Peterson ME and Patnaik AK (1999) Deoxycorticosterone-secreting adrenocortical carcinoma in a dog. *Journal of Veterinary Internal Medicine* **13**, 386–390

Russell NJ, Foster S, Clark P *et al.* (2007) Comparison of radioimmunoassay and chemiluminescent assay methods to estimate canine blood cortisol concentrations. *Australian Veterinary Journal* **85**, 487–494

Schachter S, Nelson RW, Scott-Moncrieff C *et al.* (2004) Comparison of serum-free thyroxine concentrations determined by standard equilibrium dialysis, modified equilibrium dialysis and 5 radioimmunoassays in dogs. *Journal of Veterinary Internal Medicine* **18**, 259–264

Shackleton C (2010) Clinical steroid mass spectrometry: a 45-year history culminating in HPLC-MS/MS becoming an essential tool for patient diagnosis. *Journal of Steroid Biochemistry and Molecular Biology* **121**, 481–490

Torrance AG and Nachreiner R (1989) Intact parathyroid hormone assay and total calcium concentrations in the diagnosis of disorders of calcium metabolism in dogs. *Journal of Veterinary Internal Medicine* **3**, 86–89

2

Principles of interpreting endocrine test results

Peter A. Graham

General guidelines

The interpretation of endocrine test results is often viewed as daunting. To a large extent, this is because the endocrine system is extremely dynamic in its response to both external and internal challenges. Consequently, a wide range of possible laboratory test results may be physiologically appropriate but can be difficult to distinguish from those found in truly pathological states.

There is a fine line dividing 'normal' physiology from 'abnormal' pathology, and it may not always be possible to classify all endocrine test results simplistically into these two categories. However, in some circumstances, endocrine test results can be confidently classified into positive or negative categories, with little overlap between the two. For the practising veterinary surgeon, it is important to know which results to place confidence in and which to be cautious of. Such confidence develops from:

- Knowing the physiology of the endocrine system
- Appreciating the influence of other endocrine organs and non-endocrine illnesses
- Understanding the diagnostic performance properties of the tests used.

In some circumstances test results simply reinforce a diagnosis of endocrine disease already made by judgement. In other circumstances the test results help provide a definitive diagnosis. The skill in interpretation is knowing which judgements provide a satisfactory diagnosis and which may need revisiting in an individual patient as events unfold.

Often, the presence or absence of disease in an organ system is determined based on whether an individual measurement falls within or outside a given reference interval. However, in many endocrine disorders a particular test result may remain within its reference interval but still provide strong evidence for the presence or classification of disease. The key to interpreting results in these circumstances is recollection of, and reliance upon, the concept of **negative feedback**, which is a primary rule of endocrinology. Remembering this rule helps the clinician to understand endocrine test results in specific circumstances, eases interpretation, and allows the distinction between physiologically appropriate responses and pathology. Armed with a knowledge of the principles of negative feedback, it is possible, amongst other examples, to interpret reference interval parathyroid hormone (PTH) results in canine hypercalcaemia, to classify pituitary-dependent hyperadrenocorticism (HAC), and to understand why a low-dose dexamethasone suppression (LDDS) test can be immediately followed by an adrenocorticotropic hormone (ACTH) response test, but not vice versa.

Diagnostic test performance

As described above, there can be considerable overlap in endocrine test results for disorders arising from physiological and pathological responses. As a consequence, many of the hormone concentrations measured for investigating endocrine disease provide less than perfect diagnostic performance. For example, the hypothalamic–pituitary–adrenal response to stress and other illness is frequently associated with test results expected in canine HAC, resulting in poor diagnostic specificity (many false positives). Similarly, the total thyroxine (T4) response to non-thyroidal illness makes this individual measurement poorly specific for canine hypothyroidism.

Diagnostic sensitivity and specificity
Once the *analytical* performance (see Chapter 1) of a laboratory test has been established or an appropriate response to a dynamic endocrine test has been determined, the next step is to determine a test's *diagnostic* performance. This provides information on how well the test distinguishes the presence of a given disease from its absence.

To assess diagnostic performance, dichotomized outcomes are generally used, i.e. the test result is either positive or negative, and the pathological condition or disease is either present or absent. However, while this is the best understood and most commonly used approach, it is a system of two extremes (not diseased or diseased). It does not allow for 'grey area' results, nor does it take into account the varying degrees of pathology that are often a feature of endocrine disorders, particularly those that take time to develop.

Diagnostic sensitivity
The diagnostic sensitivity (not to be confused with analytical sensitivity) is the proportion of patients

with the disease that are correctly identified by the test. The derivation of this proportion requires a diseased population of reasonable size that has been well characterized as having the disorder, usually by an independent and gold-standard diagnostic method or technique.

Dixon and Mooney (1999) derived the diagnostic sensitivity of free T4 by equilibrium dialysis (fT4d) by measuring it in 30 dogs confirmed as hypothyroid using thyroid-stimulating hormone (TSH) response test results. Of these 30 dogs, 24 yielded fT4d results below a diagnostic cut-off of 5.42 pmol/l.

Diagnostic sensitivity = 24/30 = 0.80 (80%)

Because this attribute is a proportion based on a sample, confidence intervals for the population proportion can be estimated as ± 1.96 x estimated standard error of the proportion.

95% confidence limits for sensitivity = sensitivity ± 1.96 x √ [sensitivity x (1 – sensitivity) / n]

Consequently, the larger the size of the diseased study group, the narrower the confidence intervals will be and, therefore, the more reliable the estimated sensitivity. Diagnostic sensitivity studies based on a small number of animals will generate very wide confidence intervals, meaning that they are a less reliable source of sensitivity than studies based on larger numbers. In the above example, the 95% confidence interval ranged from 0.61 (61%) to 0.92 (92%).

The diagnostic sensitivity is synonymous with the true positive rate. As sensitivity is derived from within the diseased population, the higher the sensitivity, the lower the false negative rate. Greater confidence can be placed on negative results being true, because false negatives are rare. Therefore, tests of high diagnostic sensitivity are particularly useful for ruling out disease (Figure 2.1).

Test result in diseased animals	Number of animals in each category	
	Example a	*Example b*
Positive (TP)	80	99
Negative (FN)	20	1
Totals	100	100

2.1 The derivation of diagnostic sensitivity. In example a, diagnostic sensitivity is 80% and the false negative rate is 20%. In example b, diagnostic sensitivity is 99% and the false negative rate is 1%. FN = false negatives; TP = true positives.

A commonly used memory aid is 'SnOut' (sensitivity is good for ruling-out disease).

The derived diagnostic sensitivity can be swayed, to some extent, by the selection of the diseased group. Often the diseased group contains cases that are easily categorized and, consequently, may have 'severe' or 'obvious' disease. 'Mild' or 'early' cases that are more difficult to categorize may be omitted. As a consequence, sensitivity may be overestimated in studies that do not include a representative range of degrees of presentation. If a high diagnostic sensitivity is quoted for a new test, it is prudent to check whether the diseased group represents the complete range or continuum of presentations appropriately.

Diagnostic specificity

The diagnostic specificity (not to be confused with analytical specificity) is the proportion of patients without the disease that are correctly identified by the test. The derivation of this proportion requires a well characterized population that is known **not** to have the pathology in question. Ideally, this should not simply be a healthy group, but instead should include animals of a similar signalment that have some attribute or clinical sign suggestive of the disease in question. Specificity is calculated in the same manner as sensitivity except in the non-diseased group.

Dixon and Mooney (1999) derived the diagnostic specificity of fT4d by measuring it in 77 dogs confirmed as euthyroid (i.e. not hypothyroid) using TSH response test results. Of these 77 dogs, 72 yielded results greater than or equal to 5.42 pmol/l.

Diagnostic specificity = 72/77 = 0.935 (93.5%)

Confidence intervals for diagnostic specificity are derived in an identical manner to those for sensitivity. In the above example, the 95% confidence interval ranged from 0.85 (85%) to 0.98 (98%).

The diagnostic specificity is synonymous with the true negative rate. As specificity is derived from within the non-diseased population, the higher the specificity, the lower the false-positive rate. Greater confidence can be placed on positive results being true because false positives are rare. Therefore, tests of high diagnostic specificity are particularly useful for ruling in disease (Figure 2.2).

Test result in non-diseased animals	Number of animals in each category	
	Example c	*Example d*
Positive (FP)	7	1
Negative (TN)	93	99
Totals	100	100

2.2 The derivation of diagnostic specificity. In example c, diagnostic specificity is 93% and the false positive rate is 7%. In example d, diagnostic specificity is 99% and the false positive rate is 1%. FP = false positives; TN = true negatives.

A commonly used memory aid is 'SpIn' (specificity is good for ruling-in disease).

Estimates of diagnostic specificity can be swayed by the choice of subjects in the non-diseased population. As already mentioned, it is important that the chosen subjects are appropriately under investigation for the disorder in question. For example, a study on the specificity of a test for canine HAC, using very young animals with no compatible clinical or presenting signs, is likely to overestimate diagnostic specificity significantly. If a high diagnostic specificity is quoted for a new test, it is prudent to check whether the non-diseased group is representative of the signalment and various presentations appropriate to the disease in question.

Ideally, the choice of diagnostic test should give the best available diagnostic sensitivity when the main aim is to rule out or exclude disease and the best specificity when the aim is to rule in or confirm disease (Figures 2.3 and 2.4).

Tests ranked by most sensitive	Published sensitivities (%)
TT4	89–100
TgAA	86–100
fT4d	80–98
TT4/TSH	63–91
TSH	63–87
fT4d/TSH	74–80
Tests ranked by most specific	**Published specificities (%)**
TgAA	94–100
TT4/TSH	92–100
TSH	82–100
fT4d/TSH	97–98
fT4d	78–94
TT4	73–82

2.3 Tests for canine thyroid disease ranked by sensitivity and specificity. TgAA is a test for canine thyroid pathology rather than thyroid dysfunction. TT4 = total thyroxine; TgAA = thyroglobulin autoantibody; ft4d = free thyroxine by dialysis; TT4/TSH = total thyroxine/thyroid stimulating hormone; TSH = thyroid-stimulating hormone; fT4d/TSH = free thyroxine by dialysis/thyroid stimulating hormone.

Tests ranked by most sensitive	Published sensitivities (%)
LDDS	85–100
UCCR	75–100
ACTH stimulation	80–95
Tests ranked by most specific	**Published specificities (%)**
ACTH stimulation	86–91
UCCR	24–77
LDDS	44–73

2.4 Tests for canine hyperadrenocorticism ranked by sensitivity and specificity. ACTH = adrenocorticopropic hormone; LDDS = low-dose dexamethasone suppression; UCCR = urine cortisol:creatinine ratio.

Positive and negative predictive value and the effect of prevalence

The diagnostic sensitivity and diagnostic specificity provide useful information on how a test performs in populations of well defined disease status. However, in clinical practice a well defined disease status is an uncommon luxury. Indeed, very often the reason for performing a test is to attempt to define more clearly a patient's disease status. After performing the test, a result is generated and it is important to know the likelihood (probability) that the test result is indicating a correct diagnosis.

To determine the probability of correct diagnosis, positive predictive value (PPV) and negative predictive value (NPV) are used. The PPV and NPV are derived from sensitivity (Se) and specificity (Sp) combined with prevalence (Figure 2.5).

In most situations, the true prevalence of the condition within the population of animals under test is unknown. However, understanding the behaviour of the test in different circumstances of prevalence can alter the weight placed on the result, and can influence the type of animals upon which the test is performed.

Another way to consider prevalence is the probability that the disease is present before the test is performed (pre-test probability). Pre-test probability can be significantly improved by performing the test only on animals that already have a high likelihood of having the disease (appropriate age, breed or sex, compatible clinical signs and routine clinico-pathological abnormalities, other differential diagnoses ruled out, etc).

As illustrated in Figure 2.6, prevalence (pre-test probability) has a dramatic effect on predictive values, particularly when the diagnostic sensitivity or specificity is relatively poor; as is often the case for tests for endocrine diseases.

- Tests of low diagnostic sensitivity have a poor negative predictive value in high-prevalence (high pre-test probability) situations, such as those where there are appropriate supporting data for the disorder in question.
- Tests of low diagnostic specificity have a poor positive predictive value in low-prevalence (low pre-test probability) situations when there is limited supporting clinical data for the diagnosis. Such a low prevalence is not uncommon when screening large populations for a relatively uncommon disease.

The effect of prevalence on PPV can be dramatic. When prevalence (pre-test probability) is as low as 5%, the PPV of a positive LDDS test for diagnosing canine HAC falls to an unacceptable 15%. Faced with a positive LDDS test result, and despite the result being 'positive', it is far more likely (85%) that the animal does not, in fact, have HAC. It is for this reason that the LDDS test is not suitable for 'screening' dogs for HAC, unless there is strong supporting evidence of such (high prevalence or pre-test probability).

Test results	Diseased animals	Non-diseased animals	Totals	Predictive values and prevalence
Positive	TP	FP	TP + FP	PPV = TP/(TP + FP)
Negative	FN	TN	FN + TN	NPV = TN/(FN + TN)
Totals	TP + FN	FP + TN		Prev = (TP + FN)/(TP + FN +FP +TN)
Sensitivity and specificity	Se = TP/(TP + FN)	Sp = TN/(FP + TN)		

2.5 The derivation of positive and negative predictive values. FN = false negatives; FP = false positives; Prev = prevalence; Se = diagnostic sensitivity; Sp = diagnostic specificity; TN = true negatives; TP = true positives.

(a) Data from Van Liew *et al.* (1997).

Test results	HAC present	HAC absent	Totals	Predictive values and prevalence
Positive	38	12	50	PPV 76%
Negative	2	29	31	NPV 94%
Totals	40	41	81	Prevalence 49%
Sensitivity and specificity	Se = 95%	Sp = 71%		

(b) Application of sensitivity and specificity derived in (a) to a situation of lower prevalence.

Test results	HAC present	HAC absent	Totals	Predictive values and prevalence
Positive	475	435	910	PPV 52%
Negative	25	1065	1090	NPV 98%
Totals	500	1500	2000	Prevalence 25%
Sensitivity and specificity	Se = 95%	Sp = 71%		

(c) Application of sensitivity and specificity derived in (a) to a situation of very low prevalence.

Test results	HAC present	HAC absent	Totals	Predictive values and prevalence
Positive	95	551	646	PPV 15%
Negative	5	1349	1354	NPV 100%
Totals	100	1900	2000	Prevalence 5%
Sensitivity and specificity	Se = 95%	Sp = 71%		

2.6 An example calculation of predictive values for the low-dose dexamethasone suppression test and the effect of different levels of prevalence (pre-test probabilities). HAC = hyperadrenocorticism.

Tests of low diagnostic specificity are common in veterinary endocrinology; hence the advice to increase pre-test probability (prevalence) before using total T4 for canine hypothyroidism or the LDDS test for canine HAC. In the case of total T4 for canine hypothyroidism, it is also important to avoid testing dogs in situations that are known to increase the risk of false positive results (e.g. non-thyroidal illness, certain drug therapies). Alternatively, confidence in the diagnosis of hypothyroidism can be improved, even in the false-positive group, by using a combination of thyroid function tests with better specificity, rather than relying on total T4 alone.

For diagnosing feline hyperthyroidism, total T4 has high specificity but lower sensitivity. It is therefore a good test for screening older cats as there is confidence in diagnosing hyperthyroidism with a positive test result. However, when prevalence (pre-test probability) is high, the NPV decreases and hyperthyroidism cannot be definitively ruled out with a reference interval TT4 value. An appropriate course of action is re-testing or combining with a higher sensitivity test, such as fT4d.

Published predictive values do not apply universally. As demonstrated in Figure 2.6, they are entirely dependent on prevalence (pre-test probability) within the test population and, as a consequence, predictive values should be mistrusted unless prevalence is also stated. For application to the clinical setting, the cited prevalence must be similar to the clinician's expectations.

Some studies quote test accuracy (all correct results as proportion of all tests). This measure of performance is affected by prevalence in the same way as predictive values and therefore should be critically evaluated in a similar manner.

Effects of non-endocrine factors

In some instances non-endocrine factors can significantly affect the interpretation of endocrine test results and can influence the tests chosen. They may even dictate whether a test is performed at all. Specific effects of non-endocrine factors on individual endocrine system test results are discussed in relevant chapters.

For many situations, the effects of non-endocrine factors are subtle. A change in test results due to a physiological factor may be seen in an individual animal or between the results of groups of animals. However, such a change is not often sufficient to cause a significant change in diagnostic category. In these situations, even when a physiological factor has 'pushed' a result over a diagnostic threshold, it is likely that the result would be 'borderline' and be viewed with an appropriately low level of diagnostic confidence, rather than being confidently misclassified as diseased or healthy. However, there are some particular situations in which non-endocrine factors can result in significant and frequent misclassification of health *versus* disease.

Breed

The physical characteristics of dogs vary greatly, and so the risk of diagnostic misclassification when using general all-breed reference intervals is unsurprising; breed-specific reference intervals may be considered more appropriate. Since wide breed variability is less of an issue in cats, this problem is of greater concern in dogs.

The necessity for breed-specific reference intervals is dependent on studies of large numbers of healthy individuals within each breed of interest. So far, only a limited number of studies have been completed and, from those, a strong case for breed-specific ranges has been made in only a few specific circumstances.

It is now widely accepted that dolichocephalic sight-hound breeds have a much lower reference interval for total T4 and, in some instances, free T4. In these dogs the lower end of their reference interval may be below the limit of detection of most commercially available assays. Outside this group, and despite insistence by some breed societies, there is little evidence that the general all-breed reference interval is inappropriate.

Circulating concentrations of insulin-like growth factor (IGF-1), produced by the liver under the influence of growth hormone (GH), are measured for suspected acromegaly and dwarfism, and to determine nutritional status. This is strongly affected by the size (and age, see below) of the dog. Smaller dogs have naturally lower IGF-1 concentrations than larger dogs and this needs to be taken into account when interpreting results.

Where a breed-specific reference interval is unavailable, it may be helpful to submit a 'control' sample from an age- and breed-matched dog.

Age

Very young and growing animals may have circulating hormone concentrations significantly different from their adult counterparts. For example, in the first few weeks of life, thyroid hormone concentrations are likely to be high; and in growing animals IGF-1 concentrations are much higher than in adults.

There may be more subtle changes in hormone concentration as adult animals age; for example, total T4 appears to decline slowly with age. However, in general, these changes are not sufficient to result in significant diagnostic misclassification when using an all-age reference interval.

Time of day

Although there may be a strong diurnal pattern for circulating concentrations of commonly measured hormones in humans and other mammals, this may be of limited or no relevance in dogs and cats, despite being frequently cited in textbooks. It has been shown that cortisol in the dog has a cyclic and pulsatile pattern of secretion, but a diurnal pattern has not been demonstrated. Consequently, advice that investigation of adrenal function be carried out at a particular time of day is unfounded and unnecessary.

The time of day (or more correctly, time since last medication) is of greater importance when using tests for therapeutic monitoring, such as thyroid hormone in the treatment of canine hypothyroidism or trilostane in the treatment of canine HAC.

Drugs

There is a long list of commonly used veterinary drugs that have been investigated for their potential to alter endocrine test results. By far the majority of such investigations discover only subtle or minimal effect, such that diagnostic misclassification is unlikely. However, there are some drugs that can exert a diagnostically significant effect. Common examples include:

- Sulphonamides, which can cause primary but reversible hypothyroidism
- Barbiturates, which suppress total T4 and, through induction of metabolic enzymes, could result in false positive ACTH response and LDDS test results
- Glucocorticoids, which suppress thyroid hormone concentrations and exert negative feedback on the pituitary–adrenal axis, influencing adrenal function tests.

Ideally, endocrine investigations should not be performed when these drug therapies are being used. If barbiturates or glucocorticoids cannot be avoided, specialist laboratory approaches (e.g. fT4d) or other diagnostic techniques should be considered.

Non-endocrine illness

Non-endocrine illness poses the greatest challenge and risk of misclassification. Non-endocrine illnesses significantly influence the results of the two most commonly investigated endocrine systems in companion animals: the thyroid and adrenal.

As discussed above, the diagnostic specificity of tests (such as total T4 for hypothyroidism and the LDDS test for HAC) and the diagnostic sensitivity of total T4 for feline hyperthyroidism are far from perfect. The most important reason for this is the effect of non-thyroidal or non-adrenal illness.

- Any significant non-thyroidal illness, either acute or chronic, has the potential to suppress total T4 concentrations below the reference interval. Thyroid testing should therefore be postponed in dogs with known non-thyroidal illness until it has abated or been stabilized with treatment. Alternatively, as the effect of non-thyroidal illness is less dramatic on fT4d results, measuring this parameter improves the chances of correctly diagnosing hypothyroidism.
- The effect of non-thyroidal illness presents a similar difficulty in the investigation of feline hyperthyroidism, whereby cats need to be re-tested after recovery from non-thyroidal illness or with the additional measurement of fT4d for correct diagnosis.
- Any illness that might be described as 'metabolically stressful' has the potential to result in false positive results for HAC testing. The simplistic explanation is that the physiological demand for glucocorticoids in stressful illness increases the production capacity, and this can be misinterpreted by dynamic endocrine testing (e.g. ACTH response and LDDS tests) as evidence for pathological excess (HAC).

Effect of endocrine disease

Although endocrine systems (e.g. thyroid, adrenal) are referred to as separate entities, it is worth emphasizing that in many circumstances they are tightly interconnected. In addition, the pathological process underlying or associated with the endocrinopathy can occasionally interfere with either the analytical validity of test results or the ability to interpret them correctly.

Concurrent endocrinopathy

The pre-existence of one endocrinopathy may affect the ability to reliably confirm or exclude the presence of another. For example, the routine clinicopathological abnormalities expected in a poorly controlled diabetic dog are similar to those expected in a dog with HAC. In this scenario, the significance of elevated liver enzymes and cholesterol in supporting a diagnosis of HAC must be discounted. Similarly, a dog with HAC is likely to have a low circulating total T4 concentration, even when truly euthyroid.

Hyperlipidaemia

Several endocrine diseases can result in hyperlipidaemia. Lipaemia is capable of interfering with the test results of some analytes, using certain methods of analysis. The degree of this effect is generally known by commercial laboratories for each particular analyte measured using their technology. When there is interference, it is often because the lipid present alters the equipment's ability to detect light or colour change in a sample. Antibody interactions with the analyte and the separation of antibody-bound hormone from free hormone are less commonly affected. In general, radioimmunoassays are free from the effects of interference, because light or colour change is not integral. However, for fT4d, the presence of increased concentrations of free fatty acids in the sample will, by displacement from binding proteins, result in an increased free hormone fraction.

Endogenous antibodies

As discussed in Chapter 1, immunoassays are almost exclusively used for the measurement of hormones. The principle of an immunoassay relies on an antibody directed against the hormone under test. By using a uniform amount of anti-hormone antibody in both samples and assay standards, the interaction is controlled and a reliable estimate of the hormone concentration in the sample can be made. However, if antibodies that can cross-react with the hormone under test are already present in the patient sample, control over the hormone–antibody interaction is lost. As a consequence, a reliable estimate of hormone concentration can no longer be made and false results are generated.

Anti-thyroglobulin

A common scenario in which false results are generated relates to the presence of anti-thyroglobulin antibodies that cross-react with triiodothyronine (T3) and T4 (T3AA and T4AA). These occur in approximately 30% and 10% of hypothyroid dogs, respectively. Whether the consequence of these antibodies is a false high or false low result depends on the intricacies of the immunoassay design. However, false highs (not necessarily above but often to within the reference interval) are the most common consequence. These antibodies have no physiological consequence for the animal in terms of the availability of thyroid hormones, but their effect on correctly measuring hormone is great.

In the case of total T4, the effect of T4AA can be avoided by measuring free T4 following pre-treatment of the sample, by either dialysis (fT4d) or immune separation. Techniques for free T4 measurement (e.g. direct RIA, analogue) that do not include such pre-treatment suffer the same interference from T4AA as does total T4 measurement.

Anti-insulin

False high results due to anti-insulin antibody interference may also be seen when measuring insulin, either before treatment or, more commonly, following treatment with insulin that is antigenically distinct from the endogenous insulin.

Anti-mouse

Assays that depend on monoclonal antibodies (MABs) derived from murine hybridomas (such as the commonly available canine TSH assay) are at risk from anti-mouse antibodies circulating in the patient. This is seen in human patients occupationally exposed to mice or mouse serum products or those treated with MAB therapeutic products. This phenomenon has yet to be convincingly recognized in dogs.

Endocrine therapy

Although the design of immunoassays for measuring hormones should be as specific as possible for the hormone in question, in some assays the antibody used will cross-react with related compounds. For example, prednisolone will cause falsely increased cortisol results but dexamethasone will not, and the steroid precursors accumulating during trilostane therapy will contribute to a more marked elevation in 17-hydroxyprogesterone concentrations than expected.

If 'symptomatic' or 'palliative' treatment is undertaken without confirmation of the underlying condition, accurate interpretation can be hindered. The treatment of calcium disorders without identifying the underlying condition can be problematic. If the treatment normalizes circulating calcium concentration, the interpretation of PTH results is compromised. Similarly, the treatment of suspect hypoadrenocorticism prior to confirmatory endocrine testing may compromise the investigation if it is later conducted after glucocorticoid administration. In such circumstances, aldosterone measurement may be more helpful.

Exogenous glucocorticoid, including topical eye, ear and skin medication will often result in suppressed ACTH response test results that should not be interpreted as evidence of adrenal deficiency.

References and further reading

Beale K and Torres S (1991) Thyroid pathology and serum antithyroglobulin antibodies in hypothyroid and healthy dogs. *Journal of Veterinary Internal Medicine* **5**, 128

Dixon RM, Graham PA and Mooney CT (1996) Serum thyrotropin concentrations: a new diagnostic test for canine hypothyroidism. *Veterinary Record* **138**, 594–595

Dixon RM and Mooney CT (1999) Evaluation of serum free thyroxine and thyrotropin concentrations in the diagnosis of canine hypothyroidism. *Journal of Small Animal Practice* **40**, 72–78

Feldman EC and Mack RE (1992) Urine cortisol:creatinine ratio as a screening test for hyperadrenocorticism in dogs. *Journal of the American Veterinary Medical Association* **200**, 1637–1641

Feldman EC, Nelson RW and Feldman MS (1996) Use of low- and high-dose dexamethasone suppression tests for distinguishing pituitary-dependent from adrenal tumor hyperadrenocorticism in dogs. *Journal of the American Veterinary Medical Association* **209**, 772–775

Iversen L, Jensen AL, Hoier R *et al.* (1998) Development and validation of an improved enzyme-linked immunosorbent assay for the detection of thyroglobulin autoantibodies in canine serum samples. *Domestic Animal Endocrinology* **15**, 525

Kaplan AJ, Petersen ME and Kemppainen RJ (1995) Effects of disease on the results of diagnostic tests for use in detecting hyperadrenocorticism in dogs. *Journal of the American Veterinary Medical Association* **207**, 445–451

Kerl ME, Peterson ME, Wallace MS, Melian C and Kemppainen RJ (1999) Evaluation of a low-dose synthetic adrenocorticotrophic hormone stimulation test in clinically normal dogs and dogs with naturally developing hyperadrenocorticism. *Journal of the American Veterinary Medical Association* **214**, 1497–1501

Nachreiner RF, Refsal KR, Graham PA, Hauptman J and Watson GL (1998) Prevalence of autoantibodies to thyroglobulin in dogs with nonthyroidal illness. *American Journal of Veterinary Research* **59**, 951–955

Nelson RW, Ihle SL, Feldman EC and Bottoms GD (1991) Serum free thyroxine concentration in healthy dogs, dogs with hypothyroidism, and euthyroid dogs with concurrent illness. *Journal of the American Veterinary Medical Association* **198**, 1401–1407

Peterson ME, Melian C and Nichols R (1997) Measurement of serum total thyroxine, triiodothyronine, free thyroxine, and thyrotropin concentrations for diagnosis of hypothyroidism in dogs. *Journal of the American Veterinary Medical Association* **211**, 1396–402

Petrie A and Watson P (2006) *Statistics for Veterinary and Animal Science*, 2nd edn. Blackwell Publishing, Oxford,

Rijnberk A, Van Wees A and Mol JA (1988) Assessment of two tests for the diagnosis of canine hyperadrenocorticism. *Veterinary Record* **122**, 178–180

Scott-Moncrieff JC, Nelson RW, Bruner JM and Williams DA (1998) Comparison of serum concentrations of thyroid-stimulating hormone in healthy dogs, hypothyroid dogs, and euthyroid dogs with concurrent disease. *Journal of the American Veterinary Medical Association* **212**, 387–391

Van Liew CH, Greco DS and Salman MD (1997) Comparison of results of adrenocorticotropic hormone stimulation and low-dose dexamethasone suppression tests with necropsy findings in dogs: 81 cases (1985–1995). *Journal of the American Veterinary Medical Association* **211**, 322–325

3

Disorders of vasopressin production

Robert E. Shiel

Introduction

Arginine vasopressin (AVP), also known as anti-diuretic hormone (ADH), is the principal hormone responsible for water homeostasis. Loss of normal AVP control can be caused either by reduced circulating concentrations of AVP or by an inadequate renal response, termed central and nephrogenic diabetes insipidus, respectively. Both conditions are characterized by the presence of marked polyuria and polydipsia (PU/PD). Conversely, excessive secretion of AVP or increased renal responsiveness results in the syndrome of inappropriate ADH secretion (SIADH), characterized by hyponatraemia and hypo-osmolality.

Primary disorders of AVP production are rare in dogs and cats. However, impaired AVP release and reduced renal responsiveness are important mechanisms in the pathogenesis of PU/PD in several disorders. The following discussion focuses on primary disorders of vasopressin production but, as primary polydipsia is closely related, a brief description is included.

Physiology

Synthesis of vasopressin

Arginine vasopressin is a nine amino acid peptide similar in structure to oxytocin. It is synthesized as preproarginine vasopressin within hormone-specific neurons in the hypothalamic supraoptic and paraventricular nuclei. This precursor protein consists of: a signal peptide; AVP; hormone-specific neurophysin; and a glycoprotein. The signal peptide is cleaved and the prohormone undergoes folding and assembly, a process guided by the interaction between the neurophysin and AVP. The prohormone is transported to the axon terminals in the posterior pituitary. Neurophysin and glycoprotein residues are cleaved from AVP during transport, but all three are stored together in secretory granules within the posterior pituitary until an appropriate stimulus for release. All three molecules are released in unison, but circulate independently. Circulating AVP has a half-life of approximately 15 minutes, allowing a rapid decline in blood concentrations once the hormone has exerted its effect.

Biological effects of vasopressin

Once released, AVP has several functions exerted through a range of different receptors. Control of water homeostasis is mediated via V2 receptors located in the basolateral membrane of principal cells in the renal collecting tubules. Binding of AVP to V2 receptors causes increased expression of aquaporin-2 water channels within the apical cell membrane, thereby increasing water permeability and resorption from the tubular lumen. Aquaporin-2 molecules are re-internalized when vasopressin dissociates from the receptor, thereby returning tubular permeability to its resting state. This process allows rapid regulation of water homeostasis in response to minor alterations in plasma osmolality. More prolonged stimulation of receptors also increases the synthesis and total number of aquaporin-2 molecules. The overall effect is increased resorption of water, decreased urine volume and eventual return of plasma osmolality to reference values. Conversely, decreased AVP secretion leads to decreased aquaporin-2 expression and increased diuresis. Vasopressin and V2 receptors also regulate urea absorption in the inner medullary collecting duct, thereby directly contributing to the maintenance of the renal interstitial concentration gradient.

Binding of AVP to vascular endothelial V2 receptors stimulates the release of von Willebrand factor (vWf) and coagulation factor VIII. Several other receptors are responsible for the additional metabolic effects of AVP, including:

- The V1a receptor, which is involved in vascular wall contraction, glycogenolysis and platelet aggregation
- The V3 receptor (also termed the V1b receptor), which is expressed within the anterior pituitary and mediates the stimulatory effect of AVP on adrenocorticotropic hormone (ACTH) secretion.

AVP has also been identified as a neurotransmitter in other areas of the brain and has an important role in behavioural responses. Many other tissues express AVP receptors, and their full biological role is not yet understood.

Stimuli for vasopressin release

The principal stimulus for release of vasopressin is an increase in plasma osmolality. Increased plasma osmolality is detected by osmoreceptors within the hypothalamus. These cells are believed to lie within the organum vasculosum of the lamina terminalis and in the anterior hypothalamus. They are surrounded by a highly fenestrated capillary network and are considered to lie outside the blood–brain barrier. Increases of only 1% in plasma osmolality result in AVP release and water resorption in the renal collecting tubule. Although AVP concentrations may increase dramatically in response to hyperosmolality, minor increases in AVP concentration are sufficient to produce near maximal urine concentration (Figure 3.1). Therefore, clinical signs of AVP deficiency are often not apparent until late in the disease process. The maximal urine concentration achieved is dependent upon the magnitude of the renal interstitial concentration gradient.

The release of AVP also occurs in response to decreased blood volume or pressure. Decreased blood pressure is detected by high pressure baroreceptors in the carotid sinus and aortic arch. Decreased blood volume is detected by low pressure receptors in the atria and pulmonary veins. Afferent fibres from these areas are carried by cranial nerves IX and X to the brainstem. It has been suggested that input from these receptors exerts a tonic inhibitory effect on AVP secretion. Reduced stimulation of these receptors in response to decreased blood volume or pressure leads to increased AVP secretion, whereas increased receptor stimulation (increased blood volume/pressure) leads to decreased AVP secretion. The combined vasoconstrictive and water-retentive effects of AVP contribute to restoration of blood volume and pressure. However, a 10–15% decrease in blood volume or pressure is necessary before AVP secretion is stimulated. Therefore, the renin–angiotensin–aldosterone and sympathetic systems are considered to be the principal means by which blood volume and pressure are maintained.

Several additional factors affect AVP secretion. In dogs, the act of drinking stimulates a volume-dependent oropharyngeal response that inhibits AVP secretion. Non-specific factors such as nausea, pain, emotion and exercise can stimulate AVP release. Numerous disorders induce altered secretion of AVP and/or responsiveness of renal tubular cells, including hyperadrenocorticism, hypercalcaemia, pyometra and hypokalaemia. In addition, numerous drugs have the capacity to increase or decrease AVP release or renal responsiveness (Figure 3.2). Such diseases must be excluded and those drugs discontinued before the diagnostic

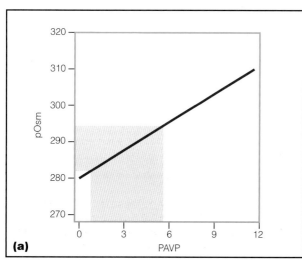

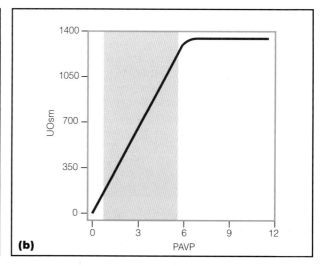

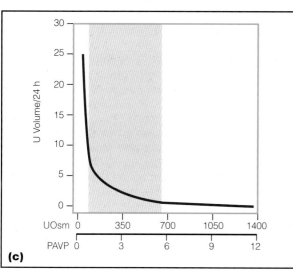

3.1 Relations between plasma osmolality (pOsm), plasma arginine vasopressin concentration (PAVP), urine osmolality (UOsm) and urine volume (U Volume/24 h). **(a)** Small changes in plasma osmolality are associated with relatively large increases in plasma AVP concentration. **(b)** Urine osmolality is increased proportional to the plasma AVP concentration, until maximal urine concentrating ability is reached (plateau). The height of this plateau is dependent upon the renal medullary concentration gradient. **(c)** Urine volume rapidly decreases in response to increases in plasma AVP concentration. The shaded area represents the reference interval for PAVP in healthy dogs. (Reproduced from Robinson and Verbalis (2008) with permission from the publisher. © Elsevier)

Increase AVP release
• Opioids • Apomorphine • Beta-adrenergic drugs • Insulin • Metoclopramide • Vinca alkaloids
Decrease AVP release
• Glucocorticoids • Alpha-adrenergic agonists • Phenytoin • Tetracyclines
Increase AVP responsiveness
• Non-steroidal anti-inflammatory drugs • Thiazide diuretics
Decrease AVP responsiveness
• Glucocorticoids • Barbiturates • Alpha-adrenergic agonists • Methoxyflurane

3.2 Common drugs known to affect the release of arginine vasopressin (AVP) or renal responsiveness to the hormone.

investigation of AVP disorders. Finally, plasma AVP concentrations increase in response to anaesthesia and surgery in dogs.

The other main factor controlling both plasma osmolality and blood volume is thirst. Increased plasma osmolality and decreased blood volume and/or pressure stimulate thirst. While a 1% increase in osmolality is sufficient to stimulate AVP secretion, a 2–3% increase is necessary to stimulate thirst in humans. Thus, thirst can be considered a second line response for maintenance of plasma osmolality and blood volume.

Central diabetes insipidus

Central diabetes insipidus (CDI) is the clinical syndrome that results from deficiency of AVP. Complete deficiency of this hormone is most common. However, partial diabetes insipidus, characterized by a subnormal AVP response, has been reported in some animals.

The disorder has been reported in both dogs and cats, but is an uncommon diagnosis in both species. True estimates of prevalence are not available, largely because the condition is frequently misdiagnosed due to failure to identify other more common causes of PU/PD.

Aetiology

As outlined above, AVP is produced within hormone-specific neurons in the hypothalamus, transported via axons to the posterior pituitary, and stored until there is an appropriate signal for its release. Abnormalities in any of these areas can result in the development of CDI. Lesions affecting

the distal pituitary stalk or posterior pituitary alone commonly result in transient CDI. This may be because of the low concentrations of AVP required to maintain osmolality, and sufficient AVP release from fibres ending in the median eminence and pituitary stalk. Pituitary tumours often extend dorsally, and prolonged compression of the overlying hypothalamus can cause irreversible damage to the supraoptic and paraventricular nuclei. If >90% of the cells within these nuclei are destroyed, CDI can develop. Proximal transection of the pituitary stalk can result in death of AVP-producing neurons by retrograde degeneration. Severe hypothalamic lesions can also result in permanent CDI by directly destroying AVP-producing cells or by altering osmoreceptor regulation of secretion.

The recognized causes of CDI in dogs and cats are listed in Figure 3.3. Neoplasia is the most common cause in dogs, of which chromophobe adenoma, chromophobe adenocarcinoma and craniopharyngioma appear to be most common. Rare reports of primary focal B cell lymphoma, meningioma or pro-opiomelanocortin secreting tumours and metastatic tumours have also been documented.

• Idiopathic
• Trauma
• Neoplasia
  – Craniopharyngioma
  – Chromophobe adenoma or adenocarcinoma
  – Metastatic neoplasia
• Surgery
  – Hypophysectomy
• Developmental structural defects
• Infection
• Inflammation
• Cysts

3.3 Recognized causes of central diabetes insipidus in dogs and cats.

Trauma-induced CDI is the most common cause in cats, and has also been reported in dogs. Trauma-induced CDI may be transient or permanent, presumably related to the degree of damage to the hypothalamic nuclei and/or site of transection of the pituitary stalk. In humans, the response to traumatic stalk transection follows a triphasic pattern: acute CDI develops within 24 hours, due to axon shock, followed by an antidiuretic period associated with unregulated AVP release from storage granules in the posterior pituitary, and eventual development of transient or permanent CDI (Robinson and Verbalis, 2008). This triphasic response has not been specifically described in dogs. The development of transient or permanent CDI has been reported as a complication of hypophysectomy in dogs, primarily performed for the treatment of pituitary-dependent hyperadrenocorticism (PDH) (Hanson et al., 2005). Transient CDI often develops within the first 1–2 weeks following hypophysectomy, but resolves within 2 weeks in most dogs with PDH (Meij et al., 1998; Hara et al., 2003). In dogs, persistent clinical signs of CDI have been reported in 53% of PDH cases treated surgically, but lifelong treatment was necessary in fewer than half of these animals (Hanson *et al.* 2005). The likelihood of developing CDI was higher in dogs with enlarged pituitary glands (pituitary to brain area ratio >0.31).

A single case of CDI associated with visceral larva migrans has been reported in a dog (Perrin *et al.*, 1986). Structural developmental disorders causing CDI have been reported rarely in both dogs and cats (Winterbotham and Mason 1983; Bagley *et al.*, 1993; Ramsey *et al.*, 1999).

In some cases of CDI, an underlying cause cannot be identified. These are generally termed idiopathic in dogs and cats, although several 'idiopathic' cases have been characterized at a molecular level in humans. Mutations in the signal peptide and hormone-specific neurophysin can result in impaired secretion of AVP. No such mutations have yet been identified in dogs or cats. However, juvenile-onset CDI has been described in two Afghan Hound littermates (Post *et al.*, 1989) without any apparent underlying defect.

Clinical features

CDI can occur at any age, and there is no apparent breed or sex predisposition. PU/PD is commonly the only presenting sign in affected animals. The onset of clinical signs is variable, ranging from acute to chronic over several weeks or months. The presence of additional clinical features should prompt thorough investigation for other potential causes of PU/PD (see Chapter 20).

In many cases, water intake and urine volume are markedly increased, up to 5–20 times normal values. Polydipsia can be so severe that water intake is preferred over food, resulting in weight loss. Some animals may drink any liquid available, including their own urine. Excessive water consumption can lead to vomiting, especially when large volumes of water are made available following a period of water restriction. Polyuria can result in nocturia and loss of house training. Urinary incontinence has been reported in several cases. This may be associated with overflow incontinence, due to large volumes of urine, or may represent owner misinterpretation of nocturia. Clinical signs are less marked in animals with partial CDI.

In dogs with underlying pituitary or hypothalamic neoplasia, additional neurological clinical signs may develop, due to invasion or compression of adjacent tissue. In the largest case series of CDI in dogs, 7 of 10 animals developed neurological signs prior to death or euthanasia, including ataxia, seizures, obtundation, altered behaviour, impaired vision and tremors (Harb *et al.*, 1996). Neurological signs can also be present in dogs and cats following head trauma, or develop due to multifocal or extensive inflammatory, infectious and developmental structural central nervous system defects.

Multiple endocrine abnormalities in addition to CDI can occur in association with congenital or acquired lesions affecting the pituitary gland. CDI was reported associated with pituitary dwarfism and likely secondary hypothyroidism in a young German Shepherd Dog, due to probable congenital structural abnormalities (Ramsey *et al.*, 1999). Central hypothyroidism, secondary hypoadrenocorticism and/or decreased growth hormone production have also been described in association with traumatic and neoplastic disorders (Barr, 1985; Smith and Elwood, 2004; Tejada *et al.*, 2008; Foley *et al.*, 2009). Cortisol and thyroid hormone deficits also develop following hypophysectomy, due to the removal of thyroid-stimulating hormone (TSH; thyrotropin) and ACTH-secreting cells within the anterior pituitary. These changes are predictable, and replacement therapy should be commenced before the development of clinical signs of such endocrinopathies (Hanson *et al.*, 2005).

Because chromophobe adenomas and adrenocarcinomas are known to result in CDI, signs of hyperadrenocorticism may be present concurrently with CDI. In such cases, dogs will present with dermatological and metabolic changes associated with hyperadrenocorticism. However, CDI should not be specifically investigated until hyperadrenocorticism is adequately controlled.

Severe and sudden water restriction in animals with CDI can lead to the syndrome of hypertonic dehydration. Hypertonicity occurs because water is lost from the circulation but electrolytes are conserved. This causes markedly increased plasma osmolality, and a fluid shift from the intracellular to extracellular compartments, preserving normal extracellular and vascular volume. Thus, substantial cellular dehydration can develop without the typical clinical signs of dehydration. Affected animals can exhibit anorexia, weakness, disorientation, ataxia and seizures. Although uncommon, severe hypertonic dehydration can rapidly develop in CDI cases with concurrent adipsia due to involvement of thirst centres within the hypothalamus (Bagley *et al.*, 1993). Conversely, similar neurological signs can develop in animals given free access to water following a period of chronic dehydration and hypernatraemia. In this case, neurological signs are due to cerebral oedema caused by a fluid shift from the extracellular to intracellular compartments. Clinically, these disorders can be difficult to distinguish in a dog or cat with suspected CDI and neurological signs. However, an accurate history and measurement of sodium concentrations and/or serum osmolality can help to differentiate these two syndromes.

Diagnosis

There is no single confirmatory test for CDI in dogs. The diagnosis is dependent upon thorough exclusion of other causes of PU/PD (see Chapter 20). The remaining differential diagnoses at the end of a complete diagnostic evaluation should consist of CDI, primary nephrogenic diabetes insipidus and primary polydipsia alone. At this point only, a modified water deprivation test, hypertonic saline infusion test or desmopressin trial may be performed to distinguish between these conditions. However, incorrect conclusions may be drawn from these tests, particularly if the preceding diagnostic workup has been inadequate.

Routine clinicopathological features

No significant haematological or biochemical abnormalities are consistently observed in dogs or cats with CDI, provided water is not restricted. If any significant abnormalities are depicted, they are more likely to be associated with another disease potentially causing PU/PD.

In animals with CDI, serum urea concentrations are frequently reduced as a result of renal medullary solute washout and the loss of AVP-dependent urea reabsorption in the renal tubule. Decreases can be more marked than in other polyuric conditions because of the severity of polyuria.

If water has been restricted, primary water loss can result in elevated haematocrit, hyperproteinaemia, hypernatraemia and prerenal azotaemia. Severe hypernatraemia and serum hyperosmolality are present in cases of hypertonic dehydration. Serum osmolality can be measured directly, or calculated using a formula based upon sodium, potassium, urea and glucose concentrations (where sodium (Na), potassium (K), urea and glucose concentrations are measured in mmol/l).

$$\text{Serum osmolality} = 2\,(Na + K) + urea + glucose$$

Calculated osmolality values usually parallel directly measured values, unless unmeasured osmoles (such as mannitol) are present. Some human studies suggest that calculated values are less reliable in animals with marked hypo- or hyperosmolality, but this has not been evaluated in dogs or cats. Osmolality ranges in healthy dogs and cats are approximately 290–310 and 290–330 mOsm/kg, respectively. In hypertonic dehydration, the largest contributor to hyperosmolality is sodium; therefore, calculation of osmolality is not necessary in markedly hypernatraemic animals in an emergency setting.

Urinalysis

Urine specific gravity (SG) values <1.030 in dogs and <1.035 in cats are consistent with PU/PD, but much lower values are detected in animals with CDI. Indeed, the only consistent clinicopathological finding in dogs with CDI is the presence of hyposthenuria or, less commonly, isosthenuria. Severe hyposthenuria (SG 1.000–1.006) is usually detected in dogs with complete CDI. Common differentials for such marked hyposthenuria include hyperadrenocorticism in dogs, hyperthyroidism in cats, liver disease, hypercalcaemia, primary polydipsia and both central and nephrogenic forms of diabetes insipidus. In some cases, isosthenuria has been noted at presentation, presumably as a result of partial CDI (Harb *et al.*, 1996).

Bacteriological culture of urine should always be performed as part of the diagnostic investigation of PU/PD, regardless of the suspected cause. Urine sediment examination alone is insufficient, because an active sediment can be difficult to recognize in animals with markedly dilute urine. Approximately 25% of dogs with CDI have urinary tract infections at presentation (Harb *et al.*, 1996).

Water deprivation test

The water deprivation test involves the sudden and complete withdrawal of water and subsequent assessment of urine and plasma osmolality and urine SG. In theory, urine will become concentrated in animals with primary polydipsia, but will remain dilute (despite increasing plasma osmolality and hypernatraemia) in dogs with both CDI and nephrogenic diabetes insipidus.

This test is not recommended because it can result in rapid alterations of water and electrolyte status that can be life-threatening. This is a particular risk in practices lacking an in-house laboratory capable of measuring osmolality and electrolyte concentrations. Renal medullary washout may limit urine concentrating capacity, regardless of the cause of polyuria and the animal's capability of producing AVP. In addition, animals with partial CDI may have results that are difficult to distinguish from both nephrogenic diabetes insipidus and primary polydipsia.

Modified water deprivation test

The modified water deprivation test is used to differentiate between CDI, nephrogenic diabetes insipidus and primary polydipsia (Mulnix *et al.*, 1976). However, it is time-consuming, unpleasant for the animal, and results can be difficult to interpret. A summary of the protocol is provided in Figure 3.4.

Stage 1: Gradual restriction of water intake: Renal medullary washout can occur in animals with PU/PD regardless of the cause. As described earlier, the magnitude of the renal medullary concentration gradient determines maximal urine concentrating ability. Therefore, in the presence of renal medullary washout, water reabsorption cannot occur even if adequate concentrations of AVP and functional V2 receptors are present.

The first step of the modified water deprivation test is gradual water restriction over a 3-day period. In theory, this allows for re-establishment of the renal medullary concentration gradient. This part of the test can be performed in the home. However, owners must be aware of the need for rapid veterinary intervention if their animal becomes depressed or dehydrated. This is more likely in those patients initially presenting with severe PU/PD. The veterinary surgeon must also be confident of compliance and restricted access to other sources of water. As a consequence, hospitalization during this period may be preferred.

Typically, in the 3-day water restriction protocol, water is restricted to 120–150 ml/kg on the first day, 80–100 ml/kg on the second day and 60–80 ml/kg on the third day, offered in small but frequent amounts. Dietary water intake should be minimized by feeding dry food. Owners should monitor their pet's bodyweight and demeanour, and the animal should be examined by the veterinary surgeon immediately if dullness or other adverse effects develop.

(a) Protocol

Stage 1: Gradual restriction of water intake

- Day 1: 120–150 ml/kg
- Day 2: 80–100 ml/kg
- Day 3: 60–80 ml/kg

Stage 2: Complete water deprivation

1. Remove water.
2. Place indwelling urinary catheter and empty bladder.
3. Obtain accurate bodyweight.
4. Measure urine specific gravity (± haematocrit, total protein, sodium, urea, plasma and urine osmolality)
5. Every 1–2 hours, assess hydration status, empty bladder, obtain accurate bodyweight, measure urine SG (± additional clinicopathological parameters).
6. Endpoints: Loss of 5% bodyweight or urine SG >1.025.
   Discontinue if the animal becomes dull or lethargic, or if marked hypernatraemia (>165 mmol/l), hyperosmolality (>350 mOsm/kg) or azotaemia develops.

Stage 3: Administration of synthetic analogues of AVP

1. Administer 2–10 µg (depending on size of animal) desmopressin intravenously.
2. Monitor urine SG (± other clinicopathological parameters) every 30 minutes for 2 hours, followed by every hour until 8 hours after the administration of desmopressin and, if necessary, at 12 and 24 hours.
3. Endpoints: Increase in SG to >1.010–1.015, for up to 24 hours after desmopressin administration. (Water can be offered at a rate of 2.5–3.0 ml/kg/h during this stage.)

(b) Expected results

	Random urine SG	Urine SG after water deprivation	Urine SG after desmopressin administration	Water consumption after desmopressin therapeutic trial
Complete CDI	1.001–1.007	<1.008	>1.010–1.015	>50% decrease
Partial CDI	1.001–1.007	1.008–1.020	>1.015	>50% decrease
Primary NDI	1.001–1.007	<1.008	<1.008	No decrease
Primary polydipsia	1.001–1.020	>1.030	–	Usually no decrease (<50% decrease)

3.4 Modified water deprivation test.

Stage 2: Complete water deprivation: Water is completely withheld during the second part of the test for a variable period. Due to the need for intensive monitoring and repeated testing, this stage of the test is performed under direct veterinary supervision. The animal is catheterized, the bladder emptied and urine SG or osmolality measured. An accurate bodyweight is obtained immediately after emptying the bladder. Baseline total protein (TP), sodium and haematocrit can also be deter mined at this time. Clinical signs, bodyweight, urine SG or osmolality and occasionally clinicopathological parameters (haematocrit, TP, sodium and urea concentrations) are monitored every 1–2 hours until a predefined endpoint is reached. This can be:

- Urine SG >1.025
- ~5% bodyweight is lost
- Dullness and/or azotaemia
- Sodium concentration >165 mmol/l.

At each time point, the bladder is completely emptied by catheterization. The risk of developing urinary tract infection secondary to insertion of an indwelling urinary catheter is low when the catheter is in place for only a few hours. However, animals with dilute urine may have an increased risk of developing such infections. Prophylactic antibiotics can be administered, but should not be commenced until after the catheter is removed, due to the higher risk of developing resistant antimicrobial infections.

The time taken to achieve 5% weight loss is variable. In dogs with complete CDI, it is usually rapid, occurring within 3–10 hours of water restriction (Feldman and Nelson, 2004). In dogs with primary polydipsia and partial CDI it can take considerably longer. The test is usually commenced early in the morning to increase the probability that it will be completed by the end of the working day. Nevertheless, overnight continuation of the test is necessary in some patients. If direct overnight supervision is not possible, maintenance water requirements (2.5–3.0 ml/kg/h) can be provided and the test resumed the following morning (Peterson and Nichols, 2004).

Animals should be closely monitored during the modified water deprivation test to prevent excessive fluid loss. Pure water loss is most common in patients with diabetes insipidus, and hypertonic dehydration can develop during the water restriction phase. As described above, significant cellular dehydration and associated signs can develop before typical signs of dehydration develop. For this reason, monitoring bodyweight is a more sensitive marker for pure water loss than assessing clinical hydration status. Given that the endpoint is a decrease of only 5% bodyweight, scales must be sufficiently accurate to detect small changes. Monitoring serum sodium concentrations is particularly useful in dogs with severe PU/PD in which rapid water loss and hypernatraemia can develop. TP and haematocrit can also be monitored over time. TP has been shown to be more reliable than haematocrit, presumably due to the effects of splenic contraction on the latter parameter.

Adequate urine concentration during this stage (SG >1.025) is consistent with primary polydipsia. No significant urine concentration occurs with complete central or nephrogenic diabetes insipidus. A moderate response (SG 1.008–1.020) is consistent with partial CDI.

***Stage 3:* Administration of synthetic analogues of AVP:** If urine SG remains <1.025 despite loss of 5% bodyweight, the synthetic AVP analogue desmopressin (1-deamino, 9-D-arginine vasopressin (DDAVP)) is administered. Maintenance volumes of fluid (2.5–3.0 ml/kg/h) can be given orally in small amounts during this stage of the test. Large single volumes should be avoided because rapid alterations of plasma sodium concentration and osmolality may precipitate neurological signs. This is a particular risk in animals in which severe hypernatraemia (>165 mmol/l) has developed. In addition, animals may drink excessively and vomit. It is preferable to administer desmopressin by the intravenous route to ensure a maximal response. Desmopressin is available as a sterile solution (4 μg/ml) for injection.

Urine SG or osmolality is monitored every 30 minutes for 2 hours, followed by every hour until 8 hours after administration of desmopressin, and if necessary after 12 and 24 hours. The maximal response to desmopressin typically occurs within 4–8 hours, but can take up to 24 hours in some animals. The test can be discontinued if urine SG increases to >1.015. If adequate urine concentration (SG >1.015) occurs, this supports a diagnosis of complete CDI. Alternatively, if urine remains unconcentrated, nephrogenic diabetes insipidus is suspected. Partial concentration, with a further increase following desmopressin administration, is most consistent with partial CDI.

In practice, interpretation of the results of the modified water deprivation test may not be clear cut. Incomplete restoration of the renal medullary concentration gradient during the first stage of the test will decrease urine concentrating ability regardless of the underlying cause of PU/PD. Renal AVP receptors may be downregulated in chronic polydipsia, resulting in a lower than expected response to desmopressin administration. Altered sensitivity and osmotic threshold for AVP release can develop as a consequence of chronic overhydration and dehydration. These factors can cause osmolality changes in

response to both dehydration and desmopressin administration that may lead to misclassification of the cause.

As described above, partial CDI results in slight to moderate urine concentration during the water deprivation stage, with a further increase in concentration following administration of desmopressin. Some animals with primary polydipsia will display identical patterns. Furthermore, hyperadrenocorticism can be associated with a similar response, emphasizing the importance of eliminating this diagnosis prior to commencement of the modified water deprivation test. In conclusion, although typical CDI and primary polydipsia responses can be readily interpreted, intermediate results cannot be assigned to any single disorder. In such cases, additional testing or trial therapy may be necessary.

Water should be gradually reintroduced following the modified water deprivation test. This prevents excessive overconsumption of water and associated vomiting or rapid alterations in plasma osmolality.

Measurement of plasma AVP
Assays for the measurement of plasma AVP concentration have been validated for use in the dog. Measurement of this hormone is problematic because it is very sensitive to proteolysis and requires immediate chilling, separation and freezing of samples. In addition, its measurement is offered by few veterinary laboratories and even then inconsistently.

In theory, measurement of AVP can allow differentiation of CDI and nephrogenic diabetes insipidus; low concentrations are expected in the former and high concentrations in the latter condition. However, the interpretation of basal AVP concentrations can be difficult. Vasopressin is secreted in a pulsatile fashion, with wide inter-individual variation in the number of pulses, pulse duration and pulse amplitude, even in healthy dogs (van Vonderen *et al.*, 2004b). This is further compounded by the effects of chronic over-hydration and under-hydration on the sensitivity and osmotic threshold for AVP release (van Vonderen *et al.*, 2004a).

Hypertonic saline infusion test
The hypertonic saline infusion test was once considered the gold standard method for differentiating CDI, nephrogenic diabetes insipidus and primary polydipsia. The test is performed by administering 20% sodium chloride intravenously via the jugular vein for 2 hours at a rate of 0.03 ml/kg. Plasma osmolality is measured every 20 minutes, and samples stored for measurement of AVP. In theory, a decreased or absent vasopressin response is consistent with CDI. A normal or exaggerated response, with failure to concentrate urine, is indicative of nephrogenic diabetes insipidus; whereas a normal vasopressin response with appropriate urine concentration indicates primary polydipsia. However, the ability of the hypertonic saline infusion test to differentiate the different causes of PU/PD has been questioned (van Vonderen *et al.*, 2004a). In this study, dogs with urine osmolality changes consistent with primary polydipsia displayed exaggerated,

subnormal and non-linear responses to hypertonic saline infusion. The test is not commonly performed in practice because an osmometer must be available on site to monitor urine and plasma osmolality. In addition, the administration of a hypertonic solution can precipitate hypertonic dehydration, particularly in animals that cannot mount an appropriate protective antidiuretic response.

Response to therapy
A simple alternative to the provocative testing protocols described above is the assessment of the clinical response to trial desmopressin therapy. This can also be used in situations where other tests have failed to yield a definitive diagnosis.

The average 24-hour water intake is determined by the owner at home over a period of 2–3 days before the test is commenced. Therapeutic doses of desmopressin are administered, typically via the conjunctival sac. Treatment is continued over a period of 5–7 days, during which time the owner continues to monitor water intake. Water consumption dramatically decreases in dogs with both complete and partial CDI. As expected, dogs with primary polydipsia and nephrogenic diabetes usually fail to respond.

The desmopressin trial is generally considered safe to perform when the diagnosis of CDI is uncertain. Desmopressin therapy is associated with minimal adverse effects when administered to healthy dogs, except when dogs are concurrently water-loaded (Hardy and Osborne, 1982; Vilhardt and Bie, 1983). However, the persistent polydipsia throughout the therapeutic trial in dogs with primary polydipsia can result in the development of water intoxication and severe hypervolaemic hyponatraemia. Clinical signs of hyponatraemia are described below. In such cases, treatment should be immediately discontinued. The resultant diuresis should rapidly improve electrolyte and osmolality values.

Diagnostic imaging
Computed tomography (CT) or magnetic resonance imaging (MRI) can be performed to identify developmental or acquired structural lesions within the hypothalamus and/or pituitary gland (Figure 3.5). In healthy humans, a hyperintense signal on MRI can be identified within the sella turcica, thought to represent secretory granules containing vasopressin or oxytocin within the neurohypophysis. The presence of this bright spot is identified in approximately 80% of healthy humans but is absent in the majority of people with CDI. This has been used to evaluate human neurohypophyseal function. Although the intensity of the posterior pituitary on T1-weighted MRI images is directly proportional to vasopressin content in dogs (Teshima *et al.*, 2008), this has not been evaluated as a diagnostic test.

Additional tests
Urinary aquaporin-2 excretion has been demonstrated to reflect exposure of renal tubular cells to AVP in healthy dogs, following hypotonic and hypertonic saline infusions (van Vonderen *et al.*, 2004c). Further studies are required to determine whether this test can be applied in a clinical setting.

Treatment
Treatment of CDI may not be necessary, provided the animal has continuous access to water and the owner is willing to accept uncontrolled PU/PD. Water restriction should not be attempted because this can result in rapid dehydration and hyperosmolality.

Synthetic arginine vasopressin analogues
The synthetic AVP analogue desmopressin is successful in controlling the clinical signs of CDI in the majority of cases. This drug has little effect on V1a receptors and does not induce significant vasoconstriction. It is available in several forms: a sterile solution for intravenous administration (4 µg/ml), a solution for intranasal use (100 µg/ml) and as tablets (0.1–0.2 mg).

Most commonly, the intranasal solution is administered at an empirical dose of 1–4 drops (approximately 1.5–4.0 µg/drop) into the conjunctival sac or nose 1–3 times daily. Injectable desmopressin can be administered subcutaneously at a dose of 2–5 µg once or twice daily. The nasal preparation has also

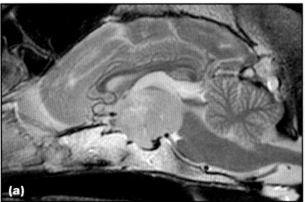
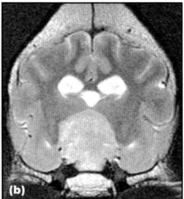

3.5 T2-weighted MRI saggital **(a)** and transverse **(b)** images from a 4-year-old male Golden Retriever with marked PU/PD. A 2 cm mass was visible in the sella turcica with a hyperintense rim and extension into the brain stem and displacement of the third ventricle dorsally. Modified water deprivation testing and response to desmopressin was consistent with central diabetes insipidus. Post-mortem examination confirmed a pituitary carcinoma with dorsal extension and associated compression of the hypothalamus.

been administered subcutaneously, but the preparation is not sterile and not specifically authorized for this route. Oral formulations can be used at an initial dose of 0.1 mg once to twice daily. However, absorption of desmopressin from the gastrointestinal tract and response to oral therapy are very variable between patients. Therefore, this route is ineffective in some animals.

In cats, conjunctival treatment is successful but is not tolerated by many in the long term. Adequate control of clinical signs in cats has also been reported with 4 μg desmopressin s.c. q24h, or 25– 50 μg orally q8–12h (Aroch et al., 2005).

Although the pharmacokinetics of desmopressin vary depending upon the method of administration, both nasal and oral routes have been reported to control clinical signs of CDI in humans. It is therefore recommended that the mode of administration should be based upon the ability of the owner to administer the drug by a particular route. Additional factors, such as high cost of the oral medication, should also be considered.

The response to desmopressin is usually rapid. Some owners elect to treat animals only at night to prevent nocturia. The absorption and duration of action of desmopressin are very variable between animals. The dose and dosing frequency should be tailored to whatever achieves best control in an individual patient. The dosing frequency is often spaced to allow slight return of polyuria between administrations. This helps to avoid adverse reactions.

Adverse effects are rare with desmopressin therapy. Hyponatraemia is very uncommon, presumably because maximal antidiuresis is not persistent with recommended treatment protocols. Desmopressin has little activity at V1a receptors, and elevated blood pressure has not been documented following desmopressin administration (Hjalmas and Bengtsson, 1993).

Other indications for desmopressin therapy: In humans, desmopressin is used to increase concentrations of vWf and coagulation factor VIII in blood, an effect mediated by V2 receptor activation. A 3–6-fold increase in circulating vWf concentration is typically observed. By comparison, the response in dogs is modest, with only a 25–70% increase in circulating vWf reported following the administration of desmopressin. However, it has been shown to decrease buccal mucosal bleeding time and to control haemorrhage and surgical bleeding more consistently in dogs with von Willebrand's disease (Brooks, 2000; Callan and Giger, 2002). For this reason, desmopressin has been recommended for the treatment and prevention of haemorrhage associated with von Willebrand's disease (Nichols and Hohenhaus, 1994). The administration of desmopressin to blood donors prior to blood collection has also been advocated. A faster clinical response has been observed in recipients with von Willebrand's disease when compared to plasma collected by conventional methods (Turrentine et al., 1988). A substantial increase in coagulation factor VIII was not detected when this drug was administered to four German Shepherd

Dogs with haemophilia A, and a clinical response was not observed (Mansell and Parry, 1991). Perioperative desmopressin has been shown to decrease disease-free interval and survival time in dogs with mammary neoplasia (Hermo et al., 2008). The mechanism is uncertain but could reflect an antimetastatic effect of vWf.

Vasopressin, acting through V1a receptors, is a potent vasoconstrictor, with preferential maintenance of perfusion to the central nervous system and heart. For this reason, it has been used in cardiopulmonary cerebral resuscitation in dogs (Plunkett and McMichael, 2008). Desmopressin is a selective V2 agonist, and has much less potent pressor effects.

Finally, the administration of desmopressin with subsequent measurement of cortisol has been described as a means of differentiating pituitary-dependent from adrenal-dependent hyperadrenocorticism (Zeugswetter et al., 2008). There is overexpression of the V3 receptor gene in pituitary corticotrope tumours. Therefore, an exaggerated ACTH and subsequent cortisol response would be expected in dogs with PDH. Using a cut-off value of 10% over baseline, a cortisol response to desmopressin administration allowed exclusion of adrenal neoplasia in 75% of dogs with hyperadrenocorticism.

Other medications
In humans, drugs such as thiazide diuretics and chlorpropamide are occasionally prescribed for the control of CDI. Use of these drugs has been described in experimental and/or naturally occurring canine cases; however, their use is rarely necessary given the high success of desmopressin therapy. They are more commonly used for the management of primary nephrogenic diabetes insipidus in this species (see below).

Dietary modification
Restricted sodium and protein diets may be used to decrease obligate water loss associated with their excretion. Dietary therapy of CDI is ineffective as the sole method of treatment, but may be beneficial in cases that are difficult to stabilize by desmopressin therapy alone.

Treatment of hypertonic dehydration
Hypertonic dehydration should be managed immediately. In affected animals, the underlying disorder is pure water loss; therefore, therapy is aimed at replacing this deficit. If the animal is capable of drinking, oral fluid should be offered. If this is not possible (e.g. the dog is obtunded or vomiting) intravenous fluid administration should be commenced. Hypotonic fluids, either 5% dextrose or 0.45% saline, can be administered. Mild hypernatraemia of acute onset can be treated rapidly. However, severe hypernatraemia should be corrected slowly, particularly if it has been present for >24 hours or if the duration is unknown. In these cases, organic osmolytes may have formed, and rapid reduction of serum osmolality could result in cerebral oedema. The decline in serum sodium concentration should not exceed 0.5 mmol/l per hour.

Prognosis

The majority of dogs and cats with CDI respond adequately to desmopressin therapy. The long-term prognosis is dependent upon the underlying cause. Idiopathic cases can be managed successfully for several years. Animals with pituitary or hypothalamic neoplasia may deteriorate, with progressive neurological signs.

Primary polydipsia

Primary polydipsia is characterized by excessive water intake with secondary polyuria. This can result from altered function of the thirst centres within the brain, or altered stimulation of these centres by osmoregulatory, neural or hormonal stimuli. In humans, primary polydipsia is most commonly described associated with various types of psychosis, especially schizophrenia. In dogs, it is usually a manifestation of a behavioural problem. In most cases the underlying abnormality is not identified. Primary polydipsia can also develop in hyperthyroid cats and in animals with hepatic insufficiency.

In theory, primary polydipsia is differentiated from CDI by demonstrating adequate urine concentrating ability during a modified water deprivation test (see above). However, the distinction between CDI and primary polydipsia is not always clear. Disorders affecting osmoreceptors may result in concurrent alteration of thirst and vasopressin responses. Prolonged primary polydipsia will lead to decreased AVP production and release. Finally, abnormal vasopressin responses to hypertonic saline infusion have been demonstrated in young dogs with suspected primary polydipsia (van Vonderen *et al.*, 2004a). The syndrome of primary polydipsia in dogs and cats requires additional study.

Nephrogenic diabetes insipidus

The broad definition of acquired nephrogenic diabetes insipidus includes several metabolic, endocrine and renal structural diseases (see Chapter 20). The most common of these include conditions structurally affecting the renal tubules and collecting ducts, such as pyelonephritis, tubular necrosis, and interstitial nephritis. However, hypercalcaemia, hypokalaemia, hyperadrenocorticism and many other diseases also interfere with V2 receptor and/or aquaporin-2 function.

As discussed above, primary nephrogenic diabetes insipidus is a rare disorder, characterized by the inability of renal tubular cells to respond to adequate plasma concentrations of AVP. In humans, primary nephrogenic diabetes insipidus is caused by mutations of either the V2 receptor or aquaporin-2. A congenital form of nephrogenic diabetes insipidus has been described in Siberian Huskies, associated with a 10-fold reduction in the responsiveness of renal tubular cells to vasopressin (Luzius *et al.*, 1992). A mutation of the V2 receptor gene was suspected. Clinical signs were reported only in male dogs, presumably because of the presence of this gene on the X chromosome.

Diagnosis

Diagnosis of primary nephrogenic diabetes insipidus is based upon exclusion of all other causes of PU/PD plus a failure to concentrate urine following 5% dehydration and administration of desmopressin.

Treatment

Chlorpropamide

Chlorpropamide (5–40 mg/kg orally q24h) increases the responsiveness of renal tubular principal cells to AVP, and may have additional direct antidiuretic effects in the loop of Henle. In humans it is more commonly used for the treatment of partial CDI. There is limited information on its use in dogs and cats, but results appear variable and commonly disappointing. Adverse effects include hypoglycaemia.

Natriuretic agents

Natriuretic agents, such as thiazide diuretics, are occasionally used in the management of human CDI. The principle of their use is that extracellular volume contraction will lead to decreased glomerular filtration rate (GFR) and increased sodium and water reabsorption in the proximal tubule. This results in decreased water delivery to the distal tubule, and consequently decreased water loss. Thiazides may also directly increase aquaporin-2 expression in renal tubule principal cells. Thiazide diuretics have been shown to have a variable antidiuretic effect in dogs with nephrogenic diabetes insipidus. Thiazides reduce urine output by 50% in some cases but are ineffective in others. The recommended dose of hydrochlorothiazide is 2.5–5.0 mg/kg orally q12h in dogs and cats.

Diet

A diet restricted in sodium and protein is often recommended, for the reasons described earlier.

Syndrome of inappropriate ADH secretion

The syndrome of inappropriate ADH secretion (SIADH) is characterized by persistent production of AVP, despite decreased plasma osmolality. The principal clinical signs are neurological, a consequence of hypo-osmolality. This is an extremely rare disorder in dogs, with <10 naturally occurring cases recorded in the literature, and reports are largely confined to single case studies. There is no sex or breed predisposition, and it has been reported at a range of ages in dogs. A single case, associated with vinblastine toxicity, has been described in the cat (Grant *et al.*, 2010).

Aetiology

Inappropriate secretion of AVP combined with unrestricted water intake results in excessive renal tubular reabsorption of water, extracellular volume expansion and hyponatraemia. Hyponatraemia is worsened and maintained by pressure natriuresis, an intrarenal protective phenomenon characterized by increased sodium excretion in response to renal arterial pressure increases. Extracellular and blood volume expansion in SIADH is mild; therefore, the condition is classified as a form of normovolaemic hyponatraemia.

Several mechanisms have been postulated for the development of SIADH, including ectopic AVP production or altered control of AVP release from the posterior pituitary. Rare gain of function mutations in the V2 receptor have been reported to cause a nephrogenic form of SIADH in humans. This has not been described in other species.

Causes of SIADH in humans include:

- Pulmonary disease
- Neoplasia
- Central nervous system disorders
- Bilateral head and neck surgery
- Drug reactions
- Acquired immunodeficiency syndrome
- Prolonged strenuous exercise
- Senile atrophy.

Hereditary and idiopathic forms are also recognized.

In dogs, SIADH has been reported in association with presumptive dirofilariasis, granulomatous amoebic meningoencephalitis, hydrocephalus, and a meningeal sarcoma affecting the thalamic and dorsal hypothalamic region (Breitschwerdt and Root, 1979; Houston et al., 1989; Brofman *et al.*, 2003; Shiel *et al.*, 2009). It has been produced experimentally in dogs by caval constriction and obstruction and has been reported as a potential complication of transsphenoidal hypophysectomy in dogs (McQuarrie *et al.*, 1978; Thrasher *et al.*, 1983; Meij *et al.*, 1998). Several cases have been described as idiopathic; however, diagnostic investigations were not always comprehensive.

The development of clinical signs in SIADH is dependent upon the magnitude of hypo-osmolality and the speed with which it develops. If plasma osmolality decreases, intracellular fluid becomes relatively hypertonic and an osmotic gradient is established that causes entry of water into cells. A 30–35 mOsm/kg gradient is sufficient to result in intracellular translocation of water in dogs. In the brain, this is of particular concern because of the limited capacity of the tissue to expand because of its enclosure within the cranial vault. To protect against this event, brain cells contains low-molecular-weight organic compounds termed organic osmolytes. The intracellular concentrations of organic osmolytes can increase or decrease in response to hypernatraemia and hyponatraemia, respectively, thereby reducing the osmotic gradient between intracellular and extracellular fluid. However, these responses take 24–48 hours to develop. As a result, relatively large alterations in plasma osmolality can be associated with minimal clinical signs, provided they develop slowly, whereas acute severe hyponatraemia is associated with more severe clinical signs because of an inability of cerebral tissue to institute a protective response. If plasma osmolality decreases to a sufficiently low level, this protective mechanism is no longer sufficient and cellular overhydration and associated signs occur. In many cases, this causes the animal to become dull and adypsic, which can lead to increased osmolality and resolution of signs.

Unlike in the human counterpart, PU/PD is common in both naturally occurring and experimental canine SIADH. PU/PD may occur due to hypothalamic lesions affecting both thirst and AVP centres, or may develop because of pressure diuresis or altered glomerular tubular balance. Studies in laboratory animals have also demonstrated decreased V2 receptor binding and renal aquaporin-2 expression in AVP-induced antidiuresis that could lead to decreased water reabsorption and polyuria.

Clinical features

The majority of clinical features of SIADH are related to severe hyponatraemia (usually <125 mmol/l). Clinical signs reported in dogs include weakness, lethargy, nausea, tremor, seizures and coma. As mentioned above, PU/PD has been reported in several cases, but it is not a consistent finding.

Diagnosis

A diagnosis of SIADH is based upon the following criteria (Feldman and Nelson, 2004):

- Exclusion of other causes of hyponatraemia
- Demonstration of concurrent plasma hypo-osmolality and inappropriately high urine osmolality
- Adequate renal and adrenal function
- Natriuresis despite hyponatraemia
- Lack of clinical evidence of hypovolaemia, ascites or oedema
- Correction of hyponatraemia with fluid restriction.

Differentials for hyponatraemia are listed in Figure 3.6.

Marked hyperlipidaemia and hyperproteinaemia result in pseudohyponatraemia, an artefactual decrease in sodium that is due to the decrease in the aqueous content of plasma. This is more common when sodium concentrations are assessed by flame photometry than with ion-specific electrode techniques.

- Pseudohyponatraemia (hyperlipidaemia, hyperproteinaemia)
- Hypoadrenocorticism
- Gastrointestinal disease
- Body cavity effusion
- Congestive heart failure
- Advanced renal disease
- Liver disease
- Primary polydipsia
- Hypothyroidism
- Exercise-associated hyponatraemia
- Diabetes mellitus
- Drug administration (diuretics, mannitol, hypotonic intravenous fluid)

3.6 Differential diagnoses for hyponatraemia in the dog.

Routine haematology is often unremarkable. Serum biochemistry shows marked hyponatraemia, and calculated or measured osmolality is low. Urinalysis results are variable. Decreased urine SG can be detected in animals with PU/PD. However, urine SG and osmolality are invariably higher than plasma values. Urine and plasma osmolality should be measured concurrently to allow correct interpretation of results. Likewise, fractional sodium excretion and serum sodium concentration should be measured concurrently.

Additional testing of thyroid, adrenal, hepatic and renal function should be performed. Hypoadrenocorticism is the major differential for severe hyponatraemia in dogs; therefore, ACTH response testing is advisable. Clinically, hypoadrenocorticism is associated with marked hypovolaemia, and the presence of normovolaemic hyponatraemia should raise suspicion that SIADH is present. Although not reported in dogs, diagnostic imaging is advised to investigate pulmonary and neoplastic causes of SIADH. MRI or CT of the brain should be undertaken, given the number of cases associated with structural central nervous system diseases.

In human medicine, the measurement of AVP is not necessary to confirm the diagnosis of SIADH. In dogs, AVP responses to hypertonic saline infusion cannot consistently differentiate various clinical syndromes associated with PU/PD. Furthermore, the pulsatile nature of AVP secretion in the dog could make interpretation of test results difficult.

Treatment

If SIADH secondary to drug therapy is suspected, the medication should be immediately discontinued. Common drugs associated with increased AVP release or response are listed in Figure 3.2.

SIADH is classified as normovolaemic hyponatraemia and is managed differently from both hypervolaemic and hypovolaemic hyponatraemia. Hypervolaemic hyponatraemia is typically managed by diuretic therapy, and hypovolaemic hyponatraemia by isotonic saline at a rate deemed appropriate to correct the fluid deficit. In contrast, isotonic saline will have little effect if SIADH is present; natriuresis and water excretion will occur, and plasma osmolality will remain unaltered.

The therapy for asymptomatic SIADH is moderate water restriction. This includes water obtained from food and other sources. Treatment is aimed at improving clinical signs rather than restoring sodium concentrations to within the reference interval. Salt should not be restricted, because patients often have ongoing natriuresis and negative total body sodium balance.

Symptomatic hyponatraemia can develop in animals with severe or rapidly developing hyponatraemia and may require more aggressive management. This can be accomplished by the judicious administration of hypertonic saline. The aim of treatment should be to resolve clinical signs by slowly increasing sodium concentrations, but it is not necessary to return the sodium concentration to within the reference interval (for further information see the *BSAVA Manual of Canine and Feline Emergency and Critical Care*).

The increase in serum sodium concentration should be carefully monitored, and the rate limited to a maximum of 0.5 mmol/l/h. Slightly higher rates may be used in seizuring or comatose patients at immediate risk of tentorial herniation, but alterations in osmolality should still not exceed 12 mmol/l in the first 24 hours. In a chronically hyponatraemic animal, the concentration of organic osmolytes within brain cells is decreased to match plasma osmolality. Rapid elevation of the serum sodium concentration results in dehydration of cerebral tissue due to inability of cells to produce organic osmolytes at a sufficient rate to counteract the newly formed osmotic gradient. This can result in a syndrome known as central pontine myelinosis or osmotic demyelination syndrome; this is a demyelinating disease with severe neurological morbidity and mortality. Clinical signs typically develop several days after osmolality changes occur. The severity of signs may improve over time, but are often permanent.

In human medicine there are a number of V2 receptor antagonists available for the treatment of SIADH. There has been a single case report on the use of one such drug (OPC-31260, a benzazepine derivative) in a dog with idiopathic SIADH (Fleeman *et al.*, 2000). Administration of this drug at a dose of 3 mg/kg orally q12h resulted in aquaresis and increased plasma osmolality, with good control of clinical signs over a follow-up period of 3 years. No deleterious effects were observed.

References and further reading

Aroch I, Mazaki-Tovi M, Shemesh O, Sarfaty H and Segev G (2005) Central diabetes insipidus in five cats: clinical presentation, diagnosis and oral desmopressin therapy. *Journal of Feline Medicine and Surgery* **7**, 333–339

Bagley R, de Lahunta A, Randolph J and Center S (1993) Hypernatremia, adypsia, and diabetes insipidus in a dog with hypothalamic dysplasia. *Journal of the American Animal Hospital Association* **29**, 267–271

Barr SC (1985) Pituitary tumour causing multiple endocrinopathies in a dog. *Australian Veterinary Journal* **62**, 127–129

Breitschwerdt EB and Root CR (1979) Inappropriate secretion of antidiuretic hormone in a dog. *Journal of the American Veterinary Medical Association* **175**, 181–186

Brofman PJ, Knostman KA and DiBartola SP (2003) Granulomatous amebic meningoencephalitis causing the syndrome of inappropriate secretion of antidiuretic hormone in a dog. *Journal of Veterinary Internal Medicine* **17**, 230–234

Brooks M (2000) von Willebrand disease. In: *Schalm's Veterinary Hematology, 5th edn*, ed. B. Feldman *et al.*, pp. 509–515. Lippincott, Williams & Wilkins, Philadelphia

Bubenik LJ, Hosgood GL, Waldron DR and Snow LA (2007) Frequency of urinary tract infection in catheterized dogs and comparison of bacterial culture and susceptibility testing results for catheterized and noncatheterized dogs with urinary tract infections. *Journal of the American Veterinary Medical Association* **231**, 893–899

Callan MB and Giger U (2002) Effect of desmopressin acetate administration on primary hemostasis in Doberman Pinschers with type-1 von Willebrand disease as assessed by a point-of-care instrument. *American Journal of Veterinary Research* **63**, 1700–1706

Cohen M and Post GS (2002) Water transport in the kidney and nephrogenic diabetes insipidus. *Journal of Veterinary Internal Medicine* **16**, 510–517

DiBartola SP (2006) Disorders of sodium and water: hypernatremia and hyponatremia. In: *Fluid, Electrolyte and Acid-base Disorders in Small Animal Practice, 3rd edn*, ed. SP DiBartola, pp. 47–79. Saunders Elsevier, St Louis

Feldman EC and Nelson RW (2004) Water metabolism and diabetes insipidus. In: *Canine and Feline Endocrinology and Reproduction, 3rd edn*, ed. EC Feldman and RW Nelson, pp. 2–44 Saunders, St Louis

Fleeman LM, Irwin PJ, Phillips PA and West J (2000) Effects of an oral vasopressin receptor antagonist (OPC-31260) in a dog with syndrome of inappropriate secretion of antidiuretic hormone. *Australian Veterinary Journal* **78**, 825–830

Foley C, Bracker K and Drellich S (2009) Hypothalamic–pituitary axis deficiency following traumatic brain injury in a dog. *Journal of Veterinary Emergency and Critical Care (San Antonio)* **19**, 269–274

Grant IA, Karnik K and Jandrey KE (2010) Toxicities and salvage therapy following overdose of vinblastine in a cat. *Journal of Small Animal Practice* **51**, 127–131

Hanson JM, van 't HM, Voorhout G *et al.* (2005) Efficacy of trans-sphenoidal hypophysectomy in treatment of dogs with pituitary-dependent hyperadrenocorticism. *Journal of Veterinary Internal Medicine* **19**, 687–694

Hara Y, Masuda H, Taoda T *et al.* (2003) Prophylactic efficacy of desmopressin acetate for diabetes insipidus after hypophysectomy in the dog. *Journal of Veterinary Medical Science* **65**, 17–22

Harb MF, Nelson RW, Feldman EC, Scott-Moncrieff JC and Griffey SM (1996) Central diabetes insipidus in dogs: 20 cases (1986–1995). *Journal of the American Veterinary Medical Association* **209**, 1884–1888

Hardy RM and Osborne CA (1982) Aqueous vasopressin response test in clinically normal dogs undergoing water diuresis: technique and results. *American Journal of Veterinary Research* **43**, 1987–1990

Hermo GA, Torres P, Ripoll GV *et al.* (2008) Perioperative desmopressin prolongs survival in surgically treated bitches with mammary gland tumours: a pilot study. *Veterinary Journal* **178**, 103–108

Hjalmas K and Bengtsson B (1993) Efficacy, safety, and dosing of desmopressin for nocturnal enuresis in Europe. *Clinical Pediatrics (Philadelphia)* **32**, 19–24

Houston D, Allen D, Kruth S *et al.* (1989) Syndrome of inappropriate antidiuretic hormone secretion in a dog. *Canadian Veterinary Journal* **30**, 423–425

Luzius H, Jans DA, Grunbaum EG *et al.* (1992) A low affinity vasopressin V2-receptor in inherited nephrogenic diabetes insipidus. *Journal of Receptors and Signal Transduction Research* **12**, 351–368

Mansell PD and Parry BW (1991) Changes in factor VIII: coagulant activity and von Willebrand factor antigen concentration after subcutaneous injection of desmopressin in dogs with mild hemophilia A. *Journal of Veterinary Internal Medicine* **5**, 191–194

McQuarrie DG, Mayberg M, Ferguson M and Shons A (1978) Reduction of free water clearance with cephalic venous hypertension. *Archives of Surgery* **113**, 573–580

Meij BP, Voorhout G, van den Ingh TS *et al.* (1998) Results of trans-sphenoidal hypophysectomy in 52 dogs with pituitary-dependent hyperadrenocorticism. *Veterinary Surgery* **27**, 246–261

Mulnix JA, Rijnberk A and Hendriks HJ (1976) Evaluation of a modified water-deprivation test for diagnosis of polyuric disorders in dogs. *Journal of the American Veterinary Medical Association* **169**, 1327–1330

Nichols R and Hohenhaus AE (1994) Use of the vasopressin analogue desmopressin for polyuria and bleeding disorders. *Journal of the American Veterinary Medical Association* **205**, 168–173

Perrin IV, Bestetti GE, Zanesco SA and Sterchi HP (1986) Diabetes insipidus centralis caused by visceral larva migrans of the neurohypophysis in the dog. *Schweizer Archiv für Tierheilkunde* **128**, 483–486

Peterson M and Nichols R (2004) Investigation of polyuria and polydipsia. In: *BSAVA Manual of Canine and Feline Endocrinology, 3rd edn*, ed. C. Mooney and M. Peterson, pp. 16–25. BSAVA Publications, Gloucester

Plunkett SJ and McMichael M (2008) Cardiopulmonary resuscitation in small animal medicine: an update. *Journal of Veterinary Internal Medicine* **22**, 9–25

Post K, McNeill JR, Clark EG, Dignean MA and Olynyk GP (1989) Congenital central diabetes insipidus in two sibling Afghan hound pups. *Journal of the American Veterinary Medical Association* **194**, 1086–1088

Ramsey IK, Dennis R and Herrtage ME (1999) Concurrent central diabetes insipidus and panhypopituitarism in a German shepherd dog. *Journal of Small Animal Practice* **40**, 271–274

Robinson A and Verbalis J (2008) Posterior pituitary. In: *Williams' Textbook of Endocrinology, 11th edn*, ed. H. Kronenberg *et al.*, p. 226. Saunders Elsevier, Philadelphia

Schwartz-Porsche D (1980) Diabetes insipidus. In: *Current Veterinary Therapy VII*, ed. R. Kirk, pp. 1005–1011. Saunders, Philadelphia

Shiel RE, Pinilla M and Mooney CT (2009) Syndrome of inappropriate antidiuretic hormone secretion associated with congenital hydrocephalus in a dog. *Journal of the American Animal Hospital Association* **45**, 249–252

Smith JR and Elwood CM (2004) Traumatic partial hypopituitarism in a cat. *Journal of Small Animal Practice* **45**, 405–409

Tejada T, Lario V, Lopez-Grado J, Borras D and Font A (2008) Central diabetes insipidus and secondary hypothyroidism associated with a pituitary macroadenoma in a dog. *European Journal of Companion Animal Practice* **18**, 161–165

Teshima T, Hara Y, Masuda H *et al.* (2008) Relationship between arginine vasopressin and high signal intensity in the pituitary posterior lobe on T1-weighted MR images in dogs. *Journal of Veterinary Medical Science* **70**, 693–699

Thrasher TN, Moore-Gillon M, Wade CE, Keil LC and Ramsay DJ (1983) Inappropriate drinking and secretion of vasopressin after caval constriction in dogs. *American Journal of Physiology* **244**, 850–856

Turrentine MA, Kraus KH and Johnson GS (1988) Plasma from donor dogs, pretreated with DDAVP, transfused into a German shorthair pointer with type II von Willebrand's disease. *Veterinary Clinics of North America: Small Animal Practice* **18**, 275

van Vonderen IK, Kooistra HS, Timmermans-Sprang EP, Meij BP and Rijnberk A (2004a) Vasopressin response to osmotic stimulation in 18 young dogs with polyuria and polydipsia. *Journal of Veterinary Internal Medicine* **18**, 800–806

van Vonderen IK, Wolfswinkel J, Oosterlaken-Dijksterhuis MA, Rijnberk A and Kooistra HS (2004b) Pulsatile secretion pattern of vasopressin under basal conditions, after water deprivation, and during osmotic stimulation in dogs. *Domestic Animal Endocrinology* **27**, 1–12

van Vonderen IK, Wolfswinkel J, van den Ingh TS *et al.* (2004c) Urinary aquaporin-2 excretion in dogs: a marker for collecting duct responsiveness to vasopressin. *Domestic Animal Endocrinology* **27**, 141–153

Vilhardt H and Bie P (1983) Antidiuretic response in conscious dogs following peroral administration of arginine vasopressin and its analogues. *European Journal of Pharmacology* **93**, 201–204

Westgren U, Wittstrom C and Harris AS (1986) Oral desmopressin in central diabetes insipidus. *Archives of Disease in Childhood* **61**, 247–250

Winterbotham J and Mason K (1983) Congenital diabetes insipidus in a kitten. *Journal of Small Animal Practice* **24**, 569–573

Wong LL and Verbalis JG (2001) Vasopressin V2 receptor antagonists. *Cardiovascular Research* **51**, 391–402

Zeugswetter F, Hoyer MT, Pagitz M *et al.* (2008) The desmopressin stimulation test in dogs with Cushing's syndrome. *Domestic Animal Endocrinology* **34**, 254–260

4

Pituitary dwarfism

Annemarie M.W.Y. Voorbij and Hans S. Kooistra

Introduction

Dwarfism or growth retardation may be caused by several endocrine and non-endocrine causes. This chapter will concentrate on congenital growth hormone deficiency.

Normal pituitary development

During embryogenesis, the adenohypophysis develops from Rathke's pouch, which arises from the roof of the primitive mouth contiguous with the primordium of the ventral diencephalon. Rathke's pouch subsequently separates by constriction from the oral cavity.

- The cells of the anterior wall of Rathke's pouch proliferate and form the anterior lobe.
- The posterior wall of Rathke's pouch is closely apposed to the neural tissue of the neurohypophysis and forms the pars intermedia.
- The pars intermedia remains separated from the anterior lobe by the hypophyseal cleft (formerly the lumen of Rathke's pouch).
- The posterior lobe is derived from neural ectoderm at the base of the developing diencephalon (Figure 4.1).

The development of the adenohypophysis is a highly differentiated process that is tightly regulated by the coordinated actions of numerous transcription factors (for a review, see Zhu *et al.*, 2007). These factors are not only involved in the formation of the adenohypophysis, but also regulate the endocrine cell specification. Following proliferation of the progenitor cells that will form the adenohypophysis, different endocrine cell phenotypes arise in a distinct temporal fashion and undergo highly selective differentiation. As for other species, in the fetal adenohypophysis of the dog, corticotropic cells are the first to differentiate from the pituitary progenitor cells (Sasaki and Nishioka, 1998). In a later stage the pituitary progenitor cells differentiate into thyrotropes, somatolactotropes, and gonadotropes. The mature pituitary anterior lobe is populated by at least five highly differentiated types of endocrine cells (Simmons *et al.*, 1990; Sasaki and Nishioka, 1998) that are classified according to the tropic hormones they produce (Figure 4.2):

- Somatotropic cells – secrete growth hormone (GH)
- Lactotropic cells – secrete prolactin (PRL)
- Thyrotropic cells – secrete thyrotropin (thyroid-stimulating hormone (TSH))
- Gonadotropic cells – secrete luteinizing hormone (LH) and follicle-stimulating hormone (FSH)
- Corticotropic cells – synthesize the precursor molecule pro-opiomelanocortin (POMC), which gives rise to adrenocorticotropic hormone (ACTH) and related peptides.

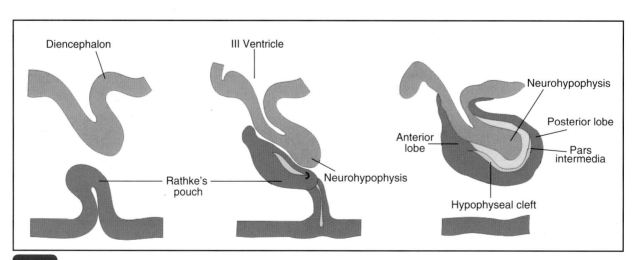

4.1 Schematic illustration of canine pituitary gland development.

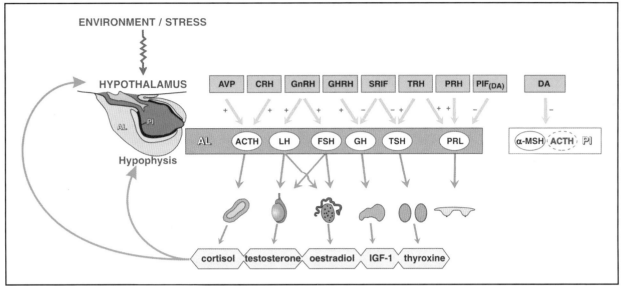

4.2 Simplified diagram of the hypophysiotrophic regulation of the secretion of hormones in the adenohypophysis (modified from Meij, 1997). ACTH = adrenocorticotropic hormone; AL = anterior lobe; AVP = arginine–vasopressin; CRH = corticotropin-releasing hormone; DA = dopamine; FSH = follicle-stimulating hormone; GH = growth-hormone; GHRH = growth hormone-releasing hormone; GnRH = gonadotropin-releasing hormone; IGF-1 = insulin-like growth factor-1; LH = luteinizing hormone; MSH = melanocyte-stimulating hormone; PI = pars intermedia; PIF = prolactin inhibitory factor; PRH = prolactin-releasing hormone; PRL = prolactin; SRIF = somatotropin-releasing factor (somatostatin); TRH = thyroid-releasing hormone; TSH = thyroid-stimulating hormone; + = stimulation; – = inhibition.

In dogs and cats, the somatotropic cells account for 50% or more of the anterior lobe cells. The other cell types each represent about 5–15% of the endocrine cells.

Growth hormone

Growth hormone (GH) is a single-chain polypeptide containing 190 amino acids. The amino acid sequence of GH varies considerably between different species.

Secretion

Like other pituitary hormones, GH is secreted in a pulsatile fashion. Pituitary GH secretion is regulated predominantly by the opposing actions of the stimulatory hypothalamic peptide GH-releasing hormone (GHRH) and the inhibitory hypothalamic peptide somatostatin (Figure 4.3). The GH pulses predominantly reflect the pulsatile delivery of GHRH, whereas GH concentration between pulses is primarily under somatostatin control.

GH release can also be elicited by synthetic GH secretagogues. These exert their effect on GH release by acting through receptors different from those for GHRH. The endogenous ligand for these receptors has been characterized and is called ghrelin (Kojima et al., 1999). This 28-amino-acid peptide is primarily expressed in enteroendocrine cells of the stomach. Ghrelin not only stimulates GH release but also stimulates food intake. In addition, ghrelin accelerates gastric and intestinal emptying. In both dogs and cats, plasma ghrelin concentration increases during fasting and decreases after food intake, while ghrelin administration increases food intake. In young dogs, ghrelin is a more potent GH secretagogue than GHRH (Bhatti et al., 2002).

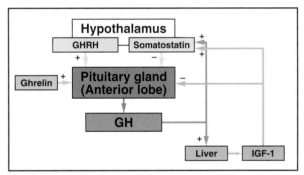

4.3 Schematic illustration of the regulation of pituitary growth hormone secretion. GH = growth hormone; GHRH = growth hormone-releasing hormone; IGF-1 = insulin-like growth factor-1; + = stimulation; – = inhibition.

Effects

The effects of GH can be divided into two main categories: rapid catabolic actions and slow (long-lasting) hypertrophic actions.

- The acute **catabolic** actions are mainly due to insulin antagonism and result in enhanced lipolysis, gluconeogenesis, and restricted glucose transport across the cell membrane. The net effect of these catabolic actions is promotion of hyperglycaemia.
- The slow **anabolic** effects are mainly mediated via insulin-like growth factors (IGFs).

Insulin-like growth factors

IGFs are produced in many different tissues, and in most they have a local (paracrine or autocrine) growth-promoting effect. The main source of circulating IGF-1 is the liver.

The chemical structure of an IGF is about 50% identical to insulin, but, in contrast to insulin, IGFs are bound to carrier proteins (insulin-like growth factor-binding proteins, IGFBPs). As a result of this binding, they have a prolonged half-life, which is consistent with their long-term growth-promoting actions.

IGFs are important determinants in the regulation of body size, as they stimulate protein synthesis, chondrogenesis and growth. However, there is some evidence that GH exerts its growth-promoting effect not only via IGFs but also via a direct effect on the cells.

IGF-1 exerts an inhibitory effect on GH release, by stimulating the release of somatostatin and by a direct inhibitory influence at the pituitary level. In addition, GH itself has a negative feedback effect at the hypothalamic level (see Figure 4.3).

Pathophysiology

Any defect in the organogenesis of the pituitary gland may result in a form of isolated or combined pituitary hormone deficiency. Congenital GH deficiency or pituitary dwarfism is the most striking example of pituitary hormone deficiency. Congenital GH deficiency has been reported in different dog breeds, including the German Shepherd Dog, Carelian Bear Dog, Czechoslovakian Wolfhound and Saarloos Wolfhound, but only rarely in cats.

Hormone deficiencies

Congenital GH deficiency is most often encountered in the German Shepherd Dog (Andresen and Willeberg, 1976). In these dogs, and in Czechoslovakian and Saarloos Wolfhounds, pituitary dwarfism is not caused by isolated GH deficiency, but is due to a combined pituitary hormone deficiency. German Shepherd dwarfs have a combined deficiency of GH, TSH and prolactin, together with impaired release of gonadotropins. By contrast, ACTH secretion is preserved in these animals (Kooistra et al., 2000).

Role of pituitary cysts

Originally, pituitary dwarfism in German Shepherd Dogs was ascribed to pressure atrophy of the anterior lobe by cyst formation in Rathke's pouch (Müller-Peddinghaus et al., 1980). Indeed, in most German Shepherd dwarfs pituitary cysts are present. However, at a young age such dogs sometimes have an absent or very small pituitary cyst, unlikely to be responsible for pressure atrophy (Kooistra et al., 2000). In addition, the fact that ACTH secretion is preserved argues against cyst formation in Rathke's pouch as the primary cause of pituitary dwarfism in this breed. The cyst formation in Rathke's pouch is probably a consequence of the underlying genetic defect rather than the cause of pituitary dwarfism in affected dogs.

Inheritance

In German Shepherd Dogs and in Czechoslovakian and Saarloos Wolfhounds the disorder is due to a simple, autosomal recessive inherited abnormality. Because ACTH secretion is preserved, it was supposed that a mutation in a gene that encodes for a developmental transcription factor that precludes effective expansion and/or differentiation of pituitary stem cells after the differentiation of the corticotropic cells is the cause of this disorder. Recent research has revealed that a mutation of the gene encoding the transcription factor *LHX3* is the most likely cause of congenital GH deficiency in German Shepherd Dogs and breeds that they have been used to produce, such as Czechoslovakian Wolfhounds, Saarloos Wolfhounds and probably also Carelian Bear Dogs (Voorbij et al., 2006).

Clinical features

Pituitary dwarfism can lead to a wide range of clinical manifestations, which are not shared by all dwarfs (Figure 4.4). During the first weeks of their

Musculoskeletal system
• Stunted growth
• Thin skeleton
• Changes in ossification centres
• Delayed closure of growth plates
• Delayed dental eruption
• Fox-like facial features
• Muscle atrophy
Dermatological features
• Soft, woolly hair coat
• Retention of lanugo hairs
• Lack of guard hairs or isolated patches
• Bilateral symmetrical alopecia of trunk, neck and proximal extremities
• Hyperpigmentation of the skin
• Thin, fragile skin
• Wrinkles
• Scales
• Comedones
• Papules
• Pyoderma
• Seborrhoea sicca
Reproductive system
• Cryptorchidism
• Flaccid penile sheath
• Failure to have oestrous cycles
Other manifestations
• Shrill, puppy-like bark
• Signs of secondary hypothyroidism
• Mental dullness
• Impairment of renal function
• Persistent ductus arteriosus
Post-mortem findings
• Pituitary cysts
• Atrophy of adenohypophysis
• Hypoplasia of thyroid gland

4.4 Clinical manifestations and post-mortem findings associated with pituitary dwarfism in dogs (modified after Nelson, 2003).

lives, pituitary dwarfs may be of normal size but after this period they grow more slowly than their littermates.

Pituitary dwarfs are usually presented to the veterinary surgeon at 2–5 months of age because of proportionate growth retardation and an abnormally soft and woolly hair coat. The latter is due to retention of lanugo or secondary hairs and lack of primary or guard hairs. The lanugo hairs are easily epilated and there is gradual development of truncal alopecia, beginning at points of wear and sparing the head and extremities (Figure 4.5). The skin becomes progressively hyperpigmented and scaly, and secondary bacterial infections are quite common. Most German Shepherd Dog dwarfs have a pointed muzzle, resembling that of a fox (Figure 4.6).

Because it is an autosomal inherited disorder, there is an equal distribution between males and

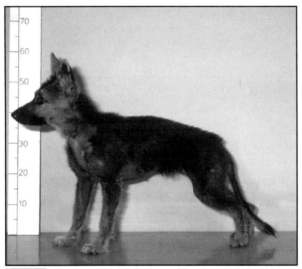

4.5 A 6-month-old German Shepherd bitch with growth retardation, retention of secondary hairs (puppy coat) and lack of primary hairs due to pituitary dwarfism.

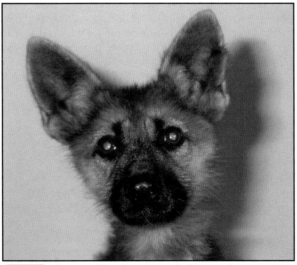

4.6 German Shepherd dwarf with the characteristic pointed muzzle, typical of these animals.

females. In male dwarfs, unilateral or bilateral cryptorchidism is a common finding. In female dwarfs, persistent oestrus is often observed, characterized by swelling of the vulva, attractiveness to male dogs, and bloody vaginal discharge of more than 4 weeks' duration. Circulating progesterone concentration remains low, often below 3 nmol/l, indicating that ovulation does not occur.

Physical examination may also reveal a continuous heart murmur due to a patent ductus arteriosus (Kooistra *et al.*, 2000).

Initially, pituitary dwarfs are usually bright and alert. With time, the animals develop inappetence and become less active. This situation usually occurs at 2–3 years of age and has been ascribed to secondary hypothyroidism and impaired renal function.

Differential diagnosis

Although the clinical signs of pituitary dwarfism may be very obvious, other endocrine and non-endocrine causes of growth retardation have to be excluded. Juvenile-onset (congenital) hypothyroidism may be the most important differential diagnosis, but other endocrine causes such as juvenile diabetes mellitus, iatrogenic hypercorticism due to glucocorticoid administration, and even hypoadrenocorticism, should also be considered.

With regard to the non-endocrine causes, malnutrition, gastrointestinal disorders, exocrine pancreatic insufficiency, liver disease (e.g. portosystemic shunting), renal disease, heart failure and skeletal disorders may be the cause of growth retardation. In addition, the apparently dwarf animal may simply be a small individual within the normal biological variation, or the result of an unexpected and unwanted mating.

Diagnosis

Routine clinicopathological features
Routine laboratory examination does not usually reveal any significant abnormalities, apart from an elevated plasma creatinine concentration. GH deficiency is associated with maldevelopment of the glomeruli, and renal function may also be impaired because of a functionally decreased glomerular filtration rate as a result of the deficiencies of GH and thyroid hormones.

Thyroid hormones
There may be evidence of secondary hypothyroidism because pituitary dwarfism is often the result of combined pituitary hormone deficiency. Consequently, a circulating thyroxine concentration below the reference interval is a common finding in pituitary dwarfs. However, instead of an elevated TSH concentration (expected with primary hypothyroidism), TSH concentrations are often at or close to the lower limit of detection of the assay because of decreased pituitary TSH secretion.

Growth hormone

The function of the somatotropic cells can be evaluated directly by measuring the circulating GH concentration. However, as the basal plasma GH concentration may also be low in healthy dogs, a definite diagnosis of GH deficiency cannot be based upon a low plasma GH concentration alone.

Because of the variation in amino acid sequence of GH in different species, GH concentrations should be determined by a species-specific, homologous radioimmunoassay. Unfortunately, validated homologous assays for measuring canine and feline GH are not widely available.

Insulin-like growth factor-1

GH deficiency results in low circulating IGF-1 concentrations. IGF-1 has a long half-life and its secretion is not episodic. The amino acid sequence of IGF-1 is less species-specific than that of GH and therefore IGF-1 can be measured using a heterologous (human) assay. Measurement of the plasma IGF-1 concentration can be used to assess the GH status of an animal indirectly.

Circulating IGF-1 concentrations are low in pituitary dwarfs, even when age and body size are taken into account. The mean (± SEM) plasma IGF-1 concentration in German Shepherd dwarfs has been reported to be 8.1 ± 1.3 nmol/l, considerably lower than the mean plasma IGF-1 concentrations in healthy adult (36.7 ± 3.0 nmol/l) and immature German Shepherd Dogs (45.2 ± 6.6 nmol/l) (Kooistra et al., 2000). Nevertheless, these IGF-1 measurements do not provide such a definitive diagnosis as do the measurements of GH after stimulation.

Pituitary function tests

Basal plasma GH values can be low in healthy animals. Consequently, the definitive diagnosis of GH deficiency is based upon the results of a stimulation test. For this purpose GH stimulants such as GHRH (1 μg/kg i.v.) or alpha-adrenergic drugs, such as clonidine (10 μg/kg i.v.) or xylazine (100 μg/kg i.v.), can be used. GH concentrations are determined at least immediately before, and 20–30 minutes after, intravenous administration of the stimulant.

In healthy dogs, circulating GH concentrations should increase at least 2–4-fold. In dogs with pituitary dwarfism, there is no significant rise in circulating GH concentrations (Figure 4.7). Administration of xylazine or clonidine may give rise to sedation, bradycardia, hypotension and vomiting.

An additional test to determine GH response is the ghrelin stimulation test. In young dogs, ghrelin is an even more potent stimulator than GHRH. Human ghrelin is administrated intravenously at a dose of 2 μg/kg. A post-ghrelin plasma GH concentration of >5 μg/l at 20–30 minutes after intravenous administration of the stimulant excludes congenital GH deficiency (Bhatti et al., 2006).

To test the secretory capacity of the other hormone-secreting pituitary cells, the adenohypophysis can be concurrently stimulated with

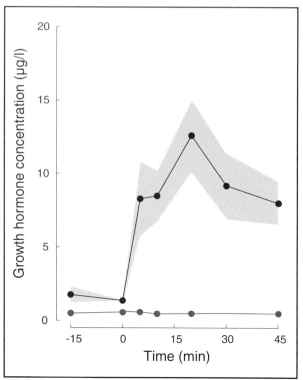

4.7 Results of a GHRH stimulation test in eight German Shepherd Dogs with pituitary dwarfism (red line) and in eight adult healthy Beagles (blue line; mean ± standard error (shaded area).

corticotropin-releasing hormone (CRH, 1 μg/kg i.v.), thyrotropin-releasing hormone (TRH, 10 μg/kg i.v.), and gonadotropin-releasing hormone (GnRH, 10 μg/kg i.v.) (Meij et al., 1996). The results of this combined pituitary anterior lobe function test in healthy dogs and German Shepherd dogs with pituitary dwarfism are depicted in Figure 4.8.

Diagnostic imaging

Imaging of the pituitary area (using CT or MRI) often reveals the presence of pituitary cysts in dogs with congenital GH deficiency (Figure 4.9). In the majority of young dogs with pituitary dwarfism, the pituitary is quite small despite the presence of cysts (Kooistra et al., 2000). This is compatible with pituitary hypoplasia. As the pituitary dwarfs grow older, the pituitary cysts become larger (Kooistra et al., 1998). When large cysts are present, the pituitary size may also increase.

It is important to note that pituitary cysts are not unusual in healthy dogs, especially in brachycephalic dogs. Consequently, the presence of pituitary cysts is not synonymous with pituitary dwarfism.

Genetic testing

The finding that German Shepherd Dogs with pituitary dwarfism have a mutation of the gene encoding the transcription factor LHX3 has resulted in the development of a genetic test. Using this genetic test, affected dogs and also carriers of the mutation can be identified. The test requires 4 ml of EDTA–blood. It is currently only performed at Utrecht University (Dr H.S. Kooistra, Yalelaan 108, 3584 CM, Utrecht, The Netherlands).

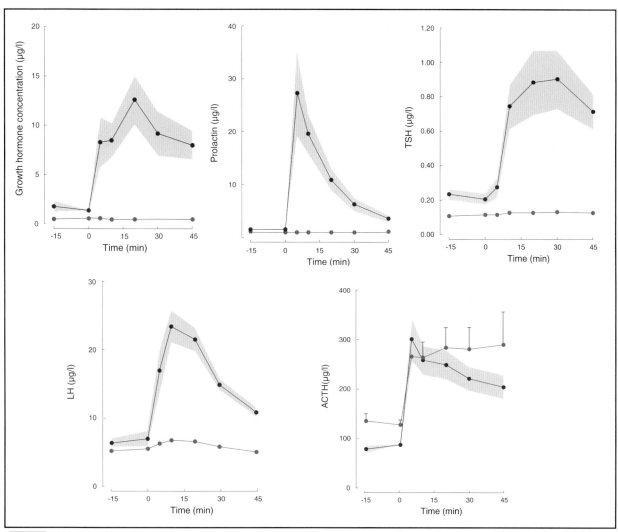

4.8 Mean (± standard error) plasma concentrations of growth hormone (GH), prolactin, thyroid-stimulating hormone (TSH), luteinizing hormone (LH) and adrenocorticotropic hormone (ACTH) during a combined pituitary anterior lobe function test in eight German Shepherd dwarfs (●) and eight healthy Beagles (●).

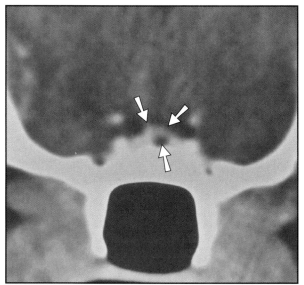

4.9 Contrast-enhanced CT image of the pituitary area of a German Shepherd dwarf at 6 months of age (pituitary height 3.6 mm, pituitary width 4.3 mm). A radiolucent area with a diameter of 1.5 mm is visible in the pituitary, suggestive of a cyst (arrowed).

Treatment

Unfortunately, canine GH is not available for therapeutic use. Attempts have been made to treat dwarfs with human GH. However, because of the differences between canine and human GH, antibody formation may preclude its use (Van Herpen *et al.*, 1994). In more recent years, porcine GH has become available for therapeutic use, but legislation forbids its use in most European countries. Administration of porcine GH will not result in the formation of antibodies, because the amino acid sequence of porcine GH is identical to that of canine GH (Ascacio-Martinez and Barrera Saldana, 1994).

The recommended subcutaneous dose for heterologous GH is 0.1–0.3 IU per kg bodyweight three times per week. This treatment may result in GH excess and, consequently, side effects such as diabetes mellitus may develop. Therefore, 3-weekly monitoring of the plasma concentrations of GH and glucose is vital.

Long-term dose rates should depend on measurements of the plasma concentration of IGF-1.

Whether or not treatment results in a significant increase in body size is dependent on the status of the growth plates at the time GH treatment is initiated. A beneficial response of the skin and hair coat usually occurs within 6–8 weeks after the start of therapy. The hair that grows back is primary lanugo hair; growth of guard hairs is variable.

Progestogens are capable of inducing expression of the GH gene in the canine mammary gland and subsequent secretion of this GH into the systemic circulation (Selman *et al.*, 1994). This has raised the possibility of progestogen treatment for congenital GH deficiency. Treatment of young German Shepherd dwarfs with medroxyprogesterone acetate at 2.5–5.0 mg/kg s.c., initially at 3-week intervals and subsequently at 6-week intervals, has resulted in some increase in body size and the development of a complete adult hair coat. Parallel with the physical improvements, circulating IGF-1 concentrations rose sharply, whereas GH concentrations rose but never exceeded the upper limit of the reference interval (Kooistra *et al.*, 1998). Similarly, proligestone treatment of pituitary dwarfs has been reported to result in the development of an adult hair coat, increased bodyweight, and elevated plasma IGF-1 concentration (Knottenbelt and Herrtage, 2002).

Progestogen treatment may be associated with several side effects, including:

- Recurrent periods of pruritic pyoderma
- Skeletal maldevelopment
- Development of mammary tumours
- Acromegaly
- Diabetes mellitus
- Cystic endometrial hyperplasia.

As with the treatment using heterologous GH, monitoring of the plasma concentrations of GH, IGF-1 and glucose are important. In bitches, ovariohysterectomy should be performed before the start of the progestogen treatment.

Thyroid hormone replacement should be started as soon is there is evidence of hypothyroidism.

Prognosis

The long-term prognosis for German Shepherd dwarfs is usually poor without proper treatment. By 3–5 years of age, affected animals are usually bald, thin and dull. These changes may be due to:

- Progressive loss of pituitary function
- Continuing expansion of pituitary cysts
- Progressive renal failure.

At this stage owners usually request euthanasia for their dog, if they have not done so long before (Rijnberk and Kooistra, 2010). Although the prognosis improves significantly when dwarfs are adequately treated with either porcine GH or progestogens (and levothyroxine), their prognosis remains guarded.

References and further reading

Andresen E and Willeberg P (1976) Pituitary dwarfism in German shepherd dogs: additional evidence of simple, autosomal recessive inheritance. *Nordisk Veterinary Medicine* **28**, 481–486

Ascacio-Martinez JA and Barrera Saldana HA (1994) A dog growth hormone cDNA codes for a mature protein identical to pig growth hormone. *Gene* **143**, 277–280

Bhatti SFM, De Vliegher SP, Mol JA, Van Ham LML and Kooistra HS (2006) Ghrelin-stimulation test in the diagnosis of canine pituitary dwarfism. *Research in Veterinary Sciences* **81**, 24–30

Bhatti SFM, De Vliegher SP, Van Ham L and Kooistra HS (2002) Effects of growth hormone-releasing peptides in healthy dogs and in dogs with pituitary-dependent hyperadrenocorticism. *Molecular and Cellular Endocrinology* **197**, 97–103

Knottenbelt CM and Herrtage ME (2002) Use of proligestone in the management of three German shepherd dogs with pituitary dwarfism. *Journal of Small Animal Practice* **43**, 164–170

Kojima M, Hosoda H, Date Y *et al.* (1999) Ghrelin is a growth-hormone-releasing acetylated peptide from stomach. *Nature* **402**, 656–660

Kooistra HS, Voorhout G, Mol JA and Rijnberk A (2000) Combined pituitary hormone deficiency in German shepherd dogs with dwarfism. *Domestic Animal Endocrinology* **19**, 177–190

Kooistra HS, Voorhout G, Selman PJ and Rijnberk A (1998) Progestin-induced growth hormone (GH) production in the treatment of dogs with congenital GH deficiency. *Domestic Animal Endocrinology* **15**, 93–102

Meij BP (1997) *Transsphenoidal hypophysectomy for treatment of pituitary-dependent hyperadrenocorticism in dogs*. Thesis, Utrecht University

Meij BP, Mol JA, Hazewinkel HAW, Bevers MM and Rijnberk A (1996) Assessment of a combined anterior pituitary function test in beagle dogs: rapid sequential intravenous administration of four hypothalamic releasing hormones. *Domestic Animal Endocrinology* **13**, 161–170

Müller-Peddinghaus R, El Eltebry MF, Siefert J and Ranke M (1980) Hypophysärer Zwergwuchs beim Deutschen Schäferhund. *Veterinary Pathology* **17**, 406–421

Nelson RW (2003) Disorders of the hypothalamus and pituitary gland. In: *Small Animal Internal Medicine*, 3rd edition, ed. RW Nelson and CG Couto, pp. 660–680. Mosby, St Louis

Rijnberk A and Kooistra HS (2010) Hypothalamus-pituitary system. In: *Clinical Endocrinology of Dogs and Cats*, 2nd edition, ed. A Rijnberk and HS Kooistra, pp. 13–54. Schlütersche, Hannover

Sasaki F and Nishioka S (1998) Fetal development of the pituitary gland in the beagle. *The Anatomical Record* **251**, 143–151

Selman PJ, Mol JA, Rutteman GR, Van Garderen E and Rijnberk A (1994) Progestin-induced growth hormone excess in the dog originates in the mammary gland. *Endocrinology* **134**, 287–292

Simmons DM, Voss JW, Ingraham HA *et al.* (1990) Pituitary cell phenotypes involve cell-specific Pit-1 mRNA translation and synergistic interactions with other classes of transcription factors. *Genes & Development* **4**, 695–711

Van Herpen H, Rijnberk A and Mol JA (1994) Production of antibodies to biosynthetic human growth hormone in the dog. *Veterinary Record* **134**, 171

Voorbij AMWY, Van Steenbeek FG, Kooistra HS and Leegwater PAJ (2006) Genetic cause of pituitary dwarfism in German shepherd dogs. Proceedings of the *16th ECVIM-CA Congress*, p.176 [Abstract]

Zhu X, Gleiberman AS and Rosenfeld MG (2007) Molecular physiology of pituitary development: signaling and transcriptional networks. *Physiological Reviews* **87**, 933–963

5

Acromegaly

Stijn J.M. Niessen, Mark E. Peterson and David B. Church

Introduction

Several specific pathological conditions in dogs and cats can result in excess production of growth hormone (GH; also known as somatotropin) as well as resulting in excess production of insulin-like growth factor-1 (IGF-1). This combination causes a broad range of adverse effects, reflecting the different biological functions of both these hormones. Ultimately, chronic excess exposure can lead to the clinical syndrome of acromegaly. Although not considered a common disorder, recent research has uncovered that acromegaly is potentially under-diagnosed in diabetic cats. Acromegaly is now becoming an increasingly important differential diagnosis when dealing with insulin-resistant diabetes in cats.

Physiology

GH is a single-chain polypeptide hormone that is synthesized, stored and secreted by the somato-tropic (acidophilic) cells within the pars distalis of the anterior pituitary gland. Normally, GH is secreted in a well regulated pulsatile fashion, subject to negative feedback control mechanisms. Two hypothalamic hormones play an essential role in this process:

- GH-releasing hormone (GHRH), which stimulates production and secretion of GH
- Somatostatin, which inhibits secretion of GH.

GH itself, together with IGF-1, provides negative feedback.

GH exerts its effects both directly and indirectly. The indirect actions of GH are mediated by IGF-1. IGF-1 is predominantly produced by the liver, provided there is sufficient portal insulin. IGF-1 has anabolic effects and can induce increased protein synthesis and soft-tissue and skeletal growth. In contrast, the direct effects of GH are predominantly catabolic, and include lipolysis and restricted cellular glucose transport. Extensive research has shown that, through a wide variety of mechanisms, GH is an important modulator of insulin sensitivity (Dominici et al., 2005). Excess GH concentrations can therefore induce insulin resistance, as well as overt diabetes mellitus.

Aetiology

In the vast majority of cases, the pathogenesis of GH excess is different in cats and dogs.

Dogs

In bitches, acromegaly is almost exclusively caused by endogenous or exogenous progestogen excess that induces overproduction (and subsequent high circulating concentrations) of GH by mammary tissue. Mature intact bitches may develop acromegaly spontaneously, because of the high endogenous progesterone concentrations characteristic of dioestrus. Alternatively, acromegaly in bitches may result from attempts to suppress oestrus by the administration of long-acting progestogens (e.g. medroxyprogesterone acetate). The development of diabetes mellitus during pregnancy (so-called gestational diabetes mellitus) may be related to progesterone-induced GH excess, and acromegaly has been described during pregnancy in some dogs (Norman et al., 2006; Fall et al., 2008).

Both endogenous and exogenous progestogen excess are able to induce the expression of the gene encoding GH in the mammary gland (Selman et al., 1994b; Mol et al., 1996). As the mammary GH gene is identical to the pituitary-expressed gene, GH secreted by the mammary gland is biochemically identical to pituitary GH.

Two cases of suspected, and one of confirmed, canine acromegaly resulting from a GH-secreting pituitary tumour (as described in humans and cats) have been reported, and represent a rare exception to the above aetiologies, but with a similar clinical presentation (Lucksch, 1923; King et al., 1962; Fracassi et al., 2007).

Cats

In cats, as in humans, acromegaly is most often caused by an adenoma of the GH-secreting cells of the pars distalis of the pituitary gland (Niessen, 2010). GH-producing hyperplasia of these cells is also recognized as a cause in a minority of acromegalic cats (Niessen et al., 2007a; Niessen, 2010). This latter process might represent a pre-adenomatous change or a separate disease process. Multi-hormonal hypersecretion (including hyperpro-lactinaemia) has been described rarely in humans but not yet in cats. However, a cat with a pituitary adenoma causing both hyperadrenocorticism and acromegaly has been described (Meij *et al.,* 2004). As in dogs, administration of progestogens to cats can induce expression of the mammary GH gene and thereby stimulate the local production of GH in mammary tissue (Mol *et al.,* 1996). In cats, this mammary gene is identical to the pituitary-expressed gene and is driven by the same promoter (Mol *et al.,* 2000). However, if local production of GH does occur, it has never been shown to result in high circulating GH concentrations nor in the clinical state of acromegaly (Peterson, 1987; Niessen, 2010).

Clinical features

Many of the clinical and laboratory findings in dogs and cats with acromegaly are similar, but there are some essential differences. Not all of the changes or signs associated with acromegaly are consistently present, especially if the disease is diagnosed early. Unlike the situation in humans, most acromegalic cats are diabetic and many present with problems of insulin resistance, with non-diabetic acromegalic cats only encountered sporadically. Diabetes mellitus may or may not be a feature in acromegalic dogs. Acromegalic cats can be morphologically indistinguishable from non-acromegalic diabetic cats at the time of diagnosis, which could at least partly explain the apparent 'under-diagnosis' of this endocrinopathy in this species (Niessen *et al.,* 2007b; Niessen, 2010). In both dogs and cats, several other specific abnormalities have been reported in various body systems and these are outlined below. The owner-reported historical and clinician-reported physical examination findings of the largest feline acromegaly case series to date are presented in Figure 5.1.

Most common owner-reported historical features
• Polyuria
• Polydipsia
• Polyphagia (often extreme)
• Weight gain
• Lameness
• Central nervous system signs
• Increase in paw size
• Broad facial features
• Abdominal enlargement
• Plantigrade stance – hindlimbs (diabetic neuropathy)

Most common clinician-reported physical examination features
• Abdominal organomegaly (liver and kidneys)
• Broad facial features
• Respiratory stridor
• Prognathia inferior, with increased distance between upper and lower canine teeth
• Multiple limb lameness
• Systolic cardiac murmur
• Clubbed (enlarged) paws
• Central nervous system signs
• Immature bilateral cataracts
• Gallop rhythm
• Plantigrade stance – hindlimbs
• Periods of open-mouth breathing and tachypnoea when stressed (due to congestive heart failure)

5.1 Historical and physical examination findings of the largest feline acromegaly case series study to date (Niessen *et al.,* 2007a).

Signalment

In humans, dogs and cats, naturally occurring acromegaly is a disease of middle to old age. In the largest group of acromegalic cats so far reported, the median age was 11 years (range, 6–17 years). There is no indication of any specific breed predisposition.

In contrast to the situation in humans, where acromegaly has no sex predilection, most acromegalic cats are males (with a reported ratio of 8:1 in one study (Niessen *et al.,* 2007b)), as are non-acromegalic diabetic cats.

The majority of dogs with naturally occurring acromegaly are entire females (Eigenmann and Venker-van Haagen, 1981; Eigenmann *et al.,* 1983). Based on the ability of dioestrus-induced progesterone to increase systemic GH concentrations from mammary tissue in this species, the female predisposition for acromegaly in dogs is understandable. However, the rare acromegalic dogs with a functional pituitary adenoma were all males.

Physical features

In humans the earliest recognizable signs of acromegaly are soft tissue swelling and hypertrophy of the face and extremities. Facial alterations in humans include a large nose, thick lips, prominent skin folds, macroglossia, prognathism and widened interdental spaces within the mandible. Many of these changes occur in acromegalic dogs and cats but, as in humans, they develop insidiously and are therefore frequently overlooked. They are not consistently present, especially early on in the disease process. Comparison with pictures of the animal when younger might prove useful to demonstrate more subtle abnormalities.

Both dogs and cats with acromegaly have been reported to exhibit mandibular enlargement resulting in prognathism, widened interdental spaces, thickening of the bony ridges of the skull, soft-tissue swelling of the head and neck and enlargement of the paws (Peterson *et al.,* 1990; Norman and Mooney, 2000; Niessen *et al.,* 2007b) (Figures 5.2 and 5.3). In dogs, the skin may become thickened and develop excessive folds, particularly around the head and neck.

GH-induced proliferation of connective tissue may cause the body to increase in size, most frequently manifested as marked weight gain and enlargement of the abdomen and face. In both dogs and cats, body condition can vary from normal to varying degrees of obesity. In one study, the median body-weight for a large cohort of acromegalic cats was 5.8 kg (range 3.5–9.2 kg) and it is generally believed that acromegalic cats are less likely to be underweight than a matched group of non-acromegalic diabetic cats. The increase in body weight can occur despite the presence of poorly regulated diabetes mellitus and such a phenomenon should prompt the consideration of acromegaly as an underlying cause of the diabetes mellitus.

Hypertrophy of all organs in the body (e.g. heart, liver, kidneys and tongue) has also been described with acromegaly, particularly in cats (Figure 5.4).

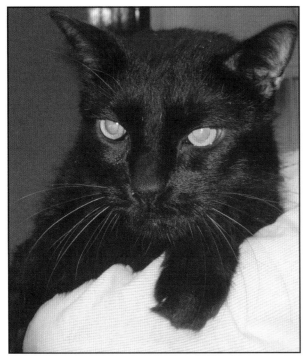

5.2 Mandibular enlargement resulting in prognathism and thickening of the bony ridges of the skull in a cat with acromegaly. While a typical finding, this is not seen in all acromegalic cats.

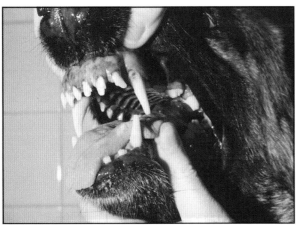

5.3 Widening of interdental spaces due to chronic exposure to excess growth hormone in a dog with acromegaly.

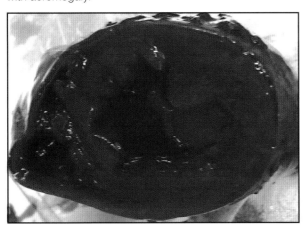

5.4 Cross-section of the myocardium from an acromegalic cat, showing generalized hypertrophy.

Diabetes mellitus

The most commonly recognized clinical manifestation of acromegaly in cats is insulin-resistant diabetes mellitus. Diabetes mellitus is also common in dogs with acromegaly but even in the absence of diabetes, acromegalic dogs may demonstrate carbohydrate intolerance (Eigenmann and Venker-van Haagen, 1981; Fracassi *et al.*, 2007).

Extensive research has shown that GH is an important modulator of insulin sensitivity. Many mechanisms appear to be involved, including hyperinsulinaemia-induced reduction of insulin receptors and impairment of insulin's kinase activity. Insulin and GH have many post-receptor events in common. Both liver and striated muscle are thought to be important sites for GH-induced insulin resistance. In striated muscle it has been suggested that GH-induced insulin resistance involves an increase in the p85 subunit of phosphatidylinositol 3-kinase, resulting in reduced insulin signalling. Growth hormone also induces suppressors of cytokine signalling and reduces insulin sensitivity by enhancing stimulation of serine phosphorylation of insulin receptor substrate 1, decreasing its affinity for the insulin receptor. Finally, GH has been shown to decrease the expression of the insulin-sensitizing adipocytokines adiponectin and visfatin (Dominici *et al.*, 2005).

In a proportion of cats, chronic overproduction of insulin results in accelerated islet apoptosis and so-called 'islet exhaustion'. The combination of decreased insulin-secreting capacity and the insulin resistance leads to clinically significant diabetes mellitus (see Chapter 13).

Large doses of insulin are frequently required during treatment, although adequate control can prove impossible to obtain with insulin injections alone. In one large study, the insulin requirement of acromegalic diabetic cats was markedly higher than that of non-acromegalic diabetic cats (median of 7 IU q12h (range 1–35 IU q12h) compared to a median of 3 IU q12h for non-acromegalic diabetic cats) (Niessen *et al.*, 2007b).

Although polyphagia is a recognized symptom of uncontrolled diabetes mellitus, excess GH is also likely to play an important role in this phenomenon. This is substantiated by the frequent observation of persistent, and often extreme, polyphagia, despite apparent reasonable control of the diabetes mellitus in acromegalic cats treated with insulin.

Respiratory system

In dogs with acromegaly, the soft tissue proliferation in the oropharyngeal region may be so profound that they exhibit panting, exercise intolerance and inspiratory stridor due to compression of the upper airway. Inspiratory stridor due to upper airway narrowing also occurs relatively frequently (>50%) in acromegalic cats. Dyspnoea may develop in cats with long-standing untreated acromegaly as a result of pulmonary oedema or pleural effusion from assumed GH-induced cardiac failure.

Skeletal system
In some cats with acromegaly, articular changes (associated with degenerative arthritis) are severe and crippling (Peterson *et al.*, 1990). The articular changes initially result from fibrous thickening of the joint capsule and related ligaments, as well as bony overgrowth and articular cartilage proliferation. Features more typical of degenerative joint disease develop later as a result of the distorted joint architecture.

Radiographic evidence of acromegalic arthropathy includes an increase in joint space secondary to thickening of the articular cartilage, cortical thickening, osteophyte proliferation, periarticular periosteal reaction and collapse of the joint. Similar arthropathy has not been observed in dogs with acromegaly.

Bony changes that may occur in cats and dogs with acromegaly include the aforementioned enlargement of the mandible, leading to prognathism and an overbite by the lower incisors. The spacing between the teeth may increase, a common change in acromegalic dogs. In acromegalic cats there may be an increase in the distance between the upper and lower canine teeth. Finally, the bony ridges of the calvarium may be thickened, and marked spondylosis deformans of the spine may be evident in some patients, leading to gait abnormalities such as chronic progressive stiffness and rigidity. These changes are more likely to be the consequence of chronic acromegaly and as such are less likely to be encountered if the disease is diagnosed early.

Cardiovascular system
A true increased prevalence of cardiac disease in acromegalic cats compared to a control group of middle aged to older non-acromegalic cats needs to be objectively established, especially in light of a perceived high prevalence of cardiovascular disease in diabetic cats in general (Little and Gettinby, 2008). Nevertheless, earlier reports suggested the possibility of GH-induced cardiomyopathy resulting in various abnormalities including a systolic murmur, gallop rhythm, and possibly signs of congestive heart failure (e.g. dyspnoea, muffled heart sounds and ascites) (Peterson *et al.*, 1990; Norman and Mooney, 2000). Radiographic findings may be normal or may include mild to severe cardiomegaly, pleural effusion and pulmonary oedema. Echocardiography frequently reveals left ventricular and septal hypertrophy, but can also be normal. ECG findings are generally unremarkable. Similar cardiac changes have not been observed in dogs with acromegaly.

Hypertension, common in humans with acromegaly, has also been proposed to contribute to cardiac hypertrophy in cats. However, in the largest case series of acromegalic cats reported to date, hypertension was not more prevalent than would be expected in a group of age-matched control cats (Niessen *et al.*, 2007b). Although the likelihood of a link between hypertension and acromegaly is therefore low, it is nevertheless good practice to determine blood pressure in any older cat and institute treatment if necessary.

Nervous system
In cats, central nervous system (CNS) signs can develop as a result of expansion of the pituitary tumour beyond the sella turcica. However, the tumours tend to be both benign and slow growing, and overt neurological signs are rare, even when a large pituitary tumour is compressing and invading the hypothalamus (Peterson *et al.*, 1990; Niessen *et al.*, 2007b).

If they do occur, neurological signs may include stupor, somnolence and poor appetite. The vast majority of dogs with acromegaly do not have pituitary tumours, and consequently CNS signs do not occur.

Renal system
Polyuria and polydipsia are common signs of acromegaly in cats and dogs and appear to develop primarily because of the associated diabetic state.

Dogs
A case of non-diabetic canine acromegaly and extreme polyuria and polydipsia during dioestrus was previously described and transient presence of diabetes insipidus was demonstrated, by documenting an inadequate rise of arginine–vasopressin (AVP) concentration after water deprivation and stimulation with hypertonic saline. Clinical signs, except for bony changes, completely disappeared in this bitch following ovariohysterectomy (Schwedes, 1999).

In addition to polyuria and polydipsia, acromegaly has been reported to cause alterations in renal function. Renal failure has however not been observed in dogs with acromegaly.

Cats
Cats with long-standing acromegaly have been reported to develop azotaemia, proteinuria and clinical signs of renal failure. However, in a recent study comparing serum biochemistry values of acromegalic diabetic cats with non-acromegalic diabetic cats, renal azotaemia proved to be no more prevalent in the acromegalic group (Niessen *et al.*, 2007b). Histologically, the kidneys of acromegalic cats can show mesangial thickening of the glomeruli, changes similar to those described in human patients with diabetic nephropathy. Additionally, periglomerular fibrosis, adipose and hydropic change with epithelial degeneration and regeneration of tubules have been recorded in acromegalic cats. Several questions remain, however, including whether renal disease is genuinely or coincidentally associated with the acromegalic state or is merely an age-related phenomenon, and what the underlying pathophysiological mechanism is.

Reproductive system
In dogs with progesterone-induced acromegaly, concomitant mammary gland nodules, cystic endometrial hyperplasia, or pyometra may develop. The pathogenesis of the mammary gland nodules involves progestogen-induced GH production by the mammary gland tissue; GH then acts locally in an autocrine or paracrine manner to promote mammary

tumorigenesis by stimulating proliferation of susceptible mammary epithelial cells.

By contrast, the pathogenesis of the uterine changes of cystic endometrial hyperplasia probably involves a direct effect of the progestogen excess rather than GH, since local (uterine) production of GH does not occur in dogs (Kooistra *et al.*, 1997).

Iatrogenic hypoadrenocorticism

Dogs with acromegaly caused by the chronic administration of progestogens may develop iatrogenic hypoadrenocorticism, characterized by low serum cortisol concentrations (both basal and adrenocorticotropic hormone (ACTH) stimulated cortisol) and atrophy of the adrenal cortex. The intrinsic glucocorticoid-like activity of these progestogens suppresses ACTH secretion, causing the secondary hypoadrenocorticism (Selman *et al.*, 1994a).

Administration of high doses of progestogens to cats also suppresses the pituitary–adrenal axis and leads to iatrogenic, secondary hypoadrenocorticism. However, cats that develop iatrogenic hypoadrenocorticism secondary to progestogen administration do not develop acromegaly.

Pancreatic disease

Pancreatic disease has been reported in feline acromegaly. Specific macroscopic and microscopic lesions have included pancreatic enlargement (Figure 5.5), cysts, diffuse hyperplasia with fibrous tissue and lymphoid follicles. It remains to be determined whether pancreatic disease is indeed more common in acromegalic compared with non-acromegalic diabetic cats, particularly as only small numbers have been studied and there is potentially a high prevalence of pancreatic disease in diabetic cats

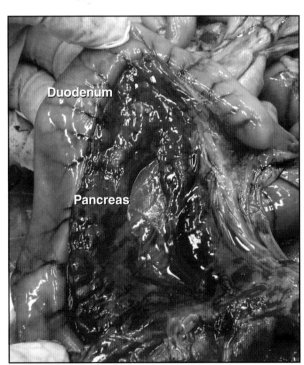

5.5 Macroscopic abnormalities, specifically pancreatic enlargement and cysts, in a pancreas from a cat with acromegaly.

in general (Forcada *et al.*, 2008). Pathology of the pancreas could represent a secondary effect of long-term insulin-resistant diabetes or direct effects of GH and IGF-1.

Neoplasia

Acromegaly has been associated with colorectal cancer in humans. As relatively few cases of feline acromegaly have been described thus far, it is difficult to make such an assessment for acromegalic cats. Nevertheless, in the authors' experience a significant number of acromegalic cats have had concomitant neoplasia, particularly of the pharynx or oesophagus, on post-mortem examination.

Diagnosis

The diagnosis of acromegaly consists of evaluating abnormalities in serum GH and/or IGF-1 concentrations in animals with suggestive clinical signs.

- Acromegaly should be suspected in bitches receiving progestogens and in intact bitches that develop diabetes mellitus or laryngeal stridor during dioestrus or pregnancy
- Acromegaly should be suspected in any cat that has insulin-resistant diabetes mellitus (i.e. persistent hyperglycaemia despite total daily insulin doses of >2 IU/kg) or poorly controlled diabetes mellitus
- Acromegaly should not be completely excluded in male dogs with appropriate clinical signs.

Routine clinicopathological analyses

Routine biochemistry may reveal elevated total protein concentrations and haematocrit, in addition to diabetes-associated changes (elevations in cholesterol, alanine aminotransferase (ALT) and alkaline phosphatase (ALP)). Hyperphosphataemia has been reported anecdotally in acromegalic animals. Nevertheless, in the only study comparing routine clinicopathological changes in acromegalic *versus* non-acromegalic diabetic cats, hyperproteinaemia was the only genuinely over-represented parameter amongst the acromegalic cats (Niessen, 2010). While azotaemia has been assumed to be a common sequel of untreated feline acromegaly, the most recent and largest case series showed no indication of such an increased prevalence.

Growth hormone and IGF-1 measurement

Confirmation of the diagnosis requires demonstration of a high circulating GH concentration. Unfortunately, an adequate assay for feline and canine GH levels is not currently commercially available in the UK.

Determination of serum IGF-1 concentrations contributes to the diagnosis of acromegaly by indirectly evaluating GH concentration. The IGF-1 concentration reflects the magnitude of GH secretion over the previous 24 hours and has been reported to be high in both dogs and cats with acromegaly. An *abnormally elevated* serum IGF-1 concentration strongly suggests acromegaly, but the disease should not be excluded if values are within the upper half of the reference interval. Portal insulin is necessary for hepatic IGF-1 production, which means that in an acromegalic diabetic cat before or at the start of insulin therapy, IGF-1 can prove falsely low. However, with insulin treatment, portal concentrations increase and the IGF-1 concentration may eventually increase into the acromegalic range. In addition, elevated serum IGF-1 concentrations have recently been reported in diabetic cats *without* acromegaly, and therefore false-positive test results can also occur (Lewitt *et al.,* 2000; Niessen *et al.,* 2007a). The reasons for this are not clear, although there is some evidence that, in cats, insulin administration results in an increased proportion of one of the IGF binding proteins, IGFBP3, being present in a high affinity state and thus increasing total serum IGF-1 concentrations (Lewitt *et al.,* 2000).

If the serum or plasma GH or IGF-1 concentration cannot be measured, most dogs with acromegaly are tentatively diagnosed on the basis of a characteristic set of clinical and laboratory findings, together with a history of recent dioestrus or exposure to a progesterone source, plus improvement in clinical signs after withdrawal of progesterone or ovariohysterectomy.

In view of the more variable clinical picture and the high prevalence of the disease in cats with diabetes mellitus, diagnosing feline acromegaly probably represents a bigger challenge. Determining basal feline GH concentration is the most accurate method of confirming a diagnosis. A confirmed case with a normal GH concentration has yet to be described, while a recently validated feline GH radio-immunoassay proved useful in distinguishing healthy cats from acromegalic cats, with no overlap occurring between the two groups studied (Niessen *et al.,* 2007a). Additionally, stability studies showed that feline GH concentrations remained stable following overnight transport at room temperature, making estimation of serum feline GH concentrations a potentially practical method of confirming the diagnosis. However, currently the assay's limited availability means the diagnosis is based on the demonstration of a markedly elevated basal IGF-1 concentration in a cat with clinical signs consistent with acromegaly.

Additional documentation of a pituitary mass by CT (Figure 5.6) or MRI is further support for the diagnosis, with the latter being a more sensitive method for this particular condition. However, normal intracranial imaging does preclude a diagnosis of feline acromegaly (Niessen *et al.,* 2007a).

Differential diagnoses

In dogs, the signalment, history and physical examination findings are highly suggestive of acromegaly. In cats, other common causes of true or apparent insulin-resistant diabetes mellitus or poor glycaemic control must be initially considered. These include: management-associated causes (incorrect

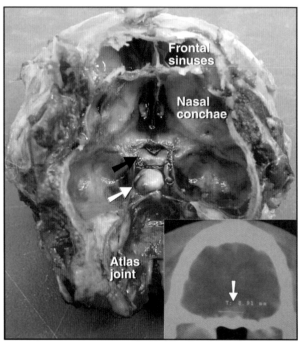

5.6 Post-mortem and CT findings in an acromegalic cat. The white arrows (in both pictures) indicate the enlarged pituitary gland. The black arrow indicates the optic chiasm, illustrating the rare potential for visual abnormalities to occur when a large pituitary tumour is present.

insulin administration or storage, use of inactive insulin preparations, hypoglycaemia-induced hyperglycaemia, short duration of insulin action); infectious disease (e.g. urinary tract infection, dental disease); inflammatory disease (e.g. pancreatitis, inflammatory bowel disease, gingivostomatitis); concurrent endocrinopathies (hyperthyroidism, hyperadrenocorticism); iatrogenic hormone administration (corticosteroids, megestrol); other disorders (including obesity, neoplasia, nephropathy and cardiovascular disease); and stress hyperglycaemia mimicking true insulin resistance. The investigation of the unstable feline diabetic patient is outlined in greater detail in Chapter 23.

Treatment

Dogs

In dogs, treatment for progesterone-induced acromegaly is via ovariohysterectomy or discontinuation of progestogen-based medication. Circulating GH concentrations normalize rapidly after ovariohysterectomy but more slowly after withdrawal of progestogens. This is accompanied by resolution of the soft tissue proliferation and signs of respiratory stridor. However, skeletal changes may persist indefinitely.

The insulin requirement for GH-induced diabetes mellitus will also decline, but the reversibility of the diabetes depends on the insulin reserve of the pancreatic islet beta cells. Consequently, it is advisable to start insulin therapy as soon as possible in an effort to preserve beta cell function and maximize the chances of diabetic remission.

Should ovariohysterectomy not be immediately possible or permitted, or should a long-acting exogenous progestogen have been administered, treatment with aglepristone, a progesterone receptor antagonist, has recently been suggested. A study in Beagles with acromegaly induced by exogenous progestogens documented a significant temporary decrease in plasma GH and IGF-I concentrations. Cessation of aglepristone administration resulted in a return of the elevated plasma IGF-I concentrations (Bhatti *et al.,* 2006).

Cats

In cats, three potential treatment modalities are available: radiation therapy; hypophysectomy; and medical therapy. Of these, radiotherapy is currently considered to be the most effective, although the response can vary in individual animals.

Radiation therapy

The reported response to radiation therapy ranges from poor to excellent. In cats that show a good to excellent response to external radiation therapy, there is shrinkage in tumour size, normalization of high circulating concentrations of GH, resolution of insulin resistance, improvement in diabetic control and, at times, remission of the diabetic state. However, disadvantages of this treatment are not inconsiderable and include limited availability, extended time in hospital, frequent anaesthesia, high expense, unpredictable outcome and frequent persistence of high IGF-1 concentrations (and its biological consequences), despite decreased GH concentrations (so-called GH-IGF-1 discordance) (Niessen, 2010). This latter situation is also recognized in humans. Consequently, serum IGF-1 concentrations are not a suitable marker for control of the acromegalic state or the associated insulin-resistant diabetes mellitus. Although earlier reports of the efficacy of radiotherapy suggested a disappointingly variable response, a more recent study suggested 13 of 14 insulin-resistant diabetic acromegalic cats responded favourably to the administration of an average total radiation dose of 3,700 cGY, administered as an incremental, hypofractionated dosage protocol of 10 doses (Dunning *et al.,* 2009).

However, since acromegaly is principally a disease of autonomous endocrine activity, it seems counterintuitive to hope that a therapeutic modality aimed principally at reducing tumour size is likely to be the optimum management strategy. Consequently, efforts to develop alternative treatment methods that are more suited to directly dealing with the hormonal disturbances are an area of ongoing research.

Hypophysectomy

Surgical hypophysectomy is the therapeutic modality of choice for human patients with a GH-secreting microadenoma or well circumscribed small macroadenoma, because it has traditionally provided the best cure rate. However, human patients with a large invasive macroadenoma commonly have residual disease following surgery and require additional therapeutic intervention.

Both experience with, and access to, transsphenoidal hypophysectomy in acromegalic cats is currently limited. The procedure has been described in a small number of cats (Meij *et al.,* 2001) but proved risky. Cryohypophysectomy represents an alternative and has been described in two cases to date (Abrams-Ogg *et al.,* 2002; Blois *et al.,* 2008); it requires further evaluation and longer-term follow-up before it can be confidently recommended.

Medical therapy

Medical therapy plays an important role in the management of acromegaly in human patients (Burt and Ho, 2003). Of the medical treatments available, somatostatin analogues (e.g. octreotide) improve symptoms and signs of acromegaly in the majority of human patients, with normalization of the serum IGF-1 concentration and tumour shrinkage in half of the patients.

Dopamine agonists (e.g. bromocriptine and selegiline) are effective in some human patients but are less efficacious and have more side effects than octreotide. Pegvisomant, a recently introduced GH receptor antagonist, is the most effective drug treatment for acromegaly (Stewart, 2003); however, it is likely only to have an adjuvant role as its mechanism of action is not directed at the tumour itself (i.e. the pituitary tumour would continue to grow).

Although medical treatment for acromegaly would be the most attractive type of therapy for many cat owners, neither somatostatin analogues nor dopamine agonists have been successful in lowering serum GH concentrations or improving insulin sensitivity (Peterson *et al.,* 1990; Abraham *et al.,* 2002). Pegvisomant has not yet been evaluated in cats with acromegaly, and the drug would only be expected to be effective if there is sufficient homology between feline and human GH receptors.

A recent study demonstrated a decrease in serum GH concentration following intravenous octreotide administration (Slingerland *et al.,* 2008), suggesting that some affected patients may be suited to such treatment. However, a recent trial with lanreotide (a novel long-acting somatostatin-analogue) conducted by the authors produced disappointing results.

Regardless of the chosen treatment modality, a detailed and continued assessment of quality of life should regularly be performed with the owner. A recently developed standardized and validated quality of life measurement tool for diabetic cats could prove essential in such objective assessment and may stimulate and guide a productive discussion between clinician and owner, ensuring that the impact of the cat's acromegaly on the owner's life does not remain unaddressed (Niessen *et al.,* 2010).

Prognosis

Dogs

In dogs with progesterone/progestogen-induced GH excess, the prognosis is excellent if the source can be eliminated. Diabetes mellitus resulting from GH excess is sometimes reversible after removal of its source. Even in dogs where the diabetic state persists after elimination of progestogen excess, the insulin resistance that commonly accompanies the acromegaly will resolve, and the diabetes will be easier to control. Too few cases of pituitary adenoma-induced canine acromegaly have been described to generalize on prognosis.

Cats

In cats, even without definitive treatment for acromegaly, the short-term prognosis is relatively good. Associated insulin-resistant diabetes mellitus can generally be managed with large, divided daily doses of insulin. Reported survival times of both aggressively and conservatively managed acromegalic cats vary enormously, with some cats surviving for only a few months and others living for many years and dying from causes unlikely to be related to acromegaly. An objective direct comparison between survival times of both aggressively and conservatively treated cats is still to be performed.

References and further reading

Abraham LA, Helmond SE, Mitten RW, Charles JA and Holloway SA (2002) Treatment of an acromegalic cat with the dopamine agonist l-deprenyl. *Australian Veterinary Journal* **80**, 479–483

Abrams-Ogg A, Holmberg DL, Quinn RF et al. (2002) Blindness now attributed to enrofloxacin therapy in a previously reported case of a cat with acromegaly treated by cryohypophysectomy. *Canadian Veterinary Journal* **43**, 53–54

Abrams-Ogg A, Holmberg DL, Stewart WA and Claffey FP (1993) Acromegaly in a cat: diagnosis by magnetic resonance imaging and treatment by cryohypophysectomy. *Canadian Veterinary Journal* **34**, 682–685

Berg RI, Nelson RW, Feldman EC et al. (2007) Serum insulin-like growth factor-I concentration in cats with diabetes mellitus and acromegaly. *Journal of Veterinary Internal Medicine* **21**, 892–898

Bhatti SF, Duchateau L, Okkens AC et al. (2006) Treatment of growth hormone excess in dogs with the progesterone receptor antagonist aglepristone. *Theriogenology* **66**, 797–803

Blois SL and Holmberg DL (2008) Cryohypophysectomy used in the treatment of a case of feline acromegaly. *Journal of Small Animal Practice* **49**, 596–600

Burt MG and Ho KK (2003) Comparison of efficacy and tolerability of somatostatin analogs and other therapies for acromegaly. *Endocrine* **20**, 299–305

Concannon P, Altszuler N, Hampshire J, Butler WR and Hansel W (1980) Growth hormone, prolactin, and cortisol in dogs developing mammary nodules and an acromegaly-like appearance during treatment with medroxyprogesterone acetate. *Endocrinology* **106**, 1173–1177

Dominici FP, Argentino DP, Muñoz MC et al. (2005) Influence of the crosstalk between growth hormone and insulin signaling on the modulation of insulin sensitivity. *Growth Hormone IGF Research* **15**, 324–336

Dunning MD, Lowrie CS, Bexfield NH, Dobson JM and Herrtage ME (2009) Exogenous insulin treatment after hypofractionated radiotherapy in cats with diabetes mellitus and acromegaly. *Journal of Veterinary Internal Medicine* **23**, 243–249

Eigenmann JE, Eigenmann RY, Rijnberk A et al. (1983) Progesterone-controlled growth hormone overproduction and naturally occurring canine diabetes and acromegaly. *Acta Endocrinologica* **104**, 167–176

Eigenmann JE and Venker-van Haagen AJ (1981) Progestogen-induced and spontaneous canine acromegaly due to reversible growth hormone overproduction: clinical picture and pathogenesis. *Journal of the American Animal Hospital Association* **17**, 813–822

Elliott DA, Feldman EC, Koblik PD, Samii VF and Nelson RW (2000) Prevalence of pituitary tumors among diabetic cats with insulin resistance. *Journal of the American Veterinary Medical Association* **216**, 1765–1768

Fall T, Kreuger SJ, Juberget A, Bergstrom A and Hedhammar Å (2008) Gestational diabetes mellitus in 13 dogs. *Journal of Veterinary Internal Medicine* **22**, 1296–1300

Forcada Y, German AJ, Steiner JM et al. (2008) Determination of fPLI concentrations in cats with diabetes mellitus. *Journal of Feline Medicine and Surgery* **10**, 480–487

Fracassi F, Gandini G, Diana A et al. (2007) Acromegaly due to a somatroph adenoma in a dog. *Domestic Animal Endocrinology* **32**, 43–54

Goossens MM, Feldman EC, Nelson RW et al. (1998) Cobalt 60 irradiation of pituitary gland tumors in three cats with acromegaly. *Journal of the American Veterinary Medical Association* **213**, 374–376

Gunn-Moore D (2005) Feline endocrinopathies. *Veterinary Clinics of North America: Small Animal Practice* **35**, 171–210

Kaser-Hotz B, Rohrer CR, Stankeova S et al. (2002) Radiotherapy of pituitary tumours in five cats. *Journal of Small Animal Practice* **43**, 303–307

King JM, Kavanaugh JF and Bentinck-Smith J (1962) Diabetes mellitus with pituitary neoplasms in a horse and in a dog. *Cornell Veterinarian* **52**, 133–145

Kooistra HS, Okkens AC, Mol JA et al. (1997) Lack of association of progestin-induced cystic endometrial hyperplasia with GH gene expression in the canine uterus. *Journal of Reproduction and Fertility (Suppl.)* **51**, 355–361

Lewitt MS, Hazel SJ, Church DB et al. (2000) Regulation of insulin-like growth factor-binding protein-3 ternary complex in feline diabetes mellitus. *Journal of Endocrinology* **166**, 21–27

Lichtensteiger CA, Wortman JA and Eigenmann JE (1986) Functional pituitary acidophilic adenoma in a cat with diabetes mellitus and acromegalic features. *Veterinary Pathology* **23**, 518–521

Little CJ and Gettinby G (2008) Heart failure is common in diabetic cats: findings from a retrospective case-controlled study in first-opinion practice. *Journal of Small Animal Practice* **49**, 17–25

Lucksch F (1923) Über Hypophysentumoren beim Hunde. *Tierärztliche Archiv* **3**, 1–16

Meij BP, Van der Vlugt-Meijer RH, van den Ingh TS and Rijnberk A (2004) Somatotroph and corticotroph pituitary adenoma (double adenoma) in a cat with diabetes mellitus and hyperadrenocorticism *Journal of Comparative Pathology* **130**, 209–215

Meij BP, Voorhout G, Van Den Ingh TS and Rijnberk A (2001) Transsphenoidal hypophysectomy for treatment of pituitary-dependent hyperadrenocorticism in 7 cats. *Veterinary Surgery* **30**, 72–86

Middleton DJ, Culvenor JA, Vasak E and Mintohadi K (1985) Growth hormone-producing pituitary adenoma, elevated serum somatomedin C concentration and diabetes mellitus in a cat. *Canadian Veterinary Journal* **26**, 169–171

Mol JA, Lantinga-van Leeuwen I, van Garderen E and Rijnberk A (2000) Progestin-induced mammary growth hormone (GH) production. *Advances in Experimental and Medical Biology* **480**, 71–76

Mol JA, van Garderen E, Rutteman GR and Rijnberk A (1996) New insights in the molecular mechanism of progestin-induced proliferation of mammary epithelium: induction of the local biosynthesis of growth hormone (GH) in the mammary glands of dogs, cats and humans. *Journal of Steroid Biochemistry and Molecular Biology* **57**, 67–71

Niessen SJ (2010) Feline acromegaly: an essential differential diagnosis for the difficult diabetic. *Journal of Feline Medicine and Surgery* **12**, 15–23

Niessen SJ, Khalid M, Petrie G and Church DB (2007a) Validation and application of a radioimmunoassay for ovine growth hormone in the diagnosis of acromegaly in cats.*Veterinary Record* **160**, 902–907

Niessen SJ, Petrie G, Gaudiano F et al. (2007b) Feline acromegaly: an underdiagnosed endocrinopathy. *Journal of Veterinary Internal Medicine* **21**, 899–905

Norman EJ and Mooney CT (2000) Diagnosis and management of diabetes mellitus in five cats with somatotrophic abnormalities. *Journal of Feline Medicine and Surgery* **2**, 183–190

Norman EJ, Wolsky KJ and MacKay GA (2006) Pregnancy-related diabetes mellitus in two dogs. *New Zealand Veterinary Journal* **54**, 360–364

Peterson ME (1987) Effects of megestrol acetate on glucose tolerance and growth hormone secretion in the cat. *Research in Veterinary Science* **42**, 354–357

Peterson ME, Taylor RS, Greco DS et al. (1990) Acromegaly in 14 cats. *Journal of Veterinary Internal Medicine* **4**, 192–201

Schwedes CS (1999) Transient diabetes insipidus in a dog with acromegaly. *Journal of Small Animal Practice* **40**, 392–396

Selman PJ, Mol JA, Rutteman GR and Rijnberk A (1994a) Progestin treatment in the dog. II. Effects on the hypothalamic–pituitary–adrenocortical axis. *European Journal of Endocrinology* **131**, 422–430

Selman PJ, Mol JA, Rutteman GR, Van GE and Rijnberk A (1994b) Progestin-induced growth hormone excess in the dog originates in the mammary gland. *Endocrinology* **134**, 287–292

Slingerland LI, Voorhout G, Rijnberk A and Kooistra HS (2008) Growth hormone excess and the effect of octreotide in cats with diabetes mellitus. *Domestic Animal Endocrinology* **35**, 352–361

Stewart PM (2003) Pegvisomant: an advance in clinical efficacy in acromegaly. *European Journal of Endocrinology* **148**, S027–S032

6

Hyperparathyroidism

Barbara J. Skelly

Introduction

Primary hyperparathyroidism (PHPT) is an uncommon disease in dogs and is rare in cats but must still be considered as a possible cause of hypercalcaemia, particularly in an older, relatively asymptomatic dog. PHPT develops when one or more of the parathyroid glands begins to function autonomously. Hyperparathyroidism may also develop because of non-endocrine disruption to calcium homeostasis, such as that associated with renal disease or nutritional imbalance. This chapter will discuss all recognized forms of hyperparathyroidism and their appropriate management strategies.

Physiology of the parathyroid glands

The parathyroid glands and parathyroid hormone

Parathyroid hormone (PTH; parathormone) is a small polypeptide hormone (84 amino acids) produced and secreted by the chief cells of the four parathyroid glands. In dogs and cats the parathyroid glands are arranged in two pairs: the cranial or external glands, situated outside the thyroid capsule adjacent to the thyroid gland; and the caudal or internal glands, located within thyroid tissue (Figure 6.1). Parathyroid tissue, like thyroid tissue, can be ectopic, and accessory glands are usually situated alongside the trachea. The parathyroid glands are different in structure from the thyroid glands in that they consist of cords or nests of cells around capillaries (Figure 6.2), rather than of the distinctive thyroid colloid-filled follicles.

The parathyroid glands synthesize PTH continuously, but the number of secretory granules is low. This is because much of the active synthesized PTH is immediately broken down within the parathyroid chief cells, so that secretory granules contain active hormone plus carboxy-terminal fragments of the polypeptide. The active part of the polypeptide is the 34 amino acid *N*-terminal, the structure of which is conserved across species, whilst the carboxy-terminal fragment is required to allow PTH to progress along the cellular secretory pathway.

- Calcium mediates the rate at which degradation occurs, so that reduced serum calcium concentrations slow the degradation rate and

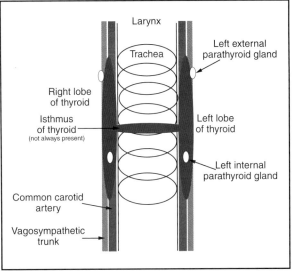

6.1 Schematic representation of the anatomical position of the parathyroid glands.

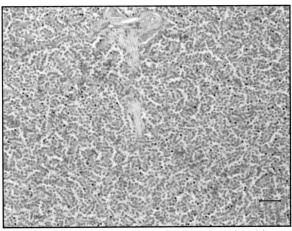

6.2 Histological appearance of the parathyroid glands from a healthy dog, showing cords or nests of cells around capillaries. H&E stain; bar = 50 μm. (Courtesy of Fernando Constantino-Casas)

increase intact PTH secretion, and increased serum calcium concentrations speed up the degradation rate and decrease intact PTH secretion.
- The active form of vitamin D, 1,25-dihydroxycholecalciferol (1,25(OH)$_2$-vitamin D; calcitriol) and phosphate also regulate PTH

secretion. High concentrations of vitamin D reduce PTH gene transcription and thus reduce the levels of PTH synthesized. High phosphate acts in a similar way to low serum calcium concentration, by reducing intact PTH breakdown and increasing its release.

PTH acts on bone, the kidney and the gastrointestinal tract to increase calcium mobilization or reuptake (Figure 6.3). Negative feedback occurs from raised serum calcium concentrations, such that PTH secretion is switched off once the required calcium concentration is reached.

The importance of calcium

Calcium plays an important role in neuromuscular conductivity and muscle contraction, and is also a second messenger, regulating and mediating cellular responses to different stimuli in a range of contexts (endocrine system, coagulation cascade, etc). Calcium concentrations are highest in the extracellular fluid, while intracellular concentrations are low. Increases in the intracellular calcium concentration lead to cell dysfunction and death.

Electrolyte concentrations are tightly controlled, and calcium is no exception.

- The reference interval for total calcium in the dog and cat varies according to the laboratory used but is generally in the range of 2.3–2.8 mmol/l for dogs and 2.1–2.8 mmol/l for cats. Total calcium includes calcium bound to albumin, chelated calcium and ionized or free calcium. Relatively small increases are clinically significant (Figure 6.4).
- Although total calcium measurement can give an indication that there is a disorder of calcium regulation, ionized calcium concentrations are

Severity of hypercalcaemia	Serum concentration of total calcium (mmol/l)
Mild	2.9–3.2
Moderate	3.3–3.7
Severe	>3.7

6.4 The relative severity of serum calcium concentration.

more useful and pertinent, as only calcium in its ionized form is physiologically active. The reference interval for ionized calcium is generally in the range of 1.2–1.4 mmol/l for dogs and cats.

Calcium homeostasis

Calcium is the most abundant cation in the body, with 99% stored in skeletal bone in the form of hydroxyapatite. This skeletal reservoir acts as a store for calcium that can be remobilized (Figure 6.5) through the action of osteoclasts on the bone, whereas calcium storage is mediated by osteoblasts. Thus, the homeostatic control of calcium in the body involves movement between the skeleton and extracellular fluids and soft tissues, but also involves calcium uptake or loss through the kidneys and gastrointestinal tract (see Figure 6.3).

The hormones involved in calcium homeostasis are:

- PTH
- Vitamin D
- Calcitonin.

PTH acts directly on target cells in the kidney and in bone, and also indirectly via the synthesis of $1,25(OH)_2$-vitamin D, to influence intestinal calcium uptake. The effects of PTH are:

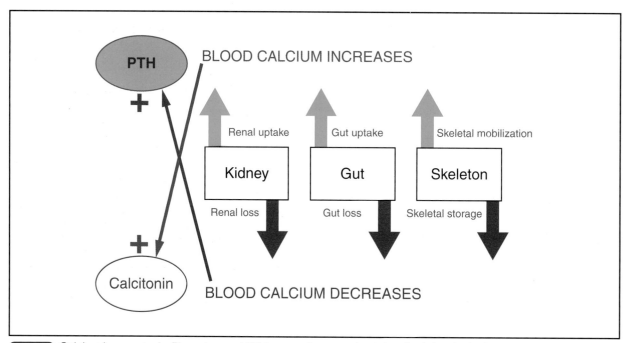

6.3 Calcium homeostasis. The release of PTH causes increased uptake of calcium in the kidney and gut, and mobilization from the skeleton.

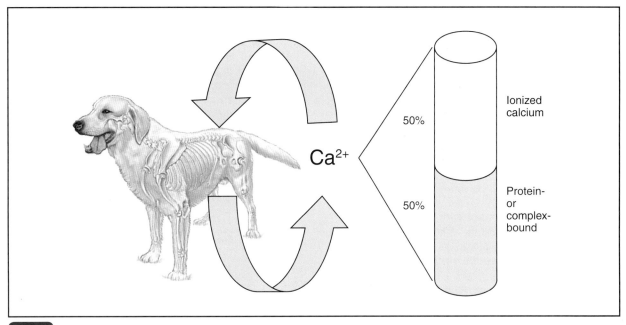

6.5 The skeletal calcium acts as a reservoir, so that calcium can be stored or mobilized, depending on need.

- To increase tubular absorption of calcium
- To increase bone resorption and the number of osteoclasts on the surface of bones
- To promote the synthesis of the active form of vitamin D by the kidney through the synthesis and activation of the enzyme 1α-hydroxylase.

Primary hyperparathyroidism

Hyperparathyroidism is defined by hypercalcaemia in the face of inappropriately high concentrations of PTH (either above or within the reference interval). Hyperparathyroidism is one of the many diff-erential diagnoses for hypercalcaemia, as described in Chapter 21. Hyperparathyroidism may be primary or secondary. In primary hyperparathyroidism (PHPT) there is hypercalcaemia and high or high-normal PTH with no other identifiable underlying cause.

Prevalence
PHPT is an uncommon disease in dogs; it is very rare in cats, where there are only a few case reports and no large case series as there are in dogs (Kallet *et al.,* 1991; Den Hertog *et al.*, 1997; Savary *et al.*, 2000).

Aetiology and pathophysiology
PHPT is caused by adenoma, carcinoma or adenomatous hyperplasia of one or more parathyroid glands. As a consequence the glands function autonomously, independent of the effects of serum calcium concentration. In contrast, secondary hyperparathyroidism is expected to be caused by hyperplasia of more than one parathyroid gland in response to a more generalized stimulus to produce PTH. In reality, both primary and secondary hyperparathyroidism often become blurred, particularly in light of the description of the pathological changes in the parathyroid glands. Hyperplasia may not affect each gland uniformly and, though most frequently associated with secondary disease, has been described as a cause of PHPT in the cat and dog (Thompson *et al.,* 1984; DeVries *et al.*, 1993; Savary *et al.*, 2000).

Parathyroid adenomas
In humans, a spectrum of disorders is described. These include:

- Familial isolated hyperparathyroidism (FIH)
- Familial hypocalciuric hypercalcaemia (FHH)
- Multiple endocrine neoplasia type 1 (MEN1) and type 2A (MEN2A)
- Hyperparathyroidism–jaw tumour syndrome (HPT–JT).

In all but one of these disorders (FIH), hyperparathyroidism exists as part of a complex syndrome.

FIH has been associated with mutations in three of the genes more usually associated with other phenotypes: *CaSR*, *MEN1* and *HRPT2* (Warner *et al.*, 2004). A diagnosis of FIH is therefore reached if the diagnostic criteria for any of the other phenotypes are not met when using standard, non-molecular genetic tests. When human patients with FIH are investigated, the *CaSR* and *MEN1* genes are assessed initially, as *HRPT2* mutation is a less common cause of isolated hyperparathyroidism (Simonds *et al.*, 2004).

In dogs the Keeshond is the only breed in which PHPT is inherited. The mode of inheritance was investigated by Goldstein *et al.* (2007) and by

Skelly and Franklin (2007). Keeshonds have an autosomal dominant form of PHPT that has partial, age-dependent penetrance. This means that a Keeshond need only have one copy of the mutated allele to develop the disease, and those dogs carrying the mutation will go on to develop the disease if they live long enough. No dogs have been identified that have two copies of the mutated allele and it is speculated that this would be incompatible with survival to birth. A genetic test is available for PHPT in the Keeshond but the mutation and the identity of the gene involved have not yet been published. The genetic test for PHPT is available from Cornell University (www.vet.cornell.edu/labs/goldstein/). This test enables breeders to limit their use of mutation-carrying animals and choose replacement breeding stock on the basis of being negative for the disease-causing mutation.

Clinical features

Signalment
PHPT is a disease of older dogs (mean age 11.2 years; range 6–17 years). There is no sex predisposition but there is a breed predilection in that Keeshonds are over-represented. In one review of cases, Keeshonds were found to have the highest breed-associated odds ratio, at 50.7 (Refsal *et al.*, 2001). Neonatal hyperparathyroidism was reported in a litter of German Shepherd Dog puppies (Thompson *et al.*, 1984) but there have been no other reports since.

Clinical signs
The clinical signs of hyperparathyroidism are summarized in Figure 6.6.

Renal and urinary tract signs
• Polyuria • Polydipsia • Urinary incontinence • Stranguria • Pollakiuria • Urolithiasis
Neuromuscular signs
• Depression • Exercise intolerance • Shivering • Facial pain and discomfort when eating
Gastrointestinal signs
• Vomiting • Inappetence • Constipation
Other
• Dental pain • Difficulty in eating • Stiff gait • Lameness

6.6 Clinical signs of hyperparathyroidism.

PHPT is not a dramatic disease; rather, it is slow in development and insidious in nature. As such, changes are subtle and can occur over a long period. As affected dogs tend to be older, many of the clinical signs are attributed to ageing changes and owners do not seek veterinary advice until late in the course of the disease. PHPT is frequently identified when blood samples are taken for other reasons (e.g. as a pre-anaesthetic screen). In one study of 210 cases, 42% of dogs were identified as having PHPT when they were presented for other reasons, such as routine geriatric checks, or when pre-anaesthetic blood testing was performed for procedures such as dental treatment (Feldman *et al.*, 2005). The most common reason for seeking veterinary advice was for the investigation of clinical signs related to urolithiasis or urinary tract infection (50% of the 210 cases). Urolithiasis can also present as acute urinary outflow obstruction in a dog with PHPT.

Polyuria and polydipsia were noticed by <10% of owners of dogs with PHPT; this is a surprisingly small number, given that calcium acts as an antagonist to vasopressin (antidiuretic hormone, ADH) in the collecting ducts of the kidney and thereby inhibits the urine-concentrating mechanism. The result is that affected dogs are polyuric with a secondary, compensatory polydipsia.

The presence of hypercalcaemia can also affect the kidneys in other ways. Dogs that are hypercalcaemic are at an increased risk of developing renal failure. It is difficult to understand the mechanism of failure, and why this condition affects some dogs and not others. For dogs with PHPT, it has been suggested that calculating the calcium phosphate product may help to predict the likelihood of the development of renal failure; dogs with PHPT that have a low phosphate and a relatively low calcium phosphate product are thought to be less likely to develop renal failure. In the large case series of 210 dogs, the risk of renal failure was deemed to be low, while in a smaller case series (29 dogs) from the UK (Gear *et al.*, 2005), approximately 25% developed renal insufficiency. In that study, the calcium phosphate product was a poor predictor of renal impairment.

Phosphate concentrations should be at the low end of, or below, the reference interval in a dog with PHPT. If this were not the case, renal insufficiency might already be developing, albeit before overt azotaemia is recognized. In these cases, closer monitoring and a more guarded prognosis should be given.

It is interesting to examine the genetically homogeneous Keeshond population and the incidence of renal failure in those carrying the mutation linked to PHPT. It is this author's experience that some dogs left untreated die of other causes with normal renal function while having prolonged, in some cases severe, hypercalcaemia (>4.0 mmol/l). Other dogs succumb to renal failure with much more modest calcium elevations, whilst at least one dog developed a large nephrolith and urolithiasis (Figure 6.7) and died of renal failure

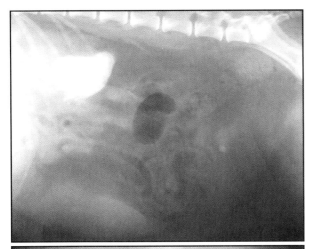

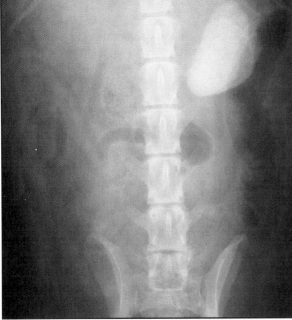

6.7 Lateral and ventrodorsal abdominal radiographs showing a large nephrolith in the left kidney and multiple smaller uroliths.

after disease management had seemingly been successful. It is therefore clear that predicting long-term outcome with or without treatment is fraught with problems. Erring on the side of caution when managing hypercalcaemia is recommended.

Relevant findings on physical examination are few and non-specific. They may include stiffness and gait abnormalities, dull mentation, weakness and muscle wastage. There are no characteristic changes. Little information is gathered from palpation of the ventral neck area as any parathyroid abnormalities are usually beyond the most sensitive palpation skills.

Urolithiasis: Urolith formation is common in dogs with hyperparathyroidism due to the increased concentrations of calcium that are filtered by the kidney and lost in urine. Although PTH causes increased calcium uptake from renal tubules, in cases of PHPT there is overt hypercalciuria, presumably as re-uptake is unable to match the amount of calcium that is filtered. Conditions in urine are such that there is an increased tendency to precipitate calcium salts within the urinary tract. Dogs with PHPT have hypercalciuria but also have increased phosphate excretion. Urine is therefore supersaturated with both calcium and phosphate, and it is unsurprising that this leads to calcium phosphate precipitation and stone formation.

The incidence of calcium oxalate urolithiasis is also increased in dogs with PHPT. Dietary oxalate uptake from the gut is reduced when there is abundant intraluminal calcium, because calcium oxalate is not absorbable from the intestine. If intestinal calcium absorption increases, oxalate absorption will also increase and the kidney will filter higher levels of both calcium and oxalate, again leading to supersaturation in the urine.

Clinicopathological features

The degree of hypercalcaemia is largely dependent on the duration of the disease before its identification. If PTH is mediating the hypercalcaemia then, in the presence of normal renal function, hypophosphataemia should also be evident. Keeshonds from families with PHPT generally start to show mild to moderate hypercalcaemia (up to 3.3 mmol/l) when they are 6–8 years of age, and this gradually worsens over subsequent years. Some untreated dogs continue to experience increased calcium concentrations until severe hypercalcaemia is reached (>4.0 mmol/l). As the genetic basis for PHPT in other breeds is not known, it is not clear how reproducible this pattern is between breeds, but in all breeds the disease appears to be slow and insidious in development.

Upon identification of hypercalcaemia, other parameters should be measured to characterize the origin of electrolyte disturbance. The critical parameters to measure in animals with PHPT include total and ionized calcium, phosphate, PTH and parathyroid hormone-related protein (PTHrp).

PTH

PTH is found in the blood as both intact hormone and carboxyl-terminal fragments that are the result of hormone degradation. To measure PTH concentrations, intact assays that measure the biologically active hormone (amino acids 1—84) are used. However, such assays may also detect truncated PTH (amino acids 7–84), considered biologically inactive. Whole PTH assays that measure amino acids 1–84 have been developed for human use but have not been fully evaluated in dogs or cats (see Chapter 1). Currently, ELISA is the predominant method used to measure PTH in the UK. A canine-specific intact ELISA (Canine Intact PTH ELISA Kit, Immutopics), which has also been validated for cats, is available, and some laboratories have validated human-specific intact PTH testing kits for use in the dog and cat. Samples of EDTA plasma are preferred for PTH measurement.

The reference interval for PTH is approximately 20–65 pg/ml in the dog and <40 pg/ml in the cat but may differ depending on the laboratory and assay used. Expected results in PHPT are a PTH elevation above the reference interval or, although within the reference interval, inappropriately high for the concurrent serum calcium (i.e. in the upper half of the reference interval, >35 pg/ml for dogs).

PTHrp

PTHrp is measured by two-site IRMA and by *N*-terminal radioimmunoassay (RIA). There are several circulating forms of PTHrp that have biological activity, including intact PTHrp (amino acids 1–141), an *N*-terminal fragment (1–36) and an *N*-terminal plus mid-region fragment (1–86). The roles of the different forms are not completely understood. Like PTH, PTHrp is not stable and is measured preferentially in plasma, using EDTA as an anticoagulant. The reference interval for PTHrp is generally <0.5 pmol/l in both dogs and cats.

Other

Biochemical parameters may be otherwise unremarkable. Urea and creatinine concentrations may be elevated, due to pre-existing renal damage or prerenal factors, along with phosphate concentrations. This complicates diagnosis, in that the changes associated with PHPT with secondary renal failure can mimic those of primary renal disease with secondary PTH elevation and hypercalcaemia (Figure 6.8).

Parameter	PHPT	Secondary renal hyperparathyroidism
Total calcium	↑	↓ or normal or ↑
Ionized calcium	↑	↓ or normal
Phosphate	↓	↑
PTH	↑ or high normal	↑ or high normal
PTHrP	normal	normal or ↑

6.8 A comparison of the clinicopathological features of PHPT and renal secondary hyperparathyroidism.

Haematological parameters show no consistent changes, although anaemia of chronic disease may be identified, particularly if hypercalcaemia has been present for some time.

Pathology

Three different types of pathological change are reported from autonomously secreting parathyroid glands: carcinoma, adenoma and hyperplasia. To some extent, the subdivision is subjective and may vary between pathologists. This is because, as with many functional endocrine tumours, differentiation is difficult, especially if only one gland is excised and examined. In parathyroid carcinomas where malignant criteria are identified, metastatic disease is rare. Disease recurrence, where there is involvement of another gland, is possible with all three pathological classifications.

Diagnostic imaging

Ultrasonography of the ventral neck is the most useful imaging modality when investigating parathyroid adenomas, with 90–95% positively identified by experienced imagers (Feldman *et al.*, 2005). A high-frequency transducer of 7.5–10 MHz is required for adequate resolution. In healthy dogs and cats the parathyroid glands are so small that they are rarely recognized. When they are either hyperplastic or enlarged and adenomatous, or when there is a parathyroid carcinoma, the parathyroid glands are identified as small (2–20 mm), round to oval, hypoechoic nodules within the thyroid tissue (Figure 6.9) (Wisner and Nyland, 1998).

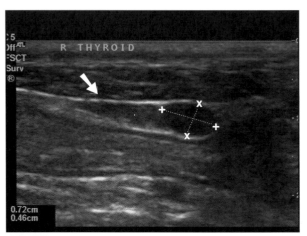

6.9 Ultrasonographic image of the ventral neck showing the right thyroid gland (arrow) containing a large, hypoechoic parathyroid nodule (dimensions delineated by dotted lines).

Scintigraphy using technetium-99m sestamibi has been used in dogs as an aid to parathyroid identification but, unlike in humans, it lacks sensitivity and specificity and is therefore unreliable (Matwichuk *et al.*, 1996).

Abdominal radiographs may be useful, as they may reveal calcium-containing renal or cystic calculi (see Figure 6.7) that are not yet causing any clinical signs.

Treatment

Pre-treatment management of hypercalcaemia

Once hypercalcaemia has been recognized in a patient it is important to institute treatment to lower the calcium concentrations whilst other diagnostic tests are underway. Renal damage, caused by persistent hypercalcaemia due to PHPT, is uncommon but is impossible to predict. All affected animals must therefore be considered at risk if they are significantly hypercalcaemic.

Fluid therapy is the cornerstone of the management of hypercalcaemia. Diuresis, using 0.9% sodium chloride at rates of 5 ml/kg/h, increases renal calcium loss and lowers serum calcium concentrations. Fluid therapy should aim to correct any dehydration and then additionally expand the extracellular fluid volume so that the glomerular filtration rate is increased. Sodium chloride is the fluid of choice, because extra sodium ions are able to compete with calcium and reduce tubular calcium re-uptake. When an animal is considered to be optimally hydrated, furosemide (2 mg/kg q8–12h) can potentiate renal calcium loss by reducing tubular calcium re-uptake still further. When using sodium chloride at high rates, particularly coupled with furosemide, serum potassium must be monitored to avoid inducing hypokalaemia.

If this treatment is not sufficient to lower serum calcium levels, other medications can be used. These include:

- Glucocorticoids
- Bisphosphonates
- Calcitonin
- Plicamycin.

Glucocorticoids: The use of glucocorticoids (in the dose range of approximately 1 mg/kg bodyweight) to lower serum calcium levels should be restricted to those cases where there is a clear diagnosis and a delay to rational treatment. They are most effective when used in cases of hypercalcaemia of malignancy, as they cause rapid tumour lysis and reduction in the production of the mediators of hypercalcaemia, e.g. PTHrp. When used in undiagnosed patients there is a real risk of masking and complicating the diagnosis of neoplasia. Glucocorticoids work by increasing renal calcium loss, decreasing intestinal calcium uptake and decreasing bone resorption. They do not have a great effect in cases of PHPT and do not achieve significantly lowered calcium concentrations.

Bisphosphonates: Bisphosphonates are potent inhibitors of bone resorption; they act through the inhibition of osteoclastic activity and by inducing osteoclast apoptosis. Several different bisphosphonates have been used in veterinary medicine; those used most often include clodronate, etidronate and pamidronate. Although clodronate and etidronate can be administered orally, this route is not very effective, with <1% of a dose being absorbed in some cases (Plumb, 2005). An intravenous infusion of pamidronate is more reliable (1.3–2 mg/kg in 150 ml of 0.9% saline, given over 2 hours (Plumb, 2005). Pamidronate is approximately 100 times more potent than etidronate. The effects last up to 3 weeks, although this is variable between patients and the dose can be repeated as required. This drug is generally well tolerated (Hostutler *et al.*, 2005) but can cause gastrointestinal side-effects and hypocalcaemia, particularly if overdosed. Pamidronate has been frequently used to treat human patients with hypercalcaemia of malignancy, but a newer, more potent bisphosphonate, zoledronate, is now superseding pamidronate as the drug of choice. Zoledronate is 100–850 times more active than pamidronate and can be infused more rapidly, but has not been used extensively in dogs and this author has no personal experience of the use of this drug.

Calcitonin: Salmon calcitonin is commercially available to treat hypercalcaemia. Like bisphosphonates, it inhibits osteoclastic activity, and additionally inhibits the renal reabsorption of calcium. It is useful as an emergency treatment to decrease calcium concentrations. A disadvantage of this treatment when compared to bisphosphonates such as pamidronate is that after an initial intravenous infusion (4 IU/kg), treatment must continue daily (4–8 IU/kg s.c.) every 12–24 hours (Nelson and Elliott, 2003). Calcitonin therapy can cause anorexia and vomiting. It is an expensive treatment and is rarely used. Animals may become resistant to the effects of calcitonin after a few days of treatment.

Plicamycin (mithramycin): There are few reports of this being used in dogs. A dose rate of 25 μg/kg i.v. in 5% dextrose over 2–4 hours q2–4wk has been suggested (Schenk *et al.*, 2006).

Definitive treatment options

Surgical parathyroidectomy: Surgery is the treatment of choice at many referral institutions, and is also preferred if the parathyroid nodule is >12 mm in size (Rasor *et al.*, 2007). Good visualization of the thyroid glands is essential during surgical exploration of the neck; this is achieved using a ventral midline cervical approach. Parathyroid adenomas are usually easily identified compared to normal parathyroid glands, and appear darker and larger. When the internal parathyroid glands are affected, they can be identified by palpation and are visible through the ventral or dorsal aspect of the thyroid gland. Their identification is aided greatly if the surgeon knows where to look after ultrasonography has identified an abnormal gland.

Parathyroid adenomas can be removed either by dissection of the enlarged gland from the adjacent thyroid tissue or by partial thyroidectomy, where the parathyroid and part of the thyroid gland are removed *en bloc*. The intraoperative appearance of a parathyroid adenoma is illustrated in Figure 6.10. In cases of PHPT, only one gland is usually affected. If more than one gland is found to be enlarged, then up to three glands may be removed at one time. At least one parathyroid gland should be left *in situ* so that calcium homeostasis can be maintained. When multiple glands are enlarged then it is more likely that the glands are hyperplastic rather than adenomatous, and therefore secondary rather than primary hyperparathyroidism is suspected.

Percutaneous, ultrasound-guided ethanol ablation: In order for parathyroid nodules to be effectively treated using ethanol injection they must be successfully identified by ultrasound examination, and must also be >3 mm in diameter, so that a 27 gauge needle can be inserted accurately. Animals must be under general anaesthesia. The technique works because ethanol induces coagulation necrosis and thrombosis in the parathyroid nodule (Long *et al.*, 1999). The success of the technique is operator-dependent, in that skill is needed for accurate

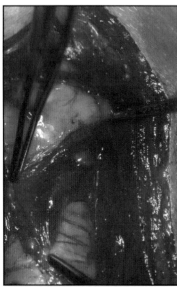

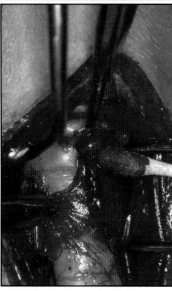

6.10

Removal of a parathyroid adenoma. The thyroid (dark red) is visible overlying the trachea with a smaller, paler, parathyroid nodule (at tip of cotton bud). (Courtesy of Ed Friend)

needle placement and injection so that the carotid artery and vagosympathetic trunk, which pass close by, are not compromised. When the three techniques for treating PHPT were compared, ethanol ablation was the least successful, with a positive outcome achieved in 13/18 procedures (72%), compared with 45/48 (94%) for surgery and 44/49 (90%) for heat ablation (Rasor *et al.*, 2007). However, only a small number of cases were treated by ethanol ablation; perhaps greater experience is required with this technique. In a recent review, a success rate of >90% in 30 dogs was reported (Schaefer and Goldstein, 2009).

Percutaneous, ultrasound-guided heat ablation: This technique is the least frequently used of the three, mainly because the number of institutions offering this therapy is so small. There are no referral centres in the UK using this method and in the USA it is offered only at the University of California, Davis (Pollard *et al.*, 2001; Rasor *et al.*, 2007). The technique depends on inserting a needle into a parathyroid nodule and causing thermal

necrosis at the needle tip. To do this, the animal is anaesthetized and positioned on an electrocautery ground pad; a 20 gauge catheter is inserted into the affected parathyroid gland and radiofrequency applied at 10–20 W until the entire gland becomes hyperechoic.

Pre- and post-treatment considerations

When PHPT is treated successfully, using one of the three techniques described above, PTH and therefore calcium concentrations should decrease rapidly and, in some circumstances, a hypocalcaemic crisis may be encountered. This usually happens if the pre-treatment calcium has been severely elevated for some time prior to treatment. Generally, hypocalcaemia is more likely to be encountered if the pre-treatment calcium exceeded 3.5 mmol/l for more than a few months, although this is variable. When a parathyroid adenoma is functioning autonomously, the remaining parathyroid glands become atrophied and are unable to support normal calcium homeostasis once the affected tissue has been removed. Such a crisis can be averted by giving vitamin D ± oral calcium supplements in the immediate post-treatment period. Vitamin D is available in several different preparations but it is important to use a preparation that will have a relatively rapid onset of action. The two preparations most frequently recommended are:

- $1,25(OH)_2$-vitamin D is the active form of vitamin D and therefore does not require further metabolism to become active when given. It has a rapid onset of action (1–4 days) and a short half-life. Toxic effects would be expected to resolve in 2–7 days. Calcitriol comes in capsules of 0.25 or 0.5 µg. The dose rate used is 20–30 ng/kg orally q12h (Chew and Nagode, 2000). *This product is not authorized for veterinary use.*
- Alfacalcidol is the formulation most commonly used by this author. This needs to undergo 25-hydroxylation by the liver before it is active. This process occurs rapidly in a relatively unregulated fashion, so this does not significantly alter the time to maximal effect compared to calcitriol. The drug is available as 0.25, 0.5 and 1 µg capsules and also as drops (2 µg/ml), so is useful in small dogs and cats. A dose of 0.01–0.03 µg/kg q24h is used. However, these doses have some flexibility and may be titrated upwards and downwards to effect to suit any individual animal. *This product is not authorized for veterinary use.*

These preparations may be used with or without oral calcium supplementation. The following are options and dose rates:

- Calcium gluconate at 25–50 mg/kg/day divided twice or three times daily
- Calcium lactate at 25–50 mg/kg/day divided twice or three times daily
- Calcium carbonate 25–50 mg/kg/day divided twice daily.

These doses are calculated on the basis of **elemental** calcium present in the preparation, **not** on the mg size of tablet, thus all the dose rates are the same once the elemental calcium content has been taken into account, e.g. 1 mg elemental calcium = 11.2 mg calcium gluconate = 7.7 mg calcium lactate = 2.5 mg calcium carbonate.

Often, and particularly when postoperative hypocalcaemia has been severe and symptomatic, calcium supplementation will be used in the short term for patient stabilization. For longer-term management it is rarely necessary to use extra dietary calcium, as most pet foods contain more than adequate amounts, so long as the means of absorption (enough vitamin D) is present.

Emergency or short-term treatment of hypocalcaemia: Intravenous calcium supplementation may be required for dogs that become hypocalcaemic after surgery, either symptomatically or asymptomatically. The clinical signs of hypocalcaemia are listed in Figure 6.11.

Signs associated with neuromuscular excitability
• Muscle fasciculation or tremors • Face rubbing • Hypersensitivity to external stimuli • Stiff, stilted gait • Tetanic seizures • Respiratory arrest
Behavioural changes
• Agitation • Anxiety • Vocalization • Aggression
Other
• Panting • Pyrexia

6.11 Clinical signs of acute hypocalcaemia.

Dogs that are hospitalized and are not being exercised or unduly stressed may be stable with calcium concentrations below the reference interval but require supplementation and careful monitoring to avoid a hypocalcaemic crisis. When required, intravenous calcium gluconate in a 10% solution is the treatment of choice. Symptomatic patients can be given 0.5–1.5 ml/kg i.v. slowly over 20–30 minutes until clinical signs have subsided and the patient is considered to be stable. An ECG should be used to monitor cardiac effects and the infusion stopped if there is ST segment elevation, QT shortening or if arrhythmias develop. Thereafter, a continuous rate infusion can be used at 10–15 mg/kg/h (10–15 ml/kg over 24 hours) until oral therapy allows better control.

The use of subcutaneous calcium supplementation is controversial. Sterile abscess formation and skin sloughing has been reported when calcium salts are used subcutaneously (Feldman and Nelson, 2004); however, some authors recommend that calcium gluconate be administered using this route, as it is not likely to cause a problem. Although it is true that calcium gluconate may be given subcutaneously with no adverse effects, it is also true that in some cases even calcium gluconate can cause dramatic skin sloughing. For this reason, only the intravenous and oral routes of administration are recommended.

When the pre-treatment calcium concentration is >3.5 mmol/l, and particularly when it is in the severe range (>3.8 mmol/l), it is advisable to begin vitamin D supplementation 24–36 hours before surgery so that dramatic decreases in calcium do not occur. This is always something of a balancing act, as it is not advisable to exacerbate the pre-existing hypercalcaemia. However, given the known delay in onset of activity of the vitamin D preparations, pre-treatment for one day is not expected to be detrimental.

Prognosis

The short- to mid-term (<2 years) prognosis for PHPT is excellent in all breeds. In all breeds except the Keeshond the long-term prognosis also appears to be good. In Keeshonds, as in many human forms of PHPT, recurrence is a distinct possibility. This is not surprising, given the mechanisms of pathogenesis of the disease and the role of tumour suppressor genes in the evolution of hyperparathyroidism. When PHPT is managed surgically in humans, a subtotal parathyroidectomy is carried out, where only a small amount of parathyroid tissue remains *in situ* for ongoing calcium homeostasis. Keeshonds have a genetic drive to develop parathyroid adenomas, and after one has been removed more may follow if the dog lives long enough. Keeshonds that have had PHPT should be monitored throughout life for disease recurrence, particularly if first surgery was performed at a relatively young age (<9 years).

Secondary hyperparathyroidism

Three forms of secondary hyperparathyroidism are described:

- Renal secondary hyperparathyroidism
- Nutritional secondary hyperparathyroidism
- Adrenal secondary hyperparathyroidism.

Renal secondary hyperparathyroidism

An animal with functional renal compromise and hypercalcaemia can be diagnostically challenging, as it may have primary renal disease driving the hypercalcaemia or may have another condition causing hypercalcaemia with secondary renal disease. The diagnostic dilemma is further complicated by the fact that, in many cases, PTH is the driving force for hypercalcaemia. Figure 6.8 illustrates the clinicopathological similarities between

PHPT and chronic renal failure with secondary hyperparathyroidism. If an animal with PHPT has hypercalcaemia-induced renal failure and phosphate concentrations rise, then another differentiating parameter is lost. Ionized calcium is always raised in PHPT, whereas, in renal failure, <10% of dogs have elevated ionized calcium levels. Therefore, most dogs with azotaemia and significantly raised ionized calcium in conjunction with high PTH levels will have PHPT; however, a careful diagnostic work-up is still necessary. The pathophysiological changes leading to renal secondary hyperparathyroidism are described in Figure 6.12.

Phosphate retention
• Reduced capacity of the kidneys to excrete phosphate as glomerular filtration rate (GFR) falls
Decreased concentrations of calcitriol
• Damage to renal tubules further lowers renal capacity to synthesize calcitriol • Increased phosphate concentrations in proximal tubular cells inhibit 1α-hydroxylase activity and so reduce calcitriol synthesis
Ionized hypocalcaemia
• Relative calcitriol deficiency reduces calcium uptake from the intestine • Formation of complexes with phosphate, leading to soft tissue calcification • Skeletal resistance to the action of PTH
Abnormal parathyroid gland function
• PTH synthesis and secretion increases, stimulated by low ionized calcium, lack of calcitriol and possibly hyperphosphataemia • Set point for ionized calcium control of PTH secretion is raised such that PTH secretion occurs at higher concentrations of ionized calcium, allowing excessive PTH secretion even at normal blood ionized calcium concentrations • Parathyroid gland hyperplasia

6.12 Pathophysiology of renal secondary hyperparathyroidism.

The management of renal secondary hyperparathyroidism is summarized in Figure 6.13. The use of vitamin D to normalize PTH concentrations is controversial and not proven to be of benefit, while there is a significant risk of causing soft tissue calcification. Phosphate restriction is pivotal, however,

Phosphate restriction

• Dietary phosphate restriction:
  – Commercial restricted phosphate 'renal' diets
  – Home made 'renal' diets
• Intestinal phosphate-binding agents:
  – Aluminium hydroxide 30–100 mg/kg/day, divided with meals
  – Calcium carbonate 30–100 mg/kg/day, divided with meals
  – Form non-absorbable salts of phosphate in food and intestinal secretions, therefore, best mixed with food or given immediately prior to meal
  – Adverse effects: Unpalatable; Nausea and anorexia; Constipation; Hypophosphataemia; Aluminium toxicity or hypercalcaemia.

6.13 Treatment of renal secondary hyperparathyroidism. (continues) ▶

Vitamin D therapy
1,25(OH)₂-vitamin D 1.5–3.5 ng/kg/day Alfacalcidol 1.5–3.5 ng/kg/day
• Directly inhibits PTH secretion but beneficial effects unproven • Serum calcium concentrations should be monitored closely (at least weekly) • Adverse effects: Hypercalcaemia and hyperphosphataemia.

6.13 (continued) Treatment of renal secondary hyperparathyroidism.

and has been shown to reduce renal secondary hyperparathyroidism (Elliott *et al.*, 2000). A recent review details current thinking on the management of chronic renal disease using an evidence-based approach (Roudebush *et al.*, 2010).

Nutritional secondary hyperparathyroidism

Nutritional secondary hyperparathyroidism is the consequence of an imbalance between calcium and phosphate that occurs when an animal is fed a predominantly meat diet. Such diets are low in calcium and high in phosphate; low vitamin D intake may also compound the problem. BARF diets (biologically appropriate raw food, or bones and raw food) may be associated with this condition (DeLay and Laing, 2002), but it is rare that pet owners feeding a complete dog or cat food that meets all dietary requirements would ever encounter this condition. The features of the condition usually manifest in young animals where skeletal problems are present, with low bone density and fibrous osteodystrophy. Nutritional secondary hyperparathyroidism tends to exert its effects on the long bones, and pathological fractures can occur.

Severe malabsorption, where vitamin D and calcium uptake are impaired, can lead to a similar biochemical profile. Low ionized calcium then stimulates PTH release to try to restore normocalcaemia. This has been seen in, for example, Yorkshire Terriers with lymphangiectasia, and is reported in two dogs with protein-losing enteropathies (Mellanby *et al.,* 2005).

Adrenal secondary hyperparathyroidism

It has long been recognized that hyperadrenocorticism (HAC, Cushing's disease) can cause signs of dysregulation of calcium homeostasis, and that affected animals can show soft tissue calcification (calcinosis cutis, bronchial tree calcification), but the reasons for this are still unclear. More recently, a syndrome of increased circulating concentrations of PTH has been identified in animals with HAC and this has been termed adrenal secondary hyperparathyroidism (Ramsey *et al.*, 2005). The majority (92%) of 68 dogs with HAC had PTH levels above the reference interval, although total and ionized calcium concentrations were unaffected. The effects of HAC should be taken into account when reaching a diagnosis of PHPT, particularly in dogs. PTH concentrations responded to treatment of HAC, declining to reference values (Tebb *et al.*, 2005).

Case 1: 10-year-old male neutered Keeshond, 23.5 kg

The dog was investigated for possible primary hyperparathyroidism purely because of his breed (close family members had been found to be hypercalcaemic). Although considered healthy by his owners, his water intake was high. Low activity levels were attributed to advancing age. Three total calcium measurements performed over the previous 6 months had been 3.24 mmol/l, 3.75 mmol/l and 3.43 mmol/l.

History and physical examination
Physical examination was unremarkable.

Clinical pathology

Parameter	Concentration	Reference interval
Total calcium	3.45 mmol/l	2.30–2.80 mmol/l
Ionized calcium	1.73 mmol/l	1.18–1.40 mmol/l
Phosphate	0.70 mmol/l	0.60–1.30 mmol/l
PTH	136 pg/ml	10–60 pg/ml
Urea	5.9 mmol/l	3.3–8.0 mmol/l
Creatinine	74 µmol/l	45–150 µmol/l

Urinalysis

- Specific gravity 1.017
- Trace of protein
- 5–10 red blood cells per high power field
- No bacterial growth when cultured
- Frequent calcium phosphate crystals

Imaging
A left-sided parathyroid nodule was identified ultrasonographically.

Diagnosis
Primary hyperparathyroidism.

Medical and surgical management
The dog received 24 hours of fluid therapy at 8 ml/kg/h initially for 6 hours, reducing to 6 ml/kg/h until surgery.

Surgery was performed mid-morning on day 1. A small nodule 0.3 x 0.5 cm was identified and removed from the cranial pole of the left lobe of the thyroid gland. Therapy with 0.5 µg of alfacalcidol began at 8 am on day 1.

The post-surgery calcium dropped rapidly to within the reference interval on the afternoon of the same day. Thereafter, it remained high normal, but began to rise above the reference interval on day 3. On day 4, the dose of alfacalcidol was decreased by 50% to 0.25 µg per day. After day 2, only ionized calcium was measured. The dog was discharged from the hospital on day 10 with ionized calcium of 1.20–1.30 mmol/l.

Calcium concentration	Day							
	1 (8am)	1 (4pm)	2	3	4[a]	5	6	7
Total calcium (mmol/l)	3.40	2.85	2.90					
Ionized calcium (mmol/l)	1.70	1.35	1.40	1.54	1.56	1.60	1.49	1.42

[a] Dose of alfacalcidol decreased to 0.25 µg from 0.5 µg per day.

Initially, further calcium measurements were carried out every 3 days. After three measurements that stayed in the range 1.30–1.40 mmol/l, measurements were taken weekly. After 3 weeks the alfacalcidol dose was dropped to 0.25 µg every other day. After a further month, this dose was further reduced to 0.25 µg every third day. This supplementation was stopped after one month at the every third day dose.

Case discussion
This dog was never hypocalcaemic and never suffered clinical signs attributable to hypocalcaemia. The decision was made to administer vitamin D supplementation even though the pre-treatment calcium did not exceed 3.5 mmol/l. This decision was based on the observation that calcium had increased but had also been relatively variable over the past few months and that at times it had been measured to be as high as 3.75 mmol/l. In this case, the treatment choice erred on the side of caution. The aim of supplementation is to avoid extremes of hypercalcaemia and hypocalcaemia and to maintain the serum calcium concentration in the low normal to slightly low range. This is beneficial because it stimulates the remaining parathyroid glands to become active again and reduces the time required for supplementary vitamin D. The initial dose of 0.5 µg was perhaps a little high and this dose was reduced fairly quickly. The dose was reduced again after 3 weeks. It is this author's recommendation that rapid reductions in medication should be avoided and at least 2–3 weeks allowed between dose changes.

This dog's recovery was problem-free and by 3 months post-surgery there was no need for further medication.

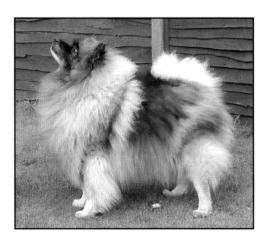

Case example 2: 11-year-old male Beagle, 17 kg

This dog was investigated for total anorexia over 2 days and occasional anorexia previous to this. Occasional vomiting as well as vomiting associated with drinking were reported. Weight loss, trembling and chronic skin and ear problems were present. Polyuria and polydipsia were not apparent, although the vomiting reported after drinking may have been associated with overdistension of the stomach with water.

Physical examination
Physical examination findings included chronic otitis externa and chronic erythema in the axillae and inguinal region. Trembling and muscle fasciculation were noted in the hind legs.

Clinical pathology

Parameter	Concentration	Reference interval
Total calcium	4.60 mmol/l	2.30–2.80 mmol/l
Ionized calcium	2.60 mmol/l	1.18–1.40 mmol/l
Phosphate	0.81 mmol/l	0.60–1.30 mmol/l
PTH	>600 pg/ml	10–60 pg/ml
PTHrp	0.7 pmol/l	0.0–0.5 pmol/l
Urea	13.6 mmol/l	3.3–8.0 mmol/l
Creatinine	173 µmol/l	45–150 µmol/l

Further diagnostic tests

- Rectal examination
- Thoracic and abdominal radiography
- Abdominal ultrasonography
- Fine needle aspiration of liver and spleen
- Cervical ultrasonography

A right-sided parathyroid nodule was identified ultrasonographically, measuring 0.45 x 0.56 cm. Small, radiodense uroliths were identified in the bladder.

Rectal examination (performed to identify a possible anal sac adenocarcinoma) was unremarkable, as was FNA of the liver and spleen (performed to identify possible lymphoma within these organs).

Diagnosis
Primary hyperparathyroidism with concurrent renal insufficiency.

Medical and surgical management
The dog received 3 days of fluid therapy at a rate of 6 ml/kg/h until taken to surgery. On the day before the operation medication with 0.25 µg of alfacalcidol was begun. At surgery, a small nodule 0.3 x 0.5 cm was identified and removed from the cranial pole of the left lobe of the thyroid gland.

Alfacalcidol therapy continued until 4 days after surgery, whereupon the dose was increased to 0.25 µg q12h. In addition, 600 mg elemental calcium, in the form of calcium gluconate, was administered q12h, starting from the evening of the day of parathyroidectomy.

Calcium concentration	Day							
	1 (8am)	*1 (4pm)*	*2*	*3 [a]*	*4 [a,b]*	*5 [a]*	*7*	*9*
Total calcium (mmol/l)	3.90	2.65	2.45			2.09	2.13	2.44
Ionized calcium (mmol/l)	2.28	1.32	1.38	1.02	1.06	0.96	1.12	1.17
Urea (mmol/l)	9.5	12.5						15.7
Creatinine (µmol/l)	161	139						178

[a] Dog received 20 ml of 10% calcium gluconate i.v. over 20 minutes twice on each of these days. [b] Dose of alfacalcidol increased to 0.25 mg q12h.

Case discussion
This patient was presented when disease was advanced and had presumably been present for some time. There was severe hypercalcaemia and the risk of post-surgical hypocalcaemia was significant. However, the dog was also showing signs of renal disease and was marginally azotaemic at the time of diagnosis. It was important, therefore, to bring the calcium concentration down quickly and to maintain it in the low-normal range to minimize ongoing renal damage. A fairly low dose of alfacalcidol was chosen (0.01 µg/kg), but this was shown to be insufficient for the maintenance of a stable postoperative calcium concentration and the dose was increased to 0.25 µg q12h on day 4. The main signs of hypocalcaemia seen in this dog were odd vocalization and agitation. Signs of tremors and stiffness were noted when the dog was taken out to urinate and pass faeces.

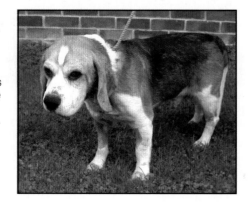

The dog remained stable on 0.25 µg of alfacalcidol for 1 month before gradual reduction in medication was instituted and all medication was withdrawn at around 5 months after surgery. Mild renal insufficiency remained but was stable and the dog was doing well until lost to follow-up.

References and further reading

Barber PJ, Elliot J and Torrance AG (1993) Measurement of feline intact parathyroid hormone: assay validation and sampling handling studies. *Journal of Small Animal Practice* **34**, 614–620

Chew D and Nagode L (2000) Treatment of hypoparathyroidism. In: *Kirk's Current Veterinary Therapy: XIII: Small Animal Practice*, ed. J Bonagura, pp.340–345. WB Saunders, Philadelphia

DeLay J and Laing J (2002) Nutritional osteodystrophy in puppies fed a BARF diet. *Animal Health Laboratory Newsletter, University of Guelph* **6**, 23

Den Hertog E, Goossens MMC, van der Linde-Sipman JS and Kooistra HS (1997) Primary hyperparathyroidism in two cats. *Veterinary Quarterly* **19**, 81–4

DeVries SE, Feldman EC, Nelson RW and Kennedy PC (1993) Primary parathyroid hyperplasia in dogs: six cases (1982–1991). *Journal of the American Veterinary Medical Association* **202**, 1132–1136

Elliott J, Rawlings JM, Markwell PJ and Barber PJ (2000) Survival of cats with naturally occurring chronic renal failure: effect of dietary management. *Journal of Small Animal Practice* **41**, 235–242

Feldman EC, Hoar B, Pollard R and Nelson RW (2005) Pretreatment clinical and laboratory findings in dogs with primary hyperparathyroidism: 210 cases (1987–2004). *Journal of the American Veterinary Medical Association* **227**, 756–761

Feldman EC and Nelson RW (2004) Hypercalcaemia and primary hyperparathyroidism. In: *Canine and Feline Endocrinology and Reproduction, 3rd edn*, ed. Feldman EC and Nelson RW, pp. 661–713. WB Saunders, St. Louis

Gao P, Scheibel S, D'Amour P *et al.,* (2001) Development of a novel immunoradiometric assay exclusively for biologically active whole parathyroid hormone 1–84: implications for improvement of accurate assessment of parathyroid function. *Journal of Bone and Mineral Research* **16**, 605–614

Gear RN, Neiger R, Skelly BJ and Herrtage ME (2005) Primary hyperparathyroidism in 29 dogs: diagnosis, treatment, outcome and associated renal failure. *Journal of Small Animal Practice* **46**, 10–16

Goldstein RE, Atwater DZ, Cazolli DM *et al.* (2007) Inheritance, mode of inheritance and candidate genes for primary hyperparathyroidism in Keeshonden. *Journal of Veterinary Internal Medicine* **21**, 199–203

Habener JF, Rosenblatt M and Potts JT Jr (1984) Parathyroid hormone: biochemical aspects of biosynthesis, secretion, action and metabolism. *Physiological Reviews* **64**, 985–1053

Hostutler RA, Chew DJ, Jaeger JQ *et al.* (2005) Uses and effectiveness of pamidronate disodium for treatment of dogs and cats with hypercalcaemia. *Journal of Veterinary Internal Medicine* **19**, 29–33

Kallet AJ, Richter KP, Feldman EC and Brum DE (1991) Primary hyperparathyroidism in cats: seven cases (1984-1989). *Journal of the American Veterinary Medical Association* **199**, 1767–1771

Lim SK, Gardella TJ, Baba H, Nussbaum SR and Kronenberg HM (1992) The carboxy-terminus of parathyroid hormone is essential for hormone processing and secretion. *Endocrinology* **131**, 2325–2330

Long CD, Goldstein RE and Hornof WJ (1999) Percutaneous ultrasound-guided chemical parathyroid ablation for treatment of primary hyperparathyroidism in dogs. *Journal of the American Veterinary Medical Association* **215**, 217–220

Matwichuk CL, Taylor SM and Wilkinson AA (1996) Use of technetium Tc99m sestamibi for detection of a parathyroid adenoma in a dog with primary hyperparathyroidism. *Journal of the American Veterinary Medical Association* **209**, 1733–1736

Mellanby RJ, Mellor PJ, Roulois A *et al.* (2005) Hypocalcaemia associated with low serum vitamin D metabolite concentrations in two dogs with protein-losing enteropathies. *Journal of Small Animal Practice* **46**, 345–351

Nelson R and Elliott D (2003) Metabolic and electrolyte disorders. In: *Small Animal Internal Medicine, 3rd edn*, ed. R. Nelson and C. Couto, pp. 816–846. Mosby, St. Louis

Plumb DC (2005) *Plumb's Veterinary Handbook, 5th edn.* Blackwell Publishing Professional, Iowa

Pollard RE, Long CD, Nelson RW, Hornof WJ and Feldman EC (2001) Percutaneous ultrasonographically guided radiofrequency heat ablation for treatment of primary hyperparathyroidism in dogs. *Journal of the American Veterinary Medical Association* **218**, 1106–1110

Ramsey I, Tebb A, Harris E, Evans H and Herrtage ME (2005) Hyperparathyroidism in dogs with hyperadrenocorticism. *Journal of Small Animal Practice* **46**, 531–536

Rasor L, Pollard R and Feldman EC (2007) Retrospective evaluation of three treatment methods for primary hyperparathyroidism in dogs. *Journal of the American Animal Hospital Association* **43**, 70–77

Refsal KR, Provencher-Bolliger AL, Graham PA and Nachreiner RF (2001) Update on the diagnosis and treatment of disorders of calcium regulation. *Veterinary Clinics of North America: Small Animal Practice* **31**, 1043–1096

Rosol TJ and Capen CC (1997) Calcium regulating hormones and diseases of abnormal mineral (calcium, phosphorus, magnesium) metabolism. In: *Academic Clinical Biochemistry of Domestic Animals*, ed. JJ Kaneko *et al.*, pp. 619–702. San Diego Press, San Diego

Roudebush P, Polzin DJ, Adams LG, Towell TL and Forrester SD (2010) An evidence-based review of therapies for canine chronic kidney disease. *Journal of Small Animal Practice* **51**, 244–252

Savary KCM, Price GS and Vaden SL (2000) Hypercalcaemia in cats: a retrospective study of 71 cases (1991–1997). *Journal of Veterinary Internal Medicine* **14**, 184–189

Schaefer C and Goldstein RE (2009). Canine primary hyperparathyroidism. *Compendium on Continuing Education for Practicing Veterinarians* **31**, 382–389

Schenk PA, Chew DL, Nagode LA and Rosol TJ (2006) Disorders of calcium: hypercalcaemia and hypocalcaemia. In: *Fluid, Electrolyte and Acid-Base Disorders in Small Animal Practice, 3rd edn*, ed. S DiBartola, pp. 122–194. Saunders Elsevier, USA

Simonds WF, Robbins CM, Agarwal SK *et al.,* (2004) Familial isolated hyperparathyroidism is rarely caused by germline mutation in HRPT2, the gene for the hyperparathyroidism–jaw tumour syndrome. *Journal of Clinical Endocrinology and Metabolism* **89**, 96–102

Skelly BJ and Franklin RJM (2007) Mutations in genes causing human familial isolated hyperparathyroidism do not account for hyperparathyroidism in keeshond dogs. *Veterinary Journal* **174**, 652–654

Tebb AJ, Arteaga A, Evans H and Ramsey IK (2005) Canine HAC effects of trilostane on parathyroid hormone, calcium and phosphate concentrations. *Journal of Small Animal Practice* **46**, 537–542

Thompson KG, Jones LP, Smylie WA *et al.,* (1984) Primary hyperparathyroidism in German shepherd dogs: a disorder of probable genetic origin. *Veterinary Pathology* **21**, 370–376

Torrance AG and Nachreiner R (1989) Human-parathormone assay for use in dogs: validation, sample handling studies and parathyroid function testing. *American Journal of Veterinary Research* **50**, 1123–1127

Warner J, Epstein M, Sweet A *et al.,* (2004) Genetic testing in familial isolated hyperparathyroidism: unexpected results and their implications. *Journal of Medical Genetics* **41**, 155–160

Wisner ER and Nyland TG (1998) Ultrasonography of the thyroid and parathyroid glands. *Veterinary Clinics of North America: Small Animal Practice* **28**, 973–991

7

Hypoparathyroidism

Barbara J. Skelly

Introduction

Hypoparathyroidism is an uncommon disease that can affect both dogs and, rarely, cats. In dogs the disease is most frequently an idiopathic primary hypoparathyroidism that results from immune-mediated destruction of the parathyroid glands. Although this aetiology is also described in cats it is rare, with few cases reported (Peterson *et al.*, 1991). Hypoparathyroidism is characterized by low circulating ionized and total calcium concentrations in combination with a low parathyroid hormone (PTH; parathormone) concentration and an elevated phosphate concentration.

Anatomy and physiology

The anatomy of the parathyroid glands is described and illustrated in Chapter 6. In summary, there are two parathyroid glands, an external and an internal parathyroid, associated with each thyroid lobe. These are responsible for the synthesis and release of PTH, which is pivotal in calcium homeostasis. Calcium regulation in the body is governed by the activities of PTH, 1,25-dihydroxycholecalciferol ($1,25(OH)_2$-vitamin D; calcitriol) and calcitonin. The activities and effects of PTH and $1,25(OH)_2$-vitamin D are illustrated in Figure 7.1.

The role of PTH

- Increases the rate of calcium release from the skeleton by increasing osteoclast activity on bony surfaces.
- Increases reuptake of calcium through renal tubules, thus limiting renal calcium loss. This occurs via a direct effect on the distal convoluted tubule and also an indirect effect on the thick ascending loop of Henle.
- Increases the rate of phosphate excretion through the kidneys.
- Stimulates the release of magnesium from bone and resorption through the renal tubules. PTH, in conjunction with $1,25(OH)_2$-vitamin D, mediates magnesium uptake through the intestinal wall.

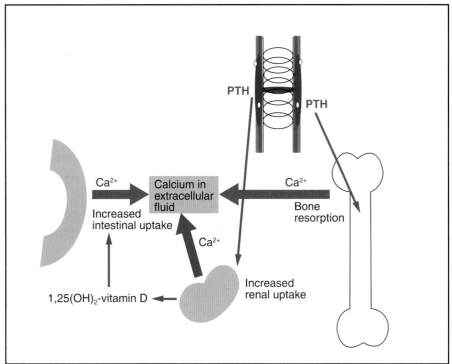

7.1 Calcium homeostasis: the role of parathyroid hormone (PTH) and $1,25$-$(OH)_2$-vitamin D in the maintenance of adequate serum calcium.

- Accelerates the formation of the active metabolite of vitamin D in the kidney by inducing synthesis and also activating 1α-hydroxylase in the mitochondria of the renal epithelial cells of the proximal convoluted tubule.

The role of vitamin D

Vitamin D is a steroid hormone, the active form of which is synthesized from cholecalciferol in two steps. Initially, 25-hydroxycholecalciferol is produced in the liver. This is the major circulating form of vitamin D, as the conversion step in the liver is relatively uncontrolled and is not influenced significantly by PTH concentrations. This form of vitamin D is then activated by the enzyme 1α-hydroxylase in the kidney under the control of PTH, or is catabolized by 24-hydroxylation to 24,25-dihydroxycholecalciferol. The activation step is antagonized by the elevated phosphate concentrations encountered in renal insufficiency and also by hypoparathyroidism.

Dogs and cats do not synthesize vitamin D efficiently in skin (in contrast to humans) and are therefore dependent on dietary intake to maintain adequate concentrations.

Vitamin D increases calcium and phosphate concentrations via an effect on its major target organ – the intestine. It also has effects on the kidney and on bone to increase calcium reuptake or release. Vitamin D is involved in the regulation of PTH synthesis, so that high vitamin concentrations will reduce PTH synthesis and secretion by the parathyroid gland.

Signalment

Hypoparathyroidism most commonly affects middle-aged female dogs and male cats. In a series of 735 dogs with hypoparathyroidism, 62% were female and 38% male (Refsal et al., 2001). In cats, the age range may be somewhat younger. Affected cats range between 5 months and 7 years (Gunn-Moore, 2005), and no breed predisposition has been observed (Feldman and Nelson, 2004). However, in dogs terrier breeds, Schnauzers, Dachshunds and Poodles may be more commonly affected, and in Australia and New Zealand the St Bernard appears to be predisposed (Kornegay et al., 1980; Jones and Alley, 1985; Refsal et al., 2001; Russell et al., 2006).

Aetiology and pathophysiology

Hypoparathyroidism is defined as an absolute or relative deficiency in PTH secretion that can be permanent or transient. Many forms of transient hypoparathyroidism are iatrogenic in nature and may be caused as a result of one of the following:

- Thyroidectomy in cats with hyperthyroidism, and in both dogs and cats with thyroid carcinoma
- Parathyroidectomy in both dogs and cats

- Ethanol or heat ablation of the parathyroid glands in dogs.

In cats, postoperative hypocalcaemia typically occurs 1–3 days after the surgical removal of a thyroid adenoma. This can be common, depending on the surgical technique chosen (Flanders et al., 1987) but is less frequently seen nowadays, as techniques have been modified to minimize the risk of parathyroid damage. Chapter 10 discusses postoperative hypocalcaemia in cats in greater detail. Eucalcaemia can be maintained as long as one functional parathyroid gland remains.

The recalcification that occurs after parathyroidectomy in human patients with hyperparathyroidism is referred to as the 'hungry bone syndrome'. This is caused by a rapid increase in bone remodelling. Hypocalcaemia can occur if the rate of skeletal mineralization exceeds the rate of osteoclast-mediated bone resorption. This syndrome can be associated with severe and diffuse bone pain. A similar phenomenon may be seen in dogs but is not well characterized.

Permanent hypoparathyroidism is caused by inflammatory destruction of the parathyroid glands, presumably due to an immune-mediated mechanism. Thus, hypoparathyroidism is similar to other endocrinopathies caused by underproduction due to immune-mediated damage (including some forms of diabetes mellitus, hypoadrenocorticism and hypothyroidism). When affected parathyroid glands are examined, an inflammatory cell infiltrate is identified, consisting mainly of lymphocytes with some plasma cells and neutrophils. Glands are fibrotic, have an increase in the number of small capillaries and a loss of normal secretory cells (Bruyette and Feldman, 1988; Peterson et al., 1991). In one review of 17 cases, only 2 dogs had gross and histopathological examinations of the parathyroid glands (Russell et al., 2006). In both cases, the gross appearance and histopathological examination of the parathyroid glands were normal, suggesting that either another mechanism was responsible for hypoparathyroidism or that microscopic changes correlate weakly with functional activity.

A further, rare cause of hypoparathyroidism has been reported in two cases. In these dogs, parathyroid gland tumours caused hypercalcaemia, but spontaneous infarction occurred and acute hypocalcaemia was the result (Rosol et al., 1988).

A link is reported between the incidence of hypomagnesaemia and hypoparathyroidism, in that severe hypomagnesaemia can cause functional hypoparathyroidism (Schenk, 2005). Magnesium depletion is reported in dogs, particularly Yorkshire Terriers, with small intestinal malabsorption; this can lead to a syndrome of reduced PTH concentrations. Inappropriately low PTH contributes to hypocalcaemia in these patients, although the primary cause of hypocalcaemia appears to be mediated through intestinal vitamin D malabsorption (Kimmel et al., 2000; Bush et al., 2001). It is recommended, therefore, that the concentration of ionized magnesium is checked in dogs and cats with reduced parathyroid function.

Clinical features

The clinical signs of hypoparathyroidism are listed in Figure 7.2 and are caused by the presence of hypocalcaemia. The differential diagnoses for hypocalcaemia are described in greater detail in Chapter 21.

The severity of clinical signs depends on the magnitude of the hypocalcaemia, with most animals not showing clinical signs until total calcium falls below 1.5 mmol/l and ionized calcium falls below approximately 0.8 mmol/l. These numbers vary according to the acid–base balance of the animal, as the presence of alkalosis reduces the ionized component and makes clinical signs more likely at a higher calcium concentration. Clinical signs are more likely if the calcium concentration has decreased rapidly (e.g. over hours to days in the case of surgical removal of a parathyroid adenoma), compared to the slow development of hypocalcaemia seen with idiopathic primary hypoparathyroidism. Ionized hypocalcaemia, ranging from mild to severe, is common in conjunction with hyperkalaemia in cats with urinary tract obstruction. In this situation, hyperkalaemia is more likely to cause bradyarrhythmias, as calcium has an important cardioprotective role.

Signs associated with neuromuscular excitability
• Muscle fasciculation or tremors • Face rubbing • Biting and licking at paws or body • Hypersensitivity to external stimuli • Stiff, stilted gait • Ataxia • Tetanic seizures • Respiratory arrest • Weakness
Behavioural changes
• Agitation • Anxiety • Vocalization • Aggression
Other
• Panting • Hyperthermia • Cataracts • Lengthening of ST segment and QT interval on ECG • Third eyelid prolapse in cats

7.2 Clinical features of hypoparathyroidism.

The majority of the diseases that cause hypocalcaemia are associated with a mild to moderate hypocalcaemia, whereas primary hypoparathyroidism and puerperal tetany (eclampsia) are most likely to result in severe hypocalcaemia. Since puerperal tetany most commonly occurs 1–4 weeks postpartum or in the latter stages of gestation, it is easily recognized and its diagnosis is relatively straightforward. Hypoparathyroidism is therefore the most likely cause of symptomatic hypocalcaemia in the dog and cat.

The signs of hypocalcaemia are intermittent and may be induced by exercise, excitement and stress. The reasons for this are twofold: the requirement for calcium increases during muscular activity and therefore a deficit is felt most keenly at this time; and panting leads to rapid alkalinization of the blood and induces a fall in the proportion of ionized calcium available. The most obvious signs to be precipitated in this way are those associated with the neuromuscular system, such as muscle tremors or fasciculation.

Neuromuscular system

Signs are often initially observed around the facial muscles but may then progress to whole body involvement and seizures. Champing was frequently reported in one case series as a manifestation of the increased excitability of the muscles of mastication (Russell *et al.*, 2006). In the same case series, facial pruritus was recorded in 4/17 (24%) of dogs. Seizures caused by hypocalcaemia are, unlike epileptic seizures, most frequent during periods of activity, not rest. Animals retain consciousness and do not tend to urinate. They often resolve spontaneously and do not respond to anticonvulsant therapy. Interestingly, the stress and excitement of a visit to a veterinary surgeon and the physical examination may precipitate overt neuromuscular signs of hypocalcaemia such as muscle tremors, cramping or seizures. In addition, handling may be resented as it may be painful and animals may become aggressive.

Gastrointestinal system

Some reports of hypoparathyroid dogs list gastrointestinal signs as frequent (Russell *et al.,* 2006). Vomiting and inappetence were reported as common findings in that case series, but the aetiopathogenesis of these signs is not clear. In dogs exhibiting inappetence, the mean circulating phosphate concentration was significantly higher than in dogs with a normal appetite, suggesting hyperphosphataemia as a possible contributing factor for the development of inappetence.

Ocular changes

Cataracts (Figure 7.3) may be found in patients with chronic and relatively severe hypocalcaemia and are described as bilaterally symmetrical punctate to linear opacities in the anterior and posterior subcapsular region of the lens (Feldman and Nelson, 2004). The mechanism of cataract formation is unclear. Typically in human hypoparathyroidism, progression is halted if serum calcium is stabilized. In one review of canine cases, however, three were described as developing cataracts after the initiation of therapy (Bruyette and Feldman, 1988). Other ocular manifestations reported in hypoparathyroid dogs include blepharospasm, blepharitis and keratoconjunctivitis sicca (Jones and Alley, 1985). These findings were reported from a hypoparathyroid St Bernard and it was unclear whether they were necessarily manifestations of the primary disease or concurrent, independent ocular changes.

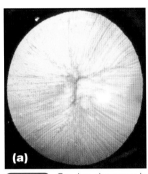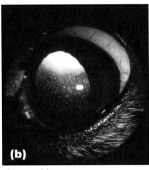

7.3 Ocular changes in dogs with hypoparathyroidism. **(a)** This lens in a Border Collie shows marked linear opacities in the anterior and posterior subcapsular cortex as well as anterior and posterior suture lines. Visual acuity would be expected to be affected, although the dog was still able to negotiate obstacles. (Courtesy of David Williams) **(b)** Punctate opacities in a lens from a different case. (Courtesy of David Gould)

Cardiac changes

In human cases severe hypocalcaemia can cause a prolongation of the QT interval on ECG, and either sudden death, because of the development of arrhythmia, or congestive heart failure. Severe chronic hypocalcaemia is described as a cause of dilated cardiomyopathy and consequent heart failure in humans. This is most frequently reported in infants with rickets, but may also affect older people with hypoparathyroidism (Brown *et al.,* 2009; Mavroudis *et al.,* 2010). Cardiac manifestations of hypocalcaemia secondary to hypoparathyroidism are uncommon in dogs, and are not emphasized in the two largest case series (Bruyette and Feldman, 1988; Russell *et al.*, 2006).

Diagnosis

Routine clinicopathological features

Hypocalcaemia is most frequently identified in animals that are hypoalbuminaemic and not displaying any significant clinical signs. A low total calcium measurement is often caused by concurrently low albumin and this does not pose a clinical problem, as the ionized calcium (physiologically available calcium) is maintained within the reference interval. Chapter 21 explains why previously used calculations to correct calcium concentrations for alterations in albumin concentration are no longer thought to be useful.

Ionized calcium

The measurement of ionized calcium allows an accurate assessment to be made of calcium homeostasis, particularly in animals with concurrent disease. Samples for measurement of ionized calcium need to be protected from air exposure and analysed rapidly for accurate results (see Chapter 21).

Depiction of hypoparathyroidism

The diagnosis of primary hypoparathyroidism is based on the following:

- Low total calcium (<1.5 mmol/l)
- Low ionized calcium (<0.8 mmol/l)
- Low concurrent PTH concentration. An expected result in primary hypoparathyroidism is for PTH to decrease to below the reference interval (20–65 pg/ml in the dog) or, even when within the reference interval, to be inappropriately low for the concurrent serum calcium (i.e. within the lower half of the reference interval <30 pg/ml). In cats where the reference interval is <40 pg/ml, a low result would be in the range of 0–20 pg/ml
- High reference interval to elevated phosphate concentration
- Adequate renal function.

PTH increases calcium uptake in the kidney whilst also reducing phosphate loss; hyperphosphataemia is thus a feature of hypoparathyroidism.

As renal failure is a differential diagnosis for hypocalcaemia and for hyperphosphataemia, renal parameters should be assessed. However, renal secondary hyperparathyroidism is frequently present in cases of renal failure, so although calcium concentrations may be reduced, PTH is high normal or above the reference interval.

In animals with hypoparathyroidism, the fractional excretion of calcium is increased in the face of hypocalcaemia, whilst the fractional excretion of phosphate is decreased. Urinary fractional excretion values can be measured relatively easily but can be difficult to interpret due to the wide variability in values both between and within individuals. In one case series, fractional excretion did not correlate well with final diagnosis (Russell *et al.*, 2006).

Diagnostic imaging

Radiography or ultrasonography of hypoparathyroid dogs is generally unhelpful. The parathyroid glands may be atrophied, but they are normally difficult to find in healthy individuals.

Treatment

The treatment of acute, subacute and chronic hypocalcaemia is summarized in Figure 7.4.

Treatment of acute symptomatic hypocalcaemia

Intravenous calcium salts are the initial treatment of choice. Calcium gluconate or calcium borogluconate is most frequently recommended, as calcium chloride solutions are caustic when extravasated. The following are guidelines.

- 0.5–1.5 ml/kg of 10% calcium gluconate slowly i.v. over 20–30 minutes until clinical signs have subsided and the patient is considered to be stable (equivalent to 4.65–13.95 mg elemental calcium/kg, as 10% calcium gluconate solution contains 9.3 mg elemental calcium per ml). An ECG may be used to monitor cardiac effects and the infusion stopped if there is ST segment

Drug	Dose	Precautions
Acute hypocalcaemia		
10% Calcium gluconate	0.5–1.5 ml/kg over 20–30 minutes	Monitor heart by auscultation, pulse palpation or ECG for bradycardia, shortened QT interval and ST segment elevation
10% Calcium borogluconate	0.3–0.9 ml/kg over 20–30 minutes	
10% Calcium chloride	0.16–0.5 ml/kg over 20–30 minutes	
Subacute hypocalcaemia		
10% Calcium gluconate	6.5–1.0 ml/kg over 24 hours in 0.9% NaCl	Do not give subcutaneously
10% Calcium borogluconate	4–6.5 ml/kg over 24 hours in 0.9% NaCl	
10% Calcium chloride	2–3.5 ml/kg over 24 hours in 0.9% NaCl	
Chronic hypocalcaemia		
Calcium carbonate Calcium gluconate Calcium lactate	25–50mg/kg of elemental calcium [a]	Can be stopped once vitamin D dose is appropriate.
Calcitriol	20–30 ng/kg/day orally divided twice a day	Time to maximum effect <4 days
Alfacalcidol	0.01–0.03 µg/kg q24h	Time to maximum effect <4 days
Dihydrotachysterol	0.02–0.03 mg/kg q24h reducing to 0.01–0.02 mg/kg q24–48h as required	Time to maximum effect <7 days

7.4 Treatment of acute, subacute and chronic hypocalcaemia. [a] 1 mg calcium = 11.2 mg calcium gluconate = 7.7 mg calcium lactate = 2.5 mg calcium carbonate.

elevation, QT shortening or if arrhythmias develop. In an emergency situation, however, calcium can be administered slowly and the heart rate auscultated or pulse monitored by digital palpation to avoid inducing bradycardia. Thereafter, a continuous rate infusion can be used at 2.5–3.75 mg/kg/h (60–90 mg/kg/day, equivalent to 6.5–10 ml/kg/day) until oral therapy has reached maximum effect. As a guide, the elemental dose of calcium required is achieved using 25 ml of 10% calcium gluconate, diluted in 250 ml of 0.9% saline and infused at a rate of 2.5 ml/kg/h.

- The commonly available solution of 200 mg/ml calcium borogluconate contains the equivalent of approximately 15 mg/ml elemental calcium. It is therefore approximately 1.6 times as concentrated as 10% calcium gluconate and can be administered as described above, using the dose at the lower end of the dose range, 0.3–0.9 ml/kg. The same precautions are required when administering this treatment.
- 10% calcium chloride solution contains three times the elemental calcium per ml (27.2 mg/ml elemental calcium) as 10% calcium gluconate solution. Thus, the dose is reduced by one-third to 0.16–0.5 ml/kg of 10% calcium chloride. This solution is extremely irritating if injected perivascularly and should be administered using a catheter only.
- It is useful to calculate the dose required and then dilute the volume up into a larger volume (in 0.9% saline); this will make it easier to achieve a slow administration rate.

- Precipitation may occur if calcium solutions are mixed with bicarbonate-containing solutions.

The use of subcutaneous calcium supplementation is controversial. Sterile abscess formation and skin sloughing (Figure 7.5) has been reported when calcium salts are used subcutaneously (Feldman and Nelson, 2004); however, some authors still recommend that calcium gluconate is given by this route, as it is not likely to cause a problem. It is true that 10% calcium gluconate diluted in a 1:1 ratio with 0.9% saline may be given subcutaneously with no adverse effects, but it is also true that, in some cases, even calcium gluconate can cause dramatic skin sloughing. For this reason only the intravenous and oral routes of administration are recommended.

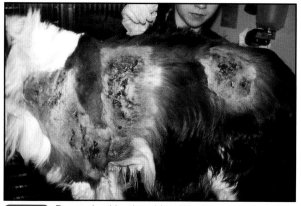

7.5 Dramatic skin sloughing in a Border Collie that had received subcutaneous calcium gluconate in several sites. (Courtesy of Andria Cauvin)

Treatment of chronic hypocalcaemia

- 1,25(OH)$_2$-vitamin D is the active form of vitamin D; it does not, therefore, require further metabolism to become active when given. It has a rapid onset of action (1–4 days) and a short half-life. Toxic effects would be expected to resolve in 2–7 days. Calcitriol comes in capsules of 0.25 or 0.5 µg. The dose rate used is 20–30 ng/kg/day orally divided twice a day, but may be decreased to 5–15 ng/kg/day long term (Chew and Nagode, 2000). *This product is not authorized for veterinary use.*
- Alfacalcidol is the formulation most commonly used by this author. This drug needs to undergo 25-hydroxylation by the liver before it is active. This process occurs rapidly in a relatively unregulated fashion so this does not significantly alter the time to maximal effect compared to calcitriol. The drug is available as 0.25, 0.5 and 1 µg capsules and also as drops (2 µg/ml), so is useful in small dogs and cats. A dose of 0.01– 0.03 µg/kg q24h is used. However, these doses have some flexibility and may be titrated upwards and downwards to suit the individual animal. *This product is not authorized for veterinary use.*
- Dihydrotachysterol is a useful vitamin D supplement because it comes in a liquid formulation as a 0.25 mg/ml solution. It requires hydroxylation by the liver to reach the active form but does not need to be hydroxylated again in the kidney. The onset of action occurs within 24 hours and reaches peak activity within 7 days.

The dose rate used is 0.02–0.03 mg/kg q24h for initial treatment. The dose can be reduced for longer-term management to 0.01–0.02 mg/kg q24–48h or as required. *This product is not authorized for veterinary use.*

The dose of elemental calcium required per day as an oral supplement is between 25 and 50 mg/kg/ day (divided into two or three doses), although initially higher doses may be used. However, calcium preparations vary in the amount of elemental calcium and doses must be adjusted to take this into consideration: 1 mg elemental calcium = 11.2 mg calcium gluconate = 7.7 mg calcium lactate = 2.5 mg calcium carbonate.

Early treatment with calcium supplementation is helpful to ensure high intestinal luminal calcium concentrations that will encourage passive calcium absorption over the period of time it takes for vitamin D to begin to work.

Long-term management

Once an animal has been stabilized on a dose of vitamin D, calcium supplementation can usually be stopped and the diet relied upon as a source of calcium. The long-term prognosis is good, but regular monitoring is advisable, particularly if other medical conditions occur that may have an impact on the intestinal absorption of calcium, e.g. chronic diarrhoea. Hypercalcaemia should also be avoided, as this will have a negative impact on renal function if allowed to persist long-term. The aim should be to keep calcium concentrations within the low–normal reference interval.

Case 1: 10-year-old, male Border Collie, 18 kg

The dog was presented with a 4-month history of frequent short-duration seizures. The seizures were described as occurring when the dog was excited or had not eaten. Blood glucose and fructosamine had been measured and had been found to be within reference limits.

Physical examination
The dog was in slim body condition, considered normal for his breed. The only significant finding was the presence of bilateral cataracts (see Figure 7.3a).

Clinical pathology

Parameter	Concentration	Reference interval
Mild elevation in ALT	155 IU/l	10–118 IU/l
Low total calcium	1.43 mmol/l	2.30–2.80 mmol/l
Low ionized calcium	0.67 mmol/l	1.18–1.40 mmol/l
High phosphate	3.64 mmol/l	0.78–1.41 mmol/l
Renal function was normal		
PTH	18.0 pg/ml	18–130 pg/ml

Imaging
No significant findings.

Diagnosis
Primary hypoparathyroidism

Treatment
1.5 µg alfacalcidol daily
1 Calcichew 500 mg tablet daily (Shire Pharmaceuticals Ltd). Per tablet: calcium carbonate 1250 mg, equivalent to 500 mg of elemental calcium.

Follow-up
Although the dog did well over the short term, the serum calcium concentration gradually increased on this dose of medication until he became hypercalcaemic. The calcium supplement was discontinued and the alfacalcidol dose decreased to 0.5 µg daily. This resulted in a total calcium concentration that was stable at around 2.50–2.60 mmol/l with the dog experiencing no clinical signs.

References and further reading

Brown J, Nunez S, Russel M and Spurney C (2009) Hypocalcaemic rickets and dilated cardiomyopathy: case reports and review of literature. *Pediatric Cardiology* **30**, 818–823

Bruyette DS and Feldman EC (1988) Primary hypoparathyroidism in the dog. Report of 15 cases and review of 13 previously reported cases. *Journal of Veterinary Internal Medicine* **2**, 7–14

Bush WW, Kimmel SE, Wosar MA and Jackson MW (2001) Secondary hypoparathyroidism attributed to hypomagnesaemia in a dog with protein-losing enteropathy. *Journal of the American Veterinary Medical Association* **219**, 1732–1734

Chew D and Nagode L (2000) Treatment of hypoparathyroidism. In: *Kirk's Current Veterinary Therapy: XIII: Small Animal Practice,* ed. J Bonagura, pp.340–345. WB Saunders, Philadelphia

Feldman EC and Nelson RW (2004) Hypocalcaemia and primary hypoparathyroidism. In: *Canine and Feline Endocrinology and Reproduction, 3rd edn,* ed. Feldman EC and Nelson RW, pp. 716–742. WB Saunders, St. Louis

Flanders JA, Harvey HJ, Erb HN *et al.* (1987) Feline thyroidectomy: a comparison of post-operative hypocalcaemia associated with three different surgical techniques. *Veterinary Surgery* **16**, 362–366

Gunn-Moore D (2005) Feline endocrinopathies. *Veterinary Clinics of North America: Small Animal Practice* **35**, 171–210

Jones BR and Alley MR (1985) Primary idiopathic hypoparathyroidism in St Bernard dogs. *New Zealand Veterinary Journal* **33**, 94–97

Kimmel SE, Waddell LS and Michel KE (2000) Hypomagnesaemia and hypocalcaemia associated with protein-losing enteropathy in Yorkshire terriers: five cases (1992–1998). *Journal of the American Veterinary Medical Association* **217**, 703–706.

Kornegay JH, Greene CE, Martin C, Gorgacz EJ, Melcon DK (1980) Iodiopathic hypocalcaemia in four dogs. *Journal of the American Animal Hospital Association* **16**, 723–734

Mavroudis K, Aloumanis K, Stamatis P *et al.* (2010) Irreversible end-stage heart failure in a young patient due to severe chronic hypocalcaemia associated with primary hypoparathyroidism and celiac disease. *Clinical Cardiology* **33**, 72–75

Meuten DJ, Chew DJ, Capen CC and Kociba GJ (1982) Relationship of serum total calcium to albumin and total protein in dogs. *Journal of the American Veterinary Medical Association* **180**, 63–67

Peterson ME, James KM, Wallace M *et al.* (1991) Idiopathic hypoparathyroidism in 5 cats. *Journal of Veterinary Internal Medicine* **5**, 47–51

Refsal KR, Provencher-Bollinger AL, Graham PA and Nachreiner RF (2001) Update on the diagnosis and treatment of disorders of calcium regulation. *Veterinary Clinics North America: Small Animal Practice* **31**, 1043–1062.

Rosol TJ, Chew DJ, Capen CC *et al.* (1988) Acute hypocalcaemia associated with infarction of parathyroid gland adenomas in two dogs. *Journal of the American Veterinary Medical Association* **192**, 212—214

Russell NJ, Bond KA, Robertson ID, Parry BW and Irwin PJ (2006) Primary hypoparathyroidism in dogs: a retrospective study of 17 cases. *Australian Veterinary Journal* **84**, 285–290

Schenk PA (2005) Serum ionized magnesium concentrations in dogs and cats with hypoparathyroidism. *Journal of Veterinary Internal Medicine* **19**, 462

Schenk PA and Chew DJ (2003) What's new in assessing calcium disorders – Part 1. *ACVIM Proceedings* pp. 517—518

Schenk PA, Chew DJ and Brooks CL (1995) Effects of storage on serum ionized calcium and pH values in clinically normal dogs. *American Journal of Veterinary Research* **56**, 304–307

8

Canine hypothyroidism

Carmel T. Mooney and Robert E. Shiel

Introduction

Hypothyroidism is considered a common endocrine disorder of dogs, yet its true prevalence is largely unknown. In the past it was commonly over-diagnosed, as the clinical features are vague and non-specific, and diagnostic tests frequently gave false positive results for the disorder in euthyroid animals. Recently, many of the challenges of diagnosis have been recognized and new tests, with more appropriate advice on their accurate interpretation, have been developed. As a result, understanding of the type of dog affected, knowledge of the associated and common clinical features, and appreciation of the most suitable tests to select have all dramatically changed and improved. A probable diagnosis is more confidently a definitive one and there has been a move from simply diagnosing clinical cases to screening dogs, with the potential aim of decreasing the prevalence of hypothyroidism in specific populations. If appropriately diagnosed, hypothyroidism is one of the most satisfying endocrine disorders to treat, with an excellent long-term prognosis. Naturally occurring hypothyroidism in cats is rare (see Chapter 11).

Aetiology

In dogs, the thyroid gland is divided into two distinct lobes, each located lateral to the proximal tracheal rings. Thyroid tissue is responsible for the production of the two active thyroid hormones, thyroxine (T4) and triiodothyronine (T3). Hormone production is controlled by thyroid-stimulating hormone (TSH, thyrotropin) from the pituitary gland, which is in turn controlled by thyrotropin-releasing hormone (TRH) from the hypothalamus. Hypothyroidism results from a decrease in the production of T4 and T3, and potentially arises from a defect in any part of the hypothalamic–pituitary–thyroid axis. In dogs, spontaneous hypothyroidism usually develops because of irreversible loss of thyroid tissue, so-called primary disease, largely as a consequence of either lymphocytic thyroiditis or idiopathic thyroid atrophy. Only a small proportion of cases arise from disorders of the pituitary gland or hypothalamus, so-called central hypothyroidism.

Primary hypothyroidism

Lymphocytic thyroiditis

Lymphocytic thyroiditis, a presumed autoimmune disorder, accounts for approximately 50% of cases of adult-onset hypothyroidism (Graham et al., 2007). Affected dogs experience either multifocal or diffuse infiltration of the thyroid tissue by lymphocytes, macrophages and plasma cells (Figure 8.1b), along with the formation of lymphoid nodules, irreversible destruction of thyroid follicles and progressive replacement of normal glandular tissue by fibrous connective tissue. The associated clinical signs of hypothyroidism only develop after approximately 75% of the gland is destroyed. This process may take months to years, varying in progression from dog to dog, and may not result in hypothyroidism in all cases. This means that there are variable periods of time during which there is significant thyroid pathology, and a potentially suboptimal or failing gland, but when a clinical state of hypothyroidism has not yet become apparent.

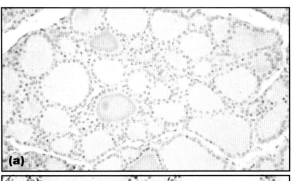
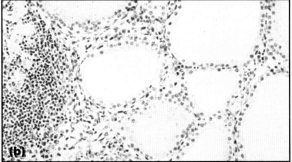

8.1 Thyroid gland histology. **(a)** Healthy canine thyroid tissue. **(b)** Lymphocytic thyroiditis. Note the inflammatory component replacing normal thyroid tissue. H&E stain. (continues) ▶

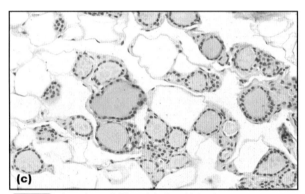

8.1 (continued) Thyroid gland histology.
(c) Idiopathic thyroid atrophy. Note the loss of normal thyroid parenchyma but without an inflammatory component. H&E stain.

Although the definitive diagnosis of lymphocytic thyroiditis requires thyroid biopsy, its existence can be inferred by demonstrating the presence of circulating autoantibodies against thyroid antigens. Commercially available tests include those for T4, T3 and, more commonly, anti-thyroglobulin autoantibodies (TgAAs). The latter are detected in approximately 50% of hypothyroid dogs (Graham *et al.,* 2007). Anti-thyroid peroxidase antibodies, common in human patients, have been demonstrated in only a small proportion of affected dogs, generally in association with other thyroid autoantibodies. Studies of thyroid autoimmunity in large numbers of dogs suggest a progression through the following stages (Figure 8.2):

- Silent thyroiditis – antibody-positive; euthyroid (all thyroid hormones within reference intervals)
- Subclinical (compensating) thyroiditis – T4 and T3 antibody-positive; euthyroid (T4 and T3 within reference intervals but with high endogenous TSH concentration)
- Clinical disease – antibody-positive; overtly hypothyroid.

Over time, antibody-positive dogs may become antibody-negative. There is a presumed eventual decline in the inflammatory process as thyroid tissue is destroyed and, consequently, autoantibodies disappear from the circulation.

The recognition of these different stages has significant implications, both for the progression of the disease and for choosing the most appropriate diagnostic tests. One study followed TgAA-positive euthyroid dogs for a 1-year period (Graham *et al.,* 2007). Approximately 1 in 5 dogs developed thyroid hormone abnormalities suggestive of declining thyroid function (usually experiencing an increase in circulating TSH values) and 1 in 20 became overtly hypothyroid.

Autoimmune thyroid disease in dogs is likely to arise out of a combination of multiple genetic and environmental factors, as it is in humans. It has long been demonstrated that lymphocytic thyroiditis is more prevalent in certain breeds of dog and in particular family lines. Familial inheritance has been demonstrated in Borzois, Great Danes and Beagles. Lymphocytic thyroiditis is also reported to be highly prevalent in such breeds as Golden Retrievers, Cocker Spaniels, Boxers, Shetland Sheepdogs, Giant Schnauzers and Hovawarts (Graham *et al.,* 2007; Ferm *et al.,* 2009). Genetic risk factors for the development of autoimmune thyroid disease have been identified in humans, although none confer increased susceptibility in all cases. Susceptibility genes include those in the major histocompatibility complex (MHC), as well as other regulators of immune and thyroid function. For a number of dog breeds, genetic susceptibility to hypothyroidism and lymphocytic thyroiditis is associated with certain haplotypes and alleles of the canine MHC dog leucocyte antigen (DLA) complex. These include the Dobermann, Rhodesian Ridgeback, English Setter and Giant Schnauzer (Kennedy *et al.,* 2006a,b; Wilbe *et al.,* 2010).

Idiopathic thyroid atrophy

Idiopathic thyroid atrophy accounts for most of the remaining non-thyroiditis cases of hypothyroidism, and is characterized by the following:

- Degeneration of follicular cells
- Reduction in follicular size
- Replacement of the normal parenchymal tissue with adipose connective tissue, but without significant inflammatory infiltration (see Figure 8.1c).

Category	Histopathological changes	Laboratory tests	Clinical signs
Silent thyroiditis	Evidence of mild inflammatory infiltration	Total T4, free T4 and cTSH within reference intervals; TgAA-positive	No clinical signs of thyroid dysfunction
Subclinical (compensating) hypothyroidism	More marked inflammatory infiltration, with unaffected follicles exhibiting changes indicative of TSH stimulation	Total T4 and free T4 within reference intervals; cTSH increased; TgAA-positive	
Clinical hypothyroidism	Marked inflammatory response with associated destruction and replacement of >75% of the thyroid gland	Total T4 and free T4 decreased; cTSH increased; TgAA-positive	Clinical signs of hypothyroidism
	Decreased active inflammation, with loss of most of the thyroid tissue	Total T4 and free T4 decreased; cTSH increased but may decline over time; TgAA-negative	

8.2 The stages of lymphocytic thyroiditis. The disease does not always progress to overt hypothyroidism in all affected dogs. The rate of progression is variable.

The underlying cause of this process is unknown. Histopathologically, it appears quite distinct from lymphocytic thyroiditis. However, it is unclear whether the two diseases are truly distinct or, in some cases, they represent different stages of the same disease process.

Theoretically, complete destruction of thyroid tissue potentially leads to a reduction in immune stimulation and response, and eventual loss of thyroiditis and conversion from TgAA-positive to TgAA-negative status. Such a theory is supported by the prevalence of both forms of hypothyroidism in certain breeds, and the tendency for lymphocytic thyroiditis to be diagnosed at an earlier age (Graham *et al.*, 2007). In addition, the progression from lymphocytic thyroiditis to thyroid atrophy has been documented in some individual dogs. However, such a theory may be too simplistic, given that there appears to be a wide variation in the prevalence of TgAA-positive and TgAA-negative hypothyroidism across different breeds, suggesting a different rate of progression of thyroiditis or a different aetiology for idiopathic atrophy.

Other causes of primary hypothyroidism
Other causes of primary hypothyroidism include neoplastic destruction, antithyroid medication (particularly potentiated sulphonamides), radiation therapy and congenital defects (see below), although these are uncommon in dogs.

Central hypothyroidism
Central hypothyroidism is caused by the failure of normal TSH secretion by the thyrotropic cells of the pituitary gland. The absence of such stimulation results in atrophic degeneration, characterized by follicular distension and flattening of the follicular epithelium, which is readily distinguishable from the changes typical of idiopathic thyroidal atrophy. It is commonly reported that central hypothyroidism accounts for approximately 5% of all spontaneous cases of hypothyroidism. However, spontaneous central hypothyroidism has rarely been reliably documented in dogs.

The most common cause of central hypothyroidism is suppression of pituitary TSH secretion by exogenous glucocorticoid administration or spontaneous hyperadrenocorticism. However, this is usually a temporary and reversible condition for which treatment of the underlying cause is curative, and thyroid hormone supplementation is not indicated. Central hypothyroidism may also result from congenital TSH deficiency (see below) or be a consequence of pituitary neoplasia. Deficiency of TRH, although reported in humans, has only once been definitively diagnosed in a dog, as a result of the growth of a pituitary tumour (Shiel *et al.*, 2007a).

Congenital hypothyroidism
Congenital hypothyroidism is reported, albeit uncommonly, both as single case reports and within families. It is possible that the true prevalence is higher than reported, as many affected puppies die early in life and may be misclassified as suffering from 'fading puppy' syndrome. Most cases are thought to be caused by thyroid hypoplasia, thyroid aplasia, dysgenesis or dyshormonogenesis. The latter has been described in Fox Terriers and Rat Terriers, where it is inherited as an autosomal recessive trait (Fyfe *et al.*, 2003; Pettigrew *et al.*, 2007). A small number of dogs, including a family of Giant Schnauzers, have also been reported with congenital central hypothyroidism.

Congenital hypothyroidism typically causes disproportionate dwarfism, helping to differentiate it from pituitary dwarfism caused by growth hormone deficiency (see Chapter 4). The abnormal physical appearance in congenital hypothyroidism develops as a consequence of epiphyseal dysgenesis and delayed epiphyseal maturation, one of the hallmarks of the condition. Affected puppies (Figure 8.3) have disproportionately wide skulls, macroglossia and delayed dental eruption. They may also exhibit some of the signs typical of the adult-onset disease. Chronic osteoarthritis is a common long-term complication in surviving dogs, due to developmental joint abnormalities. Impaired mental function is also common, particularly if instigation of treatment is delayed.

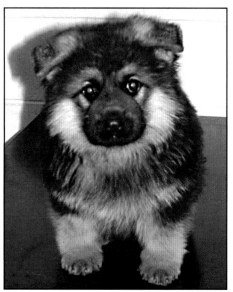

8.3 A 5-month-old male German Shepherd Dog with disproportionate dwarfism as a consequence of congenital hypothyroidism. Note the short legs, broad trunk and wide skull.

If congenital hypothyroidism is suspected, interpretation of thyroid hormone concentrations must take account of the higher values encountered in puppies compared with adult values. Healthy puppies up to 3 months of age typically have circulating total T4 values two to five times higher than those in adult dogs.

Prevalence and signalment

Adult-onset hypothyroidism is undoubtedly one of the more common endocrine disorders of dogs. Historically, epidemiological studies of the condition have been complicated by inconsistencies in the diagnostic criteria used to confirm the disease, particularly the use of tests now considered unreliable. Consequently, estimation of the prevalence of hypothyroidism varies greatly between studies. It has been suggested that the true prevalence is between 0.2 and 0.6% of the general canine population (Panciera, 1994).

Any breed can develop hypothyroidism. However, purebred dogs are most commonly affected overall, reflecting, at least in part, the genetic influence on the development of the condition, particularly for lymphocytic thyroiditis. Hypothyroidism (unspecified aetiology) has been broadly reported to occur with increased frequency in Dobermanns, Great Danes, Poodles, Golden Retrievers, Boxers, Schnauzers, Hovawarts, spaniels (particularly Cockers), setters and terriers. Many of these breeds are specifically at risk of lymphocytic thyroiditis (see above).

The disease is most common in middle-aged dogs and is only rarely recognized in animals <2 years old. Overall, the mean age at the time of diagnosis is approximately 7 years. Breeds at risk of lymphocytic thyroiditis tend to develop the condition at an earlier age.

Males and females, whether neutered or entire, appear to be at a broadly similar risk of developing hypothyroidism (Dixon *et al.,* 1999). Previous studies suggesting a female bias, or an increased risk associated with neutering, can be criticized due to small sample size and loose diagnostic criteria for hypothyroidism.

Clinical features of hypothyroidism

Thyroid hormones influence the function of almost all organ systems within the body, and, when deficient, a wide range of clinical signs is possible (Figure 8.4). Thyroid hormones act mainly as transcription factors to modify gene expression. At a cellular level, they influence multiple metabolic processes, from the regulation of mitochondrial oxygen demand to the control of protein synthesis. As a consequence, the onset of the disease is insidiously progressive and, although the clinical signs can be varied and extensive, most are non-specific.

The most common clinical signs (approximately 70% of cases) relate to a decline in metabolic rate, together with a variety of dermatological changes (Panciera, 1994; Dixon *et al.,* 1999). However, in some dogs only one abnormality is present, while in others clinical signs involving the neuromuscular, cardiovascular, reproductive, ophthalmological and gastrointestinal systems develop, and may even predominate. Consequently, hypothyroidism is a differential for many presenting complaints in practice.

Metabolic features

Hypothyroidism is associated with a decline in metabolic rate. Related clinical signs, including weight gain, lethargy, exercise intolerance and weakness, occur in the majority of hypothyroid dogs. In hypothyroid humans, basal metabolic rate reduces by up to 40%; a decline in resting energy expenditure has also been demonstrated in hypothyroid dogs. The

Metabolic
• **Lethargy** • **Weight gain** • **Exercise intolerance** • Cold intolerance
Dermatological
• **Poor quality, dry and brittle hair coat** • **Hair thinning** • **Endocrine alopecia** • **'Rat tail'** • **Hyperpigmentation** • **Myxoedema and tragic facial expression** • **Secondary pyoderma** • **Seborrhoea sicca or oleosa ± *Malassezia***
Neurological
• Various neuropathies • Central vestibular disease • Myxoedema coma
Cardiovascular
• Bradycardia • Low voltage R waves • Reduced myocardial contractility
Reproductive
• Galactorrhoea • Decreased fertility in bitch • Prolonged parturition • Reduced pup survival
Others
• Corneal lipidosis • Reduced tear production • Small intestinal bacterial overgrowth

8.4 Clinical features associated with hypothyroidism in dogs. Those noted in bold are more common.

onset of metabolic signs in dogs is typically insidious and, consequently, often missed or dismissed by owners. However, the clinical response following appropriate therapy can be dramatic, retrospectively confirming the extent of the problem. At least one 'metabolic' sign is recognized in approximately 85% of hypothyroid dogs.

Lethargy
Lethargy is the most common metabolic change, affecting up to 80% of cases. The duration of the underlying illness appears to correspond with the severity of lethargy. In some cases lethargy is profound. Unusually, some affected dogs appear unperturbed by veterinary examination and may fall asleep during a consultation.

Exercise intolerance
Exercise intolerance affects just over 25% of all cases, although many owners confuse lethargy with exercise intolerance. Frequently, dogs appear to have a normal capacity for short-term exercise, or when excited will behave appropriately. However, this is relatively short-lived, and recovery is prolonged, as shown by a need for excessive rest or sleep thereafter.

Weight gain and obesity

There is no doubt that weight gain is a common finding in hypothyroidism, occurring in approximately 40% of cases during the few months prior to initial presentation. Weight gain occurs despite a normal or slightly reduced appetite, and may be exacerbated by a concurrent unwillingness to exercise. In some affected dogs, weight gain can be marked with recorded weights >75% above the expected breed average. Despite this, a large proportion of hypothyroid dogs do not gain significant weight, and hypothyroidism cannot be ruled out based on a lack of this finding alone. In addition, whilst obesity is extremely common in dogs, most cases relate to simple overfeeding, with hypothyroidism only accounting for a small proportion of cases. Thus the presence or absence of obesity is of little diagnostic consequence for hypothyroidism.

Cold intolerance

Cold intolerance or heat seeking is reported in approximately 10% of hypothyroid dogs, and affected dogs may be noted as shivering excessively. However, the presence of heat seeking is non-specific as it is also a common feature of euthyroid dogs.

Dermatological features

Thyroid hormones play an important role in the maintenance of dermal health. Dermatological abnormalities can be extensive and more worrying to owners than the more subtle metabolic signs. They are reported in approximately 80% of affected dogs. The particular dermatological signs vary and reflect the severity and duration of the disease.

Scaling and scurfing

Hyperkeratosis causing scaling and scurfing of the skin, and poor quality hair coat, is common. Excessive dandruff or a dry dull coat is often noted in the early stages of the disorder. Otitis externa is reported in a number of hypothyroid dogs, and dryness and scaling of the external ear canal may be noted.

Alopecia

Thyroid hormones are necessary for the initiation of the anagen phase of hair growth. Absence of thyroid hormones results in persistence of the telogen phase; hairs become easily epilated, with resultant alopecia, and there is a failure of regrowth after clipping. Hair loss commonly begins in areas undergoing friction, such as on the neck in dogs that wear collars (Figure 8.5a) and on the tail, resulting in the typical 'rat-tail' appearance of hypothyroidism (Figure 8.5b). Affected animals commonly develop a bilaterally symmetrical non-pruritic 'endocrine' alopecia, with progressive hair loss along the flanks and on the trunk, usually sparing the head and extremities (Figure 8.6). However, focal, multifocal and asymmetrical alopecia can also occur, and larger breeds may develop alopecia of the extremities (presumably as a result of friction) whilst the trunk remains relatively unaffected. Dorsal nasal alopecia has been reported to be a particular feature of hypothyroidism in retrievers but also occurs in other breeds and other endocrine disorders (Figure 8.7).

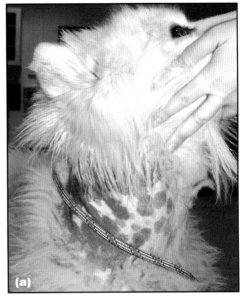

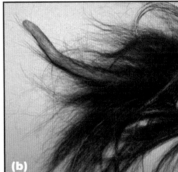

8.5
The hair loss of hypothyroidism typically begins in areas of friction such as **(a)** the neck in dogs that wear collars and **(b)** the tail ('rat tail').

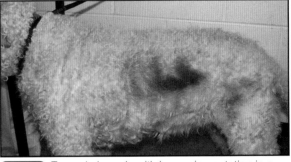

8.6 Truncal alopecia with hyperpigmentation in a hypothyroid dog.

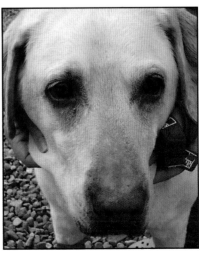

8.7
Nasal alopecia in a hypothyroid dog.

Myxoedema

Accumulation of mucopolysaccharides and hyaluronic acid in the skin occurs due to an imbalance in their normal thyroid-controlled production and degradation. It results in myxoedematous non-pitting thickening of the skin. This thickening is most pronounced over the head where it can give rise to a tragic facial expression with thickening of the lips, thickened skin over the forehead and drooping of the eyelids (Figure 8.8).

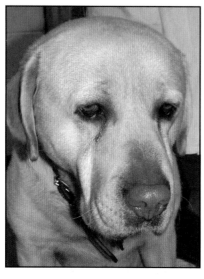

8.8
Tragic facial expression associated with hypothyroidism.

Secondary infection

Thyroid hormones assist the humoral and cellular immune responses, and consequently hypothyroidism reduces resistance to infection. Secondary recurrent and persistent superficial and deep bacterial and *Malassezia* infection are reported in 10–20% of hypothyroid dogs. Such disorders may be poorly responsive to standard therapy until the hypothyroidism is controlled. Pruritus may occur, resulting in self-excoriation and trauma, which can complicate the clinical and histopathological appearance.

Other changes

The remaining hair coat in affected dogs is usually dry and brittle, and may become lighter in colour due to environmental bleaching. Hyperpigmentation is common and is particularly noticeable over alopecic regions. Comedones may also be noted, particularly on the ventrum, and seborrhoea (sicca or oleosa) affects up to 40% of hypothyroid dogs.

Breed-related differences in hair cycle and type may be responsible for some differences in clinical features. Arctic breeds typically lose primary hairs, giving the remaining hair coat a coarse woolly appearance. Hypertrichosis, rather than hair loss, is reported in Boxers and Irish Setters.

Histopathological appearance

The dermatohistopathological features of hypothyroidism are generally considered non-specific and are consistent with a number of endocrine diseases. These commonly include predominance of telogen phase hair follicles (atrophic or hyperkeratotic), dermal thickening and, more specifically, myxoedema and vacuolation of the arrector pili muscles. Inflammatory lesions may be present, with concurrent skin infection. Irritation associated with seborrhoea may also contribute to its development. Inflammatory changes generally consist of dermal and periadnexal accumulation of neutrophils, macrophages, lymphocytes and plasma cells. Folliculitis is generally the consequence of a secondary infection. If severe, these inflammatory changes have the ability to obscure some of the more subtle histopathological findings associated with hypothyroidism, and skin biopsy samples should preferably be collected from areas that are not obviously infected or inflamed.

Neuromuscular features

Hypothyroidism causes a variety of neurological and muscular disorders in humans, which are reported in as many as 75% of patients. However, while hypothyroidism has been implicated in canine myopathies, peripheral neuropathies and central nervous system (CNS) disorders, only some have been confirmed and the causal relationship in others remains unproven or controversial.

The pathological basis for most central or generalized neuromuscular abnormalities is complex and probably multifactorial. A general reduction of the sodium–potassium ATPase capacity plays a role. Accumulation of myxoedematous fluid within the dural sheaths may contribute to peripheral neuropathies. CNS signs may occur because of atherosclerotic vascular disease or severe hyperlipidaemia, although a range of other metabolic derangements are possible.

Clinical manifestations

Clinical features of myopathy, lower motor neuron disease, megaoesophagus, laryngeal paralysis, peripheral and central vestibular disease, and myxoedema coma have all been reported in hypothyroid dogs. None is common. They are rarely specifically cited in surveys of hypothyroid dogs, and hypothyroidism is uncommonly implicated as a cause in large cases of the specific abnormalities. In the past, seizures and isolated cranial nerve neuropathies were attributed to hypothyroidism, but it is now considered unlikely that they are causally related.

Myopathy: Myopathy as a distinct clinical entity is not well defined in hypothyroid dogs. However, experimentally, hypothyroid dogs develop electromyographic and morphological evidence of myopathy (Rossmeisl *et al.*, 2009). These myopathic changes are consistent with altered muscle energy metabolism and carnitine depletion. The changes remain subclinical but may contribute to the non-specific signs of lethargy and exercise intolerance more commonly reported in hypothyroidism.

Lower motor neuron disease: This is probably the most well documented neurological abnormality of hypothyroidism, though it remains uncommon. It may initially present as generalized weakness.

Subsequent progression is variable, ranging from subtle gait alterations (often dragging or knuckling of feet and excessive wear of toenails (Figure 8.9)) to paraparesis and tetraparesis. Proprioceptive deficits are usually noted in fore- or hindlimbs, or both, and segmental reflexes may be diminished (Jaggy *et al.*, 1994).

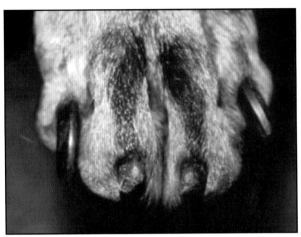

8.9 Excess wear of middle digits in the foreleg of a dog with hypothyroidism, presumably as a result of lower motor neuron disease.

Laryngeal paralysis and megaoesophagus: Both of these disorders have been associated with hypothyroidism, albeit rarely. However, based on the limited response to the appropriate thyroid hormone supplementation in most cases, there is little evidence of a true causal relationship. Consequently, hypothyroidism should only be considered when other more common causes have been excluded and/or there are additional clinical and clinicopathological features suggestive of thyroid dysfunction.

Peripheral and central vestibular disease: In the past, peripheral vestibular disease has been associated with hypothyroidism. However, this has been based partly on the response to thyroid hormone supplementation, and has not taken into account the fact that many affected dogs recover without any specific treatment.

Central vestibular disease is better described in hypothyroidism, albeit rarely. Affected dogs exhibit progressive central vestibular dysfunction that is rapidly and largely reversible with appropriate thyroid hormone supplementation (Higgins *et al.*, 2006). Other clinical signs of hypothyroidism appear to be uncommon in affected dogs, suggesting that it should be evaluated in all cases presenting for persistent or progressive central vestibular disease when other potential causes are not apparent.

Myxoedema coma: The most striking acute presentation of hypothyroidism is myxoedema coma, a rare complication of advanced hypothyroidism. Affected dogs are profoundly dull and present as stuporous or comatose, with hypothermia, bradycardia, hypotension and hypoventilation. Hypothyroidism is likely to have pre-existed for some time and

other clinical features (e.g. skin thickening) may be readily apparent. In many cases there is evidence of a precipitating disease, such as cardiac failure, or overwhelming sepsis that may or may not be related to the thyroid disease. Treatment consists of thyroid hormone supplementation (see below) alongside appropriate medical supportive care. The prognosis is more guarded but recovery can be expected with aggressive treatment.

Cardiovascular features

Thyroid hormones have direct positive chronotropic and inotropic effects on the heart. In addition they stimulate myocardial hypertrophy, and indirectly affect the cardiovascular system by increasing responsiveness to adrenergic stimulation. Thyroid hormone deficiency can therefore impair cardiac function. However, it is doubtful whether hypothyroidism truly causes significant clinical cardiac disease. Nevertheless, in dogs with pre-existing heart disease, cardiac function may be complicated by concurrent hypothyroidism, and potentially results in the progression from compensating to decompensated heart failure.

Dilated cardiomyopathy

The most widely favoured link between cardiac disease and hypothyroidism in dogs is purportedly dilated cardiomyopathy (DCM). However, there is no clear evidence of a causal relationship, and the main link is likely to be similar breed predispositions for both diseases. Studies have documented the presence of both conditions concurrently in a large number of Dobermanns (Calvert *et al.*, 1998); however, DCM was equally reported in euthyroid individuals of the same breed, suggesting that the two disorders are not causally related. Reduced myocardial contractility (as opposed to DCM) has certainly been documented in hypothyroid dogs, with improvement following appropriate treatment for the hypothyroidism.

Other changes

Other cardiovascular abnormalities associated with hypothyroidism include bradycardia, a weak apex beat and arrhythmias. Electrocardiographic abnormalities include small QRS complexes, inverted T waves and sinus bradycardia. These changes are usually reversible with appropriate therapy. A cholesterol-based pericardial effusion was suggested to result from hypothyroidism in one dog (MacGregor *et al.*, 2004).

Reproductive features

A wide range of reproductive abnormalities has been suggested to result from hypothyroidism, including persistent anoestrus, galactorrhoea, infertility, prolonged interoestrous interval, decreased male libido, abortion and stillbirth. However, as the ability to confirm hypothyroidism accurately improves, the incidence of reproductive signs appears to be reducing.

Experimentally, short-term hypothyroidism (median of 19 weeks duration) has no effect on interoestrous interval, litter size or gestation length.

However, it is associated with prolonged parturition and reduced puppy survival in the periparturient period (Panciera *et al.*, 2007). More long-term disease is also associated with decreased fertility in the bitch but has no deleterious effect on male reproduction (Johnson, 1994; Panciera *et al.*, 2008). Reproductive abnormalities are expected to resolve on restoration of euthyroidism.

Inappropriate galactorrhoea is a recognized but uncommon feature of hypothyroidism. Although previously presumed to be a consequence of increased circulating prolactin concentrations resulting from TRH stimulation, it is probably more complex. Prolactin secretion decreases in experimental hypothyroidism (Diaz-Espineira *et al.*, 2008b). However, in naturally occurring disease prolactin concentrations do not decline, but are only significantly increased (potentially resulting in galactorrhoea) in the luteal phase of the oestrous cycle in the intact bitch (Diaz-Espineira *et al.*, 2009).

Hypothyroidism is often blamed by dog breeders for poor reproductive performance, and the pressure to prescribe treatment without confirming a diagnosis may be considerable. However, whilst hypothyroidism may be one of the considerations in such cases, it is undoubtedly one of the more uncommon causes and should only be considered for the specific abnormalities described above.

Other clinical features

Corneal lipidosis (Figure 8.10) occurs in a small number of hypothyroid dogs as a consequence of alterations in the lipid profile of affected animals. Its response to appropriate therapy appears to be variable, despite the normalization of lipid values after successful thyroid hormone supplementation. Keratoconjunctivits sicca has also been reported in association with hypothyroidism, although tenuously. Controversy arises because of similar breed predispositions for both disorders, problems with diagnosis of hypothyroidism and the possibility of simply reflecting a wider autoimmune disorder. Tear production appears to be reduced in hypothyroid dogs, although whether this progresses to overt clinical disease is unclear (Williams *et al.*, 2007).

In recent years, it has been suggested that hypothyroidism is a possible cause of behavioural abnormalities, particularly aggression. However, even within published case reports, the aggression was present for many months before a diagnosis of

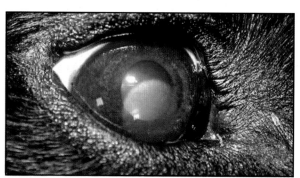

8.10 Corneal lipidosis associated with hypothyroidism.

hypothyroidism and did not completely resolve with appropriate treatment, bringing a causal relationship into disrepute.

Hypothyroidism has been reported in association with small intestinal bacterial overgrowth in a small number of dogs. This is presumed secondary to reduced gastrointestinal motility, a feature also recognized in human hypothyroid patients in whom constipation is a known complication.

Hypothyroidism may be encountered in association with other immune-mediated disorders. The most common polyendocrinopathies reported include hypothyroidism in association with diabetes mellitus or hypoadrenocorticism. However, such syndromes are not as well defined in dogs as they are in humans. The clinical presentation reflects the combination of diseases present. Commercial laboratories are frequently requested to perform thyroid function tests for dogs that exhibit polyuria and polydipsia; however, these signs are not true features of hypothyroidism unless caused by the subsequent complications of concurrent glomerulonephritis, and this is rare (Mansfield and Mooney, 2006).

Diagnosis

The following principles should be taken into consideration before diagnostic testing (Dixon, 2004):

- The diagnosis of hypothyroidism is a *clinical* diagnosis and should not be based on laboratory tests alone
- None of the existing endocrine tests is 100% accurate and some are substantially less. Performance frequently varies from highly sensitive and poorly specific to highly specific and poorly sensitive
- The influence of commonly used medications and non-thyroidal illnesses (NTIs) on thyroid function and test results can be significant. A range of medications commonly used in veterinary practice and a number of clinically similar NTIs give rise to thyroid function test results easily misinterpreted as indicating hypothyroidism.

Keeping these factors under consideration will undoubtedly help improve the ability to confirm or refute a diagnosis of hypothyroidism more accurately.

General approach

The recommended steps in investigating suspected hypothyroidism are depicted in Figure 8.11 and summarized as follows.

1. The dog should be of an appropriate age and breed.
2. Clinical signs of hypothyroidism must be present. If there are clinical signs unlikely to be associated with hypothyroidism (e.g. polyuria/polydipsia, hepatomegaly), investigation for other disorders takes precedence.

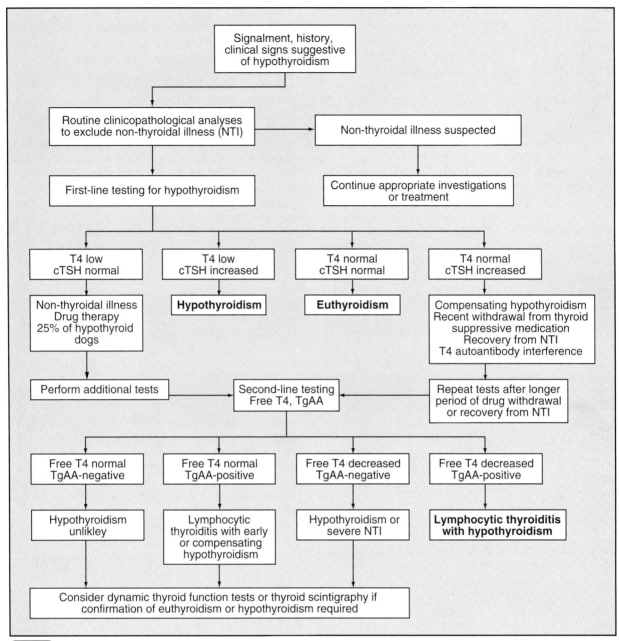

8.11 Schematic representation of the steps for diagnosing hypothyroidism.

3. Each case should be evaluated for previous and current drug therapy and testing postponed until a suitable withdrawal period has elapsed.
   - The effect of drug therapy is of serious concern. This is confounded by the fact that in many cases there is a long-standing history, particularly in dermatological disease where a wide variety of medications may have been prescribed before thyroid disease is even considered. Glucocorticoid and potentiated sulphonamide use is common. These drugs not only interfere with tests of thyroid function but can result in clinical signs attributed to hypothyroidism.
   - The withdrawal period for such drugs will clearly vary from drug to drug, and with dose and length of treatment. Often a 6-week

   withdrawal for glucocorticoids, potentiated sulphonamides and any other drugs known to interfere with thyroid function is advised. If drug withdrawal is impossible, the likely impact of the drugs used should be considered and the most appropriate test, or the one least likely to be affected, selected.
4. NTI should be excluded as far as is practical, by performing routine clinicopathological investigations and any additional appropriate diagnostic tests. Exclusion of NTI is the single most useful factor in reliably interpreting tests of thyroid function. If NTI is diagnosed, there may be no need to investigate thyroid function further. However, it is recognized that in some instances, hypothyroidism may be considered a complicating feature of another illness and in

such cases interpretation of thyroid function tests should take the NTI into consideration. The effects of NTI on thyroid tests vary depending on the nature, severity and stage of the illness.

5. Once thyroid testing is considered feasible, first-line diagnostic thyroid tests should be performed (total T4 and endogenous canine TSH (cTSH)).
6. If results are equivocal second-line diagnostic tests should be performed (free T4 by dialysis and/or TgAA).
7. If results remain equivocal more advanced diagnostic tests should be considered, such as a TSH response test or thyroid imaging.

Routine clinicopathological features

The most common abnormalities associated with hypothyroidism include hyperlipidaemia and anaemia (Figure 8.12); their presence helps to provide supportive evidence of hypothyroidism.

However, because of the high prevalence of similar abnormalities in dogs with NTI, the predictive value of most routine parameters for hypothyroidism is relatively poor (Dixon *et al.,* 1999). Despite this, routine clinicopathological tests are of immense value in helping to exclude significant NTI. In one study comparing hypothyroid dogs and sick euthyroid animals presenting with similar clinical signs, the most useful predictive findings were an increase in circulating cholesterol concentration and gamma-glutamyl transferase (GGT) activity, and a reduction in red blood cell (RBC) and neutrophil counts (Dixon *et al.,* 1999).

Hyperlipidaemia

Hypothyroidism is associated with both a reduction in the rate of lipid degradation and a reduction in lipid synthesis. The former is affected to the greater extent and thus there is an accumulation of lipids within the circulation. The principal changes are increases in high density lipoproteins (HDL), low density lipoproteins (LDL) and possibly very low density lipoproteins (VLDL) (see Chapter 28).

Hypercholesterolaemia is commonly reported, occurring in up to 80% of affected dogs. Hypertriglyceridaemia is additionally present in a similar proportion of cases. Whilst hyperlipidaemia is also a common feature of other endocrine disorders, notably diabetes mellitus and hyperadrenocorticism, the magnitude of the cholesterol increase in hypothyroidism is typically greater, and circulating cholesterol concentrations >20 mmol/l are not uncommon.

Thus, whilst hypercholesterolaemia is not specific for hypothyroidism, an unusually exaggerated increase should prompt its consideration.

Anaemia

A mild normocytic and normochromic anaemia affects approximately 40–50% of hypothyroid dogs. This is a consequence of reduced peripheral metabolic activity and a reduction in tissue oxygen demand. The severity of the anaemia generally reflects the chronicity of the hypothyroidism. Typically it is mild (e.g. red blood cell (RBC) values $5.0–5.5 \times 10^{12}/l$) or RBC values are at the low end of the laboratory reference interval.

Traditionally, hypothyroidism was thought to be associated with a variety of haemostatic abnormalities, in particular von Willebrand's disease. It is now clear that coagulopathies are not a feature of hypothyroidism *per se,* although undoubtedly certain breeds, notably Dobermanns, commonly suffer from both conditions. Moreover, thyroxine treatment has no effect on increasing production of von Willebrand factor or improving haemostatic function in affected dogs. Anaemia with evidence of regeneration should prompt consideration of another underlying cause.

Muscle enzyme activities

Increased creatine kinase (CK) activity is considered a feature of hypothyroidism attributable to decreased clearance from the circulation. However, the subclinical myopathy described in experimental cases (see above) may also play a role, as it is associated with modest increases in CK, aspartate aminotransferase (AST) and lactate dehydrogenase (LDH) activities. A mild increase in CK activity is reported in up to 35% of hypothyroid dogs. However, such prevalence is comparable to that in euthyroid dogs presenting with similar signs, highlighting its poor specificity for diagnosing hypothyroidism. Elevated AST and LDH activities are rarely reported in cases of naturally occurring canine hypothyroidism.

Liver enzymes

Mild increases in liver enzyme activities, particularly alkaline phosphatase (ALP) and GGT, are present in approximately 30% of hypothyroid dogs. This is presumed to be a consequence of mild hepatic lipid deposition associated with hypothyroidism. The diagnostic utility of increased liver enzyme results is limited, as similar increases are a common finding in a wide range of NTI. However, marked increases

Abnormality	Percentage of cases	Severity	Pathophysiology
Hyperlipidaemia (including hypercholesterolaemia and hypertriglyceridaemia)	80%	Can be marked	Reduced lipid degradation
Anaemia	40–50%	Usually mild normochromic normocytic	Reduced oxygen-carrying capacity
Increased creatine kinase	35%	Rarely exceeds twice reference interval	Decreased clearance; subclinical myopathy

8.12 Routine clinicopathological features of canine hypothyroidism.

in liver enzymes, particularly ALP, should prompt consideration of NTI, hyperadrenocorticism being the most obvious example.

Fructosamine

In human hypothyroid patients, circulating fructosamine concentrations increase when protein turnover is reduced, rather than as a result of any change in glycaemic control. Because of its widespread use as a monitoring tool for diabetic dogs, there has been much interest in the effect of other illnesses on the circulating concentration of fructosamine. Following exclusion of dogs with diabetes mellitus, fructosamine had a diagnostic specificity for hypothyroidism in excess of 80% (Dixon *et al.*, 1999). Given the relative ease with which diabetes mellitus can usually be excluded, fructosamine is therefore a useful additional screening test for suspected hypothyroidism. However, the magnitude of the increase is much less noticeable than in diabetes mellitus. Typical results from hypothyroid dogs are at the top end of the reference interval (approximately 300 mmol/l) rather than markedly above it (Reusch *et al.*, 2002). Whilst the diagnosis of hypothyroidism cannot be based on fructosamine measurements alone, it may be as valuable, if not more valuable, than other routine clinicopathological parameters in supporting a diagnosis of hypothyroidism. In diabetic dogs with concurrent hypothyroidism, fructosamine should be interpreted cautiously as an indicator of glycaemic control.

Endocrine tests

Thyroid physiology

Knowledge of the normal production and control mechanisms of thyroid hormones is essential in order to understand the performance of individual diagnostic tests.

Thyroid hormone production: The thyroid gland is responsible for the production of the two active thyroid hormones, T3 and T4. The principal product of the thyroid gland is T4, which is entirely derived from thyroidal synthesis. By contrast, only approximately half of all circulating T3 originates from thyroidal production, the remainder being produced by peripheral deiodination of T4 in the skin, liver, skeletal muscle and kidneys. Most T3 is located intracellularly, with only approximately 20% present in the circulation. T3 is three to five times more metabolically active than T4; therefore T4 can be considered to act essentially as a pro-hormone.

Transport of thyroid hormones: For transportation in the circulation, thyroid hormones are usually bound to the plasma proteins thyroxine-binding globulin (TBG), albumin, and thyroxine-binding prealbumin (TBPA, transthyretin). A minor fraction of T3 and T4 is also carried by circulating lipoproteins. The protein-bound fraction acts as a reservoir to maintain adequate free hormone concentrations. In dogs, the unbound (free) fraction of T4 accounts for approximately 0.1% of the total hormone, compared to approximately 1% of T3, which circulates unbound. These values are higher than the corresponding human values due to lower binding affinities and lower concentrations of the major carrier proteins in dogs. This is of particular relevance because whilst absolute free T4 concentrations are similar in both species, total T4 concentrations are considerably lower in dogs. Thus it is well recognized that assays designed for human use must be modified to measure total T4 concentrations in dogs. As a consequence of reduced affinity of the thyroid hormones for their carrier proteins, hormone turnover is more rapid than in humans. The half-life of T4 is only 10–16 hours in dogs, compared with about 7 days in humans.

Control of thyroid hormone production: Circulating thyroid hormone concentrations are regulated through a classical negative feedback mechanism (Figure 8.13). The main stimulus for their synthesis and secretion is a rise in serum TSH concentrations. TSH is synthesized and secreted from the pars distalis of the pituitary gland under the tonic stimulation of TRH. The secretion of TSH, and TRH, is mainly inhibited by the negative feedback effect of circulating free T4. A complicated network of neuropeptides and neurotransmitters, including dopamine and somatostatin, also modulate TSH release.

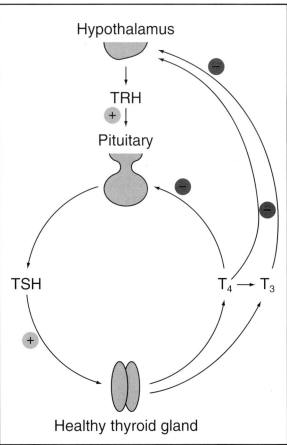

8.13 Control of thyroid function. TRH = thyrotropin-releasing hormone; TSH = thyroid-stimulating hormone; T3 = triiodothyronine; + = stimulation; – = inhibition.

Total T4

Basal serum total T4 estimation has traditionally been the mainstay for the diagnosis of canine hypothyroidism and remains an excellent first-line diagnostic test for the disease. Its advantages and disadvantages are summarized in Figure 8.14.

Advantages
• Inexpensive, widely available and easily measured • Highly sensitive marker for hypothyroidism • Reference interval values suggest hypothyroidism is unlikely
Disadvantages
• Low values do not confirm hypothyroidism • Decreased in certain breeds and in elderly dogs • Subnormal at random times during the day • Decreased by most non-thyroidal illnesses • Decreased by a range of drugs

8.14 The advantages and disadvantages of total thyroxine (T4) measurements for the diagnosis of hypothyroidism in dogs.

Diagnostic performance: There is universal agreement that circulating total T4 is usually subnormal in hypothyroidism. In most studies <5% of hypothyroid dogs have shown reference interval or increased values (Peterson *et al.*, 1997; Scott-Moncrieff *et al.*, 1998; Dixon and Mooney, 1999). Unfortunately, whilst the diagnostic sensitivity (i.e. the percentage of affected dogs with subnormal values) is undoubtedly high (>95%), the specificity (i.e. the ability of the test to exclude unaffected animals) is much lower, at approximately 75% (Figure 8.15).

Test characteristic	Test			
	Total T4	Free T4	cTSH	Combined total T4 and cTSH
Sensitivity	95%	>80%	75%	75%
Specificity	75%	>90%	80%	>90%

8.15 Comparison of the test performance for different hormones for diagnosing hypothyroidism in the dog. All values are approximate. cTSH = canine thyroid stimulating hormone; T3 = triiodothyronine; T4 = thyroxine.

Low total T4 values in euthyroid dogs: The specificity of total T4 concentration is particularly poor, largely because of the potentially profound suppressive effects of NTI and certain drug therapies. The cause of this reduction is probably multifactorial, but includes TSH suppression, decreased intrinsic thyroid synthetic activity, reduced serum thyroid hormone protein binding and altered peripheral hormone metabolism. Glucocorticoids and circulating cytokines, including interleukins and tumour necrosis factor, may play a role in the development of some of these changes in NTI.

The effect of NTI is widely recognized but is particularly common in hyperadrenocorticism (Ferguson and Peterson, 1992), neoplastic diseases (Vail

et al., 1994), diabetes mellitus, hypoadrenocorticism, renal failure, hepatic disease, pyoderma (Hall *et al.*, 1993), infectious diseases (Schoeman and Herrtage, 2007, 2008) and a variety of medical illnesses requiring intensive care (Elliott *et al.*, 1995). As a general rule, the magnitude of suppression reflects the severity of illness, and less metabolically severe illnesses may in fact have little impact on thyroid function (Kantrowitz *et al.*, 2001). Furthermore, the likelihood of recovery from NTI is inversely proportional to the degree of suppression of total T4 concentrations (Mooney *et al.*, 2008). As a general rule, any illness should be considered capable of suppressing total T4 concentrations.

Numerous categories of drugs interfere with thyroid hormone metabolism through a variety of mechanisms and can suppress total T4 values (Daminet and Ferguson, 2003) (Figure 8.16). These include glucocorticoids, anticonvulsants, non-steroidal anti-inflammatory drugs (NSAIDs) (Daminet *et al.*, 2003) and potentiated sulphonamides (Hall *et al.*, 1993). Withdrawal of these drugs should be considered prior to testing for hypothyroidism (see above). A variety of other drugs are capable of suppressing total T4 concentrations in humans but have not yet been specifically tested in dogs. As for NTI, any drug should be considered capable of such suppression unless proven otherwise.

Drugs	Effects
Glucocorticoids	Decrease total and free T4
Non-steroidal anti-inflammatory drugs	Decrease total T4 concentration
Potentiated sulphonamides	Decrease total and free T4 Increase cTSH
Barbiturates	Decrease total and free T4 Mildly increase cTSH
Clomipramine	Decreases total and free T4 Decreases total T3
Thyroid hormone replacement therapy	Decreases cTSH through negative feedback and thus inhibits spontaneous thyroid function

8.16 Some of the common drug therapies known to affect thyroid function tests in dogs. cTSH = canine thyroid stimulating hormone; T3 = triiodothyronine; T4 = thyroxine.

In addition to these 'abnormal' causes, normal physiological mechanisms can also result in subnormal total T4 concentrations.

- Daily variation: Healthy dogs exhibit fluctuation in total T4 values below the reference interval on a daily basis. Unfortunately there is no circadian pattern to this fluctuation and no recommendations on the timing of samples can be given.
- Size: Larger and medium-sized breeds generally have lower normal circulating total T4 values than do small breeds. However, obese dogs have

significantly higher total T4 values than non-obese members of the same breed.

- Breed: There is considerable evidence that total T4 concentrations vary between different breeds (Shiel *et al.*, 2007b; Shiel *et al.*, 2010). In most cases this difference is small. However, total T4 values are generally low and often below the reference interval in many sighthounds, including Greyhounds, Whippets, Irish Wolfhounds and Salukis. Consequently, measurement of total T4 in some of these breeds cannot be used for investigating hypothyroidism. Sled dogs also have lower T4 values when compared to standard reference intervals.
- Age: Total T4 concentrations progressively decline from the mid-normal in middle-aged animals, to low-normal values in elderly patients. This is an ordinary physiological feature that is of importance because a high percentage of dogs evaluated for hypothyroidism are older.
- Gender: The influence of gender on thyroid hormone concentrations has been evaluated in several large studies, with conflicting results. Males and females show similar results, but total T4 values appear to increase during progesterone-dominated phases of the oestrous cycle. However, given that values tend to remain within reference interval, these changes are unlikely to have any clinical significance.

Given the range of factors that can result in a subnormal T4 value, this measure cannot be used to confirm hypothyroidism, but can be used to rule in such a diagnosis. By contrast, reference interval values are more likely to rule out hypothyroidism, with few exceptions.

Reference interval/high total T4 values in hypothyroid dogs: In dogs, the presence of circulating autoantibodies can interfere with actual total T4 measurements using most commercial methodologies. These autoantibodies develop against a specific epitope on the thyroglobulin molecule corresponding to T4 (T4AA) (or T3 (T3AA)) in a subset of dogs with lymphocytic thyroiditis. Their exact effect is variable, but in most cases T4AAs tend to cause an artefactually higher measurement for total T4. In one study, of over 280,000 samples submitted for thyroid evaluation, T3AA was detected in 5.67% of all samples, compared with ›1.66% for T4AA (Nachreiner *et al.*, 2002). Although this prevalence appears relatively low, another study identified T4AA in 8% of 11,606 hypothyroid dogs (Graham *et al.*, 2007).

T4AA and T3AA have no apparent clinical effect but are important because of their potential to interfere with the measurement of hormone concentrations. In some hypothyroid dogs, markedly elevated total T4 concentrations are found. These usually pose few diagnostic problems in a dog under investigation for hypothyroidism, as such results raise suspicion of the presence of T4AA. However, their potential artefactually to increase low values to within the reference interval poses a greater diagnostic challenge. In many of these cases, a diagnosis of hypothyroidism may be ruled out erroneously. T4AAs presumably account for the less than perfect sensitivity of total T4 for diagnosing hypothyroidism. Often the possibility of T4AA is only considered because of other abnormal thyroid function test results (e.g. cTSH) or a persistent clinical suspicion. Some, but not all, commercial laboratories are capable of measuring actual T4AA. An alternative is to measure TgAA, as almost all dogs that are T4AA-positive are also positive for TgAA and such assays are more widely available.

Canine TSH

Measurement of cTSH concentrations has revolutionized the testing for canine hypothyroidism. In primary hypothyroidism, there is a loss of normal regulatory feedback on pituitary synthesis and secretion of cTSH. As the vast majority of hypothyroid dogs have primary hypothyroidism, increased circulating cTSH concentration is expected. The advantages and disadvantages of this test are summarized in Figure 8.17.

Advantages
• Helps differentiate low T4 of hypothyroidism from other causes

Disadvantages
• Should not be interpreted alone • Increased by certain drugs and recovery from non-thyroidal illness • Within reference interval in a high proportion of hypothyroid dogs • Increased in compensating hypothyroidism

8.17 The advantages and disadvantages of canine thyroid stimulating hormone (cTSH) measurements for the diagnosis of hypothyroidism in dogs.

When elevated above the reference interval (>approximately 0.6 μg/l), values are typically between 1 and 3 μg/l. Occasionally, marked increases in cTSH concentrations to values >10 μg/l are identified. The reasons for such dramatic increases are unclear, but it has been suggested that they may be particularly prominent in the early stages of thyroid dysfunction. In accordance with this, there is a marked increase in cTSH concentration within 2–4 months of experimental induction of hypothyroidism, prior to a gradual decline over the next 2–3 years (Diaz-Espineira *et al.*, 2008b).

Diagnostic performance: Measurement of circulating cTSH in isolation is not recommended, as it has a diagnostic sensitivity of approximately 75% and a specificity of 80% (Peterson *et al.*, 1997; Scott-Moncrieff *et al.*, 1998; Dixon and Mooney, 1999) (see Figure 8.15). It is therefore usually recommended as a first-line test, together with total T4 estimation (Figure 8.18). The specificity of combined decreased total T4 and increased cTSH exceeds 90% in most published studies. This combination of tests has therefore become the hallmark for the initial laboratory diagnosis of hypothyroidism. Together

	Total T4 decreased	Total T4 within reference interval
cTSH normal	*Interpretation*	*Interpretation*
	Non-thyroidal illness Drug therapy Approximately 25% hypothyroid dogs	Euthyroid
	Options	*Options*
	Treat non-thyroidal illness and re-test Withdraw drugs and retest Perform second-line diagnostic tests such as free T4 and TgAA	Hypothyroidism precluded
cTSH increased	*Interpretation*	*Interpretation*
	Hypothyroid	Potentiated sulphonamide therapy Recovery from NTI Compensating hypothyroidism T4 autoantibody interference
	Options	*Options*
	T4 therapy	Withdraw sulphonamide therapy and retest Wait until recovery complete and retest Perform free T4 measurement or TgAA to exclude antibody interference

8.18 Use and interpretation of total thyroxine (T4) and canine thyroid stimulating hormone (cTSH) as 'first line' endocrine tests. NTI = non-thyroidal illness; TgAA = thyroglobulin autoantibody.

with the use of free T4 and TgAA as second-line diagnostic tests, the vast majority of dogs can reliably be categorized as either hypothyroid or euthyroid.

Reference interval cTSH values in hypothyroid dogs: Whilst circulating cTSH concentrations are increased above the reference interval in the majority of hypothyroid dogs, a significant proportion have reference interval values. A variety of possible explanations have been proposed:

- Although not documented in all studies, there is some evidence that concurrent NTI can decrease cTSH concentrations into the reference interval in hypothyroid dogs. In order to avoid any possible interference, the concurrent illness should be treated, or at least stabilized, prior to testing for hypothyroidism
- Concurrent drug therapy, particularly glucocorticoids, is known to suppress cTSH values, and may decrease concentrations into the reference interval in hypothyroid dogs. Drug withdrawal should be attempted before cTSH measurement
- Some studies have suggested potential fluctuation of cTSH into the reference interval in some hypothyroid dogs with marginally elevated cTSH values. This is supported by the demonstration of pulsatile ultradian secretion of cTSH in experimental hypothyroidism (Kooistra *et al.,* 2000)
- Inappropriately low cTSH values are expected in central hypothyroidism. However, in contrast to the situation in humans, the current cTSH assay is incapable of distinguishing low from reference interval values. However, given that <5% of

hypothyroid cases are centrally mediated, such a diagnosis could not account for the much higher proportion of dogs with low total T4 and concurrent reference interval cTSH values
- The existence of varying isoforms of cTSH has been postulated to explain inappropriately reference interval cTSH values in hypothyroid dogs, although this is yet to be reliably documented in dogs
- It has also been suggested that pituitary exhaustion may occur in longstanding cases of hypothyroidism with consequent reduction in cTSH secretion. This has recently been supported by experimental studies. Over time, cTSH concentrations apparently decline and responsiveness to TRH decreases (Diaz-Espineira *et al.,* 2008b).

While the explanation for a reference interval value may be readily apparent in some dogs, in the majority it is not. The development of newer cTSH assays may help solve this diagnostic conundrum. Currently, the poor sensitivity of cTSH measurement for hypothyroidism precludes its use as a screening test for the disease.

Elevated cTSH values in euthyroid dogs: Elevated cTSH values in euthyroid dogs are not such a concern as reference interval values in hypothyroid dogs. However, they can and do occur for a variety of reasons.

- cTSH may be increased in the early stages of thyroid disease for some time before total T4 values decline and clinical signs become apparent. This so-called compensating hypothyroidism may explain increased cTSH in some euthyroid dogs. However, by definition such dogs should not be exhibiting clinical signs and are unlikely to undergo routine testing in practice. Despite this fact, these animals are being increasingly recognised during routine screening programmes such as those used by a number of breed clubs. Current statistics suggest 1 in 20 TgAA-positive euthyroid dogs becomes hypothyroid within 1 year, and regular re-testing is therefore recommended (Graham *et al.*, 2007).

- A variety of drugs potentially result in increased cTSH concentrations, particularly the potentiated sulphonamides (Hall *et al.*, 1993). These drugs interfere with thyroid hormone synthesis within the thyroid gland itself and potentially cause a temporary reversible state of thyroid hormone deficiency associated with increased circulating cTSH values. There appears to be some variation in effect depending on the specific preparation, dose and the duration of therapy, but it is clear that total T4 values can decrease and cTSH values increase within 1 and 2 weeks of starting therapy, respectively. The suppressive effect can be profound, and prolonged treatment may induce a clinical state of hypothyroidism. Withdrawal of the drug usually results in complete resolution within weeks. A transient rebound period, during which TSH is temporarily increased after cessation of glucocorticoid therapy, is recognised in humans and may occur in dogs. Certainly, increased cTSH concentrations have been reported in dogs with hyperadrenocorticism treated with trilostane (Kenefick and Neiger, 2008). A mild increase in cTSH has also been reported as a consequence of phenobarbital-containing anticonvulsant treatment, but the increase has no diagnostic significance.

- The recovery phase of NTI has also been associated with temporary increases in circulating TSH concentrations in both humans and dogs. This is presumed to reflect increased demand for thyroid hormone production with the progressive return to euthyroidism. Testing thyroid function during known recovery from NTI should therefore be avoided until the animal is clinically stable.

Free T4

Free T4 is the metabolically active portion of T4 and represents the hormone fraction that is available for tissue uptake. Theoretically, its measurement provides the most accurate assessment of cellular thyroid status. The advantages and disadvantages of this test are summarized in Figure 8.19.

Assay methods: The method used to measure free T4 concentrations is important. Only one method currently in routine use, which employs equilibrium dialysis, is considered to be capable of measuring true free hormone concentration. Using this technique, measurement of free T4 is a two-step procedure. The test takes longer to complete (24–48

Advantages
• Less affected by non-thyroidal illness and drug therapies than is total T4 • Decreased values more specific for hypothyroidism than is total T4

Disadvantages
• Must be measured by 'equilibrium dialysis' • More expensive than total T4 measurement • More prone to transport effects • Can also be decreased in severe non-thyroidal illness or by certain drugs • May be low normal in early hypothyroidism

8.19 The advantages and disadvantages of free thyroxine (T4) measurements for the diagnosis of hypothyroidism in dogs.

hours) and is correspondingly more expensive than methods for total hormone analysis. The first step involves the dialysis of the test sample across a membrane impermeable to protein-bound T4 and anti-T4 antibodies. Only free hormone can cross the membrane into the dialysate, which is then subjected to an ultrasensitive T4 radioimmunoassay.

Most non-dialysis methods are not true free hormone assays, but attempt to estimate free hormone concentration indirectly. The most common of these methods are analogue-based and provide no more information than a total T4 estimation alone. These assays are designed for human serum and are based upon separation techniques reliant upon the presence of high-affinity thyroid hormone-binding proteins. Canine thyroid hormone-binding proteins have lower affinity for T4 and are present at a lower concentration; these methods are therefore unreliable in dogs, particularly when additional factors (such as NTI) further decrease thyroid hormone binding affinity.

Diagnostic performance: Free T4 is theoretically less affected by the variety of factors that affect total T4, including but not limited to NTI and T4AAs. The diagnostic specificity of free T4 is >90% (Dixon and Mooney, 1999), which is significantly better than for total T4 (i.e. it is less likely to result in a false positive diagnosis of hypothyroidism) (see Figure 8.15). The sensitivity of free T4 for hypothyroidism is approximately 80%, which is lower than the corresponding value for total T4. Overall, it is the most accurate single test for hypothyroidism. However, its expense, poorer availability, potential for sample handling errors (see Chapter 1) and poorer sensitivity preclude its widespread use as a first-line diagnostic test. If used as a second-line diagnostic test, its poorer sensitivity is relatively unimportant. It is particularly useful in cases in which total T4 is decreased and cTSH remains within the reference interval. In these cases, a free T4 concentration may help differentiate genuine hypothyroidism (low values) from NTI (reference interval values).

Reference interval free T4 values in hypothyroid dogs: A small proportion of hypothyroid dogs maintain free T4 values within the reference interval, albeit at the low end. This probably reflects an attempt to maintain adequate free T4 concentrations in the face of early hypothyroidism. There is some evidence that hypothyroid dogs with low-normal free T4 values have more thyroidal reserve than those with subnormal free T4 values.

Low free T4 values in euthyroid dogs: There is no doubt that free T4 is also affected by certain drug therapies and NTI, albeit to a lesser extent than total T4. Free T4 concentrations do decrease with NTI, but are typically maintained within the reference interval in all but the most severe diseases (Kantrowitz et al., 2001; Mooney et al., 2008). Certain drugs, including glucocorticoids and phenobarbital-containing anticonvulsant medications, are also associated with decreased free T4 concentrations (Kantrowitz et al., 1999). Testing for hypothyroidism should be delayed until after such therapy is withdrawn. However, given the nature of the cases receiving such medications, complete withdrawal of these drugs is often unachievable. Efforts should be made to reduce the dose, but ultimately the results from dogs receiving such therapies should be interpreted with caution.

Anti-thyroglobulin autoantibodies

Thyroglobulin is a large molecular weight glycoprotein and a normal component of the thyroid gland. The spontaneous development of antibodies to normal thyroid tissue, including thyroglobulin, is well recognized in dogs with lymphocytic thyroiditis. TgAAs are only one of several antibodies produced during the progression of lymphocytic thyroiditis in dogs (see above). However, they are the most important because a reliable canine-specific method for their estimation is commercially available. The advantages and disadvantages of this test are summarized in Figure 8.20.

Advantages
• Reliable method for measurement now available
• A positive result is suggestive of thyroid pathology

Disadvantages
• Provides no assessment of thyroid function
• A negative result does not rule out hypothyroidism

8.20 The advantages and disadvantages of anti-thyroglobulin autoantibody measurements for the diagnosis of hypothyroidism in dogs.

Diagnostic performance: The principal limitation of TgAA measurement is that not all dogs with hypothyroidism have lymphocytic thyroiditis, and even in those that do, TgAA-positive dogs may eventually become TgAA-negative given time (see above). Therefore, whilst a positive TgAA result provides strong evidence of thyroid disease, a negative result does not rule it out.

Identification of TgAA provides no information on thyroid function. The test is therefore not recommended for use alone, but is of value when used alongside other tests such as total or free T4 and cTSH. TgAA measurement is of particular value in cases with discordant T4 and cTSH results. Since the presence of TgAA is highly specific for lymphocytic thyroiditis, a positive result is of particular help in those cases with the anticipated decrease in total or free T4 values but unexpected reference interval cTSH results. Another advantage of TgAA estimation is that it is unaffected by concurrent drug therapy. The use of TgAA as a second-line test is frequently recommended in both these situations.

Positive TgAA results in hypothyroid dogs: Approximately half of all hypothyroid dogs have a positive TgAA result. However, epidemiological analysis of the prevalence of TgAA has shown considerable breed and age variation (Graham et al., 2007). Positive TgAA results peak in dogs between 4 and 6 years of age. This subsequently declines, presumably as thyroid tissue is destroyed. Elderly dogs >10 years of age are much less likely to have positive TgAA results, making testing of less value in older animals. Certain breeds are over-represented for lymphocytic thyroiditis, and TgAA estimation is of particular value in these animals (see above). The age at which the peak prevalence is observed also varies between breeds. The likelihood of identifying a positive result increases significantly when testing a predisposed breed of the appropriate age-range, and this should be considered when selecting a second-line test, and perhaps choosing between free T4 and TgAA.

Positive TgAA results in euthyroid dogs: Measurement of TgAA may also be used as a marker of thyroiditis in clinically healthy dogs. This is now used by a large section of the dog breeding community to identify animals predisposed to lymphocytic thyroiditis prior to breeding. Whilst more extended studies are required, TgAA appears to be a potentially useful marker for the subsequent development of thyroid dysfunction.

Other diagnostic tests

Total T3: The diagnostic accuracy of total T3 is poorer than that of total T4 and as such offers no real practical advantages. Consequently, total T3 measurement is not recommended. The poor diagnostic performance of total T3 reflects several factors:

- In early hypothyroidism, there may be increased peripheral conversion of T4 to the more metabolically active T3, thereby maintaining circulating concentrations within the reference interval
- T3AAs are more common than T4AAs, with the same potential for interfering with measured concentrations
- In addition, the effect of NTI is a progression from suppression of total T3 concentrations alone, through lowering total T3 and total T4 concentrations and occasionally free T4 concentrations (Mooney et al., 2008). Thus, the

overlap between total T3 values from hypothyroid dogs and those with NTI is more marked than is the case for total T4.

Free T3: Measurement of serum concentrations of free T3 is offered by a small number of commercial endocrine laboratories. The diagnostic utility of this test for the diagnosis of hypothyroidism has not been evaluated. Therefore, measurement is of little value in the investigation of thyroid function.

Dynamic thyroid function tests: A number of dynamic thyroid function tests have been used in the past. However, the development of assays for cTSH, free T4 and TgAA has largely obviated the need for such tests in routine general veterinary practice. They tend to be reserved for specific circumstances in which a diagnosis cannot be confirmed in any other way.

The **TSH response test** was traditionally considered the 'gold standard' for diagnosing canine hypothyroidism. Intravenous administration of a supraphysiological dose of exogenous TSH results in maximal stimulation of the thyroid gland. Measurement of circulating total T4 values before and after administration provides an assessment of the functional reserve capacity of the thyroid, and minimal stimulation is expected in hypothyroidism. This test is considered to be more reliable than any other single individual test for canine hypothyroidism. In early studies, TSH of bovine origin was used but this product is no longer available as a pharmaceutical preparation. Several studies have demonstrated comparable results using human recombinant TSH (Boretti *et al.,* 2006; Daminet *et al.,* 2007). Unlike bovine TSH, adverse reactions have not been reported following the administration of human recombinant TSH to dogs. However, it is very expensive.

The **TRH response test**, whereby total T4 is measured before and after TRH administration, was once recommended as a useful alternative to the TSH response test. Unfortunately the TRH response test is considerably less reliable than the combined use of the currently available baseline tests, and is therefore not recommended. At best, a good response to TRH can confidently exclude hypothyroidism. However, the lack of T4 response to TRH is not confirmatory of hypothyroidism, being a common finding in both a wide variety of NTI and in dogs receiving certain medications (Frank, 1996).

Several investigators have evaluated the **response of TSH to TRH** administration (Diaz-Espineira *et al.,* 2008b; Diaz-Espineira *et al.,* 2009). A number of protocols have been used, but relatively low doses of TRH appear to be capable of causing significant pituitary TSH stimulation whilst minimizing any side effects. Circulating cTSH peaks approximately 20 minutes following administration of intravenous TRH in euthyroid dogs. Humans with primary hypothyroidism exhibit an exaggerated and prolonged TSH response to TRH compared with healthy humans. However, there is limited TSH response to TRH in hypothyroid dogs.

Diagnostic imaging

Thyroid imaging has a well established role in the investigation of thyroid masses in humans, dogs and cats. In recent years there has been growing interest in the use of imaging techniques for the diagnosis of canine hypothyroidism. In general, imaging findings are less affected by NTI and drug administration than are basal hormone concentrations. Although imaging techniques can be of value during the investigation of complex hypothyroidism cases, additional studies are warranted before their use can be recommended in a wider clinical setting.

Radiography

Radiography has no value in the investigation of acquired primary hypothyroidism. However, characteristic changes in the axial and appendicular skeleton are apparent in dogs with congenital hypothyroidism and disproportionate dwarfism. These changes include long bone shortening and valgus deformities, epiphyseal dysgenesis and delayed ossification, shortening and broadening of the skull, and shortened vertebral bodies with scalloped ventral borders (Figure 8.21). Secondary degenerative joint disease can develop over time in affected animals. These changes can be particularly useful to differentiate this disorder from the proportionate dwarfism associated with pituitary dwarfism.

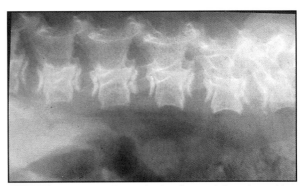

8.21 Lateral lumbar spinal radiograph in a dog with disproportionate dwarfism associated with congenital hypothyroidism. Note the shortened vertebral bodies with scalloped ventral borders.

Thyroid ultrasonography

The ultrasonographic appearance of the thyroid gland has been described in both euthyroid and hypothyroid dogs (Bromel *et al.,* 2005; Taeymans *et al.,* 2007). In euthyroid dogs, individual thyroid lobes are described as fusiform in longitudinal section and triangular in cross-section, with a smooth capsule. Echogenicity is homogeneous, and isoechoic or hyperechoic compared to the adjacent sternothyroid muscle. Thyroid volume can be calculated by applying the ellipsoid formula (vol (ml) = $\pi/6$ x length (cm) x width (cm) x height (cm)) to measured length, width and height. Maximal cross-sectional area can also be calculated. There is no apparent difference in thyroid lobe measurements between healthy dogs and euthyroid dogs with NTI.

By comparison, the thyroid lobes of TgAA-positive and TgAA-negative hypothyroid dogs display significantly decreased echogenicity, and are typically heterogeneous in appearance in thyroglobulin-negative cases but homogeneous in dogs with positive TgAA status (Figure 8.22). Thyroid lobes are often round or oval in shape, and have decreased length, width, height, volume and maximal cross-sectional area when compared to euthyroid dogs. Thyroidal volume has been suggested to be the most useful parameter to differentiate between hypothyroid and euthyroid individuals.

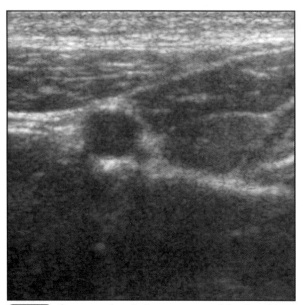

8.22 Cross-sectional ultrasonogram of the thyroid gland from a euthyroid dog (triangular shape, homogeneous and hyperechoic compared to adjacent muscle).

Although ultrasonographic results from hypothyroid dogs are statistically different from those obtained in euthyroid individuals, there is considerable overlap of all parameters between both groups. In addition, euthyroid dogs of different breeds display marked differences in thyroid lobe measurements (Bromel *et al.*, 2006). This has led to the suggestion of normalization of values to body surface area. However, this method has not been probably assessed, and studies of interbreed variability independent of body size have not been performed. Thyroid ultrasonography has high inter-observer variability, even when performed by trained diagnostic imaging specialists; a factor that is likely amplified when performed by less skilled individuals with suboptimal equipment. Therefore, further studies are warranted to evaluate a larger range of NTI and subclinical thyroid disease.

Computed tomography and magnetic resonance imaging

The CT and MRI features of thyroid glands in healthy dogs have been documented (Taeymans *et al.*, 2008a,b). In theory, alterations in size and parenchymal features could allow differentiation between euthyroid and hypothyroid individuals, as has been described in human medicine. Enlargement of the pituitary gland, secondary to thyrotropic hyperplasia

and formation of thyroid deficiency cells, has been detected by CT in dogs with experimental primary hypothyroidism, but this change is not specific for hypothyroidism (Diaz-Espineira *et al.*, 2008b). Given the high relative cost of these procedures and requirement for general anaesthesia, it is unlikely that they will ever play a significant role in the assessment of primary hypothyroidism in dogs. However, they continue to play an important role in the investigation of central hypothyroidism associated with structural pituitary and/or hypothalamic lesions.

Thyroid scintigraphy

The use of nuclear medicine techniques for the assessment of thyroid function has been described for many years, pre-dating the introduction of immunoassays. These procedures involve the administration of either technetium-99m (as pertechnetate ($^{99m}TcO_4^-$) or radioactive iodine (^{123}I or ^{131}I) with subsequent quantification of thyroidal uptake using a scintillation counter or camera. The use of pertechnetate is preferred because of its shorter half-life, lower cost, more rapid uptake and lower radiation dose when compared to radioactive iodine.

Whilst undoubtedly valuable for investigating thyroid masses in dogs, very few studies have assessed the technique for the investigation of canine hypothyroidism. The most common procedure involves the intravenous administration of 140–160 MBq of $^{99m}TcO_4^-$. This is followed by thyroid imaging 40–60 minutes later (Diaz Espineira *et al.*, 2007). Calculation of $^{99m}TcO_4^-$ uptake has been shown to differentiate reliably truly hypothyroid dogs from euthyroid animals with low total T4 concentrations (Figure 8.23). Scintigraphy has also shown promise in confirming euthyroidism in specific breeds where diagnosis of thyroid disease is complicated by the decreased concentrations of multiple thyroid hormones in healthy animals (Pinilla *et al.*, 2009).

In human medicine, however, altered radioisotope uptake has been described in association with several non-thyroidal illnesses and medications, and

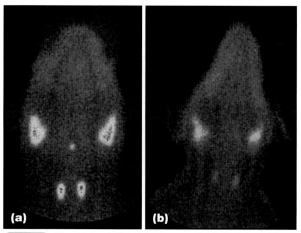

(a) (b)

8.23 Thyroid scintigraphy images in **(a)** euthyroidism and **(b)** hypothyroidism. Thyroidal uptake measurements were 0.5% and 0.05% (reference interval 0.39–1.86%).

the scintigraphic appearance of inflammatory thyroid disease is variable. There is a dearth of information on the effect of a wide range of such factors on thyroid scintigraphy results in dogs. In addition, the procedure requires specialist equipment and radiation isolation facilities. Therefore, although it is certainly a useful technique for the assessment of thyroid function, it is not a first-line test, and results should be interpreted in conjunction with clinical and clinicopathological findings.

Therapeutic trial as a diagnostic test

The use of a T4 therapeutic trial as a diagnostic method has proved popular amongst some clinicians, but should be avoided as much as possible. The principal disadvantages of a therapeutic trial are: the subsequent diagnostic problems that thyroid hormone supplementation cause if the clinical response is suboptimal; coupled with the fact that its pharmacological actions may improve some clinical signs in euthyroid dogs non-specifically. Thyroid hormone supplementation suppresses thyroid function through negative feedback. Consequently, prolonged treatment in a euthyroid dog essentially creates a state of functional hypothyroidism, which can take weeks or months to resolve after withdrawal of treatment. The use of a therapeutic trial is only appropriate when the index of suspicion for hypothyroidism remains high but diagnostic testing has repeatedly proven equivocal. Therapeutic trials should be considered a 'last resort' in these situations.

A true therapeutic trial for diagnostic purposes involves setting an objective, quantifiable target by which success or failure of therapy will be judged, starting treatment and then withdrawing therapy, subject to confirming adequate dosing and satisfying the pre-defined targets. This cessation is performed to ensure that any clinical resolution is genuinely a consequence of the treatment. Cessation of therapy should, of course, coincide with a return of clinical signs, which are then expected to resolve if therapy is reinstituted. A protocol for use of a therapeutic trial as a diagnostic test is shown in Figure 8.24.

Genetic tests for hypothyroidism and lymphocytic thyroiditis

Given the hereditary nature of hypothyroidism in certain breeds, there is substantial interest in tests capable of identifying animals at increased risk for developing the disease. Such tests are highly desirable to dog breeders. Screening for hypothyroidism is insensitive because most animals will not have developed clinical disease by the time of their first breeding. Measurement of TgAA may provide some useful information, as its peak prevalence occurs at an earlier age than hypothyroidism. It is typically recommended for the test to be performed from 12 months of age, and repeated every 1–2 years thereafter. Genetic tests depicting certain DLA haplotypes and alleles known to increase risk of hypothyroidism are also likely to become more widely available in the

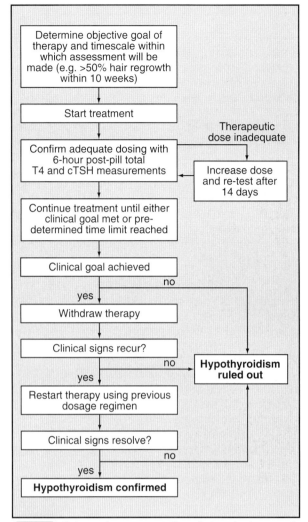

8.24 Schematic representation of steps in the use of a therapeutic trial for diagnosing hypothyroidism.

future. However, overall it is difficult to recommend specific breeding practices based on such results. The development of hypothyroidism is complex and multifactorial. Not all recognized DLA haplotypes and alleles confer significant risk in all breeds and not all TgAA-positive dogs become hypothyroid.

Effect of hypothyroidism on the diagnosis of other endocrine diseases

Hypothyroidism has recently been reported to affect a number of other hormone measurements. In both experimental and naturally occurring hypothyroidism, basal and TRH-stimulated growth hormone concentrations increase (Lee *et al.*, 2001; Diaz-Espineira *et al.*, 2008a,b). This is thought to be related to transdifferentiation of pituitary somatotropic cells to thyrosomatotropic cells. Concomitant elevation in IGF-1 concentration has been noted. Hypothyroidism is also associated with significant increases in circulating leptin and insulin concentrations (neither of which is attributable to obesity alone), confirming the role of hypothyroidism in insulin resistance (Mazaki-Tovi *et al.*, 2010).

Treatment and therapeutic monitoring

Choice of preparation

All hypothyroid dogs require chronic thyroid hormone replacement therapy (THRT) and a variety of preparations are available. Crude thyroid products derived from desiccated porcine, ovine or bovine thyroid glands have been used, but synthetic products are preferable as they are more predictable and have a longer shelf life. The use of generic products is not advised since, licensing issues aside, these products are reported to have a more variable hormone content, and result in peak thyroid hormone concentrations that are lower and more variable than that achieved with proprietary products.

Both T3- and T4-containing products, as well as combination products, are available for the treatment of hypothyroidism. Synthetic sodium levothyroxine therapy is the treatment of choice, as T4 is the principal secretory product of the thyroid gland and is the physiological prohormone for the more potent T3. Re-establishment of normal circulating T4 and T3 concentrations is therefore best achieved by administration of T4.

T3 administration circumvents the normal physiological process of T4 deiodination to T3. Consequently, whilst circulating total and free T3 concentrations may be within the therapeutic range after T3 administration, total and free T4 concentrations remain subnormal. Administration of purely T3-containing products may result in adequate concentrations in organs such as the liver, kidneys and heart which derive their T3 from the circulation. However, the brain and pituitary gland may be deficient in T3 if circulating concentration of free T4 is subnormal. Conversely, it has been suggested that administration of sufficient T3 to provide adequate brain and pituitary concentrations may result in excessive concentrations in other organs.

Combination products, containing both T4 and T3, are available for human use. These are not recommended for dogs, as they do not reflect the thyroid production ratio in this species, providing excess T3.

In Europe there are several authorized products for the treatment of hypothyroidism. They all contain T4 alone, as either tablets or liquid for oral administration (see *BSAVA Small Animal Formulary*) and are the drugs of choice for canine hypothyroidism.

Choice of dosing regime

Numerous therapeutic strategies have been recommended for the treatment of hypothyroid dogs, ranging from doses as low as 10 μg/kg q8–12h to 44 μg/kg q12h. Today there is almost general agreement that a dose of approximately 20–22 μg/kg q24h suffices in most cases, at least initially (Dixon *et al.,* 2002; Le Traon *et al.,* 2009). The clinical response to once-daily therapy is usually excellent, as long as adequate peak circulating hormone concentrations are achieved. This approach significantly improves owner compliance and is less expensive long term. Whilst the use of divided dosing certainly results in less fluctuation of circulating T4 concentrations compared to administration of the same total dose as a single daily bolus, the biological action of thyroid hormones far exceeds that of their plasma half-life. This presumably explains the clinical success of once-daily therapy.

Although the time of treatment is irrelevant, as there is no circadian release of T4 in dogs, morning dosing is recommended. This is to assist with the subsequent collection of monitoring samples, which are required 6 hours after treatment. It is important to bear in mind that administration in food significantly delays and inhibits T4 absorption by approximately 45% (Le Traon *et al.,* 2008). This does not mean that administration in food should be avoided; instead, the temporal relation between feeding and drug administration must be standardized in each individual patient, to avoid marked variations in T4 absorption from day to day.

Clinical monitoring

Adequately treated hypothyroid dogs should be clinically indistinguishable from healthy euthyroid animals. However, the time taken before all signs resolve varies between body system affected and the adequacy of therapy.

Clinical signs

Generally, metabolic signs such as mental dullness and lethargy are among the first to improve, usually appearing dramatically better within days of starting treatment (Figure 8.25). Often, it is only after treatment commences that the extent of the clinical

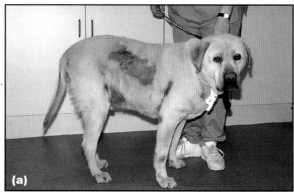
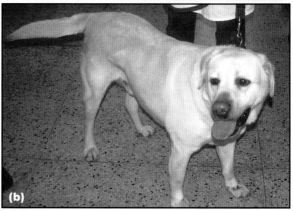

8.25 Appearance of a dog with hypothyroidism before **(a)** and after **(b)** thyroid hormone replacement therapy.

problem is retrospectively noted by owners. Improvements in cardiovascular function and ECG changes should occur during the first 8 weeks of starting treatment, although some cases will take longer. Weight loss is a consistent feature of successful treatment, and a 10% weight reduction can be expected within 3 months of starting therapy. Treated dogs can also be expected to become more active and athletic, presumably as a consequence of the combination of improved mental alertness and weight loss.

Dermatological improvements are expected to occur within a month of starting treatment, though it is common for a period of increased hair loss to precede regrowth. This apparent worsening may concern some owners, but it reflects increased follicular turnover and hair shedding in advance of normal hair replacement and should be considered as a positive sign during the early phase of treatment. Significant hair regrowth should be obvious within 3 months of starting treatment, although complete resolution may take a further 2–3 months.

The response of neurological signs to adequate THRT is more variable, and sometimes poorer, than that of other affected systems. In human hypothyroid patients, some neurological abnormalities take several years to resolve completely, and the same may be true for dogs. However, peripheral neuropathies typically improve within 1–3 months of starting treatment. CNS signs are expected to take longer to resolve, although some, if not complete, improvement can be expected within 6 months. There is limited evidence of improvement in laryngeal paralysis and megaoesophagus in affected dogs, but this probably reflects the dubious causal links between these conditions and hypothyroidism.

Laboratory monitoring

The ultimate goal of therapy is the complete resolution of clinical abnormalities. However, there are now also well defined laboratory goals that can be expected to correspond to good clinical resolution. These are important given the wide inter-individual variation in absorption of T4. Therapeutic monitoring can be performed within 2 weeks of starting therapy or after making subsequent dosage alterations, allowing fairly rapid progress towards identification of a final maintenance dose of THRT (Dixon *et al.,* 2002). Once this is achieved, monitoring every 6 months thereafter is probably adequate. It is estimated that at least one dose adjustment is required in up to 45% of cases. Generally, an increased rather than a decreased dose is required. Only a small number of dogs require two or more dose adjustments. Fewer dose adjustments may be required using the liquid formulation, and this may be related to its greater bioavailability compared with tablet formulations (Le Traon *et al.,* 2008).

Total T4

Laboratory monitoring is aimed primarily at identification of peak circulating total T4 concentration, and confirmation of the expected decrease in cTSH values. Total T4 measurements are currently preferred

over free T4 measurements for monitoring purposes, for the simple reason that clinical resolution has been correlated with specific therapeutic ranges for total T4 but not free T4 values. Whilst it is probable that free T4 fluctuation is less marked following treatment than total hormone concentration, peak circulating total T4 measurement is satisfactory. Total T4 determinations also have the advantage of being less expensive and more widely available.

Hypothyroid dogs receiving once-daily treatment have a marked increase in circulating total T4 values, which peak approximately 6 hours after treatment and then progressively decline until the next dose. In order to identify peak total T4 values, it is therefore essential that samples are collected approximately 6 hours after pill administration. Optimal peak circulating total T4 concentrations should be in the region of 50–60 nmol/l in dogs receiving once-daily therapy (Dixon *et al.,* 2002). Values <35 nmol/l are usually associated with an inadequate clinical response, and an increase in dosage is indicated. Marked increases in peak total T4 to 90–100 nmol/l or higher are unnecessary and, although dogs are usually resistant to severe clinical thyrotoxicosis, such values should probably prompt a decrease in the dose used. The magnitude of dose alterations is usually dictated by the next available tablet size when tablets are used. However, more accurate dose adjustment may be possible using the liquid formulation, and in these cases dose adjustments using 10 µg/kg at any one time are recommended.

The measurement of pre-pill or 'trough' total T4 concentrations remains common practice. The rationale for this is to ensure that T4 values do not fall substantially below the reference interval. However, maintenance of reference interval total T4 concentrations over 24 hours is not essential, due to the prolonged biological half-life of T4 compared with its circulating half-life. In addition, dose adjustments based on trough values may give rise to significant under or over treatment in individual cases. Given the clinical studies which have correlated clinical resolution with peak T4 values alone, there appears to be no real value in continuing to perform trough T4 measurements.

Canine TSH

Measurement of cTSH alongside total T4 inevitably increases the expense of therapeutic monitoring. However, its measurement is usually recommended, as cTSH provides a longer-term assessment of the adequacy of treatment, unlike total T4, which only provides information concerning treatment on that particular day. Measurement of cTSH can therefore assist in identification of poor owner compliance where a particular effort to administer the medication is made on days corresponding to the monitoring visit. Unfortunately in the proportion of hypothyroid dogs that do not have increased pre-treatment cTSH values, measurement during THRT is unlikely to be of any additional value.

Circulating cTSH values usually decrease quickly to the reference interval after the institution of THRT. Circulating cTSH appears to be highly sensitive to the suppressive effects of THRT, such that suppression of cTSH may be achieved without also achieving optional clinical control. Therefore, whilst maintenance of an increased or high-normal cTSH value is strong evidence of suboptimal therapy, suppression of cTSH does not necessarily confirm adequate treatment.

Routine clinicopathology

Improvements in the routine clinicopathological abnormalities associated with hypothyroidism following the instigation of THRT can be expected to occur broadly in parallel with the clinical response. Circulating cholesterol and triglyceride values decrease dramatically, and within just 2 weeks of starting therapy may be within or approaching the reference interval. Whilst RBC values also start to improve quickly, this change is ongoing, and RBC values continue to increase during at least the first 3 months of THRT. Fructosamine concentration decreases significantly following the start of THRT as protein turnover increases (Dixon et al., 2002; Reusch et al., 2002). Mild reductions in ALP activity are also reported. It is presumed that this reflects the progressive normalization of hepatic metabolism including the mobilization of hepatic lipid deposits once THRT starts and weight loss begins.

Therapeutic failure

Failure to achieve therapeutic circulating hormone concentrations, or absence of the expected clinical improvement, should prompt consideration of an underlying cause, and an increase in drug dosage if appropriate, followed by monitoring after 2 weeks. This process should be repeated until hormone concentrations and/or clinical improvements are acceptable. Dogs with underlying gastrointestinal disease may demonstrate an increased THRT dose requirement to achieve adequate circulating hormone concentrations. Similarly, dogs receiving concurrent glucocorticoid therapy may require a slight increase in dosage to achieve optimal control. However, there is normally wide variation in individual dose requirements between individual hypothyroid dogs in any case, and no alternative to appropriate clinical and laboratory monitoring followed by review of the THRT dosage regime.

Potential complications of therapy

It is known that dogs are particularly resistant to the thyrotoxic effects of excessive T4 supplementation, with some studies requiring up to 20 times the standard dose of T4 to induce clinical thyrotoxicosis. When it does occur, the clinical signs include polydipsia, polyuria, polyphagia, panting, weight loss, hyperactivity, tachycardia and pyrexia. Most signs should resolve within a few days of withdrawing therapy.

A gradual introduction of THRT has been recommended in dogs with decreased ability to metabolize T4 and which may be at increased risk of thyrotoxicosis, such as those that are elderly or suffer from hypoadrenocorticism or cardiac disease. However, such guidelines emanate usually when the THRT dose is considerably higher than the standard

applied here. Overall, there is little published evidence of complications associated with THRT in dogs with concurrent illness. Nevertheless, care is advised in patients with hypoadrenocorticism, by first ensuring that glucocorticoid replacement therapy has been established and any life-threatening complications attended to. The treatment of hypothyroid dogs with concurrent insulin dependent diabetes mellitus may result in a reduction in the animal's insulin requirement and alterations in the insulin dose should be anticipated before starting thyroid hormone replacement.

Thyroid hormone supplementation in myxoedema coma

In addition to the necessary symptomatic treatment (intravenous fluids, electrolyte replacement, warming, etc.) in cases of myxoedema coma, thyroid hormone supplementation is also required. Due to the decreased metabolic rate and potential hypovolaemia/dehydration, oral, subcutaneous and intramuscular routes of administration are inadequate, at least initially. Sodium levothyroxine should therefore be administered intravenously, at a dose of 5 µg/kg q12h. Once stabilized, oral administration can be substituted. Resolution of abnormal mentation, ambulation and systolic hypotension should be expected within 30 hours (Pullen and Hess, 2006).

References and further reading

Boretti FS, Sieber-Ruckstuhl NS, Favrot C et al. (2006) Evaluation of recombinant human thyroid-stimulating hormone to test thyroid function in dogs suspected of having hypothyroidism. American Journal of Veterinary Research 67, 2012–2016

Bromel C, Pollard RE, Kass PH et al. (2005) Ultrasonographic evaluation of the thyroid gland in healthy, hypothyroid, and euthyroid Golden Retrievers with nonthyroidal illness. Journal of Veterinary Internal Medicine 19, 499–506

Bromel C, Pollard RE, Kass, PH et al. (2006) Comparison of ultrasonographic characteristics of the thyroid gland in healthy small-, medium-, and large-breed dogs. American Journal of Veterinary Research 67, 70–77

Calvert CA, Jacobs GJ, Medleau L et al. (1998) Thyroid-stimulating hormone stimulation tests in cardiomyopathic Doberman pinschers: a retrospective study. Journal of Veterinary Internal Medicine 12, 343–348

Daminet S, Croubels S, Duchateau L et al. (2003) Influence of acetylsalicylic acid and ketoprofen on canine thyroid function tests. The Veterinary Journal 166, 224-232

Daminet S and Ferguson DC (2003) Influence of drugs on thyroid function in dogs. Journal of Veterinary Internal Medicine 17, 463–472

Daminet S, Fifle L, Paradis M, Duchateau L and Moreau M (2007) Use of recombinant human thyroid-stimulating hormone for thyrotropin stimulation test in healthy, hypothyroid and euthyroid sick dogs. Canadian Veterinary Journal 48, 1273–1279

Diaz-Espineira MM, Galac S, Mol JA, Rijnberk A and Kooistra HS (2008a) Thyrotropin-releasing hormone-induced growth hormone secretion in dogs with primary hypothyroidism. Domestic Animal Endocrinology 34, 176–181

Diaz Espineira MM, Mol JA, Peeters ME et al. (2007) Assessment of thyroid function in dogs with low plasma thyroxine concentration. Journal of Veterinary Internal Medicine 21, 25–32

Diaz-Espineira MM, Mol JA, Rijnberk A and Kooistra HS (2009) Adenohypophyseal function in dogs with primary hypothyroidism and nonthyroidal illness. Journal of Veterinary Internal Medicine 23, 100–107

Diaz-Espineira MM, Mol JA, van den Ingh TS et al. (2008b) Functional and morphological changes in the adenohypophysis of dogs with induced primary hypothyroidism: loss of TSH hypersecretion, hypersomatotropism, hypoprolactinemia, and pituitary enlargement with transdifferentiation. Domestic Animal Endocrinology 35, 98–111

Dixon R (2004) Canine hypothyroidism. In: BSAVA Manual of Canine *and Feline Endocrinology, 3rd edn*, ed. C. Mooney and M. Peterson, pp 76–94. BSAVA Publications, Gloucester.

Dixon RM and Mooney CT (1999) Evaluation of serum free thyroxine and thyrotropin concentrations in the diagnosis of canine hypothyroidism. *Journal of Small Animal Practice* **40**, 72–78

Dixon RM, Reid SW and Mooney CT (1999) Epidemiological, clinical, haematological and biochemical characteristics of canine hypothyroidism. *The Veterinary Record* **145**, 481–487

Dixon RM, Reid SW and Mooney CT (2002) Treatment and therapeutic monitoring of canine hypothyroidism. *Journal of Small Animal Practice* **43**, 334–340

Elliott D, King L and Zerbe C (1995) Thyroid hormone concetrations in critically ill canine intensive care patients. *Journal of Veterinary Emergency and Critical Care* **5**, 17–23

Ferguson DC and Peterson ME (1992) Serum free and total iodothyronine concentrations in dogs with hyperadrenocorticism. *American Journal of Veterinary Research* **53**, 1636–1640

Ferm K, Bjornerfeldt S, Karlsson A *et al.* (2009) Prevalence of diagnostic characteristics indicating canine autoimmune lymphocytic thyroiditis in giant schnauzer and hovawart dogs. *Journal of Small Animal Practice* **50**, 176–179

Frank LA (1996) Comparison of thyrotropin-releasing hormone (TRH) to thyrotropin (TSH) stimulation for evaluating thyroid function in dogs. *Journal of the American Animal Hospital Association* **32**, 481–487

Fyfe JC, Kampschmidt K, Dang V *et al.* (2003) Congenital hypothyroidism with goiter in toy fox terriers. *Journal of Veterinary International Medicine* **17**, 50–57

Graham PA, Refsal KR and Nachreiner RF (2007) Etiopathologic findings of canine hypothyroidism. *Veterinary Clinics of North America: Small Animal Practice* **37**, 617–631

Hall IA, Campbell KL, Chambers MD and Davis CN (1993) Effect of trimethoprim/sulfamethoxazole on thyroid function in dogs with pyoderma. *Journal of the American Veterinary Medical Association* **202**, 1959–1962

Higgins MA, Rossmeisl JH Jr. and Panciera DL (2006) Hypothyroid-associated central vestibular disease in 10 dogs: 1999–2005. *Journal of Veterinary Internal Medicine* **20**, 1363–1369

Jaggy A, Oliver JE, Ferguson DC, Mahaffey EA and Glaus T Jr. (1994) Neurological manifestations of hypothyroidism: a retrospective study of 29 dogs. *Journal of Veterinary Internal Medicine* **8**, 328–336

Johnson CA (1994) Reproductive manifestations of thyroid disease. *Veterinary Clinic of North America: Small Animal Practice* **24**, 509–514

Kantrowitz LB, Peterson ME, Melian C and Nichols R (2001) Serum total thyroxine, total triiodothyronine, free thyroxine, and thyrotropin concentrations in dogs with nonthyroidal disease. *Journal of the American Veterinary Medical Association* **219**, 765–769

Kantrowitz LB, Peterson ME, Trepanier LA, Melian C and Nichols R (1999) Serum total thyroxine, total triiodothyronine, free thyroxine, and thyrotropin concentrations in epileptic dogs treated with anticonvulsants. *Journal of the American Veterinary Medical Association* **214**, 1804–1808

Kenefick SJ and Neiger R (2008) The effect of trilostane treatment on circulating thyroid hormone concentrations in dogs with pituitary-dependent hyperadrenocorticism. *Journal of Small Animal Practice* **49**, 139–143

Kennedy LJ, Huson HJ, Leonard J *et al.* (2006a) Association of hypothyroid disease in Doberman Pinscher dogs with a rare major histocompatibility complex DLA class II haplotype. *Tissue Antigens* **67**, 53–56

Kennedy LJ, Quarmby S, Happ GM *et al.* (2006b) Association of canine hypothyroidism with a common major histocompatibility complex DLA class II allele. *Tissue Antigens* **68**, 82–86

Kooistra HS, Diaz-Espineira M, Mol JA, van den Brom WE and Rijnberk A (2000) Secretion pattern of thyroid-stimulating hormone in dogs during euthyroidism and hypothyroidism. *Domestic Animal Endocrinology* **18**, 19–29

Le Traon G, Brennan SF, Burgaud S *et al.* (2009) Clinical evaluation of a novel liquid formulation of L-thyroxine for once daily treatment of dogs with hypothyroidism. *Journal of Veterinary Internal Medicine* **23**, 43–49

Le Traon G, Burgaud S and Horspool LJ (2008) Pharmacokinetics of total thyroxine in dogs after administration of an oral solution of levothyroxine sodium. *Journal of Veterinary Pharmacology and Therapeutics* **31**, 95–101

Lee WM, Diaz-Espineira M, Mol JA, Rijnberk A and Kooistra HS (2001) Primary hypothyroidism in dogs is associated with elevated GH release. *Journal of Endocrinology* **168**, 59–66

MacGregor JM, Rozanski EA, McCarthy *et al.* (2004) Cholesterol-based pericardial effusion and aortic thromboembolism in a 9-year-old mixed-breed dog with hypothyroidism. *Journal of Veterinary International Medicine* **18**, 354–358

Mansfield CS and Mooney CT (2006) Lymphocytic–plasmacytic thyroiditis and glomerulonephritis in a boxer. *Journal of Small Animal Practice* **47**, 396–399

Mazaki-Tovi M, Feuermann Y, Segev G *et al.* (2010) Increased serum leptin and insulin concentrations in canine hypothyroidism. *The Veterinary Journal* **183**, 109–114

Mooney CT, Shiel RE and Dixon RM (2008) Thyroid hormone abnormalities and outcome in dogs with non-thyroidal illness. *Journal of Small Animal Practice* **49**, 11–16

Nachreiner RF, Refsal KR, Graham PA and Bowman MM (2002) Prevalence of serum thyroid hormone autoantibodies in dogs with clinical signs of hypothyroidism. *Journal of the American Veterinary Medical Association* **220**, 466–471

Panciera DL (1994) Hypothyroidism in dogs: 66 cases (1987–1992). *Journal of the American Veterinary Medical Association* **204**, 761–767

Panciera DL, Purswell BJ and Kolster KA (2007) Effect of short-term hypothyroidism on reproduction in the bitch. *Theriogenology* **68**, 316–321

Panciera DL, Purswell BJ and Kolster KA (2008) Effect of hypothyroidism on reproduction in bitches *(Abstract)*. *Journal of Veterinary Internal Medicine* **22**, 726

Peterson ME, Melian C and Nichols R (1997) Measurement of serum total thyroxine, triiodothyronine, free thyroxine, and thyrotropin concentrations for diagnosis of hypothyroidism in dogs. *Journal of the American Veterinary Medical Association* **211**, 1396–1402

Pettigrew R, Fyfe JC, Gregory BL *et al.* (2007) CNS hypomyelination in Rat Terrier dogs with congenital goiter and a mutation in the thyroid peroxidase gene. *Veterinary Pathology* **44**, 50–56

Pinilla M, Shiel RE, Brennan SF, McAllister H and Mooney CT (2009) Quantitative thyroid scintigraphy in greyhounds suspected of primary hypothyroidism. *Veterinary Radiology and Ultrasound* **50**, 224–229

Pullen WH and Hess RS (2006) Hypothyroid dogs treated with intravenous levothyroxine. *Journal of Veterinary Internal Medicine* **20**, 32–37

Reusch CE, Gerber B and Boretti FS (2002) Serum fructosamine concentrations in dogs with hypothyroidism. *Veterinary Research Communications* **26**, 531–536

Rossmeisl JH, Duncan RB, Inzana KD, Panciera DL and Shelton GD (2009) Longitudinal study of the effects of chronic hypothyroidism on skeletal muscle in dogs. *American Journal of Veterinary Research* **70**, 879–889

Schoeman JP and Herrtage ME (2007) The response of the pituitary-adrenal and pituitary-thyroidal axes to the plasma glucose perturbations in *Babesia canis rossi* babesiosis. *Journal of the South African Veterinary Association* **78**, 215–220

Schoeman JP and Herrtage ME (2008) Serum thyrotropin, thyroxine and free thyroxine concentrations as predictors of mortality in critically ill puppies with parvovirus infection: a model for human paediatric critical illness? *Microbes and Infection* **10**, 203–207

Scott-Moncrieff JC, Nelson RW, Bruner JM and Williams DA (1998) Comparison of serum concentrations of thyroid-stimulating hormone in healthy dogs, hypothyroid dogs, and euthyroid dogs with concurrent disease. *Journal of the American Veterinary Medical Association* **212**, 387–391

Shiel R, Acke E, Puggioni A, Cassidy J and Mooney C (2007a) Tertiary hypothyroidism in a dog. *Irish Veterinary Journal* **60**, 88–93

Shiel RE, Brennan SF, Omodo-Eluk AJ and Mooney CT (2007b) Thyroid hormone concentrations in young, healthy, pretraining greyhounds. *The Veterinary Record* **161**, 616–619

Shiel RE, Sist M, Nachreiner RF, Ehrlich CP and Mooney CT (2010) Assessment of criteria used by veterinary practitioners to diagnose hypothyroidism in sighthounds and investigation of serum thyroid hormone concentrations in healthy Salukis. *Journal of the American Veterinary Medical Association* **236**, 302–308

Taeymans O, Daminet S, Duchateau L and Saunders JH (2007) Pre- and post-treatment ultrasonography in hypothyroid dogs. *Veterinary Radiology and Ultrasound* **48**, 262–269

Taeymans O, Dennis R and Saunders JH (2008a) Magnetic resonance imaging of the normal canine thyroid gland. *Veterinary Radiology and Ultrasound* **49**, 238–242

Taeymans O, Schwarz T, Duchateau L *et al.* (2008b) Computed tomographic features of the normal canine thyroid gland. *Veterinary Radiology and Ultrasound* **49**, 13–19

Vail DM, Panciera DL and Ogilvie GK (1994) Thyroid hormone concentrations in dogs with chronic weight loss, with special reference to cancer cachexia. *Journal of Veterinary Internal Medicine* **8**, 122–127

Wilbe M, Sundberg K, Hansen IR *et al.* (2010) Increased genetic risk or protection for canine autoimmune lymphocytic thyroiditis in Giant Schnauzers depends on DLA class II genotype. *Tissue Antigens* **75**, 712–719

Williams DL, Pierce V, Mellor P and Heath MF (2007) Reduced tear production in three canine endocrinopathies. *Journal of Small Animal Practice* **48**, 252–256

9

Canine hyperthyroidism

Carmel T. Mooney

Introduction

Hyperthyroidism, while relatively common in cats (see Chapter 10) is uncommon in dogs. It is almost always associated with thyroid carcinoma, and only rarely with thyroid adenoma. As a consequence, canine hyperthyroidism cannot be discussed in isolation but is considered in the context of thyroid neoplasia, as it is the existence of the tumour rather than its functional state that dictates the diagnostic work-up, treatment and prognosis.

The development of thyroid dysfunction plays a minor role in the dog compared with the cat, although specific therapy may be required in individual cases. Overall, thyroid tumours in the dog are non-functional, invasive carcinomatous masses, whereas in the cat they are generally functional, non-invasive, relatively small adenomatous masses. In dogs, the prognosis is therefore more guarded, and aggressive therapy warranted.

Tumour types

Thyroid tumours account for 1.2–3.8% of all tumours, and approximately 10–15% of all head and neck neoplasms, in the dog.

Adenomas

In pathological studies, benign adenomas account for approximately 30–50% of all thyroid tumours (Brodey and Kelly, 1968; Leav et al., 1976). However, benign thyroid tumours are usually small focal lesions that are not commonly detected during life. Occasionally these tumours, particularly if cystic, may be obvious by palpation, as mobile ovoid masses within the cervical area. Clinical signs referable to compression of surrounding organs may be apparent on rare occasions. In most cases only one thyroid lobe is affected, although bilateral involvement is possible.

Carcinomas

Carcinomas, while responsible for approximately 50–70% of all thyroid tumours diagnosed postmortem, account for up to 90% of thyroid tumours detected during life, and therefore all thyroid masses are presumed malignant until proven otherwise. Carcinomas are usually larger than adenomas, coarsely multinodular and non-mobile. They occasionally have necrotic or haemorrhagic centres or, even more rarely, focal areas of mineralization. Unilateral involvement is more than twice as common as bilateral involvement, and when the latter occurs the neoplastic process is usually extensive. It is therefore difficult to determine whether the tumour arose in both thyroid lobes or metastases occurred from one lobe to the other. Ectopic thyroid tissue, arising from thyroglossal duct remnants and located anywhere from the base of the tongue to the base of the heart, can occasionally become neoplastic. Thyroid tumours must therefore be included in a range of differential diagnoses for oral, cervical and thoracic masses. Hyperfunctioning thyroid tissue within the right ventricle proximal to the pulmonary valve has also been recently described in a dog, although whether the tissue was neoplastic remains unclear (Olson et al., 2007).

Thyroid carcinomas are poorly encapsulated and commonly extend into or around the trachea, cervical muscles, oesophagus, larynx, nerves and local blood vessels; although invasion into the oesophageal or tracheal lumen is unusual. The major lymphatic drainage of the thyroid gland is in the cranial direction and metastatic spread to the retropharyngeal, cranial cervical and mandibular lymph nodes is common. However, early invasion into the cranial and caudal thyroid veins, with the formation of tumour cell thrombi, leads to multiple pulmonary metastases, often before involvement of regional lymph nodes. Other reported, but rare, sites of metastatic spread include kidney, adrenal gland, liver, spleen, spinal cord, bone and brain, including the pituitary gland.

Histopathologically, thyroid carcinomas are usually well differentiated and classified as follicular, compact (solid), papillary or mixed.

In humans, papillary carcinoma is the most common type of thyroid carcinoma. It has a low grade of malignancy and therefore a more favourable prognosis. This type of tumour is rare in the dog, and the majority are mixed, follicular or, less commonly, compact. The correlation between this histopathological classification and the ultimate prognosis is unclear.

Undifferentiated (anaplastic) thyroid tumours appear to be highly malignant but are uncommon. Medullary (parafollicular, C-cell) carcinoma is also considered rare but may be difficult to distinguish from other thyroid carcinomas by light microscopy alone. When specific immunocytochemical stains are used, the incidence of medullary thyroid carcinoma exceeds one-third of cases (Carver *et al.,* 1995). These tumours may have a more favourable prognosis, as distant metastatic spread is uncommon. They also appear to be well encapsulated and easily resectable at the time of surgical thyroidectomy, but further studies are required in this area.

Despite the lack of clear correlation between prognosis and histopathological classification, the probability of metastases increases in proportion to the size of the tumour. Dogs with small thyroid tumours (<20 cm^3) have a <20% incidence of metastatic disease, whereas nearly all dogs with large tumours (>100 cm^3) have metastases.

Thyroid function

In general, canine thyroid tumours are non-functional, and euthyroidism is maintained throughout the course of the disease. It has been suggested that up to 35% of dogs with detectable thyroid tumours are hypothyroid (Feldman and Nelson, 2004). Hypothyroidism may arise because of destruction of all normal thyroid tissue by aggressive bilateral carcinomas. Alternatively, large tumours could potentially produce excessive inactive thyroid hormones capable of pituitary thyroid-stimulating hormone (TSH; thyrotropin) suppression and eventual atrophy of normal thyroid tissue, although this has never been substantiated. A diagnosis of hypothyroidism must be approached with caution because of the suppressive effect of non-specific illness on circulating thyroid hormone concentrations. In the author's experience, hypothyroidism is uncommon in dogs with thyroid carcinoma. If it does occur it may be coincidental, although in certain breeds there is some evidence of hypothyroidism predisposing to thyroid carcinoma. Hyperthyroidism occurs in approximately 10–20% of thyroid carcinomas. Prognosis is not influenced by thyroid functional status *per se,* except to indicate a possible aggressively destructive carcinoma or the need for additional therapies. However, although not clearly defined because of small numbers of cases, functional tumours tend to be unilateral, of small to medium size and mobile, with less compressive effects on adjacent structures. This may be related to the existence of metabolic signs prompting earlier veterinary intervention.

There are only sporadic isolated reports of hyperthyroidism associated with thyroid adenoma in the dog.

Aetiology

In humans, ionizing radiation (therapeutic irradiation or ingestion of iodine radioisotopes following nuclear fallout), dietary iodine intake (iodine-deficient and high iodine diets), and chronic TSH stimulation have all been implicated in the pathogenesis of thyroid carcinoma. Molecular studies have depicted activation of receptor tyrosine kinases (RET and TRK; papillary carcinoma), activating mutations in *RAS* (follicular carcinomas) and inactivation of *p53* (anaplastic carcinomas). The causes of thyroid neoplasia have not been as extensively studied in dogs, although an increased risk of thyroid neoplasia from ionizing radiation has been reported (Benjamin *et al.,* 1997). The influence of dietary iodine is largely unknown, although it has been implicated in one study of dogs with a high prevalence of thyroid carcinoma in an endemic area of iodine deficiency (Aupperle *et al.,* 2003). Thyroid carcinomas retain the ability to respond to TSH, and a high prevalence of thyroid carcinoma has been reported in a closed breeding colony of untreated hypothyroid Beagles (Benjamin *et al.,* 1996). Somatic mutations in the *p53* gene have been studied in dogs, but appear to be less common than in humans (Devilee *et al.,* 1994).

In humans, thyroid tumours also form part of the multiple endocrine neoplasia (MEN) syndromes, where neoplasia or hyperplasia develops in several different endocrine organs simultaneously. MEN syndromes are classified as type 1 or type 2, with the latter further divided into type 2A and 2B. The MEN syndromes tend to involve one or more specific polypeptide- and biogenic amine-producing cell types, exhibit a histological progression from hyperplasia to adenoma and, in some cases, to carcinoma, and each has an autosomal dominant pattern of inheritance. MEN type 1 syndrome involves parathyroid, pancreatic islet and pituitary hyperplasia or neoplasia. MEN type 2A is associated with the development of bilateral phaeochromocytomas, medullary thyroid carcinomas and, less commonly, parathyroid hyperplasia or adenoma. The association of medullary thyroid carcinoma and phaeochromocytoma with multiple mucosal neuromas is termed MEN type 2B. Patients do exist with unusual manifestations of these syndromes, but these are less well characterized. Although rare, it has been suggested that MEN syndromes exist in dogs (Feldman and Nelson, 2004). However, this premise is based on numerous and often isolated case reports, or anecdotal reference to thyroid tumours occurring in association with adrenocortical carcinoma/adenoma, pituitary adenoma, parathyroid hyperplasia and phaeochromocytoma, where the thyroid tumour is more commonly defined as an adenoma or mixed or follicular carcinoma, rather than the medullary carcinoma reported in humans. A recent study described medullary thyroid carcinoma in four related Alaskan Malamute cross dogs, one of which also developed unilateral adrenal hyperplasia (Lee *et al.,* 2006). However, activating mutations in the *RET* gene, responsible for MEN 2 syndrome in humans, were not detected. Thus, while MEN syndromes may exist in dogs, they manifest differently than in humans and are poorly defined. The existence of neoplastic or hyperplastic changes in multiple endocrine organs may be coincidental in individual dogs.

Clinical features

Signalment

Thyroid tumours occur in middle-aged and older dogs with an average age at onset of approximately 10 years. Almost all dogs are >4 years old at the time of diagnosis. There is no sex predilection, unlike the situation in humans where females are more than twice as likely to develop thyroid cancer as males at most ages. Beagles and Golden Retrievers appear predisposed to the development of thyroid carcinomas, and Boxers to the development of both adenomas and carcinomas.

Clinical signs

Occasionally, thyroid tumours are coincidentally found as freely mobile masses when grooming, petting or during a general health check. They may not be associated with any discomfort.

Most dogs are presented because of a visible mass in the neck and/or its associated consequences (Figures 9.1 and 9.2). The mass is usually felt in the region of the thyroid gland, below the larynx, but occasionally, larger tumours may descend towards the thoracic inlet. As they grow in size they may become more firmly fixed to the surrounding tissues and give rise to clinical signs because of compression, displacement or, less commonly, invasion of the larynx, oesophagus and trachea. The duration of these signs varies from weeks to months. Large invasive tumours have, on rare occasions, been associated with facial oedema (precaval syndrome) and the development of Horner's syndrome (through damage to the cervical trunk). Acute severe haemorrhage arising from arterial invasion has also been described.

Clinical signs referable to regional (enlarged lymph nodes or cording of local lymphatic and blood vessels) or distant (dyspnoea from pulmonary metastases) metastatic spread may be apparent. A few dogs may present with the additional clinical signs of hypothyroidism (Chapter 8) or hyperthyroidism. Dogs with hyperthyroidism exhibit similar clinical signs to those in cats (weight loss, polyphagia, polyuria/polydipsia, restlessness, tachycardia, hypertension, etc.) but tend to be less symptomatic (Chapter 10).

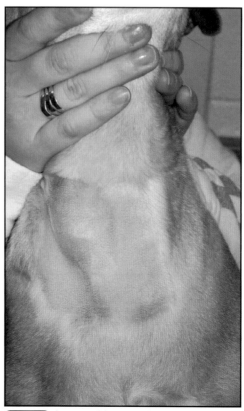

9.2 Large mid-cervical mass in a dog with thyroid carcinoma.

Diagnosis

Differential diagnosis

The differential diagnoses for large cervical swellings include abscess, granuloma, haematoma, lipoma, thyroid tumour, other tumours including carotid body tumours, and salivary mucocele. Given that thyroid tumours may be solid, necrotic, cystic or haemorrhagic, there are no consistent features that reliably differentiate them from the other possibilities.

Cytology

Fine needle (21–23 gauge) aspiration may be helpful in reliably distinguishing many of the differentials. Unfortunately, because of the vascular nature of thyroid tissue, samples are often heavily contaminated with blood, and exfoliation of neoplastic cells can be poor (Thompson *et al.*, 1980). Consequently, cytological examination may not confirm the thyroid origin of the sample. Aspiration methods that avoid haemorrhage caused by undue suction or repositioning, and the careful examination of the feather edge of the prepared sample, may prove useful in identifying thyroid cells. Alternatively, a total thyroxine (T4) estimation of any fluid removed (if adequate) will help confirm the thyroidal origin of the sample. Despite these precautions, a definitive diagnosis of malignancy is not often possible. Wide-bore needle biopsy, while of greater diagnostic yield, significantly increases the risk of haemorrhage and should only be carried out under ultrasound guidance. Even with such

Clinical feature	Common	Less common
Visible/palpable mass in neck	Unilateral	Bilateral
Local effects		Enlarged regional lymph nodes Retching/gagging Dysphonia Dysphagia/regurgitation
Metastatic effects		Coughing Dyspnoea
Other effects		Anorexia Weight loss

9.1 Presenting features associated with thyroid neoplasia in dogs. There may be additional signs related to thyroid hyper- or hypofunction.

samples, there may still be difficulty in distinguishing benign from malignant tumours, and the latter is often only confirmed by demonstration of vascular or capsular invasion in samples taken at the time of surgical thyroidectomy. As a consequence, excisional biopsy specimens should always be sent for histopathological diagnosis, particularly in animals in which metastatic spread has not yet been depicted.

Diagnostic imaging

Radiography
Radiography of the cervical area may help to assess the size of the mass and the extent of local invasion (Figure 9.3), but does not definitively diagnose the lesion as being thyroidal in origin.

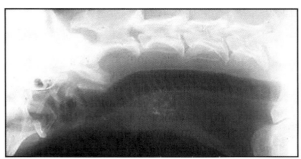

9.3 Cervical radiograph of a dog with a thyroid carcinoma, showing dorsal displacement of the trachea by a large calcified soft tissue swelling.

Ultrasonography
Cervical ultrasonography may prove useful in differentiating the origin of cervical masses. Generally, thyroid lobes can be depicted using a 7.5–10.0 MHz transducer, although those between 11 and 15 MHz will provide greater resolution and finer detail. The cervical area must be clipped for ultrasonography, but the procedure itself is simple and sedation is rarely required. Appropriate care should be given to those dogs with large masses already resulting in upper airway obstruction, as this may be exacerbated by placement in dorsal recumbency and the further compression of the airway through the use of the transducer. Abscesses, haematomas and salivary gland tissue are usually readily differentiated from thyroid tumours. Small nodules may be identified within a thyroid lobe and appear heterogeneous and hypoechoic compared to normal thyroid tissue. However, many neoplastic cervical masses undergoing investigation are large and distort the normal cervical anatomy such that their location to the thyroid is difficult. Finding two normal thyroid lobes does not exclude thyroid neoplasia, as ectopic tissue may be involved. Consequently, cervical ultrasonography cannot replace cytology and histopathology for a definitive diagnosis. It remains helpful, however, in depicting vascularity, local invasion and metastatic spread to regional lymph nodes.

Scintigraphy
As in cats, thyroid scintigraphy using radioactive iodine or technetium may be useful, as most thyroid tumours and their metastases retain the ability to trap iodine. Such scans do not provide any information with regard to thyroid function but are helpful in depicting location of the tumour and regional metastases (Marks *et al.*, 1994). Some thyroid tumours fail to adequately concentrate radioisotopes, and it has been suggested that these are less likely to respond to radioactive iodine administration.

Assessing metastatic spread
Results of post-mortem studies show that up to 80% of dogs have evidence of distant metastatic spread, although this decreases to just over 60% in clinical cases (Miles *et al.*, 1990). Thus, it is imperative that once a mass is identified as thyroid, a systematic search for metastatic spread is instigated. The clinical staging of thyroid tumours is shown in Figure 9.4. Routine haematological and biochemical examinations may be helpful in identifying secondary

Stage	Primary tumour (T)	Regional lymph nodes (N)	Distant metastases (M)
I	T1a,b	N0	M0
II	T0 T1a,b T2a,b	N1 N1 N0 or N1a	M0 M0 M0
III	T3 Any T	Any N N1b or N2b	M0 M0
IV	Any T	Any N	M1

9.4 Clinical staging of canine thyroid tumours. T0–T3 represents tumour size (0, <2cm, 2–5 cm and >5 cm, respectively) with substages a and b representing freely mobile or fixed, respectively. N0–N2 represents regional (mandibular and cervical) lymph node involvement from none to bilateral, with substages a and b representing freely mobile to fixed, respectively. M0 and M1 indicate whether or not distant metastases have been detected.

organ involvement or concurrent problems which may ultimately affect the prognosis. Local lymph nodes should be carefully examined and biopsied as necessary. Three-view thoracic radiography or, if necessary, computed tomography (CT) should always be employed to look for evidence of pulmonary spread, even in the absence of clinical signs. Given that most pulmonary metastases involve the interstitial rather than the alveolar or bronchial portions of the lung, clinical signs are less likely, even with advanced disease. Thoracic scintigraphy is not considered to be as useful as thoracic radiography for the depiction of pulmonary masses. Abdominal radiography and ultrasonography may be useful in cases where hepatic metastasis is suspected.

Assessment of thyroid function
It is necessary to measure serum total T4 concentration in dogs with appropriate clinical signs of thyrotoxicosis. Elevations are generally moderate, compared with the marked elevations that may be seen in hyperthyroid cats. Measurement of circulating endogenous TSH concentration is not particularly

useful in reliably depicting hyperthyroidism, due to the poor sensitivity of the assays currently available, although maintenance of mid to high reference interval values precludes hyperfunction. However, a measurement of total T4, in combination with canine TSH (cTSH) or free T4 measurements, will provide the most useful information to support hypothyroidism if clinical signs are suggestive.

Treatment

There are several possible treatment options currently available for thyroid carcinoma. The selection of any one option is complicated by poorly defined prognostic indicators, inconsistencies in case selection and reporting criteria amongst the different studies, and the variety and number of treatments attempted in individual patients. In spite of this, the prognosis is excellent for small, mobile, non-fixed tumours. Local control may halt metastatic spread and pre-existing metastatic spread may not ultimately affect outcome with certain treatment options. In addition, functional state appears irrelevant and clinical signs of hyperthyroidism can easily be controlled using carbimazole or methimazole at 5 mg orally q8–12h initially, and subsequently adjusted for effect.

Surgical thyroidectomy

Surgical thyroidectomy is approached as for cats (see Chapter 10). However, most tumours in dogs are unilateral, and it is therefore unnecessary to preserve parathyroid glands on the affected side. Surgical thyroidectomy allows gross examination for local invasion and submission of adequate tissue for histopathological examination, which is helpful in differentiating adenoma from carcinoma.

The surgical technique is similar to that described for cats. Adenomas and relatively small, mobile carcinomas are easy to remove (Figure 9.5).

In dogs with operable thyroid tumours and no evidence of metastatic spread, resection alone results in long-term control without subsequent development of metastases and with a median survival time (MST) of >36 months (Klein *et al.,* 1995).

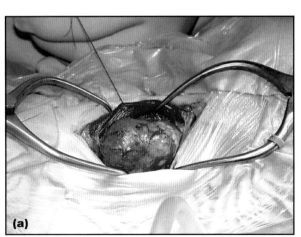

9.5 The appearance of a small, mobile thyroid tumour in a dog: **(a)** at the time of surgical incision. (continues) ▶

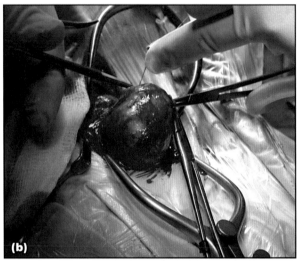

(b)

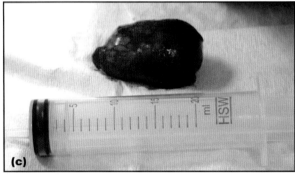

(c)

9.5 (continued) The appearance of a small, mobile thyroid tumour in a dog: **(b)** exposed; and **(c)** after removal.

However, in many cases extensive local tumour invasion precludes complete removal, and aggressive surgical attempts significantly increase the risk of extensive haemorrhage and damage to the recurrent laryngeal nerves and parathyroid glands. In such cases, surgery alone is associated with a survival rate of only 25% at one year (Carver *et al.,* 1995). Surgical debulking, followed by chemotherapy with cisplatin or doxorubicin, has been recommended for such cases (Jeglum and Whereat, 1983; Finemann *et al.,* 1998). Although associated with some improvement in MST, the limited numbers studied preclude definite recommendations.

Radioactive iodine

Administration of radioactive iodine has been suggested to be helpful if iodine uptake is maintained, but generally high and multiple doses must be used, limiting its value clinically. In one study MST was significantly longer in dogs with local or regional tumours (approximately 28 months) compared with those with distant metastases (approximately 12 months) (Turrel et al., 2006). Similarly, MST of 30 and 34 months, respectively, was reported in dogs receiving radioactive iodine alone, or following attempted surgical resection (Worth et al., 2005). However, in both these reports moderate to high radioactive iodine doses were used (with a range of approximately 400 to >7000 MBq, and a median dose varying from 1600 to 3700 MBq), with many dogs requiring more than one treatment. These doses are considerably higher than required for treatment of hyperthyroid cats (usually <200 MBq) and as a consequence there are few facilities worldwide licensed to treat such cases. These doses are also associated with a risk of significant myelosuppression.

Radiotherapy

Recent studies suggest that definitive or palliative external beam radiotherapy (linear accelerator or cobalt 60) may be associated with the best chances of survival (Brearley et al., 1999; Theon et al., 2000; Pack et al., 2001). For palliative therapy, four once-weekly fractions of 9 Gy resulted in an MST of approximately 24 months for fixed invasive tumours. This was coupled with a reduction in primary tumour size or a cessation of growth. Definitive radiation protocols achieving approximately 48 Gy, administered on alternate days over 4 weeks, resulted in an MST of 24 months, with progression-free survival rates of 80% at 1 year and 72% at 3 years. In these studies, prior existence of metastatic spread did not appear to alter survival and there appeared to be a decreased risk of metastatic spread with local control of tumour progression.

Thyroxine supplementation

Standard dose T4 supplementation is necessary following bilateral thyroidectomy. In addition, T4 therapy is usually recommended after unilateral thyroidectomy. Receptor affinity and concentration, and functional response to TSH are similar in healthy and carcinomatous thyroids (Verschueren et al., 1992). Although it is unclear whether TSH has any growth-stimulating properties in thyroid neoplasia in vivo, thyroxine therapy seems a wise precaution.

References and further reading

Aupperle H, Gliesche K and Schoon HA (2003) Tumours of the thyroid gland in dogs – a local characteristic in the area of Leipzig. *Deutsche Tierärztliche Wochenshrift* **110**, 154–157

Benjamin SA, Saunders WJ, Lee AC et al. (1997) Non-neoplastic and neoplastic thyroid disease in beagles irradiated during prenatal and postnatal development. *Radiation Research* **147**, 422–430

Benjamin SA, Stephens LC, Hamilton BF et al. (1996) Associations between lymphocytic thyroiditis, hypothyroidism, and thyroid neoplasia in beagles. *Veterinary Pathology* **33**, 486–494

Brearley MJ, Hayes AM and Murphy S (1999). Hypofractionated radiation therapy for invasive thyroid carcinoma in dogs: a retrospective analysis of survival. *Journal of Small Animal Practice* **40**, 206–210

Brodey RS and Kelly DF (1968) Thyroid neoplasms in the dog. A clinicopathologic study of fifty-seven cases. *Cancer* **22**, 406–416

Carver JR, Kapatkin A and Patnaik AK (1995) A comparison of medullary thyroid carcinoma and thyroid adenocarcinoma in dogs: a retrospective study of 38 cases. *Veterinary Surgery* **24**, 315–319

Devilee P, Van Leeuwen IS, Voesten A et al. (1994) the canine *p53* gene is subject to somatic mutations in thyroid carcinoma. *Anticancer Research* **14**, 2039–2046

Feldman EC and Nelson RW (2004) Canine thyroid tumors and hyperthyroidism. In: *Canine and Feline Endocrinology and Reproduction* 3rd edn, ed. EC Feldman and RW Nelson, pp. 219–249. WB Saunders, Philadelphia

Fineman LS, Hamilton TA, de Gortari A and Bonney P (1998) Cisplatin chemotherapy for treatment of thyroid carcinoma in dogs: 13 cases. *Journal of the American Animal Hospital Association* **34**, 109–112

Jeglum KA and Whereat A (1983) Chemotherapy of canine thyroid carcinoma. *Compendium on Continuing Education for the Practicing Veterinarian* **5**, 96–98

Klein MK, Powers BE, Withrow SJ et al. (1995) Treatment of thyroid carcinoma in dogs by surgical resection alone: 20 cases (1981–1989). *Journal of the American Veterinary Medical Association* **206**, 1007–1009

Leav I, Schiller AL, Rijnberk A, Legg MA and der Kinderen PJ (1976) Adenomas and carcinomas of the canine and feline thyroid. *American Journal of Pathology* **83**, 61–93

Lee J, Larsson C, Lui W, Hoog A and Von Euler H (2006) A dog pedigree with familial medullary thyroid cancer. *International Journal of Oncology* **29**, 1173–1182

Marks SL, Koblik PD, Hornof WJ and Feldman EC (1994) [99mTc]-pertechnetate imaging of thyroid tumors in dogs: 29 cases (1980–1992). *Journal of the American Veterinary Medical Association* **204**, 756–760

Miles KG, Lattimer JC, Jergens AE and Krause GF (1990) A retrospective evaluation of the radiographic evidence of pulmonary metastatic disease on initial presentation in the dog. *Veterinary Radiology* **31**, 79–82

Olson EE, Bulmer BJ and Heaney AM (2007) Hyperthyroidism associated with probable struma cordis in a young dog. *Journal of the American Veterinary Medical Association* **21**, 332–335

Pack L, Roberts RE, Dawson SD and Dookwah HD (2001) Definitive radiation therapy for infiltrative thyroid carcinoma in dogs. *Veterinary Radiology & Ultrasound* **42**, 471–474

Theon AP, Marks SL, Feldman ES and Griffey S (2000) Prognostic factors and patterns of treatment failure in dogs with unresectable differentiated thyroid carcinomas treated with megavoltage irradiation. *Journal of the American Veterinary Medical Association* **216**, 1775–17759

Thompson EJ, Stirtzinger T, Lumsden JH and Little PB (1980) Fine needle aspiration cytology in the diagnosis of canine thyroid carcinoma. *Canadian Veterinary Journal* **21**, 186–188

Turrel JM, McEntee MC, Burke BP and Page RL (2006) Sodium iodide I 131 treatment of dogs with nonresectable thyroid tumours: 39 cases 91990-2003). *Journal of the American Veterinary Medical Association* **229**, 542–548

Verschueren CP, Rutteman GR, Vos JH, Van Dijk JE and de Bruin TWA (1992) Thyrotrophin receptors in normal and neoplastic (primary and metastatic) canine thyroid tissue. *Journal of Endocrinology* **132**, 461–468

Worth AJ, Zuber RM and Hocking M (2005) Radioiodide (^{131}I) therapy for the treatment of canine thyroid carcinoma. *Australian Veterinary Journal* **83**, 208–214

10

Feline hyperthyroidism

Carmel T. Mooney and Mark E. Peterson

Introduction

Hyperthyroidism (thyrotoxicosis) is a disorder resulting from excessive circulating concentrations of the active thyroid hormones triiodothyronine (T3) and/or thyroxine (T4). First described in cats in 1979, hyperthyroidism has become the most common endocrine disorder of this species and a disease frequently diagnosed in small animal practice. It is unclear why such a phenomenon has occurred. Undoubtedly, increased awareness of the condition by veterinary practitioners and their clients, easier availability of diagnostic tests, and a growing pet cat population all may have played a role. However, its increased prevalence is not solely the result of an ageing cat population and it may truly be a new disease.

The prevalence of hyperthyroidism varies geographically and, at least anecdotally, regionally. It is considered reasonably common in the UK, North America, Australia and New Zealand and, more recently, Japan and Germany, but appears to be less common in Spain and Hong Kong. It is difficult to compare incidence rates and prevalence estimates accurately, due to differences in study design and populations tested. However, the overall prevalence in older cats presented to veterinary practices is up to and greater than 10% in areas where it is deemed relatively common, compared to <4% where it is considered uncommon (de Wet *et al.,* 2009).

Aetiology

Benign adenomatous hyperplasia (adenoma) of one (<30% of cases) or, more commonly, both (>70% of cases) thyroid lobes is the most common pathological abnormality associated with hyperthyroidism in cats, occurring in over 98% of cases. Microscopically, the normal thyroid follicular architecture is replaced by one or more readily discernible foci of hyperplastic tissue, forming nodules ranging from <1 mm to >2 cm in diameter. By contrast, thyroid carcinoma is a rare cause of hyperthyroidism in cats, accounting for <2% of cases.

To date, the underlying aetiology remains obscure and, irrespective of the study, it is difficult to dissociate the cause of hyperthyroidism from its effects in diseased cats. Graves' disease is the most common form of hyperthyroidism encountered in human patients. In this disease, autoantibodies are produced which bind to the thyroid-stimulating hormone (TSH; thyrotropin) receptor, mimicking its activity. However, similar stimulating antibodies have not been identified in hyperthyroid cats. Increased titres of immunoglobulins with growth-stimulating properties have been demonstrated in hyperthyroid cats, but their role, if any, in the pathogenesis of the condition remains unclear (Peterson and Ward, 2007).

Histopathologically, the feline disorder most closely resembles toxic nodular goitre, the second most common cause of hyperthyroidism in human patients. Similar to affected human tissue, adenomatous thyroid tissue from hyperthyroid cats retains its histopathological appearance, and continues to grow and function in nude mice and when cultured in TSH-free media. There are a variety of known and suggested causes of toxic nodular goitre in humans. Somatic mutations of the TSH receptor gene are important in the human disease. In early studies, mutations between codons 66 and 530, allowing inclusion of the transmembrane and most of the extracellular part of the TSH receptor and corresponding to the majority of human disease, were not found in cats. However, when hyperplastic feline thyroid tissue has been used, several mutations between codons 386 and 698 have been demonstrated, some of which have also been identified in human hyperthyroidism. The interaction of TSH with its receptor results in activation of G proteins, alterations of which may also play a role in the development of hyperthyroidism. Indeed, altered expression of inhibitory G proteins and mutations in the stimulatory $G_{s\alpha}$ gene have been identified in hyperthyroid cats. Altered expression of the oncogene *c-ras* has also been identified. The role of these findings in the pathogenesis of the disease remains to be established (Peterson and Ward, 2007).

Concurrent with the studies above, several epidemiological studies have attempted to identify potential risk factors for the disease, but a single dominant factor has not yet been detected (Peterson and Ward, 2007; De Wet *et al.,* 2009; Wakeling *et al.,* 2009). Two genetically related breeds (Siamese and Himalayan) and purebred cats have been variably reported to be at decreased risk of developing hyperthyroidism, while male cats are at increased risk.

Although numerous environmental factors have been associated with an increased risk of hyperthyroidism, such as the use of cat litter, regular use of parasiticides, etc., the most commonly identified factor is the consumption of a diet composed entirely, or almost entirely, of canned cat food (Peterson and Ward, 2007). In addition, certain varieties of canned cat food (fish or liver and giblet flavour) and cans with plastic linings and easy-open 'pop-top' lids have been implicated. Because of this dietary association, iodine has been implicated in the pathogenesis of the disease. The iodine content of commercial cat food has been reported as being extremely variable and often in excess of recommended allowances. It has been postulated that wide swings in daily iodine intake may contribute to the development of thyroid disease. However, although circulating free T4 concentrations are acutely affected by varying intake, more prolonged ingestion has no apparent effect. Selenium also plays an important role in the regulation of thyroid function in many species and, although the significance is unclear, circulating values appear to be high in cats, possibly through increased intake. There are many other agents (goitrogens and endocrine disrupters) that cats may be exposed to, either through food, its packaging or in the environment, that may be of greater importance due to differences in metabolism, particularly in the glucuronidation pathway, which is slow in the cat. The potentially goitrogenic soy isoflavones, genistein and daidzein, are common constituents of commercially available cat foods and may be present in concentrations sufficiently high to exert some biological effect (Peterson and Ward, 2007).

Given the variety of abnormalities and associations described, it is likely that hyperthyroidism is a multifactorial disease. Significantly, the same risk factors appear to exist in areas where hyperthyroidism is considered relatively uncommon, emphasizing the complexity of the pathogenesis of hyperthyroidism (De Wet *et al.*, 2009).

Clinical features

Signalment

Hyperthyroidism is a disease of middle-aged and older cats, with an average age at onset of 12–13 years. Virtually all affected cats are >4 years of age, but only 5% are <10 years old at the time of diagnosis. There has been one report of hyperthyroidism in a kitten but, given that the histopathological appearance was different, it likely represents a distinct disease entity (Gordon *et al.*, 2003). Despite the previous epidemiological studies discussed above, breed or sex predispositions have not been recognized in large clinical studies.

Clinical signs

Thyroid hormones are responsible for a variety of actions, including the regulation of heat production and the metabolism of carbohydrates, proteins and lipids. They also appear to interact with the CNS by increasing overall sympathetic drive. Consequently, when thyroid hormones are in excess, virtually every organ system is affected. Most cats present with a variety of clinical signs reflecting multiple organ dysfunction, although in some cats one clinical sign may predominate. The signs vary from mild to severe, depending on the duration of the condition, the ability of the cat to cope with thyroid hormone excess, and the presence or absence of concomitant abnormalities in other organ systems. The disease is insidiously progressive and the signs, when mild, may be considered by owners as part of the generalized ageing process. For this reason, several months may elapse before veterinary attention is sought.

Increased awareness of the condition and earlier diagnosis have meant that, although presenting with similar clinical signs, affected cats are less highly symptomatic now than previously (Peterson *et al.*, 1981; Thoday and Mooney, 1992; Broussard and Peterson, 1995). Occasionally, a diagnosis is made before owners fully realize that their pet is ill. The history and clinical features are outlined in Figure 10.1.

Common features
• Weight loss • Polyphagia • Tachycardia • Systolic murmurs • Polyuria/polydipsia • Hyperactivity/irritability • Intermittent gastrointestinal signs (vomiting or diarrhoea) • Palpable goitre
Other features
• Respiratory abnormalities (tachypnoea, panting) • Other cardiac abnormalities (gallop rhythm, arrhythmias) • Skin lesions (patchy or regional alopecia, unkempt coat) • Moderate temperature elevation
Uncommon features
• Decreased activity • Decreased appetite • Congestive cardiac failure • Hypertension • Neck ventroflexion

10.1 History and clinical features of hyperthyroid cats.

Overall, there are a number of clinical signs that are highly suggestive of hyperthyroidism, including: weight loss despite a normal or increased appetite; hyperactivity; intermittent gastrointestinal disorders; tachycardia; cardiac murmur; and palpable goitre. However, the presence or absence of any one particular sign cannot confirm or exclude the disorder. In addition, because of the variety of other different signs that are potentially caused by hyperthyroidism, it is an important differential for many presenting complaints in older cats.

General features

Almost all affected cats exhibit signs of mild to severe weight loss (Figure 10.2a), despite a normal or increased appetite, reflecting an overall increase in the metabolic rate. This increase in metabolic rate may be accompanied by a mild elevation in body temperature or heat intolerance. If allowed to progress untreated, muscle weakness/wasting, fatigability, emaciation and cachexia will ultimately result, although this can take months to years. Severe muscle weakness, as demonstrated by ventroflexion of the neck, has been described, albeit rarely, and presumably relates to hyperthyroidism-induced hypokalaemia (see below). A few affected cats exhibit intermittent periods of anorexia alternating with periods of normal or increased appetite, but this is often associated with concurrent non-thyroidal illness rather than hyperthyroidism *per se*. In the absence of concurrent illness, the mechanism is unclear.

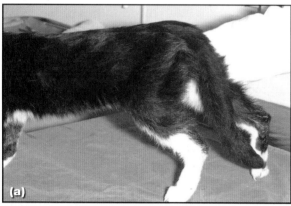

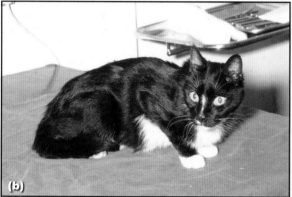

10.2 Hyperthyroid 11-year-old Domestic Shorthair cat, showing evidence of weight loss **(a)** and an anxious facial expression **(b)**. (Reproduced with permission from Thoday and Mooney, 1992)

Hyperactivity, exhibited particularly as nervousness, restlessness and aggressive behaviour, may be apparent. These signs may be more obvious when attempts are made to restrain the animal and are therefore often more noticeable to veterinary surgeons than to owners themselves.

In extreme cases tremor may be apparent and affected cats are often described as having an anxious or frantic facial expression (Figure 10.2b). There is impaired tolerance to stress, and even moderately stressful events (such as physical examination) can result in overt respiratory distress, cardiac arrhythmias, dyspnoea and eventually extreme weakness. Hyperthyroid cats should therefore be handled appropriately in the practice environment. Aimless pacing and easily interrupted

sleep patterns have been described, and this presumably reflects a state of confusion, anxiety and nervousness. Focal or generalized seizures characteristic of epilepsy have been described, albeit rarely. In such cases, there is a reduction in the severity of the seizures, or complete resolution, after treatment of the hyperthyroidism (Joseph and Peterson, 1992).

Polyuria and polydipsia

Polyuria and polydipsia occur in <50% of affected cases and can be marked in individual cats. Various mechanisms may be responsible, including concurrent primary renal dysfunction, not unexpected in a group of aged cats, decreased renal medullary solute concentration because of increased renal blood flow, electrolyte abnormalities (e.g. hypokalaemia), and primary polydipsia because of a hypothalamic disturbance associated with thyroid hormone excess.

Skin changes

In older case series, skin changes were common but were usually less of an owner concern than the metabolic changes described. Some cats presented with unkempt matted hair (Figure 10.3a), presumably because of a failure to groom. Longhaired cats particularly presented with alopecia (Figure 10.3b) (either bilaterally symmetrical or patchy), presumably resulting from excessive grooming. The latter has been suggested to reflect heat intolerance. Excessive nail growth with increased fragility has been described but is seen less frequently today.

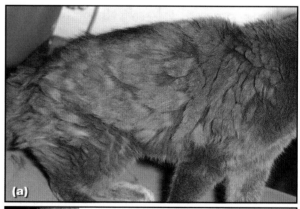

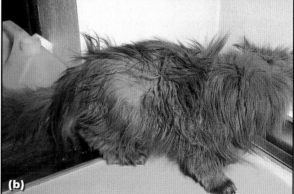

10.3 Coat changes in hyperthyroid cats. **(a)** A 13-year-old Russian Blue with extensive matting. **(b)** A 14-year-old pedigree Domestic Longhair with evidence of alopecia.

Gastrointestinal features

Gastrointestinal signs are not uncommon and usually include intermittent vomiting and, less commonly, diarrhoea. Vomiting may result from a direct action of thyroid hormones on the chemoreceptor trigger zone or from gastric stasis. It appears to be more common in cats from multi-cat households and usually occurs shortly after feeding, indicating that it may simply be related to rapid overeating. In humans, rapid gastrointestinal transit contributes to the increased frequency of defecation and diarrhoea. In addition, malabsorption and steatorrhoea may result from excess fat intake associated with polyphagia, rapid gastric emptying and intestinal transit and/or a reversible reduction in pancreatic trypsin secretion. In cats, many of these mechanisms have not been fully investigated. However, orocaecal transit time, as assessed by breath hydrogen measurements, appears to be accelerated in hyperthyroid compared to both healthy cats and those successfully treated for hyperthyroidism (Papasouliotis *et al.,* 1993; Schlesinger *et al.,* 1993).

Cardiorespiratory features

Cardiovascular signs are common and are frequently the most significant findings on initial physical examination. Tachycardia (heart rate >240 beats per minute) is frequently documented in up to 50% of cases. A powerful apex beat and systolic murmurs are also commonly encountered. Such murmurs are generally grade I to III (of VI) and vary in intensity with the heart rate. They are frequently associated with dynamic right and left ventricular outflow obstruction, rather than primary mitral or tricuspid regurgitation as previously thought. Hyperthyroidism is probably the single most important factor for the development of murmurs in older cats. Gallop rhythms attributed to rapid ventricular filling can also occur. Occasionally arrhythmias, particularly ectopic atrial and ventricular arrhythmias, have been noted.

These cardiac abnormalities are related to direct effects of thyroid hormone on cardiac muscle, indirect effects mediated through the interaction of thyroid hormone with the adrenergic nervous system, and cardiac changes that attempt to compensate for altered peripheral tissue perfusion. These effects result in a high cardiac output state and consequently cardiac hypertrophy and chamber dilation. Congestive cardiac failure associated with pleural effusion and/or pulmonary oedema (coughing, dyspnoea, muffled heart sounds, ascites) can develop, although this is uncommon. The cardiomyopathy of hyperthyroidism is usually reversible. Almost 50% of hyperthyroid cats have detectable circulating troponin I concentrations, with reduction after therapy, consistent with hyperthyroid-induced but reversible myocyte damage (Connolly *et al.,* 2005). However, in some cats cardiomyopathy persists or worsens after treatment, suggesting a pre-existing cardiac defect or thyroid hormone-related irreversible structural damage. Certainly in cats that develop congestive cardiac failure, maintenance of treatment for their cardiac disease is required even with successful resolution of the hyperthyroidism.

Mild to moderate hypertension, reversible upon induction of euthyroidism, was originally considered important in hyperthyroid cats. However, it is now clear that hyperthyroid cats are typically only mildly hypertensive, if at all, and when they are it may simply reflect the reduced tolerance of hyperthyroid cats to stressful situations such as veterinary examination ('white-coat' phenomenon). In accord with this, hypertension-associated blindness and obvious ocular abnormalities are uncommon in hyperthyroid cats, even in the presence of documented hypertension. Although hyperthyroidism is associated with increased cardiac output, there is a decrease in systemic vascular resistance mitigating against the development of significant hypertension. If moderate to severe hypertension and its effects are demonstrated in a hyperthyroid cat, other potential causes such as renal failure should be considered. Interestingly, some cats appear to develop hypertension after successful treatment of hyperthyroidism and this may result, at least in part, from the increase in systemic vascular resistance as thyroid hormone concentrations decrease, or from the associated decline in renal function (see below).

Respiratory abnormalities, chiefly tachypnoea, panting and dyspnoea at rest, are also common but tend to occur most frequently during periods of stress. In the absence of cardiac failure, respiratory muscle weakness due to chronic thyrotoxic myopathy and decreased compliance of the lungs are the most likely explanations.

Apathetic hyperthyroidism

Cats may present with apathy or depression and anorexia rather than hyperactivity and polyphagia. Similarly affected human patients usually have severe cardiac complications induced by thyroid hormone excess. In cats, apathetic hyperthyroidism has also been associated with congestive cardiac failure. However, concurrent severe non-thyroidal illness such as renal failure or neoplasia may also be complicating factors. It is important in cats presenting as apathetic cases that other illnesses are investigated as they may alter the therapeutic choice or eventual prognosis. While apathetic hyperthyroidism was previously recorded in approximately 10% of cases, this is less commonly seen today.

Palpable goitre

In healthy cats, the thyroid gland is divided into two distinct lobes positioned on either side just below the cricoid cartilage and extending ventrally for the first five or six tracheal rings. Thyroid lobes are not normally palpable. In hyperthyroid cats, either unilateral or bilateral thyroid enlargement (goitre) is invariably present. Thyroid lobes are loosely attached to the surrounding tissues and tend to migrate ventrally as they enlarge, occasionally moving through the thoracic inlet into the anterior mediastinum. Ectopic thyroid tissue located anywhere from the base of the tongue to the base of the heart is occasionally involved in the pathogenesis of the condition.

Sometimes goitre is visible, but more commonly palpation is required.

- Traditionally, to palpate for goitre the cat is restrained by holding its front legs while it is in a sitting position.
- With the neck gently extended, the thumb and forefinger are placed on either side of the trachea and swept carefully downwards from the larynx to the manubrium.
- It is important to avoid hyperextension of the neck as the thyroid lobes may become embedded in muscle or deviated retrotracheally, and therefore become more difficult to palpate.
- Goitre is usually felt as a mobile subcutaneous nodule or 'blip' that slides or slips under the fingertips.
- When there are difficulties in palpation, visualization of small nodules may be aided by clipping the ventrocervical area and moistening the skin with alcohol.

A semi-quantitative thyroid palpation technique has also been described:

- The clinician is positioned behind the standing cat and the cat's head raised and turned (45 degrees from the horizontal and vertical) alternatively to the right or left, depending on which side is being assessed.
- The tip of the clinician's index finger is placed in the groove formed by the trachea and the sternothyroideus muscle just below the larynx, and then moved ventrally down to the thoracic inlet, evaluating each side in turn (Norsworthy *et al.*, 2002).
- The degree of enlargement is assigned a score between 1 and 6, with increasing size, and is linked to the severity of hyperthyroidism.
- Although considered sensitive, such a technique is highly subjective.

In a study comparing the two different palpation techniques, the traditional technique was preferred because of greater within- and between-examiner agreement (Paepe *et al.*, 2008). However, the semi-quantitative technique was more helpful in demonstrating the side of involvement, especially in cats with large goitres crossing the midline. Whichever technique is chosen, experience is probably the most critical factor for success.

Although the likelihood of hyperthyroidism increases as goitre develops, thyroid hyperfunction is not synonymous with its presence (Boretti *et al.*, 2009). A palpable mass in this area could potentially represent lymph node enlargement or parathyroid neoplasia/hyperplasia. In addition, goitre may also be palpable in an apparently euthyroid individual, with eventual development of hyperthyroidism possible as the thyroid nodule continues to grow and secrete excessive thyroid hormone. These cats require regular re-examinations to assess thyroid function, at 6-monthly intervals, or sooner if clinical signs dictate.

Diagnosis

A variety of procedures have been recommended for investigation of hyperthyroidism. Often these simply lend support to the diagnosis but they may be particularly useful if concurrent disorders are suspected and an accurate prognosis is required. Detailed diagnostic imaging techniques are usually only required in cats in which compromised cardiac function is suspected. Specific thyroid function tests are necessary to confirm a diagnosis.

Routine clinicopathological features

Haematology

Haematological changes are of limited diagnostic value, although mild to moderate erythrocytosis (increased PCV, RBC count and haemoglobin concentration) and macrocytosis have been described (Peterson *et al.*, 1981) (see Figure 10.4). These changes presumably reflect thyroid hormone-mediated β-adrenergic stimulation of erythroid marrow, as well as the increased production of erythropoietin resulting from increased oxygen consumption. These findings have not been confirmed in all studies (Thoday and Mooney, 1992). Importantly, when they occur they are not clinically significant. Anaemia is a rare complication of hyperthyroidism which, in humans, is related to either bone marrow exhaustion or deficiencies in iron or other micronutrients. Although overt anaemia is rarely encountered, increased Heinz body formation does occur in hyperthyroid cats, and platelet size may be increased. Clinically, these abnormalities appear to have minimal effect.

Not surprisingly, a stress leucogram, as evidenced by mature neutrophilia usually accompanied by lymphopenia and eosinopenia, is common. Occasionally, there is a lymphocytosis and eosinophilia, which is thought to relate to a relative lack of cortisol induced by thyroid hormone excess.

Biochemistry

Liver enzymes: Mild to marked increases in the serum activities of alanine aminotransferase (ALT), aspartate aminotransferase (AST), alkaline phosphatase (ALP) and lactate dehydrogenase (LDH) are the most common and striking biochemical abnormalities of feline hyperthyroidism (Figure 10.4). It has been suggested that the abnormalities are caused by malnutrition, congestive cardiac failure, hepatic hypoxia, infections, and direct toxic effects of thyroid hormones on the liver. However, histopathological examination of the liver usually reveals only modest and non-specific changes (Peterson *et al.*, 1981). In addition, there are no significant abnormalities found on hepatic ultrasonography, and tests of liver function (bile acid stimulation) remain within reference interval (Berent *et al.*, 2007). Both liver and bone contribute to the increase in serum ALP activity. The bone isoenzyme usually contributes 20–30% towards total ALP activity, but its contribution can be as high as 80% (Archer and Taylor, 1996).

Haematology
• Erythrocytosis
• Macrocytosis
• Leucocytosis
• Neutrophilia
• Eosinopenia

Serum biochemistry
• Elevated ALT
• Elevated ALP
• Elevated AST
• Elevated LDH
• Azotaemia
• Hyperphosphataemia
• Mild hyperglycaemia

10.4 Common haematological and biochemical abnormalities associated with hyperthyroidism. ALP = alkaline phosphatase; ALT = alanine aminotransferase; AST = aspartate aminotransferase; LDH = lactate dehydrogenase.

Approximately 90% of affected cats have an elevation in at least one of the above enzymes. The degree of elevation is correlated with serum thyroid hormone concentrations and can be dramatic in severely thyrotoxic cats. However, the degree of elevation tends to be subtle, if present at all, in early or mild cases of hyperthyroidism. Concurrent and distinct hepatic disease should be suspected if there are marked elevations in any of ALT, ALP, AST or LDH, but only mildly elevated serum thyroid hormone concentrations.

Urea and creatinine: Undoubtedly, the effect of hyperthyroidism and its treatment on renal function in cats is of particular clinical concern, as treatment of hyperthyroidism is associated with a decline in renal function. Before treatment, mild to moderate increases in serum concentrations of urea and creatinine may be found in just over 20% of hyperthyroid cats. Such a prevalence of renal dysfunction is not unexpected in a group of aged cats. However, the abnormalities, at least in urea concentration, could be exacerbated by the increased protein intake and protein catabolism of hyperthyroidism. On the other hand, in hyperthyroid cats without azotaemia, circulating creatinine concentration is significantly lower than age-matched controls (Syme, 2007). This may be related in part to a loss of muscle mass. These effects have implications in assessing the existence of primary renal dysfunction in hyperthyroid cats (see below).

Phosphate and calcium: Increased phosphate concentration without evidence of azotaemia occurs in approximately 35–45% of cats (Archer and Taylor, 1996; Barber and Elliott, 1996). In thyrotoxic humans there is increased bone metabolism attributed to the direct effects of thyroid hormones on bone, which can lead to osteopenia and patho-logical fractures. This is associated with increased serum activity of the bone isoenzyme of ALP, increased concentrations of osteocalcin and

phosphate, and a tendency towards increased serum calcium and decreased parathyroid hormone (PTH; parathormone) and active vitamin D (1,25-dihydroxycholecalciferol; $1,25(OH)_2$-vitamin D) concentrations.

In hyperthyroid cats, serum total calcium concentration is largely unaffected, but ionized calcium is decreased and circulating PTH concentration increased. In addition, elevated osteocalcin and non-suppressed $1,25(OH)_2$-vitamin D concentrations have been found in a small number of thyrotoxic cats (Archer and Taylor, 1996; Barber and Elliott, 1996). The reasons for the differences between humans and cats, and the exact aetiology of the changes are unclear. In addition, the clinical consequences of hyperphosphataemia, ionized hypocalcaemia and hyperparathyroidism are unknown. There may be implications for skeletal integrity and renal function. The increased secretion of PTH necessary to maintain ionized calcium at the low end of or below the reference interval might contribute to or exacerbate the hypocalcaemia often encountered after surgical thyroidectomy (see below).

Other biochemical changes: A number of other clinicopathological changes have been described in hyperthyroid cats but are either clinically insignificant or rarely encountered. Blood glucose concentrations may be mildly increased, presumably reflecting a stress response. In cases with pre-existing diabetes mellitus, accelerated insulin catabolism increases requirements for exogenous insulin (Feldman and Nelson, 2004). In addition, circulating fructosamine concentration is significantly lower in hyperthyroid compared with healthy cats, probably as a result of increased protein turnover (Graham et al., 1999; Reusch and Tomsa, 1999). Caution is advised when using fructosamine as a means of monitoring diabetic cats with concurrent hyperthyroidism. Hypokalaemia has occasionally been associated with hyperthyroidism and should be suspected in any cat with evidence of severe muscle weakness (Nemzek et al., 1994). Other biochemical parameters such as cholesterol, sodium, chloride, bilirubin, ionized and total magnesium, albumin and globulin tend to remain within their respective reference intervals in hyperthyroid cats.

Urinalysis
Urinalysis is generally unremarkable but is useful in differentiating other diseases with similar clinical signs, such as diabetes mellitus. Urine specific gravity is variable. Mild proteinuria is commonly observed and may reflect glomerular hypertension and hyperfiltration or differences in tubular handling of protein (Syme, 2007). Traces of ketones in the absence of glucosuria may be found (Berent et al., 2007). Urinary tract infections occur in approximately 12% of non-azotaemic hyperthyroid cats, with no recognizable risk factors and often without classic signs of lower urinary tract disease or urinalysis changes indicating infection (Mayer-Roenne et al., 2007). As a consequence, urine culture is indicated in hyperthyroid cats.

Diagnostic imaging

Hyperthyroidism is associated with a largely reversible hypertrophic cardiomyopathy. In approximately 50% of cats, there is evidence of mild to severe cardiac enlargement on thoracic radiography. This is accompanied by evidence of pleural effusion and pulmonary oedema in cases with congestive cardiac failure. The most common echocardiographic abnormalities described have included left ventricular hypertrophy, left atrial and ventricular dilation and interventricular septum hypertrophy. However, currently, most of these changes are subtle if present at all in hyperthyroid cats, and are of questionable clinical relevance (Connolly et al., 2005; Weichselbaum et al., 2005). Increased fractional shortening remains common and invariably decreases upon successful treatment of the hyperthyroidism (Bond et al., 1988; Connolly et al., 2005).

Rarely, hyperthyroidism is associated with a dilated form of cardiomyopathy with echocardiographic evidence of reduced myocardial contractility and marked ventricular dilatation. This is usually accompanied by evidence of severe congestive cardiac failure (Jacobs et al., 1986).

Electrocardiography

Sinus tachycardia (approximately 60% of cases) and increased R-wave amplitude in lead II (approximately 30–50% of cases) were originally the most frequent electrocardiographic abnormalities recorded in hyperthyroid cats (Peterson et al., 1982). Less common abnormalities included prolonged QRS duration, shortened Q–T interval, intraventricular conduction disturbances and a variety of atrial and ventricular arrhythmias. More recent studies have reported a reduced prevalence of these disorders but an increased prevalence of right bundle branch block of unknown significance (Broussard and Peterson, 1995; Fox et al., 1999).

Thyroid function tests

The diagnosis of hyperthyroidism is confirmed by demonstrating increased thyroidal radioisotope uptake or increased production of the thyroid hormones.

In cats, T4 is the main secretory product of the thyroid gland. T3 is three to five times more potent than T4, but approximately 60% of circulating T3 is produced by extrathyroidal 5'-deiodination of T4. T4 is therefore often considered to be a pro-hormone, and activation to T3 a step autoregulated by peripheral tissues. Over 99% of circulating T4 is protein-bound, while approximately 0.1% is free and metabolically active. Overall, control of thyroid hormone production is provided by a negative feedback mechanism of circulating T4 and T3 upon thyrotropin-releasing hormone (TRH) from the hypothalamus and TSH from the anterior pituitary. In hyperthyroid cats, there is autonomous and excessive secretion of thyroid hormones from the abnormally functioning thyroid gland.

Thyroidal radioisotope uptake

Hyperthyroid cats usually exhibit increased thyroidal uptake of both radioactive iodine (^{123}I or ^{131}I) and technetium-99m as pertechnetate (^{99m}TcO$_4^-$) (Shiel and Mooney, 2007). Percentage uptake or increase in thyroid-to-salivary ratio may be calculated; both are strongly correlated with circulating thyroid hormone concentration and provide a sensitive means of diagnosing hyperthyroidism. However, apart from expense and the difficulties in dealing with radioisotopes, few have access to such equipment. In addition, caution is advised in interpreting results from cats previously treated with antithyroid drugs, as radioisotope uptake can be enhanced for several weeks after drug withdrawal (Nieckarz and Daniel, 2001). Qualitative thyroid imaging may be useful in assessment of thyroid involvement prior to surgical thyroidectomy (see below).

Thyroid hormone concentrations

Elevated circulating concentrations of total T4 and T3 are the biochemical hallmarks of hyperthyroidism and are extremely specific for its diagnosis, with no false positive results reported. Methods for their measurement are readily accessible, relatively cheap and do not involve specific sampling requirements. Radioimmunoassay (RIA) is the preferred method, but non-isotopic in-house and automated techniques are becoming increasingly popular. Generally these methods correlate reasonably well with results of RIA analysis but technique and laboratory specific reference intervals should always be used. Assays intended for human serum are acceptable, but must be fully validated for use with cat serum and, as in the dog, modified to allow for measurement of the lower circulating concentrations of hormone in this species.

Total T3 concentration: Circulating total T4 and T3 concentrations are highly correlated in hyperthyroid cats. Over 30% of hyperthyroid cats have circulating total T3 concentration within the reference interval (Peterson et al., 2001). Severe concurrent non-thyroidal illnesses (NTIs) could conceivably play a role in suppressing total T3 as it does in humans. However, the majority of hyperthyroid cats with reference interval total T3 concentrations are classified as early or mildly affected, and corresponding serum total T4 concentration is usually within or only just above its respective reference interval (usually <100 nmol/l). It is likely that T3 would increase into the thyrotoxic range in these cats if the disorder was allowed to progress untreated. A possible explanation is that as T4 production begins to increase in hyperthyroid cats, there is a compensatory decrease in peripheral conversion of T4 to the more active T3. As a consequence, measurement of total T3 is not recommended for investigation of hyperthyroidism in cats.

Total T4 concentration: Most hyperthyroid cats exhibit an elevated circulating total T4 concentration, with values up to approximately 20 times the upper limit of the reference interval reported. However, a significant proportion of hyperthyroid cats (approximately 10% of all cases and 40% of cases classified with mild hyperthyroidism) have serum total T4 concentration within the reference interval (Peterson *et al.*, 2001). Such values are usually within the mid to high end of the range. Thus while an increased total T4 value is indicative of hyperthyroidism, finding a single reference interval value does not preclude such a diagnosis.

In early or mildly affected cases, serum total T4 concentrations can randomly fluctuate from above to within the reference interval (Peterson *et al.*, 1987). Non-specific fluctuation of thyroid hormones occurs in all hyperthyroid cats, but the degree of fluctuation is of little diagnostic significance in cats with pre-existing markedly elevated hormone concentrations.

Severe NTI is also capable of significantly suppressing serum total T4 concentrations to the low end or below the reference interval in euthyroid cats and can be used as a prognostic indicator (Mooney *et al.*, 1996, Peterson *et al.*, 2001). Similarly, marginally elevated serum total T4 concentrations may be suppressed to within the mid to high end of the reference interval in cats with concurrent mild hyperthyroidism and moderate to severe NTI (Peterson *et al.*, 2001). Occasionally, serum total T4 concentrations are suppressed to the low end of the reference interval in hyperthyroid cats that are extremely ill. In such cases, the concurrent illness dictates the prognosis, and the existence of hyperthyroidism is of lesser clinical significance. Approximately 20% of hyperthyroid cats with reference interval circulating total T4 concentrations have an identifiable concurrent NTI; the remaining majority are usually classified as mild or early cases.

In early or mildly hyperthyroid cats, serum total T4 concentrations will eventually increase into the diagnostic thyrotoxic range upon retesting 3–6 weeks later. However, in some cats a longer time is required and it may be justifiable to wait until more overt clinical signs develop. Concurrent hyperthyroidism should always be suspected in severely ill cats with mid to high reference interval serum total T4 concentrations. Alternatively, other diagnostic tests may provide a means of diagnosing hyperthyroidism in these cats.

Recently, many commercial laboratories have decreased the upper limit of the total T4 reference interval, often to values as low as 30 or 40 nmol/l. Whilst this increases the sensitivity of a total T4 measurement for diagnosing hyperthyroidism, it adversely affects specificity and potentially increases the number of false positive diagnoses. Given that treatment is not without side effects and significant cost, this may be detrimental.

Free T4 concentration: Serum free and total T4 concentrations are highly correlated in hyperthyroidism. However, circulating free T4 concentrations, as measured by equilibrium dialysis, are more consistently (>98% of cases) elevated in hyperthyroid cats (Peterson *et al.*, 2001). More significantly, serum free T4 concentrations are elevated in 95% of hyperthyroid cats with reference interval total T4 values that result from mild disease and hormone fluctuation or the suppressive effect of concurrent NTI.

Although measurement of free T4 concentration is the most sensitive diagnostic test for hyperthyroidism, there are some valid arguments against its use as a replacement for total T4 estimation. Free T4 concentrations are only truly measured by techniques such as equilibrium dialysis or ultrafiltration. Controversy surrounds the validity of other methods, particularly those involving analogues, for accurately measuring free T4 concentrations, and they provide no additional information over total T4 estimations alone.

The most frequently used technique is equilibrium dialysis, but it is expensive, impractical for in-house use and is not offered by all commercial laboratories. In addition, it is more subject to errors, due to inappropriate sample handling (see Chapter 1). More importantly, however, is a loss of diagnostic specificity when free T4 concentration is measured, as up to 20% of sick euthyroid cats have elevated circulating free T4 concentrations (Mooney *et al.*, 1996; Peterson *et al.*, 2001; Wakeling *et al.*, 2008). These cats generally have corresponding total T4 values in the lower half or below the reference interval. Caution is therefore advised in using serum free T4 measurements by equilibrium dialysis as the sole diagnostic test for hyperthyroidism. It is more reliable if interpreted with a corresponding total T4 measurement. A mid to high reference interval total with elevated free T4 concentration is consistent with hyperthyroidism, whereas a low total and elevated free T4 is usually associated with NTI.

In all hyperthyroid cats with an elevated serum total T4 concentration, free T4 concentration is concurrently high and its measurement adds no further diagnostic information. Given the expense of free T4 measurement coupled with the necessity for interpretation with a total T4 estimation, and the high prevalence of elevated total T4 values in hyperthyroid cats, it is more cost effective to initially measure total T4 concentration alone. If a diagnosis is not confirmed, consideration can be given to measurement of the corresponding free T4 concentration.

TSH concentration: In humans, measurement of circulating TSH concentration is usually used as a first-line discriminatory test of thyroid function. A species-specific feline TSH assay has not yet been developed, but assays for measuring canine TSH (cTSH) are widely available, and it has been suggested that this measurement may provide some diagnostic information in cats. In one study of two separate groups of hyperthyroid and euthyroid cats, both with mild chronic kidney disease, circulating cTSH concentrations were at or below the limit of detection of the assay (0.03 ng/ml) in all hyperthyroid but only 10% of the euthyroid cats (Wakeling *et al.*, 2008). Euthyroid cats with undetectable cTSH concentrations were more likely to have histopathological evidence of thyroid nodular hyperplasia than euthyroid cats with detectable cTSH values (Wakeling *et al.*, 2007). In addition, older cats with undetectable cTSH concentrations were more likely to develop hyperthyroidism within 1 year than were those cats with detectable concentrations (Wakeling et al., 2011). As a consequence, measurement of TSH using the canine assay has been suggested to provide evidence for the existence of clinical and subclinical hyperthyroidism in cats.

Caution is advised in over-interpreting cTSH values in cats. The current canine assays only detect approximately 35% of recombinant feline TSH. Consequently, the limit of detection, already considered poor (0.03 ng/ml cTSH), equates to approximately 0.1 ng/ml of feline TSH (Ferguson et al., 2007). Such a value is inappropriate in distinguishing normal from the suppressed values expected in hyperthyroidism. In support of this, some cats with known NTI have undetectable cTSH concentrations and, similarly, not all cats with undetectable cTSH subsequently develop hyperthyroidism. Perhaps a better use for such TSH measurement would be to exclude hyperthyroidism if a value exceeded the limit of detection of the assay.

Further diagnostic tests

In the majority of hyperthyroid cats with reference interval total T4 concentration, identification of concurrent disease, repeat total T4 analysis or simultaneous measurement of free T4 allows confirmation of the diagnosis. Further diagnostic tests are rarely required. However, dynamic thyroid function tests have been recommended in the past as helpful in confirming a diagnosis of hyperthyroidism. Protocols and interpretive advice for these tests are outlined in Figure 10.5, but nowadays should only be considered for cats with clinical signs suggestive of hyperthyroidism when repeated total T4 concentration remains within reference interval or free T4 analysis is unavailable or diagnostically unhelpful. More detailed information on these tests is available elsewhere (Shiel and Mooney, 2007).

T3 suppression test: In healthy individuals T3 has a suppressive effect on pituitary TSH secretion and subsequently on T4 production by the thyroid gland. In hyperthyroidism, because of autonomous production of thyroid hormones and chronic suppression of TSH, this suppressive effect is lost. Thus, serum total T4 concentrations show minimal

or no decrease in hyperthyroid cats following exogenous T3 administration. Simultaneous measurement of serum total T3 concentrations is required to ensure compliant administration and adequate absorption of the drug, and thus avoid false positive results. Generally, the test is most useful in ruling out hyperthyroidism rather than confirming its existence.

TSH stimulation test: Due to its poor diagnostic performance this test is considered by many to be obsolete. Exogenous TSH is a potent stimulator of thyroid hormone secretion. However, serum total T4 concentration shows little or no increase following exogenous bovine TSH administration in hyperthyroid cats. This is presumably because the thyroid gland of affected cats secretes thyroid hormones independently of TSH control or because T4 is already being produced at or near maximal rate with limited reserve capacity. Cats with equivocally elevated serum total T4 concentrations tend to exhibit results which are indistinguishable from those of healthy animals, and the test is no longer recommended for evaluating hyperthyroidism. In addition, bovine TSH is no longer available for parenteral administration. Recombinant human TSH (rhTSH) is available and, although not yet specifically studied in hyperthyroid cats, appears to be a safe and effective replacement for bovine TSH. However, the interpretative limitations of this test for hyperthyroidism are probably similar and it has a significant cost implication (van Hoek et al., 2010).

TRH stimulation test: TRH is less expensive and easier to obtain than TSH. Serum total T4 concentrations increase minimally after TRH administration in mildly hyperthyroid cats. Compared to the T3 suppression test, this test is quicker and avoids tablet administration. However, TRH is associated with transient adverse reactions such as salivation, vomiting, tachypnoea and defecation. In addition, results of the test are largely the same for sick euthyroid and for hyperthyroid cats with concurrent disease and total T4 concentrations within or below the reference interval (Tomsa et al., 2001).

Therapy	Drug	Dose	Route	Sampling times	Assay	Interpretation	
						Euthyroidism	*Hyperthyroidism*
T3 suppression	Liothyronine	20 mg 8-hourly for 7 doses	Oral	0 and 2–4 hours after last dose	Total T4	<20 nmol/l with >50% suppression	>20mol/l ± <35% suppression
TSH stimulation	Bovine TSH	0.5 IU/kg	Intravenous	0 and 6 hours	Total T4	>100% increase	Minimal to no increase
	rhTSH	25 µg/cat	Intravenous	1 and 6–8 hours	Total T4	>100% increase	Minimal to no increase
TRH stimulation	TRH	0.1 mg/kg	Intravenous	0 and 4 hours	Total T4	>60% increase	<50% increase

10.5 Commonly used protocols for dynamic thyroid function tests in cats. Values quoted for interpretation are guidelines only. Each individual laboratory should furnish its own reference interval. ND = not determined; rhTSH = recombinant human TSH; TRK = thyrotropin-releasing hormone; TSK = thyroid-stimulating hormone.

Treatment

The treatment of hyperthyroidism is aimed at removing or destroying abnormally functioning thyroid tissue, pharmacological inhibition of thyroid hormone synthesis and release, or amelioration of the effects of excess thyroid hormones on peripheral tissue. Surgical thyroidectomy or thyroid ablation using radioactive iodine remain the only reasonable curative options available. Medical management is non-curative and because of this cannot be recommended as sole therapy for the rare cases of hyperfunctioning thyroid carcinoma. The major advantages and disadvantages of the main forms of therapy are outlined in Figure 10.6. Treatment is tailored to each individual cat considering the factors outlined in Figure 10.7. More recently dietary management has been advocated but results are preliminary and definitive recommendations cannot yet be given.

Medical management

Chronic medical management is a practical treatment option for many cats. It requires no special facilities and is readily available. There is a rapid return to euthyroidism, which may be desirable in severely affected cases. Anaesthesia is avoided, as are the peri- and postoperative complications associated with surgical thyroidectomy and the prolonged hospitalization often necessary after radioactive iodine administration. However, medical management is not curative, is highly dependent on adequate owner and cat compliance, and requires regular biochemical monitoring to ensure the efficacy of treatment. It is therefore often reserved for cats of advanced age or for those with concurrent diseases, and for when owners refuse either surgery or radioactive iodine, or facilities are not available.

Medical management is also necessary prior to surgical thyroidectomy to decrease the metabolic and cardiac complications associated with hyperthyroidism and may be desirable in providing symptomatic control whilst awaiting radioactive iodine therapy. Short-term medical management is often recommended as trial therapy to determine the effect of restoring euthyroidism on renal function.

- Severity of clinical thyrotoxicosis
- Presence/absence of concurrent illness
- Age of cat
- Access to/waiting list for radioactive iodine therapy
- Availability of skilled surgeon
- Adequate post-thyroidectomy care facilities
- Owner/cat compliance for drug administration
- Potential complications
- Cost

10.7 Factors for consideration prior to selecting a treatment modality for hyperthyroidism in cats.

The variety of drugs, their mode of action, dosage regimes, indications and contraindications are detailed in Figure 10.8.

Methimazole and carbimazole

The two drugs methimazole and carbimazole are recommended for both preoperative and long-term management of hyperthyroidism. They have a potent and consistently reliable effect on suppressing thyroid hormone production. A related drug, propylthiouracil, often used in human medicine, is not recommended for cats because of a high incidence of serious adverse reactions (immune-mediated haemolytic anaemia and thrombocytopenia).

Methimazole is specifically authorized for treatment of feline hyperthyroidism, both in Europe and the USA, and is presented as 2.5 and 5 mg tablets. It is available elsewhere as a drug for human use. After administration, methimazole is actively concentrated by the thyroid gland, where it inhibits thyroid hormone synthesis but not iodide trapping or release of preformed hormone. Methimazole has good oral bioavailability and a serum half-life of 4–6 hours. Despite this, the intrathyroidal residence time, where methimazole exerts its effect, is likely to be up to 20 hours, as it is in humans.

Carbimazole is available for human use in many European countries and Japan. It exerts its antithyroid effect through immediate conversion to methimazole when administered orally. Serum concentrations of methimazole achieved after carbimazole administration are less than after a similar weight of methimazole, such that a 5 mg dose of carbimazole is approximately equal to 3 mg of

Therapy	Persistent/ recurrent hyperthyroidism	Time to achieve euthyroidism	Hospitalization	Adverse reactions	Availability	Cost
Radioactive iodine therapy	Rare	1–20 weeks	2–4 weeks	Minimal	Limited	High
Surgical thyroidectomy	Possible (if inappropriate technique used)	Prior treatment recommended	1–10 days (dependent on postoperative complications)	Hypoparathyroidism	Skilled surgeon required	Intermediate
Long-term medical management	Common (dependent on owner/ cat compliance)	3–15 days	Not required	Possible	Always available	Can be significant if long-term (cost of monitoring and treatment)

10.6 The advantages and disadvantages of the three different treatment modalities for hyperthyroidism in cats.

Drug	Modes of action	Formulation	Indications	Dosage (oral)	Contra-indications
Methimazole	Inhibition of thyroid peroxidase-catalysed reactions. ?Alteration in thyroglobulin structure	2.5, 5 mg tablets	Prior to surgery	2.5 mg per cat q12h	Immediately prior to ^{131}I therapy. Severe adverse reactions
			Chronic management	2.5 mg per cat q12h or 5 mg per cat q24h	
Carbimazole	As for methimazole	5 mg tablets	Prior to surgery	5 mg per cat q12h	As for methimazole
			Chronic management	5 mg per cat q12h/q24h	
Controlled-release carbimazole	As for methimazole	10, 15 mg tablets	Prior to surgery	10–15 mg per cat q24h	As for methimazole
			Chronic management	10–20 mg per cat q24h	
Stable iodine	Inhibition of thyroid peroxidase-catalysed reactions. Inhibition of hormone release	85 mg potassium iodate tablets (50 mg free iodine)	Prior to surgery	21.25 mg per cat q8h from day 10–20	Alone, prior to surgery. Prior to ^{131}I therapy. Chronic management
Iodine plus propranolol [a]	Beta-1/beta-2 adrenoceptor blocking agent	10 mg tablets		2.5–5 mg per cat q8h for 20 days	
Atenolol	Beta-1 adrenoceptor blocking agent	25 mg tablet 5 mg/ml syrup	Prior to surgery Symptomatic control	6.25–12.5 mg per cat q24h or q12h	Alone, prior to surgery. Chronic management

10.8 Drugs used in the medical management of feline hyperthyroidism. [a] Propranolol, like atenolol, can be used alone for short-term symptomatic control of hyperthyroidism.

methimazole. Carbimazole is often touted as having a lower incidence of adverse reactions such as vomiting and anorexia. This may be because it is tasteless whereas methimazole has a bitter taste. However, methimazole, as authorized for veterinary use, is sugar-coated and, provided the tablet is not crushed, the bitter taste is presumably avoided.

Carbimazole, as a novel once-daily controlled-release formulation (10 or 15 mg tablets) was recently authorized for cats in Europe. Pharmacokinetic studies of this controlled-release formulation have shown no pronounced concentration peak and a sustained presence of methimazole in plasma (>24 hours) with an apparent terminal half-life of approximately 9 hours after oral administration (Frenais *et al.*, 2008). Based on relative bioavailability and conversion, it is estimated that 15 mg of this preparation is equivalent to approximately 7.5 mg of conventional methimazole (Frenais *et al.*, 2009). It has been shown that administration of this drug with food significantly enhances its absorption. While it is not necessary to administer it in food, in order to avoid potential variation in doses absorbed, the time between feeding and treatment should be as constant as possible (Frenais *et al.*, 2008).

The effect of prior methimazole treatment on eventual outcome of radioactive iodine therapy is controversial. It has been variably suggested to enhance, worsen or have no effect on radioiodine treatment. Although methimazole does not inhibit thyroidal iodine uptake, current administration adversely affects effective half-life of radioactive iodine and is not recommended. However, iodine uptake is enhanced in healthy cats after recent methimazole withdrawal, and this short-term rebound effect is potentially beneficial when treating with radioactive iodine (Nieckarz and Daniel,

2001). A more recent study has shown that discontinuing methimazole for <5 or >5 days prior to radioactive iodine therapy has no effect on treatment outcome (Chun *et al.*, 2002).

Dosage regimens: In early studies, methimazole was recommended orally at a dosage of 10–15 mg/cat/day divided every 8–12 hours depending on the severity of the thyrotoxicosis. This was successful in inducing euthyroidism in most hyperthyroid cats within 2–3 weeks (Peterson *et al.*, 1988). However, such cats were moderately to severely affected, unlike the milder cases seen today. It is currently recommended that 2.5 mg/cat methimazole is administered q12h.

Carbimazole was originally recommended at a dose of 5 mg/cat, administered at 8-hourly intervals (Mooney *et al.*, 1992). Again, such high doses are today rarely required and most cats will achieve euthyroidism using 5 mg/cat q12h.

The starting dose for controlled release carbimazole is 15 mg/cat q24h. In mild cases (defined as total T4 concentration 50–100 nmol/l), a lower starting dose of 10 mg/cat q24h is recommended.

The length of time to achieve biochemical euthyroidism is relatively short, with a mean of 5.7 days (range 3–15 days), at least for carbimazole (Mooney *et al.* 1992). For practical purposes and in order to ensure clinical effect, cats are usually reassessed after 10 days (controlled-release formulations) or 3 weeks (conventional tablets). A serum total T4 concentration is measured and, if within the low end or below the reference interval, thyroidectomy can be performed, administering the last dose on the morning of surgery. For severely affected cats, even if biochemical euthyroidism is achieved, a longer course of preoperative therapy may be required before the animal is considered a reasonable surgical candidate. The dose is adjusted as for long-term maintenance. If euthyroidism has not been achieved, the dose of methimazole or carbimazole can be altered in 2.5–5 mg increments, reassessing the cat again in 2–3 weeks. Lack of owner or cat compliance should first be eliminated as a reason for a failure of therapy.

For long-term management once euthyroidism has been achieved, the daily dosage is adjusted, aiming for the lowest possible dose that effectively maintains euthyroidism. Achieving this is limited by available tablet size, as neither conventional nor controlled-release formulations can be broken or crushed. Methimazole can be continued at a dose of 2.5 mg/cat q12h. Although divided doses are most effective in rapidly inducing euthyroidism, it has been reported that at 4 weeks there is no significant difference in the percentage of cats achieving euthyroidism using 2.5 mg administered q12h *versus* 5 mg administered q24h (Trepanier *et al.*, 2003). Consequently, if once-daily dosing is preferred, administering 5 mg/cat of methimazole chronically may be attempted. Experience suggests that once-daily dosing with 2.5 mg/cat is also efficacious in many cats. Conventional carbimazole has been recommended chronically at a dose of 5 mg/cat q12h, but continuing with once-daily therapy may also be effective. Further increasing the dosing interval results in recurrent hyperthyroidism. For controlled-release carbimazole, the majority (approximately 90%) can be effectively maintained on doses between 10 and 20 mg/cat daily. A few cases require lower doses (10 mg/cat every other day) and only rarely do cats require higher doses (Frenais *et al.*, 2009).

While antithyroid drugs are routinely administered orally, compliance can be problematic, particularly in fractious or inappetent cats. Drug absorption is also potentially affected by concurrent intestinal disease and there are obvious difficulties in cats that vomit. Carbimazole and methimazole can be reformulated in a pluronic lecithin organogel (PLO) for transdermal administration. This has been shown to be effective in cats when applied at a dose of 2.5 mg/cat q12h, although compared to oral administration it may take longer to attain euthyroidism (Sartor *et al.*, 2004). In addition it remains unclear whether there is sustained dermal absorption, or gastrointestinal absorption after oral ingestion through licking and grooming. The gel is applied in a thin layer to the non-haired portion of the pinnae, using a concentration approximating 5 mg/0.1 ml, which prevents excess vehicle build-up. It is purportedly associated with fewer gastrointestinal side effects than is oral therapy, but some cats resent manipulation of the ear and crusting can occur between doses, leading to erythema. Whilst transdermal products are undoubtedly an option for treating hyperthyroidism, none is specifically available for use in cats. Custom formulation increases expense of therapy, and stability of the product is not guaranteed. Both handlers and other cats in the household are at increased risk of exposure to methimazole if administered via this route.

Monitoring strategies: A serum total T4 concentration is measured 10 days to 3 weeks after commencing therapy or after each dose adjustment and, once stability has been attained, every 3–6 months or as indicated clinically. The time of sampling in relation to dosing is not important, irrespective of frequency of dosing (Rutland *et al.*, 2009). The aim is to maintain total T4 concentrations within the lower half of the reference interval, ensuring that free T4 concentrations remain within their reference interval. Clinical signs of hypothyroidism rarely develop even when total T4 is suppressed below the reference interval. This was previously thought to be because corresponding T3 concentrations tend to remain within the reference interval, thereby maintaining the metabolic rate. This may be due to increased extrathyroidal conversion from T4 or preferential thyroidal production of T3. However, the potential detrimental effect of induced hypothyroidism on renal function has recently been highlighted. In a study it was suggested that cats undergoing medical management do become hypothyroid (as defined by total T4 and cTSH concentrations below and above their respective reference intervals) and that such cats are more likely to develop azotaemia and have a shortened survival time (Williams *et al.*, 2010a). Thus, if circulating total T4 concentration is severely suppressed, the dosage of methimazole or carbimazole should, if possible, be decreased and the cat re-assessed accordingly. Regular assessment of hyperthyroid cats is necessary. Antithyroid medication has no effect on the underlying lesion and the thyroid nodules continue to grow and can enlarge, necessitating an increased dosage long-term.

Elevated serum activities of ALT and ALP decline progressively as euthyroidism is achieved (Figure 10.9). Although their measurement can be used as a non-specific indicator of therapeutic efficacy, caution is advised. In some cats with concurrent

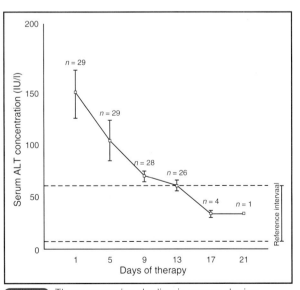

10.9 The progressive decline in serum alanine aminotransferase (ALT) concentrations in a series of hyperthyroid cats that became euthyroid with carbimazole at a dose of 5 mg/cat q8h. (Reproduced and modified with permission from Mooney *et al.*, 1992)

hepatopathies, serum activities may not decline and without simultaneous measurement of total T4, an erroneous diagnosis of poor therapeutic efficacy may be made.

Adverse reactions: Most clinical adverse reactions occur within the first 3 months of therapy. It is unclear whether all are dose-related, but aiming for the lowest possible dose appears prudent. Mild clinical side effects of vomiting, with or without anorexia and depression occur in approximately 10–15% of cats, usually within the first 3 weeks of therapy. In most cases, these reactions are transient and do not require drug withdrawal. Early in the course of therapy, mild and transient haematological abnormalities including lymphocytosis, eosinophilia or leucopenia occur in up to approximately 15% of cases treated, without any apparent clinical effect. Self-induced excoriations of the head and neck have occasionally been described, usually within the first 6 weeks of therapy. Permanent withdrawal of the drug together with symptomatic therapy is usually required, although there are anecdotal reports of recovery without drug withdrawal.

More serious haematological complications occur in <5% of cases and include agranulocytosis and thrombocytopenia, either alone or concurrently, or, more rarely, immune-mediated haemolytic anaemia. Fortnightly complete blood and platelet counts have been recommended, at least for the first 3 months of therapy, in order to detect such reactions. However, because of their rarity and unpredictability, assessment of a complete blood count, if clinical signs indicate, is a more cost effective way of dealing with such reactions. A hepatopathy, characterized by marked increases in liver enzymes and bilirubin concentration, occurs in <2% of cats. Withdrawal of the medication and symptomatic therapy is required. If such reactions occur with methimazole they are also as likely with carbimazole, and an alternative treatment for hyperthyroidism is required. Other rarely reported side effects include a bleeding tendency without thrombocytopenia or prolongation of clotting times and acquired myasthenia gravis (Trepanier, 2007).

Serum antinuclear antibodies develop in approximately 50% of hyperthyroid cats treated with methimazole for >6 months, usually in cats on high dose therapy (15 mg/day) (Peterson *et al.,* 1988). Although clinical signs of a lupus-like syndrome have not been reported, decreasing the daily dosage is recommended.

Alternative drugs
Occasionally, alternative medical therapies are required in cats because of adverse reactions to methimazole or for other specific reasons. For the most part, these therapies are short-term and only recommended prior to a more permanent treatment option.

Propranolol and atenolol: These are the most frequently used beta-adrenoceptor-blocking agents in hyperthyroid cats. They are used to control the tachycardia, tachypnoea, hypertension and hyperexcitability associated with hyperthyroidism. Although traditionally considered to have no discernible effect on serum thyroid hormone concentrations, propranolol may inhibit peripheral conversion of T4 to T3. These drugs are recommended when rapid control of clinical signs is desirable and may be used either in combination with stable iodine or methimazole. Alone, they are a useful treatment option for cats awaiting radiation therapy, or in those cases in which there is a delayed return to euthyroidism after treatment because neither has any direct effect on the thyroid gland. Propranolol is a non-selective beta-adrenoceptor-blocker and is contraindicated in cats with pre-existing uncontrolled asthma or congestive cardiac failure. Atenolol is often preferred because it is a selective beta-1-adrenoceptor-blocking agent.

Stable iodine: Large doses of stable iodine acutely decrease the rate of thyroid hormone synthesis (Wolff–Chaikoff effect) and release; these effects are erratic, inconsistent, and short-lived, and escape from inhibition can occur. In addition, stable iodine is contraindicated prior to the administration of radioactive iodine and is associated with a high incidence of adverse reactions (excessive salivation and partial to complete anorexia) purportedly because of its 'brassy' taste. For these reasons it is not used as sole therapy but usually in association with beta-adrenoceptor-blocking agents in a staged regimen for short-term preoperative treatment (Foster and Thoday, 1999). The prevalence of side effects can be reduced by placing the dose in a gelatin capsule. Using this combination results in reference interval serum total T3 concentrations in most cats and therefore clinical improvement, although serum total T4 concentrations decrease in only approximately one-third of cases. A reported advantage of stable iodine is its apparent effect on decreasing the vascularity and friability of the thyroid gland, but this is controversial.

Calcium ipodate and iopanoic acid: A number of oral cholecystographic agents (e.g. calcium ipodate and iopanoic acid) decrease T4 production, an effect presumably mediated by release of iodine as the drug is metabolized, and also acutely inhibit peripheral T4 to T3 conversion. The latter effect has been clearly demonstrated in hyperthyroid cats where administration of calcium ipodate was associated with clinical improvement and normalization of serum total T3 concentrations in >60% of cases (Murray and Peterson, 1997). Iopanoic acid has also been shown to decrease serum T3 concentrations in hyperthyroid cats (Gallagher and Panciera, 2011). Waning of the effect is possible after 3 months of therapy. Therefore, calcium ipodate and iopanoic acid are only ever likely to serve as alternatives to stable iodine in the short-term preparation for surgery. Neither drug is widely available. Similar agents such as diatrizoate meglumine have anecdotally been used.

Surgical thyroidectomy

Surgical thyroidectomy is an extremely effective treatment for hyperthyroidism; it is simple, quick, curative and cost-effective. In practice it is often considered the treatment of choice, particularly if radioactive iodine is unavailable.

Preoperative stabilization

Anaesthetizing hyperthyroid cats carries a significant risk of cardiac and metabolic complications serious enough to cause death, and it is therefore necessary to control the production or effects of excess thyroid hormone as outlined above.

Anaesthetic management

Once the hyperthyroidism is well controlled, a variety of routine anaesthetic regimens can be used – with a few exceptions. Drugs that stimulate or potentiate adrenergic activity, capable of inducing tachycardia and arrhythmias should be avoided, while drugs capable of preventing such arrhythmias are preferred. Thus, acepromazine is considered a useful premedicant, and glycopyrrolate is usually used in place of atropine. Xylazine and ketamine are avoided, while isoflurane, if available, is preferred over halothane. Minimal anaesthetic time and continual monitoring are essential. Ventricular arrhythmia is a possible complication, particularly if the hyperthyroidism is not adequately pre-controlled. If such arrhythmias persist despite routine anaesthetic management, intravenous propranolol may restore normal sinus rhythm.

Surgical technique

A ventral skin incision is made from the larynx to the manubrium. The sternohyoideus and sternothyroideus muscles are separated by blunt dissection in the midline and gently retracted. Both thyroid lobes and the external parathyroid glands can then be visualized before excision (Figure 10.10). In addition, the right recurrent laryngeal nerve, which lies in close proximity to the right thyroid gland, can be identified and avoided. Following thyroidectomy, the surgical field is carefully examined for haemostasis before closing the incision routinely. Further

details of techniques are given in the *BSAVA Manual of Canine and Feline Head, Neck and Thoracic Surgery*.

Unilateral *versus* bilateral removal

Bilateral lobe involvement occurs in >70% of cases and thus the majority of cats require bilateral thyroidectomy. In many of these cases, lobe enlargement is not symmetrical and the smaller lobe may not be clearly palpable. The decision whether to perform a unilateral or bilateral thyroidectomy is therefore often taken at the time of surgery. However, in up to 15% of bilateral cases, one thyroid lobe may appear grossly normal and if left *in situ* will result in recurrence of the condition. In unilateral cases there is atrophy of the contralateral lobe, but the distinction between what is considered normal and atrophic is not clearly defined.

Thyroid imaging, if available, is an extremely useful procedure to determine unilateral or bilateral lobe involvement and alterations in position or distant metastases from a functioning thyroid carcinoma. It is particularly useful in determining the site of hyperfunctioning ectopic/accessory tissue that may be present anywhere from the base of the tongue to the heart (Harvey *et al.*, 2009). Imaging can be carried out using ^{123}I, ^{131}I or ^{99m}TcO$_4^-$. The latter is usually preferred because of its short half-life and imaging time, relative inexpense, low radiation dose and consistent image quality (Figure 10.11), but requires access to a gamma camera. High resolution ultrasonography, in experienced hands, may be an alternative to thyroid imaging,

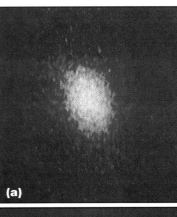
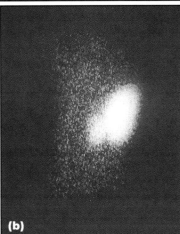

10.11 Unilateral **(a)** and bilateral **(b)** thyroid lobe involvement, as detected by thyroid imaging using pertechnetate.

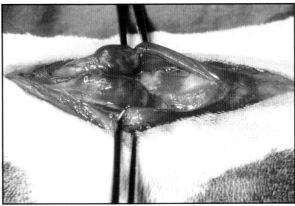

10.10 Appearance of bilateral thyroid lobe enlargement at the time of surgery. The external parathyroid glands are easily visualized as small spherical pale glands at the cranial pole of each thyroid lobe.

but larger studies are required for its evaluation (Wisner *et al.*, 1994).

In the absence of thyroid imaging, both thyroid lobes should be carefully identified and, if abnormal in any way, removed. If a unilateral thyroidectomy is carried out future monitoring for recurrence of the condition is required. Routine bilateral thyroidectomy, whilst increasing the risk of post-operative complications, obviates the need for decision making at the time of surgery. However, ectopic thyroid tissue should be considered if hyperthyroidism persists after such routine thyroidectomy.

Intracapsular *versus* extracapsular technique

Two techniques have been described for thyroidectomy, both of which attempt to preserve the cranial (external) parathyroid gland and maintain eucalcaemia (Figures 10.12 and 10.13). The choice of technique is unimportant if a unilateral thyroidectomy is being carried out, as only one parathyroid gland is necessary to maintain calcium homeostasis, but the decision requires careful consideration for bilateral thyroidectomy.

The original *intracapsular* technique involved incision through the thyroid capsule and blunt dissection of the thyroid lobe, leaving the capsule *in situ*, thereby preserving the blood supply to the cranial parathyroid gland. However, this technique is associated with a high rate of recurrence due to regrowth of tissue adherent to the capsule. The original *extracapsular* technique involved removal of the intact thyroid lobe and capsule with ligation of the cranial thyroid artery, while attempting to preserve

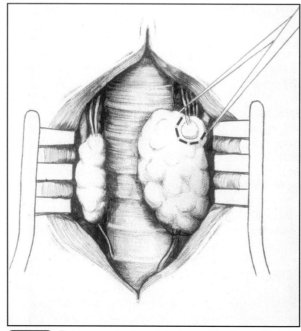

10.13 Extracapsular thyroidectomy: The thyroid lobe and capsule are removed whilst preserving vascular supply to the external parathyroid glands. For the modified technique, bipolar cautery is used instead of ligatures.

blood supply to the cranial parathyroid gland. This technique significantly decreases the rate of recurrence but is associated with an unacceptably high rate of postoperative hypoparathyroidism. Both techniques have therefore been successfully modified: the intracapsular technique by removal of the majority of the capsule after thyroid lobe removal; and the extracapsular technique by using bipolar cautery instead of ligatures, which minimizes blunt dissection around the cranial parathyroid glands. There is no significant difference in the rate of postoperative hypocalcaemia or recurrence between these two techniques and both are considered equally appropriate for bilateral thyroidectomy in cats. Haemorrhage obscuring the surgical field is a significant problem with the modified intracapsular technique; for this reason, and because of its speed, the modified extracapsular technique may be preferred.

Postoperative complications

The most significant postoperative complication is hypocalcaemia. The tendency towards ionized hypocalcaemia and hyperparathyroidism in hyperthyroidism may play some role in the development of postoperative hypocalcaemia; however, it is generally agreed that it only occurs if the parathyroid glands are injured, devascularized or inadvertently removed during the course of surgery. Since only one parathyroid gland is required to maintain function, hypoparathyroidism only develops after bilateral thyroidectomy. If removal of the cranial parathyroid glands is noted at the time of surgery, small pieces can be transplanted into a muscular pouch in the neck where revascularisation and return of function may occur. Staged thyroidectomies (three to four

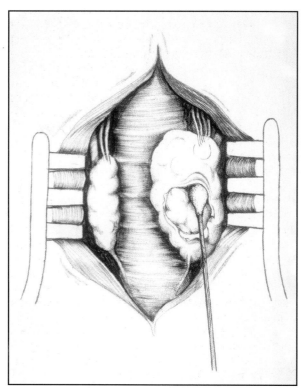

10.12 Intracapsular thyroidectomy: The thyroid capsule is incised and the thyroid lobe removed. For the modified intracapsular technique the capsule is subsequently excised.

weeks apart) exploit this phenomenon. However, any reduced risk of postoperative complications may not justify the risk and expense of two surgical procedures whichever technique is used (traditional or thyroparathyroidectomy with parathyroid autotransplantation).

Hypocalcaemia occurs within 1–5 days of surgery. Biochemical hypocalcaemia alone does not warrant treatment but should be instituted if clinical signs develop. These signs include anorexia, vocalization, irritability, muscle twitching, tetany and generalized convulsions. The treatment of postoperative hypocalcaemia is outlined in more detail in Chapter 7. Hypoparathyroidism is rarely permanent and recovery of parathyroid tissue can occur days to months after surgery. Although this may be related to reversible parathyroid damage, it is possible that calcium homeostasis is being maintained through a PTH-independent mechanism (Flanders *et al.,* 1991). If this is the case, there is always the potential risk of developing signs of hypocalcaemia in the future and care should be taken to monitor these cats appropriately.

Recurrence must also be considered a potential complication. If a unilateral thyroidectomy was originally performed, development of lesions in the contralateral gland should pose no additional surgical risk providing parathyroid function is maintained. However, repeat thyroidectomies, following recurrence after bilateral thyroidectomy, are not recommended because of a higher incidence of severe life-threatening complications. Recurrence is also more likely following surgery on ectopic thyroid tissue. In both cases, an alternative form of therapy for hyperthyroidism is indicated.

It is difficult to assign accurately a risk for hypocalcaemia and recurrence in a cat undergoing bilateral thyroidectomy, as it is highly operator-dependent. In one study of the modified intracapsular technique performed by an experienced surgeon, a low rate of postoperative hypocalcaemia (<6%) and recurrence (5%) was found (Naan *et al.,* 2006).

Other rarer but potential complications include haemorrhage, Horner's syndrome, laryngeal oedema or paralysis and voice change. These can be avoided by a meticulous surgical technique. Serum total T4 concentrations are usually low for weeks to months after surgical thyroidectomy but eventually increase into the reference interval. Treatment with exogenous thyroxine is not indicated, as permanent hypothyroidism is a rare sequel.

Radioactive iodine

Treatment with radioactive iodine is simple, safe and effective, and is the best treatment for most hyperthyroid cats. The radioisotope most commonly used is ^{131}I, which, like stable iodine, is concentrated by the thyroid gland. It has a half-life of approximately 8 days and emits both beta-particles and gamma-irradiation. The beta-particles, which cause 80% of the tissue damage, travel a maximum of 2 mm and have an average pathlength of 400 μm. They are therefore locally destructive but spare adjacent atrophic thyroid tissue, parathyroid tissue and other important cervical structures. ^{131}I can be administered intravenously or orally, but the subcutaneous route is preferred. It is equally effective, safer for personnel, is not associated with gastrointestinal side effects and can be performed under light sedation if necessary, thereby avoiding anaesthesia.

The principle of treatment is to administer a dose of ^{131}I which will restore euthyroidism whilst avoiding the onset of hypothyroidism. Traditionally, this involved the administration of a small tracer dose of ^{131}I to determine various parameters of iodine kinetics before calculation of a therapeutic dose. Whilst successful, access to sophisticated and expensive nuclear medicine equipment is required. Use of fixed high or low doses may result in over- or under-treatment of a significant number of animals. The estimation of a dose based on a scoring system, which includes the severity of the clinical thyrotoxicosis, elevation in circulating total T4 concentration and the size of the goitre as estimated by palpation, is currently the most popular method, and is successful in over 90% of cases (Mooney, 1994; Peterson and Becker, 1995). Most cats are treated with doses between 50 and 200 MBq.

Complications

There are few complications of ^{131}I therapy. Persistent hyperthyroidism, more common in severely affected cats with large goitres and extreme elevations in serum total T4 concentration can be successfully managed with a repeat injection, although in some cats euthyroidism spontaneously develops within weeks to months of treatment. Permanent hypothyroidism is rare, as is recurrence after successful treatment, and other side effects are minimal (Slater *et al.,* 1994). Several drawbacks exist. Facilities for ^{131}I are available in only a few referral centres in the UK and post-treatment hospitalization times are approximately 2–4 weeks. Due to the popularity of the treatment, waiting lists may be lengthy. This, and a possible delay in the return to euthyroidism for up to 6 months in a small number of cats, may necessitate interim symptomatic control of the thyrotoxicosis.

Prognosis

The long-term prognosis for cats treated with radio-iodine is excellent. In the largest study of 534 cats, median survival time (MST) was 24 months and 89, 72, 52 and 34% of cats were alive at 1, 2, 3 and 4 years after treatment, respectively (Peterson and Becker, 1995). In a more recent study the MST was 4.0 years compared to 2.0 years for methimazole-treated cats (Milner *et al.,* 2006). The most common causes of death in treated hyperthyroid cats are those normally associated with ageing, such as malignancy and renal disease.

Other therapies

Intrathyroidal infusion of ethanol causes tissue necrosis and eventual induction of euthyroidism. Single injections in unilateral cases, preferably using ultrasound guidance, are efficacious in inducing euthyroidism in hyperthyroid cats (Goldstein *et al.,* 2001). Staged injections in bilateral cases are less successful in treating hyperthyroidism (Wells *et al.,* 2001). However, percutaneous ethanol injection is associated with a high incidence of adverse reactions, such as transient dysphonia, Horner's syndrome, gagging and laryngeal paralysis, and cannot therefore be recommended for treatment of hyperthyroid cats.

Recent studies have indicated that use of a diet with severely restricted iodine content (Hill's Prescription Diet y/d) can result in normalization of T4 concentrations in hyperthyroid cats and provide a further option for management of this disease. However, although promising, results are as yet preliminary as only a small group of cats has been treated and all were only mildly hyperthyroid (Melendez *et al.,* 2011). It is unclear whether such treatment can be recommended alone, or as an adjunct to the more tried and tested traditional methods. To ensure efficacy, treated cats must consume only this diet long term. There are obvious difficulties in implementing such a regime in multi-cat households.

Effect of treatment on renal function

Hyperthyroidism is known to increase glomerular filtration rate (GFR), decrease circulating creatinine concentration and mask underlying renal disease. Decreased GFR, increased serum urea and creatinine concentration, and development of overt clinical signs of renal disease have all been reported after successful treatment of hyperthyroidism, irrespective of therapeutic modality (methimazole/carbimazole, surgical thyroidectomy or radioiodine). It is difficult to assess accurately the prevalence of azotaemia that potentially develops after treatment but it has been estimated at approximately 33% (Syme, 2007).

The decline in GFR is detectable within 1 month of treatment of the hyperthyroidism but remains stable for at least 6 months thereafter. Assessment of GFR before treatment can act as a predictor of post-treatment renal failure, with a low GFR in hyperthyroidism indicating an increased risk for post-treatment azotaemia. However, techniques for assessment of GFR are not widely used in practice. In their absence accurate prediction of impending renal failure is difficult. Routine pre-treatment parameters, such as serum urea or creatinine concentrations and urine specific gravity, have not been reliably useful for consistently predicting impending azotaemia (Riensche *et al.,* 2008; Williams et al., 2010b). Because of these difficulties, trial therapy using either methimazole or carbimazole has been recommended with reassessment of renal function once euthyroidism is achieved. If no marked deterioration occurs, then a more permanent therapeutic option for hyperthyroidism may be selected. However prudent this may be, its necessity is questionable given that treatment for the hyperthyroidism is required whatever the outcome. Interestingly, the survival of cats that develop azotaemia is no different from that of those that remain non-azotaemic after treatment of hyperthyroidism, provided hypothyroidism has not been induced (Williams *et al.,* 2010a).

Notwithstanding the difficulties of diagnosing hyperthyroidism, the treatment of cats with pre-existing renal insufficiency is more complicated given that it adversely affects survival significantly. Initially low and then increasing doses of methimazole have been suggested in such cats, but there is limited evidence to support this. Concurrent therapy should always be instituted for renal insufficiency and careful monitoring carried out. Maintenance of a mildly hyperthyroid state, while anecdotally recommended, is questionable given that hyperthyroidism may in itself be damaging to renal function. However, whichever treatment option for hyperthyroidism is considered it is important to avoid hypothyroidism, as it has its own detrimental effects on GFR.

Thyroid carcinoma

Functional thyroid carcinoma accounts for <2% of cases of feline hyperthyroidism and, in the authors' experience, for approximately 50% of all cases of feline thyroid carcinoma. Affected cats present with similar clinical signs to those with benign adenomatous hyperplasia. Evidence of thyroid carcinoma includes palpable large multilobulated masses in the neck, signs of distant metastases (usually intrathoracic), locally invasive appearance at the time of surgery, or rapid recurrence following either routine bilateral thyroidectomy or radioactive iodine therapy (Turrel *et al.,* 1988). While thyroid imaging often reveals multifocal, irregular and heterogeneous areas of increased uptake (Figure 10.14), such changes are also seen in cats with benign disease (Harvey *et al.,* 2009).

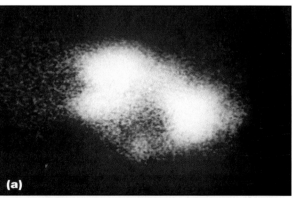

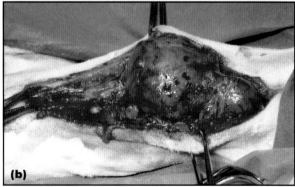

10.14 **(a)** Appearance of a pertechnetate scan in thyroid carcinoma with multiple areas of uptake. **(b)** The same gland as visualized at the time of surgery.

Cats presenting with distant metastatic disease carry a more guarded prognosis. In other cases, stabilization of the clinical signs can be achieved using methimazole/carbimazole, although as this drug is not cytotoxic the prognosis remains guarded. Removal of all affected tissue is often difficult at the time of surgery, and routine radioactive iodine therapy may not be effective because malignant tissue appears to concentrate and retain iodine less efficiently than normal or adenomatous cells. High dose (>1000 MBq) radioactive iodine provides the best option for treating cats with thyroid carcinoma, either alone or following surgical thyroidectomy. Because of the extreme doses, there are few licensed facilities available. Nevertheless, the long-term prognosis is good, with extended survival commonly achieved (Guptill *et al.*, 1995; Hibbert *et al.*, 2009).

References and further reading

Anderson D (2005) The thyroid and parathyroid glands. In: *BSAVA Manual of Canine and Feline Head, Neck and Thoracic Surgery,* ed. DJ Brockman and DE Holt, pp. 123–234. BSAVA Publications, Gloucester

Archer FJ and Taylor SM (1996) Alkaline phosphatase bone isoenzyme and osteocalcin in the serum of hyperthyroid cats. *Canadian Veterinary Journal* **37**, 735–739

Barber PJ and Elliott J (1996) Study of calcium homeostasis in feline hyperthyroidism. *Journal of Small Animal Practice* **37**, 575–582

Berent AC, Drobatz KJ, Ziemer L, Johnson VS and Ward CR (2007) Liver function in cats with hyperthyroidism before and after ^{131}I therapy. *Journal of Veterinary Internal Medicine* **21**, 1217–1223

Bond BR, Fox PR, Peterson ME and Skavaril RV (1988) Echocardiographic findings in 103 cats with hyperthyroidism. *Journal of the American Veterinary Medical Association* **192**, 1546–1549

Boretti FS, Sieber-Ruckstuhl NS, Gerber B *et al.* (2009) Thyroid enlargement and its relationship to clinicopathological parameters and T4 status in suspected hyperthyroid cats. *Journal of Feline Medicine & Surgery* **11**, 286–292

Broussard JD and Peterson ME (1995) Changes in clinical and laboratory findings in cats with hyperthyroidism from 1983 to 1993. *Journal of the American Veterinary Medical Association* **206**, 302–305

Chun R, Garrett LD, Sargeant J, Sherman A and Hoskinson JJ (2002) Predictors of response to radioiodine therapy in hyperthyroid cats. *Veterinary Radiology & Ultrasound* **43**, 587–591

Connolly DJ, Guitian J, Boswood A and Neiger R (2005) Serum troponin 1 levels in hyperthyroid cats before and after treatment with radioactive iodine. *Journal of Feline Medicine & Surgery* **7**, 289–300

Daniel GB, Sharp DS, Nieckarz JA and Adams W (2002) Quantitative thyroid scintigraphy as a predictor of serum thyroxin concentration in normal and hyperthyroid cats. *Veterinary Radiology and Ultrasound* **43**, 374–382

De Wet CS, Mooney CT, Thompson PN and Schoeman JP (2009) Prevalence of and risk factors for feline hyperthyroidism in Hong Kong. *Journal of Feline Medicine & Surgery* **11**, 315–321

Feldman EC and Nelson RW (2004) Feline hyperthyroidism (thyrotoxicosis). In: *Canine and Feline Endocrinology and Reproduction, 3rd edn*, ed. EC Feldman and RW Nelson, pp. 152–218. WB Saunders, Philadelphia

Ferguson DC, Caffall Z and Hoenig M (2007) Obesity increases free thyroxine proportionally to nonesterified fatty acid concentrations in adult neutered female cats. *Journal of Endocrinology* **194**, 267–273

Flanders JA, Neth S, Erb HN and Kallfelz FA (1991) Functional analysis of ectopic parathyroid activity in cats. *American Journal of Veterinary Research* **52**, 1336–1340

Foster DJ and Thoday KL (1999) Use of propranolol and potassium iodate in the presurgical management of hyperthyroidism. *Journal of Small Animal Practice* **40**, 307–315

Fox PR, Peterson ME and Broussard JD (1999) Electrocardiographic and radiographic changes in cats with hyperthyroidism: comparison of populations evaluated during 1992–1993 vs 1979–1982. *Journal of the American Animal Hospital Association* **35**, 27–31

Frenais R, Burgaud S and Horspool LJI (2008) Pharmacokinetics of controlled-release tablets support once daily dosing in cats. *Journal of Veterinary Pharmacology and Therapeutics* **31**, 213–219

Frenais R, Rosenberg D, Burgaud S and Horspool LJI (2009) Clinical efficacy and safety of a once-daily formulation of carbimazole in cats with hyperthyroidism. *Journal of Small Animal Practice* **50**, 510–515

Gallagher AE and Panciera DL (2011) Efficacy of iopanoic acid for treatment of spontaneous hyperthyroidism in cats. *Journal of Feline Medicine and Surgery* **13**, 441–447

Goldstein RE, Long C, Swift NC *et al.* (2001) Percutaneous ethanol injection for treatment of unilateral hyperplastic thyroid nodules in cats. *Journal of the American Veterinary Medical Association* **218**, 1298–1302

Gordon JM, Ehrhart EJ, Sisson DD and Jones MA (2003) Juvenile hyperthyroidism in a cat. *Journal of the American Animal Hospital Association* **39**, 67–71

Graham PA, Mooney CT and Murray M (1999) Serum fructosamine concentrations in hyperthyroid cats. *American Journal of Veterinary Research* **67**, 171–175

Guptill L, Scott-Moncrieff JCR, Janovitz EB *et al.* (1995) Response to high-dose radioactive iodine administration in cats with thyroid carcinoma that had previously undergone surgery. *Journal of the American Veterinary Medical Association* **207**, 1055–1058

Harvey AM, Hibbert A, Barrett EL *et al.* (2009) Scintigraphic findings in 120 hyperthyroid cats. *Journal of Feline Medicine & Surgery* **11**, 96–106

Hibbert A, Gruffydd-Jones T, Barrett EL, Day MJ and Harvey AM (2009) Feline thyroid carcinoma: diagnosis and response to high-dose radioactive iodine treatment. *Journal of Feline Medicine & Surgery* **11**, 116–124

Jacobs G, Hutson C, Dougherty J and Kirmayer A (1986) Congestive heart failure associated with hyperthyroidism in cats. *Journal of the American Veterinary Medical Association* **188**, 52–56

Joseph RJ and Peterson ME (1992) Review and comparison of neuromuscular and central nervous system manifestations of hyperthyroidism in cats and humans. *Progress in Veterinary Neurology* **3**, 114–119

Mayer-Roenne B, Goldstein RE and Erb HN (2007) Urinary tract infections in cats with hyperthyroidism, diabetes mellitus and chronic kidney disease. *Journal of Feline Medicine & Surgery* **9**, 124–132

Melendez LM, Yamka RM, Forrester SD and Burris PA (2011) Titration of dietary iodine for reducing serum thyroxine concentrations in newly diagnosed hyperthyroid cats. *Journal of Veterinary Internal Medicine* **25**, 683

Milner RJ, Channell CD, Levy JK and Schaer M (2006) Survival times for cats with hyperthyroidism treated with iodine 131, methimazole, or both: 167 cases (1996–2003) *Journal of the American Veterinary Medical Association* **228**, 559–563

Mooney CT (1994) Radioactive iodine therapy for feline hyperthyroidism: efficacy and administration routes. *Journal of Small Animal Practice* **35**, 289–294

Mooney CT, Little CJL and Macrae AW (1996) Effect of illness not associated with the thyroid gland on serum total and free thyroxine concentrations in cats. *Journal of the American Veterinary Medical Association* **208**, 2004–2008

Mooney CT, Thoday KL and Doxey DL (1992) Carbimazole therapy of feline hyperthyroidism. *Journal of Small Animal Practice* **33**, 228–235

Murray LAS and Peterson ME (1997) Ipodate as medical treatment in 12 cats with hyperthyroidism. *Journal of the American Veterinary Medical Association* **211**, 63–67

Naan EC, Kirpensteijn J, Kooistra HS and Peeters ME (2006) Results of thyroidectomy in 101 cats with hyperthyroidism. *Veterinary Surgery* **35**, 287–293

Nemzek JA, Kruger JM, Walshaw R and Hauptman JG (1994) Acute onset of hypokalaemia and muscular weakness in four hyperthyroid cats. *Journal of the American Veterinary Medical Association* **205**, 65–68

Nieckarz JA and Daniel GB (2001) The effect of methimazole on thyroid uptake of pertechnetate and radioiodine in normal cats. *Veterinary Radiology & Ultrasound* **42**, 448–457

Norsworthy GD, Adams VJ, McElhaney MR and Milios JA (2002) Relationship between semi-quantitative thyroid palpation and total thyroxine concentration in cats with and without hyperthyroidism. *Journal of Feline Medicine & Surgery* **4**, 139–143

Paepe D, Smets P, van Hoek I, Saunders J and Duchateau L (2008) Within- and between-examiner agreement for two thyroid palpation techniques in healthy and hyperthyroid cats. *Journal of Feline Medicine & Surgery* **10**, 558–565

Papasouliotis K, Muir P, Gruffydd-Jones TJ *et al.* (1993) Decreased orocaecal transit time, as measured by the exhalation of hydrogen in hyperthyroid cats. *Research in Veterinary Science* **55**, 115–118

Peterson ME and Becker DV (1995) Radioiodine treatment of 524 cats with hyperthyroidism. *Journal of the American Veterinary Medical Association* **207**, 1422–1428

Peterson ME, Graves TK and Cavanagh I (1987) Serum thyroid hormone concentrations fluctuate in cats with hyperthyroidism. *Journal of Veterinary Internal Medicine* **1**, 142–146

Peterson ME, Keene B, Ferguson DC and Pipers FS (1982) Electrocardiographic findings in 45 cats with hyperthyroidism. *Journal of the American Veterinary Medical Association* **180**, 934–937

Peterson ME, Kintzer PP, Cavanagh PG *et al.* (1981) Feline hyperthyroidism: pretreatment clinical and laboratory evaluation of 131 cases. *Journal of the American Veterinary Medical Association* **183**, 103–110

Peterson ME, Kintzer PP and Hurvitz AI (1988) Methimazole treatment of 262 cats with hyperthyroidism. *Journal of Veterinary Internal Medicine* **2**, 150–157

Peterson ME, Melian C and Nichols R (2001) Measurement of serum concentrations of free thyroxine, total thyroxine, and total triiodothyronine in cats with hyperthyroidism and cats with nonthyroidal disease. *Journal of the American Veterinary Medical Association* **218**, 529–536

Peterson ME and Ward CR (2007) Etiopathologic findings of hyperthyroidism in cats. *Veterinary Clinics of North America: Small Animal Practice* **37**, 633–645

Reusch CE and Tomsa K (1999) Serum fructosamine concentration in cats with overt hyperthyroidism. *Journal of the American Veterinary Medical Association* **215**, 1297–1300

Riensche MR, Graves TK and Schaeffer DJ (2008) An investigation of predictors of renal insufficiency following treatment of hyperthyroidism in cats. *Journal of Feline Medicine & Surgery* **10**, 160–166

Rutland BE, Nachreiner RF and Kruger JM (2009) Optimal testing for thyroid hormone concentration after treatment with methimazole in healthy and hyperthyroid cats. *Journal of Veterinary Internal Medicine* **23**, 1025–1039

Sartor LL, Trepanier LA, Kroll MM, Rodan I and Challoner L (2004) Efficacy and safety of transdermal methimazole in the treatment of cats with hyperthyroidism. *Journal of Veterinary Internal Medicine* **18**, 651–655

Schlesinger DP, Rubin SI, Papich MG and Hamilton DL (1993) Use of breath hydrogen measurement to evaluate orocecal transit time in cats before and after treatment for hyperthyroidism. *Canadian Veterinary Journal* **57**, 89–94

Shiel RE and Mooney CT (2007) Testing for hyperthyroidism in cats. *Veterinary Clinics of North America: Small Animal Practice* **37**, 671–691

Slater MR, Komkov A, Robinson LE and Hightower D (1994) Long-term follow-up of hyperthyroid cats treated with iodine-131. *Veterinary Radiology & Ultrasound* **35**, 204–209

Syme HM (2007) Cardiovascular and renal manifestations of hyperthyroidism. *Veterinary Clinics of North America: Small Animal Practice* **37**, 723–743

Thoday KL and Mooney CT (1992) Historical, clinical and laboratory features of 126 hyperthyroid cats. *Veterinary Record* **131**, 257–264

Tomsa K, Glaus TM, Kacl GM, Pospischil A and Reusch CE (2001) Thyrotropin-releasing hormone stimulation test to assess thyroid function in severely sick cats. *Journal of Veterinary Internal Medicine* **15**, 89–93

Trepanier LA (2007) Pharmacologic management of feline hyperthyroidism. *Veterinary Clinics of North America: Small Animal Practice* **37**, 775–788

Trepanier LA, Hoffman SB, Knoll M, Rodan I and Challoner L (2003) Efficacy and safety of once versus twice daily administration of methimazole in cats with hyperthyroidism. *Journal of the American Veterinary Medical Association* **222**, 954–958

Turrel JM, Feldman EC, Nelson RW and Cain GR (1988) Thyroid carcinoma causing hyperthyroidism in cats: 14 cases (1981–1986). *Journal of the American Veterinary Medical Association* **193**, 359–364

Van Hoek I, Vandermeulen E, Peremans K and Daminet S (2010) Thyroid stimulation with recombinant human thyrotropin in healthy cats, cats with non-thyroidal illness and in cats with low serum thyroxin and azotaemia after treatment of hyperthyroidism. *Journal of Feline Medicine & Surgery* **12**, 117–121

Wakeling J, Elliott J and Syme H (2011) Evaluation of predictors for the diagnosis of hyperthyroidism in cats. *Journal of Veterinary Internal Medicine* **25**, 1056–1057

Wakeling J, Everard A, Brodbelt D, Elliott J and Syme H (2009) Risk factors for feline hyperthyroidism in the UK. *Journal of Small Animal Practice*, **50**, 406–414

Wakeling J, Moore K, Elliott J and Syme H (2008) Diagnosis of hyperthyroidism in cats with mild chronic kidney disease. *Journal of Small Animal Practice* **49**, 287–294

Wakeling J, Smith K and Scase T (2007) Subclinical hyperthyroidism in cats: a spontaneous model of subclinical toxic nodular goitre in humans. *Thyroid* **17**, 1201–1209

Weichselbaum RC, Feeney DA and Jessen CR (2005) Relationship between selected echocardiographic variables before and after radioiodine treatment in 91 hyperthyroid cats. *Veterinary Radiology & Ultrasound* **46**, 506–513

Wells AL, Long CD, Hornof WJ *et al.* (2001) Use of percutaneous ethanol injection for treatment of bilateral hyperplastic thyroid nodules in cats. *Journal of the American Veterinary Medical Association* **218**, 1293–1297

Williams TL, Elliott J and Syme HM (2010a) Association of iatrogenic hypothyroidism with azotemia and reduced survival time in cats treated for hyperthyroidism. *Journal of Veterinary Internal Medicine* **24**, 1086–1092

Williams TL, Peak KJ, Brodbelt D, Elliott J and Syme HM (2010b) Survival and the development of azotemia after treatment of hyperthyroid cats. *Journal of Veterinary Internal Medicine* **24**, 863—869

Wisner ER, Theon AP, Nyland TG and Hornof WJ (1994) Ultrasonographic examination of the thyroid gland of hyperthyroid cats: comparison to $^{99m}TcO_4^-$ scintigraphy. *Veterinary Radiology and Ultrasound* **35**, 53–58

11

Feline hypothyroidism

Sylvie Daminet

Introduction

Iatrogenic, congenital and spontaneous adult-onset hypothyroidism have all been described in cats, albeit rarely. Practitioners are likely to be confronted with iatrogenic hypothyroidism as a consequence of over-treating hyperthyroidism. There are a few well documented reports of congenital feline hypothyroidism, although this is considered rare. Its true frequency remains unknown but is likely to be underestimated and/or misdiagnosed. Finally, spontaneous adult-onset feline hypothyroidism, although recognized, is even less frequently described.

Aetiology

Iatrogenic hypothyroidism

Iatrogenic hypothyroidism is a well recognized complication of all available treatment options for hyperthyroidism. It can result from an overdose of anti-thyroid drug administration, bilateral thyroidectomy or radioactive iodine (^{131}I) therapy.

The aim of anti-thyroid administration is to maintain serum total thyroxine (T4) concentrations within the lower half of the reference interval. Until recently it was assumed that cats with T4 values below the reference interval would rarely become clinically hypothyroid. This is most likely because concentrations of total triiodothyronine (T3), the biologically active hormone, tend to remain within the reference interval. However, one recent study suggests that cats with iatrogenic hypothyroidism are more likely to develop azotaemia and have reduced survival times (Williams *et al.*, 2010), suggesting that iatrogenic hypothyroidism, documented by decreased T4 and increased thyroid-stimulating hormone (TSH; thyrotropin) serum concentrations (measured using a canine TSH assay), should be avoided.

After thyroidectomy, total T4 concentrations often decrease below the reference interval for weeks to months. Most cats do not develop clinical signs of hypothyroidism and total T4 concentration usually normalizes eventually. Stimulation of the contralateral lobe (in the case of unilateral thyroidectomy) or ectopic thyroid tissue (in the case of bilateral surgery) serves to compensate for the thyroid tissue removed.

Up to 30% of hyperthyroid cats treated with ^{131}I are reported to develop iatrogenic hypothyroidism after treatment (Nykamp *et al.*, 2005). This percentage is possibly overestimated, as the diagnosis was based on decreased T4 serum concentrations alone (see diagnosis). Cats with a bilateral scintigraphic pattern on a ^{99m}Tc– pertechnetate scan appear predisposed to the development of hypothyroidism after treatment with ^{131}I (Nykamp *et al.*, 2005).

Congenital hypothyroidism

In general, congenital primary hypothyroidism can be divided into two main categories: thyroid dyshormonogenesis (a defect in the biosynthesis of thyroid hormones); and thyroid dysmorphogenesis (thyroid hypoplasia or aplasia). Both forms usually have a genetic background in humans and are inherited as autosomal recessive traits. With dyshormonogenesis, decreased negative feedback to the pituitary and hypothalamus results in increased secretion of TSH and, consequently, thyroid gland hyperplasia. Therefore, an enlarged thyroid gland (goitre) can be observed. In contrast, dysmorphogenesis leads to a non-goitrous form of congenital hypothyroidism.

Dyshormonogenesis, due to defective thyroid peroxidase activity and impaired iodine organification, has been described in related Domestic Shorthair and Abyssinian cats (Sjollema *et al.*, 1991; Jones *et al.*, 1992). Thyroid dysmorphogenesis has also been documented in related cats (Traas *et al.*, 2008). All of these reports suggest an autosomal recessive mode of inheritance.

In addition, hypothyroidism as a result of TSH resistance has been suggested in a family of Japanese cats (Tanase *et al.*, 1991). However, hypothalamic and pituitary forms of congenital hypothyroidism (central hypothyroidism) have not yet been reported in cats.

Spontaneous adult-onset hypothyroidism

Although there are anecdotal reports, only two well documented cases of spontaneous acquired primary hypothyroidism have been described (Rand *et al.*, 1993; Blois *et al.*, 2009). In one case, thyroid biopsy identified marked lymphocytic infiltration, similar to the lymphocytic thyroiditis observed in dogs. In the second case, idiopathic atrophy of the thyroid gland was suspected.

Clinical features

The most important clinical features observed in iatrogenic, congenital and spontaneous-onset hypothyroidism are outlined in Figure 11.1. Although many signs are similar to those in hypothyroid dogs, there are significant differences that must be considered. Firstly, few hypothyroid cats, irrespective of underlying cause, develop a clear alopecia. Furthermore, inappetence is possible, as is profound mental dullness. Kittens with congenital hypothyroidism can develop severe constipation.

Adult-onset hypothyroidism (iatrogenic and spontaneous)

Lethargy, inappetence and skin changes are the major clinical signs observed (Figure 11.2). Lethargy and inappetence can become severe over time. Dermatological signs are characterized by a dull, dry and unkempt haircoat (with possible matting) and seborrhoea sicca. Alopecia of the pinnae can develop in some cats. The haircoat is easily epilated and poor regrowth after clipping is possible. Hypothermia and bradycardia may be additional findings on physical examination.

In spontaneous hypothyroidism, signs are often very pronounced, which might reflect the delayed diagnosis. A puffy face, presumably resulting from myxoedema was reported in one cat (Rand *et al.*, 1993).

Congenital hypothyroidism

Many of the signs observed in adult-onset hypothyroidism can also be present in affected kittens. However, thyroid hormones are essential for normal postnatal development of the skeletal and nervous systems. Therefore, congenital hypothyroidism is characterized by disproportionate dwarfism and by neurological abnormalities.

Typically, affected kittens appear normal at birth but a decrease in growth rate, compared to their littermates, becomes evident by 2 months of age. Disproportionate dwarfism develops over the next

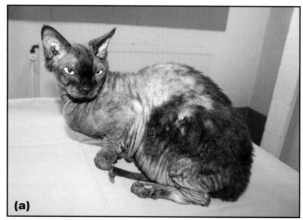

(a)

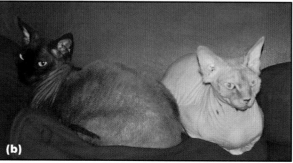

(b)

11.2 **(a)** This 5-year-old male neutered Devon Rex cat was presented with a history of lethargy, mental dullness and inappetence. The cat also had diabetes mellitus. This patient had a very low circulating total thyroxine concentration, as well as an increased canine TSH concentration, confirming primary hypothyroidism. There was a seborrhoeic hair coat that was easily epilated; note the bilateral ceruminous otitis. (Courtesy of E. Mercier and S. Daminet) **(b)** The same patient (on the left), one year before the onset of clinical signs of hypothyroidism.

few months, characterized by large broad heads, small ears, a round body and short necks and limbs. Additionally, affected kittens are generally mentally dull and may suffer from severe recurrent episodes of constipation. Sometimes dullness and retarded growth may go unrecognized by the owners, who present their cat because of recurrent

Clinical sign	Iatrogenic hypothyroidism	Congenital hypothyroidism	Spontaneous adult-onset hypothyroidism
Lethargy	+	+ (even mental dullness)	+ (even mental dullness)
Weight gain or obesity	+	+	+
Inappetence	+	+	+[a]
Constipation	+	+[a] (even megacolon)	+
Goitre	– or +	Possible	–
Disproportionate dwarfism	–	+[a]	–
Delayed closure of growth plates (on radiography)	–	+[a]	–
Dermatological signs (especially seborrhoea and ease of epilation)	+	+	+[a]

11.1 A summary of the most important clinical features observed with iatrogenic, congenital and spontaneous-onset hypothyroidism. Clinical features can be mild or severe. [a] indicates a key feature; + = usually present; – = absent.

constipation. Recently, seizures were reported as a major problem in two littermates affected by congenital hypothyroidism (Traas *et al.*, 2008).

Although hair is usually present all over the body and obvious alopecia is not present, the haircoat consists mainly of undercoat with few guard hairs. The teeth are underdeveloped and a delay in tooth eruption and the replacement of deciduous teeth is frequently observed. On physical examination, hypothermia, bradycardia and sometimes palpable goitre (with organification defects) may be detected.

Survival of untreated affected kittens depends largely on the aetiology of the congenital hypothyroidism. It is likely that many affected kittens die undiagnosed as part of the 'fading kitten' syndrome. Affected kittens can die within a few months. However, kittens suffering from a partial thyroid peroxidase activity defect can live to become adult cats without obvious clinical signs of the disease.

Diagnosis

The diagnosis of feline hypothyroidism can be challenging, regardless of the underlying cause. As in dogs, a presumptive diagnosis can be made based on a combination of compatible clinical features and occasionally supportive abnormalities on routine clinicopathological analyses (anaemia and hypercholesterolaemia). Hypothyroidism must be confirmed by hormone testing or medical imaging such as scintigraphy.

Even for iatrogenic hypothyroidism a few diagnostic pitfalls exist, despite the obvious previous or current history of therapy for hyperthyroidism. First, the concomitant presence of other diseases in those geriatric cats is not uncommon (e.g. chronic kidney disease) and can result in the so-called euthyroid sick syndrome (see below). More importantly, normalization of activity level (often manifested as a decrease) and some weight gain is expected with successful treatment of hyperthyroidism. Therefore, the clinical signs of iatrogenic hypothyroidism and the expected return to a euthyroid status can overlap somewhat. After therapy with ^{131}I, many cats develop a marked decrease in total T4, which is mostly transient, and a euthyroid status is usually expected after approximately 6 months. Some studies report up to 30% of cats with iatrogenic hypothyroidism following treatment with [131]I (Nykamp *et al.*, 2005). Many of these cats do not show relevant clinical signs of hypothyroidism; therefore, it is debatable whether they have true hypothyroidism or a transiently decreased total T4 concentration.

It is advisable to wait 6 months before making a definitive diagnosis of iatrogenic hypothyroidism after therapy with ^{131}I, especially if clinical signs of hypothyroidism are not convincing. It was recently shown that hypothyroidism in dogs leads to a decrease in glomerular filtration rate (Gommeren *et al.*, 2009); this has not yet been investigated in cats, but similar effects are expected. Treatment of hyperthyroidism already profoundly affects renal function, and it would therefore seem advisable to diagnose

hypothyroidism early in affected cats. Left untreated, hypothyroidism potentially has further adverse effects upon renal function. This underlines the importance of obtaining a definitive diagnosis in these cats.

Spontaneous (congenital and adult-onset) hypothyroidism is probably underdiagnosed because of the rarity of the disease. Kittens often appear normal at birth and the onset of typical features such as disproportionate dwarfism is often delayed. Some kittens die early or could be misdiagnosed as having idiopathic megacolon or other skeletal abnormalities.

Routine clinicopathological features

Although the exact incidence of mild normochromic normocytic anaemia and/or hypercholesterolaemia in feline hypothyroidism is not known, these changes seem to be observed more frequently with iatrogenic hypothyroidism. In congenital hypothyroidism, these changes are inconsistent (Traas *et al.*, 2009).

Thyroid hormone concentrations

Total T4

Low circulating total T4 concentrations are expected in all cases of feline hypothyroidism, and a total T4 value within reference intervals strongly supports euthyroidism.

Reference intervals for thyroid hormones have not been well established in kittens. In one study, and in contrast to puppies, kitten total T4 values approached the upper limit of the adult reference interval but did not exceed that range (Zerbe *et al.*, 1998).

As in dogs, total T4 can also be suppressed by non-thyroidal illnesses (NTIs) in cats (Peterson *et al.*, 2001). In fact, the more severe the systemic illness, the lower the total T4 concentration expected. Therefore, a decreased basal total T4 does not equate with a diagnosis of hypothyroidism. In dogs, many drugs, such as glucocorticoids, phenobarbital and sulphonamides, have been shown to suppress total T4 serum concentrations significantly (Daminet and Ferguson, 2003), but this has not yet been investigated in cats.

Because spontaneous primary hypothyroidism is rare in cats and the 'euthyroid sick syndrome' is frequently observed, the diagnosis of primary spontaneous hypothyroidism should not be based solely on basal total T4 values. Additional tests, such as serum canine TSH (cTSH) measurement, recombinant human TSH (rhTSH) response test or thyroid scintigraphy, are indicated to confirm the disease.

Free T4

In dogs, the use of free T4 measured by equilibrium dialysis has been shown to be of benefit as it has better specificity for the diagnosis of hypothyroidism compared to measurement of basal total T4. However, in cats, it has been shown that of cats with NTIs, 6–12% have increased free T4 and 3–17% have decreased free T4 concentrations, limiting the use of free T4 in investigating hypothyroidism in cats (Mooney *et al.*, 1996; Peterson *et al.*, 2001).

Endogenous TSH

In dogs with hypothyroidism, an increased TSH serum concentration confirms that the disease is primary (located within the thyroid gland). A specific assay for feline TSH measurement is not yet available, although the use of the canine immunoradio-metric assay in cats has recently been described (Wakeling *et al.*, 2008). In another recent case, and as expected, an increased cTSH concentration was observed in a cat with primary adult-onset hypothyroidism (Blois *et al.*, 2009). Although there are currently no studies that have evaluated the use of cTSH in the diagnosis of iatrogenic hypothyroidism, increased cTSH concentrations are expected. Despite the limitations of using cTSH concentrations for diagnosing hyperthyroidism (see Chapter 10), this method is already used by many endocrinologists. This is because it provides greater evidence for a diagnosis of iatrogenic hypothyroidism when levels are elevated, particularly as clinical iatrogenic hypothyroidism does not appear to be common. Additionally, the use of cTSH (and hopefully feline TSH in the near future) should be helpful in discriminating congenital primary from secondary hypothyroidism (TSH deficiency).

Dynamic thyroid function tests

In the past, bovine TSH and TRH response tests were used to diagnose hypothyroidism in cats. Nowadays, bovine TSH is no longer available. Additionally, it has been found that TRH stimulation leads to a less marked increase in total T4 than does TSH, is more prone to the influence of severe non-thyroidal illness and leads to unpleasant side effects (nausea, vomiting). Therefore, these tests are no longer recommended.

Recently, the use of the rhTSH response test has been described in cats to distinguish NTI from iatrogenic hypothyroidism following ^{131}I therapy (van Hoek *et al.*, 2009). Although it was evaluated in a limited number of feline patients, just as in dogs it appears to provide a valuable alternative to bovine TSH stimulation.

The following protocol can be used to perform rhTSH stimulation test in cats:

1. A blood sample is collected for basal total T4 measurement.
2. 25 μg rhTSH is administered i.v.
3. A second blood sample is taken 6 hours later.

rhTSH vials can be split into aliquots and stored frozen to make this test more affordable (De Roover *et al.*, 2006).

Diagnostic imaging

Radiography

As in dogs, radiography can be particularly useful to diagnose congenital hypothyroidism, as the changes observed are pathognomonic. Radiographs demonstrate retarded skeletal development, particularly epiphyseal dysgenesis of vertebral bodies and long bones.

Thyroid scintigraphy

Uptake of technetium as pertechnetate ($^{99m}TcO_4^-$) has traditionally been used for the diagnosis of canine hypothyroidism or feline hyperthyroidism. Although there are few studies, it may also become an important tool for diagnosing feline hypothyroidism. It might be especially useful in patients where the diagnosis of feline hypothyroidism is unclear, for example in cats with concomitant disease (euthyroid sick syndrome). The expected finding in adult-onset hypothyroidism is a reduction or absence of uptake of pertechnetate by the thyroid glands (Figure 11.3). Recently, thyroid scintigraphy was used as a non-invasive technique to confirm the diagnosis of spontaneous hypothyroidism in one cat (Blois *et al.*,

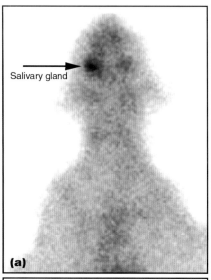

Salivary gland

(a)

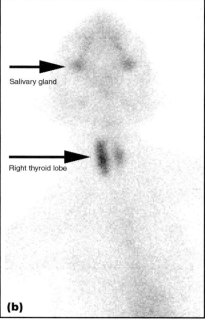

Salivary gland

Right thyroid lobe

(b)

11.3 **(a)** Ventral view of a thyroid scintigraphic scan from the cat in Figure 11.2. Note the uptake of pertechnetate in the salivary glands (arrowed) and the absence of uptake in the cervical (thyroid) region. (Courtesy of K. Peremans) **(b)** For illustration purposes, this figure shows the increased uptake of pertechnetate visible in the thyroid glands of a hyperthyroid cat (arrowed). (Courtesy of K. Peremans)

2009). Further scintigraphy with ^{123}I can be a helpful diagnostic tool to clarify the underlying mechanism in congenital hypothyroidism. In cases of dysmorphogenesis, an absence of uptake of ^{123}I is expected. Uptake of ^{123}I may be normal in cases with a thyroid peroxidase deficiency. However, organification (incorporation of iodine) is deficient and abnormal discharge of ^{123}I is observed after administration of perchlorate (perchlorate discharge test).

In the past, practitioners have often used a trial therapy with levothyroxine to diagnose feline hypothyroidism. Unfortunately, response to treatment does not mean the cat is truly hypothyroid. Using a combination of total T4 and cTSH measurements is probably the most efficient and economic way of diagnosing primary hypothyroidism. When results are equivocal, further diagnostic tests such as rhTSH stimulation test or scintigraphy should be considered before initiating trial therapy with levothyroxine.

Treatment

Although pharmacokinetic data are only available for healthy cats, recommended dosages for oral thyroxine supplementation vary between 100 µg/cat q24h and 10–20 µg/kg q24h. As in dogs, affected cats should be re-evaluated after 4–8 weeks. Further adjustment of therapy should be based on clinical response and total T4 therapeutic monitoring. With appropriate therapy, prognosis is excellent in acquired hypothyroidism. For congenital hypothyroidism, prognosis is guarded and will largely depend on the underlying aetiology of the hypothyroidism and age at diagnosis.

References and further reading

Blois SL, Abrams-Ogg ACG, Mitchell C *et al.* (2009) Use of thyroid scintigraphy and pituitary immunochemistry in the diagnosis of spontaneous hypothyroidism in a mature cat. *Journal of Feline Medicine and Surgery* **12**, 156–60

Daminet S and Ferguson DC (2003) Influence of drugs on thyroid function in dogs. *Journal of Veterinary Internal Medicine* **17**, 663–472

De Roover K, Duchateau L, Carmichael N, van Geffen C *et al.* (2006) Effect of storage of reconstituted recombinant human thyroid-stimulating hormone (rhTSH) on thyroid-stimulating hormone (TSH) response testing in euthyroid dogs. *Journal of Veterinary Internal Medicine* **20**, 812–817

Gommeren K, van Hoek I, Lefebvre HP *et al.* (2009) Effect of thyroxine supplementation on glomerular filtration rate in hypothyroid dogs. *Journal of Veterinary Internal Medicine* **23**, 844–849

Jones BR, Gruffydd-Jones TJ, Sparkes AH *et al.* (1992) Preliminary studies on congenital hypothyroidism in a family of Abyssinian cats. *Veterinary Record* **131**, 145–148

Mooney CT, Little CJL and Macrae AW (1996) Effect of illness not associated with the thyroid gland on serum total and free thyroxine concentrations in cats. *Journal of the American Veterinary Medical Association* **208**, 2004–2008

Nykamp SG, Dykes NL, Zarfoss MK *et al.* (2005) Association of the risk of development of hypothyroidism after iodine 131 treatment with the pretreatment pattern of sodium pertechnetate Tc 99m uptake in the thyroid gland in cats with hyperthyroidism: 165 cases (1990–2002) *Journal of the American Veterinary Medical Association* **226**, 1671–1675

Peterson ME, Melian C and Nichols R (2001) Measurement of serum concentrations of free thyroxine, total thyroxine, and total triiodothyronine in cats with hyperthyroidism and cats with nonthyroidal disease. *Journal of the American Veterinary Medical Association* **218**, 529–536

Rand JS, Levine J, Best SJ *et al.* (1993) Spontaneous adult-onset hypothyroidism in a cat. *Journal of Veterinary Internal Medicine* **7**, 272–276

Sjollema BE, Denhartog MT, Devijlder JJM *et al.* (1991) Congenital hypothyroidism in 2 cats due to defective organification – data suggesting loosely anchored thyroperoxidase. *Acta Endocrinologica* **125**, 435–440

Tanase H, Kudo K, Horikoshi H *et al.* (1991) Inherited primary hypothyroidism with thyrotropin resistance in Japanese cats. *Journal of Endocrinology* **129**, 245–251

Traas AM, Abbot BL, French A and Giger U (2008) Congenital thyroid hypoplasia and seizures in 2 littermate kittens. *Journal of Veterinary Internal Medicine* **22**, 1427–1431

Van Hoek IM, Vandermeulen E, Peremans K *et al.* (2009) Thyroid stimulation with recombinant human thyrotropin in healthy cats, cats with non-thyroidal illness and in cats with low serum thyroxin and azotaemia after treatment of hyperthyroidism. *Journal of Feline Medicine and Surgery* **12**, 117–121

Wakeling J, Moore K, Elliott J *et al.* (2008) Diagnosis of hyperthyroidism in cats with mild chronic kidney disease. *Journal of Small Animal Practice* **49**, 287–294

Williams TL, Elliot J and Syme HM (2010) Association of iatrogenic hypothyroidism with azotemia and reduced survival time in cats treated for hyperthyroidism. *Journal of Veterinary Internal Medicine* **24**, 1086–1092

Zerbe CA, Casal ML, Jezyk PF *et al.* (1998) Thyroid profiles in healthy kittens from birth to 12 weeks of age. *Proceedings, Forum of Veterinary Internal Medicine*, p.212 [abstract]

12

Canine diabetes mellitus

Lucy J. Davison

Introduction

Canine diabetes mellitus (DM) is a common endocrinopathy, characterized by relative or absolute deficiency of the hormone insulin. It is not a single disease, but rather can arise as the result of several different pathophysiological mechanisms, converging on a similar set of clinical signs.

The last 10 years have seen an increase in knowledge of the factors underlying canine diabetes and its pathogenesis, although many questions remain unanswered. This chapter will review current knowledge, including pathogenesis and management, with a particular focus on recent findings that have a direct clinical impact. A general protocol for management of the newly diagnosed patient will also be outlined, with investigation of the unstable diabetic dog being discussed in Chapter 22.

Prevalence and epidemiology

The most recent survey of diabetes in the UK canine population reported a prevalence of DM of 0.32%, based on insurance database records (Davison *et al.*, 2005). An increasing incidence of diabetes in the global canine population is suggested by the fact that the proportion of diabetic dogs referred to second-opinion veterinary hospitals in the USA has increased from 19 to 64 per 10,000 patients over the past 30 years (Guptill *et al.*, 2003). This, however, could also be related to improvements in diagnosis and management of diabetes by first-opinion veterinary practitioners, a greater willingness to refer problem diabetic cases and an increase in commitment by owners of diabetic dogs to pursue therapy.

Aetiology and classification of disease

Insulin is usually secreted in response to an increase in circulating concentration of glucose (and amino acids) and is antagonized by several other hormones, including glucagon. As the presence of insulin allows glucose to be transported into cells from the blood, reduction in the amount or activity of this hormone results in an impaired ability to control blood glucose and hence hyperglycaemia. In the healthy animal, insulin is produced by the pancreas, an organ that contains both exocrine and endocrine tissue. The exocrine cells produce enzymes, such as trypsin, for digestion of food in the small intestine. The endocrine tissue, found in the islets of Langerhans scattered through the pancreas, produces hormones which are released into the circulation. Pancreatic beta cells constitute 60–80% of each islet and it is these cells that are responsible for the synthesis of insulin, and whose destruction or dysfunction can lead to diabetes. Other endocrine cell types in the islets include delta cells, which secrete somatostatin, and alpha cells, which secrete glucagon – a hormone that counteracts the effects of insulin. Islet cells can become exhausted in the face of persistent hyperglycaemia, although they have a capacity to recover once blood glucose has normalized. If islet damage is sustained, however, it becomes irreversible, since pancreatic islet cells have no capacity to regenerate.

In both humans and dogs, diabetes is a multifactorial disease, thought to involve genetic factors (Redondo and Eisenbarth, 2002; Rand *et al.*, 2004) and environmental factors such as diet and infectious organisms (Fleeman and Rand, 2001; Hoenig, 2002; Catchpole *et al.*, 2005). As multiple pathological processes can lead to canine diabetes, various classification systems have been proposed, but there is no universally accepted system in veterinary medicine. Human diabetes was initially classified into insulin-dependent (IDDM) and non- insulin-dependent disease (NIDDM), according to the patient's requirement for exogenous insulin therapy, but this system has now been replaced by classification based on pathophysiology. Classification by insulin dependency is not helpful in the canine patient, since all diabetic dogs are insulin-dependent, with a few exceptions (Catchpole *et al.*, 2005). A more useful classification, therefore, is that which describes DM according to the underlying disease process (Figure 12.1) (Catchpole *et al.*, 2005, 2008). Such classification also has practical relevance, since the underlying cause of the diabetes can impact significantly on the glycaemic control that might be reasonably expected. Four of the most common categories of disease aetiology are discussed in more detail below.

Insulin deficiency diabetes
Insulin deficiency in dogs is characterized by a loss of pancreatic beta cells. The aetiology of beta cell deficiency/destruction in diabetic dogs is currently unknown but a number of disease processes are thought to be involved: • Congenital beta cell hypoplasia/abiotrophy • Beta cell loss associated with pancreatitis • Immune-mediated beta cell destruction • Beta cell exhaustion/glucose toxicity as a consequence of prolonged insulin resistance (see below).
Insulin resistance diabetes

Insulin resistance usually results from antagonism of insulin function by other hormones and can also be exacerbated by the presence of infection or inflammation.
 	
• Dioestrous diabetes.
• Other forms of hormonal antagonism:
  – Secondary to hyperadrenocorticism
  – Secondary to acromegaly (rare).
• Iatrogenic:
  – Synthetic glucocorticoids
  – Synthetic progestogens.
• Carbohydrate intolerance associated with obesity.
• Insulin receptor defects such as those seen in humans might exist in canine diabetic patients, although these have not so far been reported.

12.1 Proposed veterinary classification for canine diabetes mellitus.

Congenital or juvenile canine diabetes mellitus

There are occasional reports of DM in dogs <6 months of age. Pancreatic histopathology is variable in these cases, but usually few islets are visible and those beta cells that are present are degenerate and vacuolated (Minkus *et al.,* 1997). In a study of four dogs with juvenile-onset DM, the histopathology was consistent with congenital islet cell aplasia (Atkins *et al.,* 1979). An inherited, early-onset form of diabetes characterized by abiotrophy of pancreatic beta cells has been reported in Keeshonds. Mating studies demonstrated that the condition was likely to result from an autosomal recessive mutation, although the precise genetic defect has not been fully elucidated (Kramer *et al.,* 1988). It is also possible that insulin receptor defects exist in young canine DM patients, although these have not so far been reported. Dogs with congenital DM can be successfully managed with insulin therapy, and although the establishment of good glycaemic control in the growing animal is challenging, it is not impossible.

Hormonal antagonism

Some canine patients become clinically diabetic because of the presence of circulating hormones that are antagonistic to insulin, and comparisons with both type 2 and gestational diabetes in humans have been made. Gestational diabetes has been reported in dogs (Fall *et al.,* 2008b) but another potentially common example of hormonal antagonism is the progesterone-dominated phase of dioestrus in entire female dogs (Eigenmann *et al.,* 1983; Rijnberk *et al.,* 1993). Dogs are non-seasonally

mono-oestrous; following oestrus all normal bitches enter a luteal phase (dioestrus) lasting around 60 days. As well as the potential diabetogenic effect of progesterone during dioestrus, by a physiological mechanism unique to dogs, growth hormone is synthesized in the mammary glands and released into the circulation, also counteracting the action of insulin. This results in glucose intolerance, which can progress to overt diabetes in a proportion of patients. Although, theoretically, immediate ovariohysterectomy could result in a clinical cure in these patients, the beta cells may be left irreversibly exhausted, in which case ongoing therapy with exogenous insulin is required.

It also follows that glycaemic control is difficult to achieve with insulin therapy in entire female diabetic dogs, due to the varying degrees of insulin resistance during the oestrous cycle. It is therefore recommended that all female dogs are neutered as soon as possible after diagnosis of diabetes. In addition, it has been reported that pyometra in entire bitches and obesity in older dogs are both associated with hyperinsulinaemia and glucose intolerance, although there are no reported cases of diabetes in dogs arising as a direct result of obesity (Mattheeuws *et al.,* 1984).

Another hormone that antagonizes insulin is cortisol, a corticosteroid hormone produced by the adrenal cortex. Dogs with hyperadrenocorticism, usually associated with a tumour of the pituitary gland or adrenal gland, have elevated serum cortisol concentrations, and are at risk of concurrent diabetes (Hess *et al.,* 2003). Functional studies of the endocrine pancreas in non-diabetic dogs with hyperadrenocorticism have demonstrated elevated serum insulin concentrations before and after stimulation with intravenous glucagon (Montgomery *et al.,* 1996). Theoretically, diabetes caused by hyperadrenocorticism can be transient and the animal's glucose homeostasis could return to normal when the primary disease has been adequately controlled (Hoenig, 2002). However, diabetic dogs with well controlled hyperadrenocorticism usually still require insulin therapy, with poorly controlled hyperadrenocorticism often necessitating an increase in insulin dose.

The proportion of diabetes in dogs caused by hormonal antagonism is uncertain, since many cases of hyperadrenocorticism may be undiagnosed and the number of entire female dogs in the UK is reducing due to an increase in elective neutering. One study reported that 34% of all diabetic dogs referred to the University of Glasgow Veterinary School had hyperadrenocorticism or dioestrus diabetes (Graham, 1995). In a cohort of 221 diabetic dogs from the University of Pennsylvania, 50 dogs (22%) were reported to have evidence of concurrent adrenocortical dysfunction (abnormal low-dose dexamethasone suppression test and/or ACTH stimulation test) (Hess *et al.,* 2000a). In another study of 60 dogs with confirmed hyperadrenocorticism, 23 were hyperglycaemic with moderate to severe hyperinsulinaemia and 5 were suffering from overt DM with a relative insulin deficiency (Peterson *et al.,* 1984).

One way in which insulin resistance and hence pancreatic 'reserve' can be evaluated in newly diagnosed canine patients with suspected hormonal antagonism is to perform an intravenous glucagon stimulation test (Montgomery *et al.,* 1996; Watson and Herrtage, 2004; Fall *et al.,* 2008a). This test evaluates serum insulin or insulin C-peptide (co-secreted with endogenous insulin and not cross-reactive with injected insulin in insulin assays) secreted in response to an intravenous test dose of glucagon. A subnormal response indicates pancreatic exhaustion and insulin deficiency, whereas a supranormal response, particularly in a hyperglycaemic animal, implies insulin resistance due to hormonal antagonism.

Pancreatitis

It has become increasingly clear that the inflammation of pancreatic exocrine tissue can also result in damage to the beta cells, leading to insulin-dependent diabetes mellitus. Canine pancreatitis exists in an acute form, characterized by vomiting and abdominal pain, and a chronic form, which can be more difficult to diagnose because of its more subtle clinical signs. When the pancreas becomes inflamed, digestive enzyme precursors (e.g. trypsinogen) are cleaved inside pancreatic acinar cells rather than in the small intestine, so that active enzymes (e.g. trypsin) are released within the pancreas, causing local tissue damage. These enzymes are regulated by proteases such as α_2-macroglobulin that become depleted in pancreatitis.

Obese, older, female, small-breed dogs and spaniels are thought to be at increased risk of pancreatitis. However, the reason why some dogs suffer from acute disease whereas others suffer from chronic disease is not known (Watson *et al.,* 2007). Similarly, the reason why some dogs with pancreatitis develop diabetes whereas others maintain good glucose tolerance remains to be established. Preliminary findings indicate that some dogs suffering from chronic pancreatitis have reduced beta cell function on glucagon-stimulation testing (Watson and Herrtage, 2004), and in some patients it is possible that clinical signs of diabetes could be the first indication of a subclinical, low-grade pancreatitis.

A diagnosis of pancreatitis has an important clinical impact in a diabetic patient, as it can prove more difficult to achieve good glycaemic control in dogs whose diabetes occurs as a result of pancreatitis. As early as 1971, one study reported that 6 of 10 diabetic dogs examined postmortem had histological evidence of pancreatitis (Cotton *et al.,* 1971), and that dogs with clinical or biochemical evidence of pancreatitis in addition to their diabetes had a worse prognosis. A higher prevalence of acute and chronic pancreatitis in non-surviving diabetic patients compared to diabetic dogs who had been well controlled and were euthanased for other reasons was demonstrated in a separate study (Ling *et al.,* 1977). More recently, serum biochemical or histopathological evidence of pancreatitis has been reported to be present in 28–40% of diabetic dogs (Alejandro *et al.,* 1988), and post-mortem

histopathological studies suggest that the prevalence of chronic pancreatitis in the canine population as a whole may be underestimated by clinicians (Watson *et al.,* 2007).

Another important potential clinical implication of chronic pancreatitis is the development of exocrine pancreatic insufficiency (EPI), in which poor digestion and absorption of food can make diabetes very difficult to control and can lead to dramatic weight loss. The diagnosis can easily be missed if exocrine pancreatic disease has not previously been detected. In one study (Watson, 2003), 2 of 4 dogs with confirmed chronic pancreatitis had concurrent diabetes, which had occurred after the development of EPI in these cases. This progression is similar to that seen in humans, in whom the diagnosis of chronic pancreatitis typically pre-dates the development of EPI by several years, with diabetes usually occurring even later in the disease process than EPI. The relationship between diabetes, pancreatitis and exocrine pancreatic disease is complex, with a variable histopathological picture (Figure 12.2).

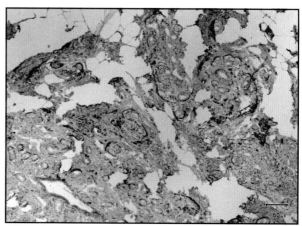

12.2 Histopathological section from the pancreas of a dog with concurrent chronic pancreatitis and diabetes. Grossly, there was very little pancreatic tissue remaining, and there is very little exocrine tissue visible histologically. A few remnants of islet tissue (dark brown) are present in this section immuno-stained for synaptophysin (monoclonal mouse anti-human clone SY38). This patient was totally insulin-dependent, despite the presence of some islet tissue, suggesting that the exocrine disease had also affected islet function. (Original magnification X40) (Courtesy of Dr Penny Watson, University of Cambridge)

One of the difficulties in establishing the prevalence of acute or chronic pancreatic inflammation in dogs with diabetes is the limited sensitivity and specificity of available diagnostic tests. In addition, chronic pancreatitis can be almost asymptomatic, and many of the signs of acute pancreatitis (e.g. lethargy and vomiting) can be attributed, mistakenly, to other conditions, including diabetic ketoacidosis. For this reason, despite its potential importance in prognosis, testing for exocrine pancreatic disease is rarely performed at the time of diagnosis of canine DM. Serum biochemical markers for pancreatitis include amylase and lipase, which are commonly, though not always, elevated with pancreatic inflammation. Many other variables affect serum amylase and lipase, including renal function, so false positive elevations are possible. Measurement of canine trypsin-like immunoreactivity (canine TLI), which is often increased during active pancreatic inflammation, can also be useful; however, serum concentration does not always correlate with the severity of disease (Mansfield *et al.*, 2003). In addition, the combination of exocrine pancreatic insufficiency (reduced TLI) and acute pancreatic inflammation (elevated TLI) has the potential to result in a TLI measurement within the reference interval. Canine pancreatic lipase immunoreactivity (cPLI) has been proposed as a more specific and sensitive marker for acute pancreatic inflammation and its measurement should be considered in any newly diagnosed diabetic patient. In a small study of diabetic dogs with no clinical signs of pancreatitis at diagnosis, a cPLI concentration above the reference interval was detected in 5 of 30 patients, although none of these was above the diagnostic cut-off value for pancreatitis (Davison *et al.*, 2003a). Ultrasound examination of the pancreas can also be valuable in some cases, but the sensitivity and specificity of this technique is variable, with a high degree of operator dependence. The gold standard for diagnosis of pancreatitis is pancreatic biopsy; however, this is an invasive procedure and difficult to justify, particularly as there is also a risk of missing a focus of inflammation confined to one area of the organ.

Autoimmunity

As diabetic dogs, almost without exception, are insulin-dependent, it was historically thought that canine DM had the same underlying autoimmune pathogenesis as human type 1 diabetes. As already discussed, chronic pancreatitis and hormonal antagonism are known to be responsible for the development of diabetes in some dogs, but it is possible that autoimmune destruction of beta cells is occurring in other dogs, although the evidence for this is less convincing than in humans and in rodent models of disease.

Human type 1 (insulin-dependent, juvenile-onset) DM is characterized by lymphocytic infiltration of the islets, known as 'insulitis', as well as the presence of serum autoantibodies to pancreatic proteins (including insulin, glutamic acid decarboxylase 65 (GAD65) and insulinoma antigen 2 (IA-2)) prior to the development of clinical signs (Taplin and Barker, 2008). In dogs, lymphocytic infiltration of pancreatic islets has been reported in a small proportion of cases (Alejandro *et al.*, 1988), but generally studies of canine pancreatic tissue in diabetes have demonstrated a more variable, heterogeneous pathology. There is some evidence of anti-beta cell antibodies in the serum of some diabetic dogs, suggesting an immune-mediated mechanism might be responsible for beta cell destruction in a proportion of cases (Haines and Penhale, 1985). The antigen-specificity of any autoimmune response in diabetic dogs is currently unknown, although recent work has suggested that a small number of diabetic dogs have autoantibodies to GAD65, IA-2 and insulin, similar to those seen in human type 1 disease (Davison *et al.*, 2008).

The potential increasing incidence of diabetes in dogs is another parallel with human type 1 diabetes. A seasonal pattern in the diagnosis of DM in dogs in the UK and the USA has been demonstrated, corresponding to the winter peak in diagnosis of type 1 diabetes in human patients (Atkins and MacDonald, 1987; Davison *et al.*, 2005). These similarities in disease onset between species have led to speculation that there may be underlying similarities in environmental factors underlying the disease. It has been suggested that such environmental triggering events could be seasonal in nature. e.g. viral infections which predominate in the winter months. Other factors proposed as being involved in human diabetes and which could also play a role in canine DM include dietary changes, vitamin D status, obesity, inactivity and climatic change.

The age at onset of canine DM, usually 'middle age', is one the features of canine diabetes that contrasts with human type 1 diabetes, which is usually diagnosed in young children. It has therefore been suggested by some authors (Fleeman and Rand, 2001; Catchpole *et al.*, 2005) that canine diabetes is more comparable to the late-onset form of human type 1 DM known as latent autoimmune diabetes of the adult (LADA).

Clinical features

Signalment

Age
Diabetes is generally a disease of middle-aged and older dogs, usually being diagnosed between the ages of 5 and 12 years, although there are some reports of patients as young as 6 months (Davison *et al.*, 2005).

Breed
In the most recent UK survey of diabetes, Labrador Retrievers, cross-breeds, collies and Yorkshire Terriers predominated (Davison *et al.*, 2005). However, as there is no compulsory dog registration scheme, it is difficult to estimate the proportions of each breed in the UK dog population. It is therefore not possible to determine whether these data indicate a genuine increase in risk of diabetes or simply reflect the popularity of these breeds. Examination of a database of insured dogs (courtesy of PetProtect UK) suggests that the relatively high proportion of some breeds in the diabetic population (e.g. Labrador Retrievers) might simply reflect their popularity. In contrast, other breeds (e.g. Cavalier King Charles Spaniel, Tibetan Terrier, Samoyed and Cairn Terrier) genuinely appear to be over-represented in the diabetic population compared to the general population. It is also interesting to note the relatively low numbers of some popular breeds in the diabetic population, such as German Shepherd Dogs, Boxers and Golden Retrievers, suggesting that such breeds might have a decreased risk of developing diabetes. A recent survey in the USA compared the number of affected dogs to the number of non-diabetic dogs of the same breed admitted to a veterinary school

hospital, concluding that Samoyeds, Miniature Schnauzers and Miniature Poodles were at greatest risk of diabetes (Hess *et al.*, 2000a).

Breed associations with disease are likely to reflect underlying genetic risk factors. Human type 1 diabetes has a strong genetic association with the genes encoding the MHC class II proteins involved in antigen presentation to the immune system (Todd *et al.*, 1987). Recent genetic studies of canine diabetes have identified certain canine MHC alleles (encoding dog leucocyte antigen (DLA) proteins) that are associated with increased diabetes risk in some breeds (Kennedy *et al.*, 2006). In addition, certain polymorphisms within other immune response genes have been identified as contributing to diabetes risk in certain breeds (Short *et al.*, 2009). Taken together, these findings implicate dysregulation of the immune response in some cases of canine DM, although many more susceptibility genes and mechanisms remain to be discovered.

Gender
Historically, a predisposition in female dogs has been reported in canine diabetes. In early surveys, around 70% of diabetic dogs were female (Marmor *et al.*, 1982); however, in more recent surveys, the female bias is less obvious (Davison *et al.*, 2005). It is thought that this is most likely related to an increased trend for neutering female dogs, leading to a reduction in the proportion of diabetes cases resulting from insulin antagonism during the progesterone-dominated phase of dioestrus.

Clinical signs
The majority of diabetic dogs are 'well' at the time of presentation, with the main complaints of the owner being polyuria, polydipsia and weight loss. Common clinical signs of diabetes are summarized in Figure 12.3.

Common	Possible
• Polyuria • Polydipsia • Weight loss • Muscle wasting • Polyphagia	• Cataracts • Smell of ketones on breath • Hepatomegaly • Reduced exercise tolerance • Recurrent bacterial infections

12.3 Clinical signs of diabetes mellitus.

Polydipsia and polyuria
The polydipsia is secondary to polyuria, which can also lead to signs of inappropriate urination, particularly if a secondary urinary tract infection is present. The polyuria arises as a result of the blood glucose concentration exceeding the renal threshold for resorption (12–14 mmol/l) and hence glucose escapes into the urine. This has a profound osmotic diuresis effect.

Polyphagia
A high proportion of canine diabetic patients are also polyphagic, as insulin is required for adequate activity of the hypothalamic satiety centre, which is involved in determining the dog's appetite.

Weight loss
Weight loss occurs partly as a result of glucosuria, but also because of metabolic changes resulting from cells being 'starved' of glucose (as insulin is not present to allow glucose into the cells). The body mobilizes fat and protein (muscle) stores for gluconeogenesis, which, as well as leading to weight loss, can also result in hyperlipidaemia, hepatic lipidosis (hepatomegaly) and muscle wasting.

Generally, signs progress fairly rapidly, but in some rare cases the disease has a gradual onset and the first sign noted by some owners may be the development of apparently 'acute' cataracts (see later). A small proportion of dogs will present acutely unwell with ketosis or ketoacidosis, particularly if there are secondary complications such as pancreatitis or a urinary tract infection. Such patients might be collapsed, tachypnoeoic (acidosis), smell of acetone (breath) and have a history of anorexia or vomiting. Ketoacidosis should be considered an emergency and requires immediate intensive treatment, which is discussed in detail in Chapter 24.

Diagnosis

A diagnosis of diabetes mellitus in dogs is usually made using a combination of clinical signs and documentation of a persistent fasting hyperglycaemia (>14 mmol/l) with glucosuria. Hyperglycaemia and glucosuria can be caused by several clinical syndromes, and differential diagnoses are listed in Figure 12.4. A variety of other tests may be performed to aid in diagnosis and assist in determining any potential underlying cause.

Hyperglycaemia

• Stress (up to 14–15 mmol/l)
 • Iatrogenic:
   – Glucocorticoid treatment
   – Progestogen treatment
   – Glucose-containing intravenous fluids
   – Alpha 2-agonist sedatives
 • Hormonal antagonism:
   – Hyperadrenocorticism
   – Dioestrus
   – Phaeochromocytoma
   – Acromegaly (rare)
 • Diabetes mellitus

Glucosuria (renal threshold 12–14 mmol/l glucose)

• Stress
 • Iatrogenic:
   – Glucose-containing intravenous fluids
 • Renal tubular dysfunction
   – Fanconi syndrome
   – Primary renal glucosuria
   – Renal failure
   – Nephrotoxins
 • Interference with test:
   – Glucose in owner's collecting jar for urine (e.g. jam jar)
   – Vitamin C or pigment in urine can affect dipstick results
 • Diabetes mellitus

12.4 Differential diagnoses for hyperglycaemia and glucosuria.

Routine clinicopathological analyses

It can be helpful to perform routine haematology and serum biochemistry in patients with suspected diabetes, to establish whether there are any other concurrent diseases and to confirm the diagnosis.

Common biochemical abnormalities in diabetes include hypercholesterolaemia and hypertriacylglycerolaemia (hypertriglyceridaemia), resulting from mobilization of fat stores and loss of inhibition of hormone-sensitive lipase in adipose tissue. Severe lipaemia can interfere with biochemical assays and, consequently, a fasting blood sample is preferred. Secondary fatty changes in the liver can also lead to persistent mild, moderate or severe elevation of liver enzymes, such as alkaline phosphatase (ALP) and alanine aminotransferase (ALT).

It is uncommon to see marked haematological changes in diabetic patients, although a stress leucogram (lymphopenia and mature neutrophilia) can be detected in some cases. Occasionally, an elevation in packed cell volume is noted, consistent with dehydration; however, in other cases a mild non-regenerative anaemia of chronic disease is seen.

Blood glucose measurement

It is very important that any equipment used to assess blood glucose in a diabetic patient is as accurate as possible. Historically, blood glucose meters designed and calibrated for human capillary blood have been employed to measure venous blood glucose in veterinary patients. There are many such devices available, several of which have been tested for accuracy with canine blood, with variable results. The most accurate device is one that is well maintained, regularly calibrated against another machine or an external laboratory gold standard and which draws up the correct volume of blood into a disposable chamber. Machines that are not well cared for, used infrequently or rely on blood being 'spotted' on to a test strip that is inserted into the machine tend to be less accurate. In addition, in the UK there are now specific veterinary glucometers available, including control calibrators for canine and feline blood, which may be more reliable (Figure 12.5). There can also

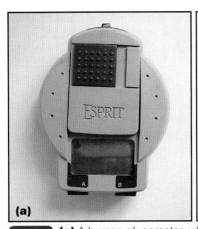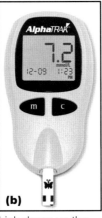

12.5 **(a)** A human glucometer, which draws up the correct volume of blood for testing into a disposable cartridge. **(b)** New glucometers are available that are specifically designed to work with the blood of veterinary species. © Abbot Animal Health.

be variability between individual glucometers of the same type; so, when performing repeated measurements, it is advisable to use the same glucometer for each measurement so that trends in blood glucose can be more accurately assessed.

Urinalysis

Urinalysis is important in the canine diabetic patient, primarily to confirm glucosuria but also to assess for evidence of concurrent urinary tract infection. In addition to assessment of haematuria, pH, proteinuria and ketonuria by dipstick, sediment analysis should always be performed for evidence of inflammation or bacterial infection. Diabetic patients are particularly at risk of such infections as the high glucose concentration in the urine favours bacterial growth. Clinical signs of urinary tract infection are very similar to those of diabetes mellitus, so a potential infection can easily be missed during history-taking. Without adequate treatment, bacterial urinary tract infection will lead to insulin resistance and make it more difficult to achieve good glycaemic control, so culture and sensitivity of a cystocentesis urine sample is recommended both routinely and particularly where there is suspicion of infection.

Any evidence of proteinuria should be followed up with quantification of urinary protein, using a urine protein:creatinine ratio. Proteinuria should also prompt measurement of blood pressure and fundic examination if this has not already been performed as part of the general clinical examination.

Fructosamine and glycosylated haemoglobin

Long-term presence of hyperglycaemia can be confirmed by measurement of glycated blood proteins, such as fructosamine or glycosylated haemoglobin, which are elevated in diabetic patients. As discussed later, these parameters are also used as a guide to glycaemic control once treatment has started, particularly in patients who are resistant to repeated blood glucose sampling. Fructosamine is a term used to describe plasma proteins, mainly albumin, that have undergone non-enzymatic irreversible glycosylation in proportion to their surrounding glucose concentration. In dogs, the serum fructosamine concentration is related to the average blood glucose concentration over the preceding 1–2 weeks, but is also influenced by the rate of plasma protein turnover in the animal. The term glycosylated haemoglobin (GHb) is used to describe haemoglobin that has become irreversibly chemically bound to glucose, which occurs in proportion to the concentration of glucose in the plasma. Studies in canine patients indicate that GHb reflects the average blood glucose concentrations over the preceding 2–3 months (Jensen, 1995). Several commercial veterinary laboratories now offer fructosamine assays and they are routinely used by most veterinary surgeons, but there is currently no commercially available assay for glycosylated haemoglobin for dogs in the UK.

Further diagnostic tests for ketosis and ketoacidosis

In any 'unwell', inappetent or newly diagnosed diabetic patient, measurement of ketones in urine or preferably blood should always be performed. Further evidence for ketoacidosis can be gained from blood gas analysis, with demonstration of reduced blood pH and bicarbonate concentration in the ketoacidotic patient as a result of metabolic acidosis. Blood or urine ketone measurement can be achieved in several ways, generally using either semi-quantitative dipsticks or biochemical analysers. The ketones produced by canine diabetic patients include acetoacetate, acetone and beta-hydroxybutyrate, with quantification of blood beta-hydroxybutyrate being considered one of the most accurate methods for detection of ketosis. It is important to note that with some semi-quantitative ketone assays, such as urine dipsticks, a negative result does not always rule out ketosis. This is because in some patients the principle ketone is beta-hydroxybutyrate and many semi-quantitative tests will detect only acetoacetate or acetone. Another clinical consequence of this limited assay sensitivity is that, as ketosis is resolving with treatment beta-hydroxybutyrate can be converted to acetoacetate, giving a paradoxical increase in ketonuria, which should not therefore always be interpreted as a sign of deterioration. The diagnosis and management of diabetic ketoacidosis are discussed in more detail in Chapter 24.

Functional testing and assessment of pancreatic inflammation

There are several other tests that can be performed at the time of diagnosis, with the specific aim of categorizing the disease as being the result of insulin resistance, insulin deficiency and/or pancreatitis. These tests include the measurement of serum amylase, lipase, TLI and cPLI, elevations of any or all of which can be indicative of exocrine pancreatic disease. As previously mentioned, a diagnosis of concurrent pancreatitis can have an impact on the management and prognosis of the patient, so it is important that the presence of pancreatic inflammation is not missed.

Additionally, where insulin resistance is suspected, beta cell reserve can be assessed in untreated diabetic dogs by measurement of serum insulin or insulin C-peptide, and glucose concentrations before and after an intravenous injection of glucagon. Further endocrine testing (e.g. adrenal and thyroid function tests) is sometimes required if a concurrent endocrinopathy is suspected, although false positive results can be obtained in stressed animals or in the case of sick euthyroid syndrome. For this reason, it is often preferable to attempt diabetic stabilization prior to further endocrine testing.

Management

Once the diagnosis of diabetes mellitus has been made, it is important that treatment is instituted as soon as possible. The time and financial commitment required from the dog's owner should not be underestimated, and it is vital to make these details clear from the outset. Management of a diabetic pet requires daily administration of insulin, a fixed routine, and enough financial support not only for insulin and consumables but also for monitoring, diagnostic tests and potential intermittent periods of hospitalization. Many owners are anxious about how they and their dog will cope with treatment and may take several days to adjust to the idea of their pet being diabetic. However, even if the owner is undecided about their commitment initially, instigation of treatment should not be delayed by longer than a few hours, as ketosis or ketoacidosis could develop and complicate the situation further. Once committed, even the most anxious owner can be taught to administer insulin to their pet and in most cases, particularly after the initial first few months of stabilization are completed, the dog's quality of life should be very good. A recent study in Sweden demonstrated a median survival time of 2 years in diabetic patients surviving more than one day beyond diagnosis (Fall *et al.*, 2007), which is encouraging, given the advanced age of most dogs at the time of diagnosis. In fact, once a diabetic dog has been stabilized on an insulin regimen, life expectancy is similar to that of non-diabetic dogs of the same age (Graham and Nash, 1995). However, it is also fair to warn owners that some dogs are more difficult to stabilize than others, and generally those dogs that have concurrent pancreatitis, ketoacidosis or hyperadrenocorticism are more likely to fall into this more 'brittle' category, with a poorer prognosis.

The aims of diabetes therapy are outlined in Figure 12.6.

- Resolution of clinical signs such as polyuria and polydipsia
- Maintenance of a good appetite and stable bodyweight
- Owner perception that the patient has a good quality of life and is able to undertake a reasonable amount of daily exercise
- Minimal complications, such as ketosis, hypoglycaemia, infections, cataracts

12.6 Aims of diabetes therapy.

Diet and exercise

The key to achieving glycaemic control in canine diabetic patients is a fixed daily routine. As the same dose of insulin is given each day, the type and amount of food should be the same and ideally there should be no large variations in the amount of exercise the dog undertakes. Whilst *ad libitum* feeding can work well in some diabetic cats, it is not recommended for dogs. Similarly, between-meal 'snacks' are best avoided, and if they must be used, for example in training, the calories should be taken from the day's energy allowance and sugary or starchy treats avoided.

Type of diet

The most important factor when selecting a diet for a diabetic dog is whether the patient finds the food palatable and will eat it consistently. This is not usually a problem, as diabetes tends to result in polyphagia. Dietary concerns relating to concurrent diseases (e.g. chronic renal failure, urolithiasis, inflammatory bowel disease) must also be considered, and often take precedence over a specific 'diabetic' diet. Several very good commercial prescription diets are available for canine diabetic patients. They are available in wet and dry formulations, broadly based on the principles that food should be palatable, nutritionally balanced and highly digestible. Additionally, to minimize postprandial hyperglycaemia, the diet should not contain large amounts of simple sugars. Calories should be provided mainly by a combination of complex carbohydrates and protein, whilst fat should be particularly restricted in patients with a history of pancreatitis. Various studies have been performed on the value of high-fibre diets in canine diabetes, with some suggesting higher-fibre diets are beneficial and others suggesting they are less appropriate for diabetic dogs in poor body condition (Fleeman and Rand, 2001; Fleeman et al., 2009). Whilst weight remains an important guide to control of the disease, it can be difficult for a thin diabetic dog to regain weight. If weight loss continues, despite satisfactory glycaemic control, measurement of canine TLI should be considered, in case of underlying exocrine pancreatic insufficiency.

Timing of feeding

Food should be divided into at least two meals a day; however, more frequent feeding is sometimes required in patients receiving twice-daily insulin. The first meal should coincide with the first insulin injection, with some clinicians preferring the insulin to precede the meal by 30 minutes, some feeding 30 minutes prior to insulin, and some recommending that insulin and food be given together. This is really a matter of personal preference, depending on the owner's routine and the dog's history or appetite. For example, it would be preferable to check before giving insulin that a dog with a history of inappetent episodes is keen to eat, to reduce the risk of hypoglycaemia occurring later in the day if the patient has been injected but does not eat. This is particularly important if the owner is not usually at home with the dog during the day. However, some dogs need the stimulus of the immediate fall in blood glucose concentration after injection (e.g. due to the soluble component of lente insulins) to stimulate their appetite and will only eat a full meal once the insulin has started to work. Such patients are best injected as early as possible in the morning, particularly if the owner is out all day, to allow time for the insulin to work and for the owner to be able to check that the dog has eaten before they leave the house. In any circumstances it is advisable to ask owners to contact the practice if their diabetic dog does not eat, since this can be a sign of more serious problems such as ketoacidosis or pancreatitis.

- If the dog is being injected once daily and fed twice daily, each meal should contain 50% of the energy requirement for that patient, and the second meal should be fed at the time of peak activity of insulin, i.e. 6–8 hours after injection.

- If patients are receiving twice-daily insulin, then they should receive a meal with both injections, each containing 30–50% of the daily energy requirements.
- Often, twice-daily treated dogs will also be hungry 6–8 hours after each injection, at the time of peak insulin activity. If this is the case, a smaller meal (10–20% of the daily energy requirements) can be provided at these times. Owners often prefer to use dry food for these smaller meals and for good control they should be provided either every day or not at all, since variation in feeding can lead to glycaemic instability.

Exercise

Exercise need not be restricted in diabetic patients, although it can take time to build up the muscle mass that is lost in the early phase of the disease. As with food and insulin, the most important factor is consistency; it is not ideal for a diabetic dog to have little or no exercise during the week and one or more very long walks at the weekend. Increasing exercise without increasing the amount of food runs the risk of hypoglycaemia but, conversely, increasing food too much without providing extra insulin can result in hyperglycaemia and osmotic diuresis. Hypoglycaemia is clearly the most dangerous of these potential complications; it is therefore sensible to advise the owner of any diabetic dog to take a sugary snack or oral glucose gel with them when on a walk, in case their dog starts to show signs of hypoglycaemia.

Types of insulin

All canine diabetic patients are insulin-dependent, almost without exception. Owners will often ask whether it is possible to control their dog's diabetes without injections, for example using oral hypoglycaemic drugs designed to control human type 2 diabetes, such as sulphonylureas. Since many oral hypoglycaemic drugs act by stimulating insulin secretion, unfortunately they are of no value in most canine patients, since their islets are irreversibly damaged by the time of diagnosis and are incapable of producing any insulin. The potential value of drugs such as alpha-glucosidase inhibitors, which delay absorption of dietary polysaccharides and therefore could be used in combination with insulin, has yet to be determined in dogs. Ongoing research is also being performed into alternative insulin delivery routes, such as mucosal or oral treatment, but problems with insulin degradation make these unacceptable for routine use at the present time, so injection remains the only effective method of insulin delivery.

Species of origin

There are currently no recombinant canine insulin preparations available for veterinary use, and the majority of dogs historically have been treated with insulin purified from bovine or porcine pancreas. In recent years, there have been two insulin preparations authorized for treatment of diabetes in dogs in the UK: one is a bovine insulin preparation available in soluble (neutral), lente or protamine zinc formulations; the other is a lente form of porcine insulin.

Since the end of 2010, however, there have been significant problems with the supply of bovine pancreas for preparation of veterinary insulins in the UK. This has led to withdrawal of authorized bovine neutral, lente and PZI preparations for the foreseeable future, leaving porcine lente insulin as the only authorized preparation with consistent availability.

Porcine insulin is homologous to canine insulin, whereas bovine insulin differs by two amino acids; however, both show similar clinical effects. Another important difference between authorized bovine and porcine preparations is their concentration. Standard human and bovine preparations are all formulated as 100 IU/ml whereas porcine lente insulin is more dilute (40 IU/ml) and hence requires different syringes. It is therefore vital to ensure that owners have the correct syringes for whichever insulin preparation is being used. Porcine lente insulin has the advantage that small dose adjustments are more accurate; however, where large doses are required for heavier dogs, the volume of insulin injected each day can become impractical for some owners. If it becomes necessary to change the insulin preparation that a patient is receiving, it is advisable to use a starting dose that is 10–30% lower than the dose of the previous preparation to avoid potential hypoglycaemia, since the kinetics of absorption of insulin will vary between preparations.

Duration of action

The duration of action of insulin depends not only on the preparation, but also on the route of delivery and the individual being injected. Bovine soluble (neutral) insulin was previously the only preparation authorized for intravenous and intramuscular injection, as well as the standard subcutaneous route. However, this product is no longer available, and there is currrently no authorized soluble insulin preparation for use in the UK. Neutral (soluble) insulin is the only preparation suitable for the intensive management of diabetic ketoacidosis, since it has the quickest onset (within 1 hour) and shortest duration (up to 4–6 hours) of activity, with the intravenous route having the most immediate and shortest effect. If the authorized veterinary product remains unavailable, then a non-veterinary soluble recombinant human or bovine neutral insulin must be used in critically ill ketoacidotic patients.

Lente preparations have a biphasic activity, with 30% of the insulin being present in a soluble form, with a more immediate effect. The remaining 70% of the insulin is in an ultralente form, which peaks in activity at around 6–8 hours and lasts up to 12–24 hours. The longest lasting insulins in medical use tend to be those in which the insulin is formulated with protamine and zinc (PZI), which have a delayed onset of activity but can have a longer peak activity and a duration of activity of up to 24 hours in some patients, although the UK authorized preparation is currently not available.

Other insulins

Other insulin therapies exist, including isophane insulin (neutral protamine Hagedorn (NPH)), semilente and ultralente recombinant human insulin (some available in semi-automated insulin 'pens'), and mixed beef/pork insulin, but none of these is authorized for use in dogs in the UK.

Of particular future interest is insulin 'glargine', a genetically engineered recombinant insulin analogue based on the human insulin amino acid sequence but with one asparagine in the insulin A chain replaced by glycine and two extra arginines on the C terminus of the B chain. This shifts the isoelectric point of the insulin, producing a solution that is completely soluble at pH4 but forms subcutaneous microprecipitates when it is injected and exposed to the physiological pH of 7.4. This allows slow release of the insulin, which can last up to 24 hours in humans, with minimal peaks and troughs in activity. Early studies of its use in diabetic cats have been encouraging, although the small number of published reports using glargine in dogs suggests that the effects in this species might be less reliable (Francassi *et al.*, 2011) and the product, along with other insulin analogues such as detemir, remains unauthorized for veterinary use in the UK at present.

Stabilization protocol

Many protocols have been described for the initial stabilization of diabetic patients and each has its particular advantages and disadvantages. No single protocol is suitable for every patient, owner or veterinary practice, but a key feature common to all is excellent communication between client and practice.

Client education

The days immediately after diagnosis are also a vital period of diabetes 'education' for the client. Important factors to be discussed include the establishment of a daily diabetic routine of diet and exercise and the practicalities of insulin storage and injection technique, as well as monitoring of clinical signs and potential diabetic emergencies, such as hypoglycaemia. It is also important to arrange to neuter entire female diabetic patients as soon as some degree of glycaemic control has been achieved. There is some possibility that if ovariohysterectomy is performed expediently, the beta cells might recover and the animal might not remain insulin-dependent. Much of this initial information can be provided in person by the veterinary surgeons and nurses within the practice; however, reinforcement by other available materials, such as DVDs, literature and websites, can also be very valuable. It can also be very useful for the owner of a diabetic animal to keep a daily diary to record the general demeanour, appetite and thirst of their pet for monitoring purposes.

The importance of making sure the insulin is stored in the refrigerator to avoid extremes of light and temperature, not used past its expiry date, gently rolled rather than shaken before each injection and administered with the correct syringes must be emphasized to the owner. Injection technique should be demonstrated to owners until they are comfortable with it, including drawing up the solution without air bubbles (Figure 12.7) and safe sites for injection. Insulin is usually injected subcutaneously

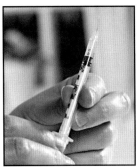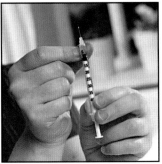

12.7 Care must always be taken to draw up insulin without any air bubbles, as this can have a significant impact on the dose. © Intervet Schering Plough.

in the region of the dorsal neck, and the owner should be encouraged to rotate injection sites within this region every few days. The UK authorized porcine lente insulin has very recently become available in an insulin 'pen' form, for semi-automated injections, which might assist those owners who struggle with syringes.

Dose and frequency
Most 'well' diabetic patients are not ketotic and have an excellent appetite so that stabilization can be performed on an outpatient basis if preferred. This decision is primarily made depending on the clinical presentation of the patient, but also considers the lifestyle of the owner, their willingness/ability to travel to the practice and their confidence at giving insulin injections. It is even possible to stabilize 'well' patients with ketonuria by this 'outpatient' method as long as they are eating well and making good clinical progress, but if they are inappetent or otherwise unwell, closer observation and more intensive treatment are recommended (see Chapter 24). Once the choice of insulin type has been made (see earlier) a decision must be reached with regard to once-daily or twice-daily treatment. PZI insulin, because of its longer duration of action, is usually given once-daily, whereas lente preparations are commonly injected every 12 hours. The recent problems with availability of an authorized PZI preparation for dogs have prevented its introduction to new patients; due to this limited availability, current recommendations are to start all newly diagnosed canine diabetic patients on porcine lente insulin, ideally twice daily. Although most owners would prefer to inject their dog only once a day, clinical evidence suggests that dogs are more stable (and the risk of hypoglycaemia is minimized) with twice-daily therapy (Hess and Ward, 2000; Fleeman and Rand, 2001), hence the recommendation. Another advantage of twice-daily treatment is that a 'missed' insulin injection, which can occur due to unexpected circumstances, is less likely to cause a problem as the dog will only be without insulin for 24 rather than 48 hours.

Where a longer-acting preparation is clinically necessary no UK authorized preparations are currently available. It is possible, however, to obtain bovine PZI, which is currently available for human use, and in North America a recombinant human

PZI preparation is marketed for use in feline diabetes; however, neither product can be considered as a first-choice insulin.

As a guide, a starting dose of insulin is usually in the region of 0.5 IU/kg, but in some cases a higher dose than this might eventually be required. However, it is preferable to start with a low dose and work upwards than to risk hypoglycaemia. Adjustments to the initial dose are often made with respect to body condition score and weight, such that very large dogs or obese dogs might receive a lower dose and very small dogs a slightly higher dose. Consideration must also be given to the presence of concurrent infection, inflammation or hormonal antagonism that might result in insulin resistance, although this should resolve with appropriate treatment of the underlying cause. It is advisable to monitor the dog carefully for several hours following the very first dose of insulin, in case the patient is more sensitive to insulin than expected and develops hypoglycaemia.

Monitoring and dose adjustments
Depending on the patient and the owner, the dog can either be stabilized at home, with the dog returning to the practice at least once daily, at the time of expected peak activity of insulin (nadir glucose), for blood glucose measurement, or be stabilized on an inpatient basis. The main purpose of nadir blood glucose monitoring is not to assess glycaemic control in any detail but to establish that the blood glucose is not falling to a dangerously low level (<4 mmol/l) if the dog is more sensitive to insulin than expected. The disadvantage of this technique is that with single blood glucose measurements, the clinician can only estimate the time at which the blood glucose is likely to be at its lowest point. As a rough guide, somewhere between 4 and 8 hours post-injection is a useful starting point for blood glucose measurement when using a lente preparation compared to the 9–12 hours post-injection which would be a more appropriate time to sample PZI-treated patients. The pharmacokinetics and pharmacodynamics of insulin will vary between dogs, hence the nadir might fall earlier or later than the blood glucose measurement, making the result potentially misleading. However, an outpatient approach is still particularly useful for dogs who do not eat well in hospital and whose owners are at home most of the day and able to monitor for signs of hypoglycaemia. Alternatively, some owners will prefer that the patient receives their first few doses of insulin in hospital, perhaps visiting their dog to learn to administer the injections under veterinary or nursing supervision. The dog can then return home once it has been established by blood glucose measurement that the insulin dose is safe.

After 4–7 days of treatment, a 12–24-hour blood glucose curve to assess progress is recommended. Blood glucose curves can vary from day to day, and can be influenced by many factors so must always be interpreted with caution (Fleeman and Rand, 2003). The main questions addressed by a blood glucose curve are discussed in more detail below, but include: whether the insulin is working consistently; how long it is lasting; and whether the nadir concentration of glucose is dangerously low. It is likely that a dose adjustment will be made at this stage, or a recommendation to change to twice-daily treatment if the insulin effect is lasting <24 hours and stabilization was initiated using only once daily treatment. Changes to management will also depend on other clinical parameters, such as appetite, thirst and general demeanour of the patient, and it is preferable not to change more than one parameter (food, insulin, exercise regime) at a time during this phase. When changing a patient from once-daily to twice-daily treatment, the dose used will depend on many factors, but it is preferable to make sure that the dose at each injection is the same and that the injections are given 12 hours apart. If a glucose curve has demonstrated that the once-daily insulin dose is safe but the effect lasts <12 hours, then the same dose should be considered for twice-daily use. If the effect appears to last slightly longer than 12 hours, but less than 24 hours, a guideline twice-daily dose would be 75% of the once-daily dose.

Once frequency of insulin treatment has been determined, dose adjustments should be small (ideally 1 IU at a time for smaller dogs and 1–2 IU for larger dogs). If larger dose adjustments are made, because of consistently high blood glucose, they should never be >10% of the dose. The exception to this is dose reduction when profound hypoglycaemia has been detected, in which case a more dramatic reduction in dose (of up to 50%) can be undertaken. This phase of slow stabilization requires patience from owner, dog and veterinary surgeon, with each dose change ideally being followed by a 3–5 day adjustment period at home and then a 12–24-hour blood glucose curve. A steady, patient and cautious approach in the immediate weeks following diagnosis increases the likelihood of a suitable dose of insulin being reached within 1–2 months, as the correct dose will not be 'overshot' by rapid and large dose adjustments. Depending on the patient and the owner, a combination of glucose curves and assessment of clinical parameters, such as 24-hour water intake and fructosamine measurement, is usually used to assess and achieve glycaemic control in the stabilization phase. If hospitalization is necessary, more frequent dose adjustments are often used; however, animals should only be discharged when dose adjustments are not required for at least 3 consecutive days.

Monitoring glycaemic control

The introduction of diagnostic tests to measure fructosamine and glycosylated haemoglobin has helped improve monitoring of glycaemic control in veterinary patients and prevent secondary complications. Changes in these parameters allow informed adjustments of insulin therapy to be made and decisions to be taken as to whether further investigations are required. In practical terms, this means that if the patient is not amenable to repeated glucose curves, an alternative, but often slower, method of adjusting insulin dose is to use serum fructosamine measurement as a guide to glycaemic control. It is important, however, that this is performed alongside observation of clinical signs, such as weight change and measurement of water intake.

Blood fructosamine

Fructosamine can be measured every 2–3 weeks using a single blood sample, with the advantage that this test can be performed at any time of day rather than the specific timings needed for a blood glucose curve. Its most useful role is for monitoring a patient's progress longitudinally, i.e. comparing a dog to itself over time and deciding whether glycaemic control is deteriorating or improving. In this situation it is vital that the same laboratory is used for testing each time, as assays and reference intervals can vary substantially. When the patient has reached a suitable dose of insulin, fructosamine concentration will be steady, bodyweight will be stable and the dog should not be drinking excessively. This route of stabilization is often more successful for dogs receiving twice-daily insulin, as it is difficult to determine whether the duration of insulin activity is adequate in once-daily treated dogs using fructosamine alone.

Although reference intervals can vary widely between laboratories, generally fructosamine concentrations <400 µmol/l are accepted to represent very good glycaemic control, whereas concentrations >550 µmol/l suggest very poor control. These values must be interpreted with caution: fructosamine measurement is not ideally suited to determining whether a patient falls into 'poor', 'acceptable', 'good' or 'very good' glycaemic control compared to the general diabetic population. This is because the values representing these degrees of control can vary between patients, as fructosamine concentration is not influenced exclusively by blood glucose but also by other factors, such as protein turnover. As a result, fructosamine should always be interpreted in the light of clinical signs and previous measurements from the same patient. It is important to note that whilst it is desirable that fructosamine concentration is consistent with adequate glycaemic control (and blood glucose concentration stays between 5 and 12 mmol/l in a blood glucose curve), this is not always completely achievable. It is more important to meet the clinical aims of therapy outlined in Figure 12.6.

For example, a reassuring fructosamine result in a patient still showing clinical signs of instability does not suggest good glycaemic control, but instead might be the average result of a combination of hypo- and hyperglycaemic periods throughout the day. Conversely, an elevation in fructosamine should not cause too much alarm in a patient who is doing well on assessment by clinical criteria (according to Figure 12.6). Rather than adjusting a regimen which is resolving clinical signs satisfactorily in such a patient, it would be preferable to maintain the same regimen and repeat the fructosamine measurement and clinical assessment in 2–4 weeks. If fructosamine is continuing to rise, further investigation might be warranted but if clinical signs and fructosamine are stable then any adjustments should be considered very carefully, as they might cause deterioration rather than improvement in an already stable animal with a reasonable quality of life.

Urine glucose

If owners are able to collect urine easily from their dog, this offers a further method of assessing glycaemic control, since semi-quantitative dipsticks allow assessment of glucosuria and ketonuria. Glucose will be present in the urine if the concentration in the blood exceeds the renal threshold (12–14 mmol/l), which is not unusual for at least some part of the day in many diabetic dogs. It is therefore important that urine glucose is assessed at the same time of day on each occasion, preferably in the morning, and that values are interpreted alongside other clinical data. A small amount of urine glucose in a morning sample is acceptable, but if this amount rises in a consistent pattern or ketones are also present, the owner should be instructed to seek veterinary advice. Conversely, if no glucose is detected in a morning urine sample, then it is possible that the dog is at risk of hypoglycaemia and the insulin dose should be reviewed. Caution must be exercised in altering insulin dose based on urine glucose alone, particularly in dogs receiving once-daily therapy, who will almost always demonstrate morning glucosuria. Increasing the dose will not resolve glucosuria if the insulin effect is lasting <24 hours, and 'chasing' the urine glucose by gradual increase of insulin dose is a common cause of insulin-induced hyperglycaemia (Somogyi overswing – discussed in Chapter 22). In dogs with a history of ketoacidosis, intermittent urinalysis at home can also prove very useful in providing early warning of ketonuria.

Blood glucose curve

Another potentially valuable method of evaluating the efficacy of insulin therapy in diabetic patients is a serial blood glucose curve, involving repeated blood sampling every 1–2 hours over a 12–24-hour period. Blood glucose curves can be an important part of the assessment of glycaemic control in some patients, but in others they provide very little useful diagnostic information, for example if a patient will not eat during a hospital stay or is difficult to blood sample repeatedly. It is clear from recent research that even in stable patients the blood glucose curve can vary from day to day, so care must be taken not to over-interpret findings. In the hours following a severe hypoglycaemic episode, for example, the presence of antagonistic hormones, such as glucagon, adrenaline and cortisol, might prevent any further hypoglycaemic values being obtained, despite the same dose of insulin being given. Stress can also contribute to elevated blood glucose values in hospitalized dogs (although not to the same extent as hospitalized cats), such that the curve obtained in hospital might be very different from the blood glucose curve that would be obtained at home. It is particularly important to avoid 'joining up' the various points on an hourly or 2-hourly curve with lines, since this makes an assumption that no peaks or troughs are occurring between samples, and can be

misleading. It is also important to wait for several days for a patient to 'equilibrate' to a new insulin dose before performing a curve, for example sending them home for a few days in between repeated curves if it is safe and practical to do so.

In an ideal diabetic patient the blood glucose concentration would stay between 4 mmol/l and 12 mmol/l all day during a blood glucose curve. However, as blood glucose curves can be confusing and rarely look like textbook examples, it is useful for both owner and clinician to be realistic in the expectation of how much will be gained from the information generated. Methodical analysis of a blood glucose curve will, however, usually allow a judgement to be made about glycaemic control and potential changes in treatment. Case selection is also important in gaining the most value from glucose curves that can be uncomfortable for the patient and require a lot of effort from practice staff. Unstable diabetic patients and newly diagnosed patients being stabilized on insulin are most likely to benefit from an hourly 12- or 24-hour curve, whereas performing a blood glucose curve simply to 'check' a patient who is already fulfilling all the aims of therapy described in Figure 12.6 is of questionable value, as it is unlikely to alter clinical management.

There are several questions that can be asked when examining a blood glucose curve, although recommendations on management changes can vary between clinicians. As a guide, the following questions should be considered:

1. **Is the insulin having any effect?** This can be confirmed if the blood glucose falls at any point in the 6–8 hours following an injection. It is also helpful to notice how long after food this effect is seen, and whether the fall in glucose had any associated effect on appetite.
2. **How long is the effect lasting?** This can be confirmed by noting the first time the blood glucose starts to rise again, which can be as short as a few hours after injection. It is particularly useful to notice whether the blood glucose rises or is still controlled when a dog eats a meal a few hours after the injection.
3. **Is the nadir (lowest blood glucose point) safe or potentially too low?** If the blood glucose falls below 3–5 mmol/l whilst the dog is being hospitalized for a blood glucose curve, the patient is at risk of clinically significant hypoglycaemia. This can occur because the dog is not eating the amount of food it would normally eat at home, but can also occur if the insulin dose is too high. If there is any concern over hypoglycaemia as the curve is being performed, the patient should be fed and the blood glucose checked again 30 minutes later, with monitoring continued and further insulin therapy withheld until blood glucose starts to rise.
4. **Are there any factors that might also be contributing to the finding seen?** A curve is unlikely to be representative of the patient's normal day-to-day glycaemic control if the dog is otherwise unwell (e.g. pancreatitis, urinary tract

infection, ketoacidosis), will not eat its usual food or has very recently had a severe hypoglycaemic episode or a change in insulin dose. Similarly, stress during blood sampling, an inaccurate glucometer or haemolysed/lipaemic samples can also affect a blood glucose curve. These factors should always be considered as possible explanations of unexpected or erratic results.

Home glucose monitoring

In some cases, particularly where patients are easy to handle but not suited to hospitalization, it can be possible for an owner to generate a blood glucose curve at home without performing venepuncture (Casella *et al.*, 2003). This can be done using an automated lancet device in an area of hairless skin, such as the underside of the pinna. Such devices use

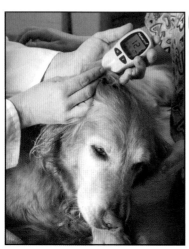

12.8 Use of a glucometer to measure glucose in a capillary blood sample obtained from the pinna with a lancet device.

a spring-loaded disposable needle, which makes a pinprick incision through the skin and allows a small volume of capillary blood to escape, sometimes with the use of a vacuum. Glucose concentration can then be measured using a glucometer, which draws up the correct volume of blood (Figure 12.8).

Care must be taken, however, to make sure that the welfare of the patient is not compromised by any such testing, as it can be painful if performed incorrectly. Problems can arise by testing being performed one of the following ways:

* Too frequently
* By a person without adequate training
* In a patient that does not tolerate the testing
* By an owner, without direct veterinary supervision of the results generated.

Home glucose monitoring may be better reserved for more established diabetic cases rather than used in the initial stabilization phase, unless the owner is already experienced in diabetes management.

Continuous glucose monitoring

The generation of a blood glucose curve by repeated venepuncture, or even using a lancet device, can be stressful and painful for the dog and there is also a risk that a significant blood glucose peak or nadir will fall between two sampling times and will not be recorded. A recent technological advance in the management of human diabetes is the development of a continuous glucose monitoring system (CGMS; Medtronic MiniMed, Northridge, USA), which has also been used successfully in dogs (Davison *et al.*, 2003b) (Figure 12.9).

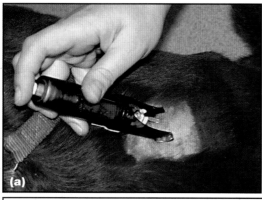
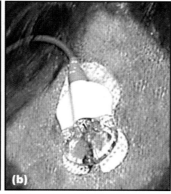
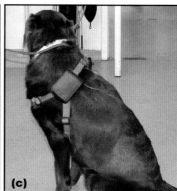

Glucose sensor profile

12.9 Use of a continuous glucose monitoring device. **(a)** The glucose monitoring sensor is inserted below the skin using a spring-loaded device. **(b)** The sensor is connected to the continuous glucose monitoring device and can be left in place for up to 72 hours. **(c)** The patient can wear the continuous glucose monitoring device attached to a harness (a wireless radiotelemetry system is also available). **(d)** The data are used to generate a continuous interstitial fluid glucose trace using the computer software.

Legend: □ Meter value ■ Paired meter value — Sensor value × Fructosamine ♦ Insulin ▲ Meal

The system requires subcutaneous implantation of a platinum glucose sensor using a spring-loaded device which can be left in place for up to 72 hours. The CGMS does not completely remove the need for blood sampling, as at least one blood glucose measurement must be taken in each 12-hour period in order to calibrate the machine and to check that the sensor is still active. Interstitial fluid glucose concentrations are measured every 10 seconds by the sensor and an average value recorded every 5 minutes. Blood and interstitial fluid glucose concentrations are in equilibrium, and experimental studies have shown that differences are generally only seen when blood glucose concentration is changing rapidly, where a lag phase of between 3 and 14 minutes might be expected. The sensor is connected either directly or wirelessly to a pager-sized monitor that is either worn by the patient or kept in close proximity (1–2 metres away). The monitor can also store information regarding insulin injections and feeding, so that they can be superimposed on the glucose curve that is generated by the associated software. Data can be downloaded to a computer for analysis or, in newer models, assessed in real time on the monitor itself. The main advantage of the CGMS is that a large amount of data can be collected and analysed without the need for repeated blood sampling. However, its use at present is limited only to centres seeing a large number of diabetic patients, because of the cost of the device and the disposable platinum sensors. The working range of the device also precludes its use in patients with blood glucose above the upper limit of detection (>22 mmol/l). This device can be particularly helpful in the investigation of unstable diabetic patients, discussed in more detail in Chapter 22.

Long-term monitoring

Regular veterinary appointments are advisable, even in seemingly well controlled cases. Unlike for cats, it is very rare for dogs to undergo a 'diabetic honeymoon' phase following insulin treatment, requiring dose reduction or discontinuation of insulin therapy. However, further insulin dose adjustments are sometimes necessary because of weight gain, concurrent disease or a change in management of the dog, such as increased exercise or a different diet. Regular planned assessment of patients decreases the likelihood of diabetic emergencies, as changes in glycaemic control can be identified and treated early. The involvement of the nursing team in the practice in the regular assessment of diabetic patients is also very valuable, sharing the responsibility of care so that several people are familiar with each case.

Ideally, a routine clinical appointment should be scheduled approximately every 2 months for a well controlled diabetic patient, with the factors listed in Figure 12.10 being addressed. In patients that are stable with an established routine, this type of appointment is an excellent opportunity for nursing staff to become involved in the care of canine diabetic patients. If the owner reports any problems or if any factors listed in Figure 12.11 become apparent, further investigations should be undertaken.

- Measure bodyweight (monthly)
- Review diary records with owner, looking for any changes:
  - Appetite
  - Thirst
  - Behaviour
- Check urine sample for evidence of infection and/or ketones
- Monitor dental hygiene
- Discuss any concerns about diet/feeding
- Review insulin injection technique if required
- Check owners are prepared for potential diabetic emergencies
- Fructosamine measurement every 4–6 months or more regularly if any concerns

12.10 Assessments to be made at a regular diabetic appointment.

- Episodes of fainting or unusual behaviour (hypoglycaemia)
- Appetite or thirst changed significantly (unstable diabetes or concurrent disease, e.g. exocrine pancreatic insufficiency, renal failure)
- Blood, protein or ketones present in the urine (cytology and bacterial culture and sensitivity should be performed in any case of haematuria in a diabetic)
- Bodyweight altered significantly
- Signs of infection, e.g. periodontal disease
- Deterioration in vision (cataracts)
- Lumps appearing at injection sites (injection reactions can result in erratic absorption of insulin)
- The animal is quiet or depressed (possibly hypoglycaemia or concurrent illness)
- There has been vomiting or diarrhoea (vomiting with no change in insulin dose might lead to dangerous hypoglycaemia)
- There has been a change in haircoat or body shape (might suggest another endocrinopathy, e.g. hypothyroidism, hyperadrenocorticism)

12.11 Findings that should prompt further investigation at a diabetic assessment appointment.

Management of concurrent illness

Any concurrent illness in a diabetic patient should be managed as swiftly as possible.

Infection

Diabetic patients are particularly at risk of bacterial and fungal infection because the higher glucose in their blood and interstitial fluid promotes growth of these organisms and because of inherent immunosuppression (Hess *et al.*, 2000b). If not recognized and treated, infection and inflammation will lead to insulin resistance, more severe hyperglycaemia and exacerbation of infection. Antibiotic use in diabetic patients should be based on the result of bacterial culture and sensitivity, with a minimum of 2–3 weeks' treatment required in most cases. In the case of fungal disease or more severe bacterial infection, prolonged treatment courses and intensive management of blood glucose may be necessary for adequate control.

Inappetence or vomiting

Any disease that reduces appetite or leads to vomiting will also have an impact on glycaemic control. As previously discussed, owners should always be advised to contact the practice if their diabetic dog does not eat or is vomiting. With reduced caloric intake for any reason, there is a risk of hypoglycaemia at the time of peak activity of the insulin. In mild disease, such as vomiting related to dietary indiscretion, a reduction of insulin dose by 50% for 1 or 2 days until recovery of appetite is acceptable. Longer periods of inappetence, such as those associated with acute pancreatitis, require further diagnostic intervention and careful monitoring of blood glucose concentrations. Management of the diabetic patient with acute pancreatitis should follow the same principles as management in a non-diabetic patient, including analgesia, small low-fat meals if the patient is not vomiting and anti-emetic treatment if necessary. In such cases it can be useful to manage blood glucose with several small doses (0.1–0.3 IU/kg) of soluble (neutral) insulin given intramuscularly throughout the day (depending on the amount of food eaten and the blood glucose measurement), rather than with the longer-acting preparation usually administered (but see earlier notes on availability). Neutral (soluble) insulin has the advantage of having a rapid onset of action but also a short duration, meaning that the animal is less at risk of hypoglycaemia if it does not eat for several hours.

Drugs

Another challenge in diabetic patients is the use of drugs that antagonize insulin or contain sugar in the form of a syrup. In particular, corticosteroids such as prednisolone will have a detrimental effect on glycaemic control and require an increase in insulin dose to compensate for this. If possible, the use of such drugs should be avoided, but this is not always practical. For example, in severe cases of allergic or immune-mediated disease it might become necessary to use corticosteroids, but their use should be avoided in diabetic patients for more minor indications. Topical treatment is less likely to cause a problem, but in some cases even eye, ear or skin preparations can result in insulin resistance. If the use of corticosteroids is unavoidable, the minimum effective dose should be used, and other appropriate 'steroid-sparing' drugs considered (e.g. azathioprine in immune-mediated disease). Injectable depot preparations of corticosteroid have a more variable duration and activity, making it very difficult to predict changes in insulin requirements that might be required, so should be avoided in favour of shorter-acting once-daily oral preparations. Ciclosporin has been proposed as an alternative immunosuppressive drug for immune-mediated disease in diabetic patients, although in humans it is known to affect blood glucose levels by inhibiting insulin secretion. This is less likely to cause a problem in diabetic dogs as they usually have no functioning islets remaining and are entirely dependent on exogenous insulin for appropriate glycaemic control.

General anaesthesia

The period of fasting required for general anaesthesia in diabetic patients can cause concern regarding glycaemic control. The most likely indications for general anaesthesia in a diabetic patient are ovariohysterectomy, cataract surgery or management of severe dental disease. Diabetic patients are at risk of developing hypoglycaemia and cerebral damage during anaesthesia, and blood glucose concentrations can remain uncontrolled for many hours after a surgical procedure.

It is advisable to perform anaesthesia on diabetic patients as early as possible in the day to allow them to recover in time to eat before the onset of peak insulin activity. Following an overnight fast from midnight, a common regime is to give the patient half of their usual insulin dose in the morning but no food. The patient should be placed on intravenous dextrose saline fluid therapy throughout the anaesthetic, and blood glucose monitored regularly throughout the procedure, with an intravenous glucose bolus (of up to 1–2 ml/kg of 25% dextrose) being administered if blood glucose falls to <5 mmol/l. On recovery, the patient should be encouraged to eat as soon as possible (preferably their usual diet) and blood glucose monitored hourly or 2-hourly. Once-daily insulin treated patients can return to their normal routine the following morning, whereas twice-daily treated patients, if recovering well, can receive their insulin and food as normal in the evening.

Long-term complications

Although insulin therapy can be used successfully to manage the majority of canine diabetic patients, suboptimal glycaemic control can lead to secondary complications, such as hypoglycaemic seizures, cataract formation, recurrent infections or diabetic ketoacidosis. Canine diabetes is also thought to be a risk factor for development of atherosclerosis, although this is usually only apparent at post-mortem examination and does not generally cause clinical signs (Hess *et al.*, 2003). Unlike human diabetic patients, diabetic dogs do not commonly suffer from clinical signs associated with diabetic nephropathy or peripheral neuropathy. It is possible that this represents a difference in pathophysiology between the two species, but is more likely related to the difference in lifespan; secondary complications can take many decades to develop in humans, and diabetic dogs usually live only for a few years following diagnosis.

Ocular disease

Ocular complications occur with variable frequency, with cataracts (Figure 12.12) being the most common. Cataracts are thought to occur as a result of osmotic disruption of the lens due to an accumulation of sorbitol (a metabolic product of excess glucose) and are more common in poorly controlled patients. Recent work has also demonstrated high activity of the aldose reductase pathway within the canine lens compared to the feline lens, which is thought to play a role in cataract development (Richter *et al.*, 2002). Even most well controlled patients are likely to develop cataracts within 2 years of diagnosis, which will eventually result in

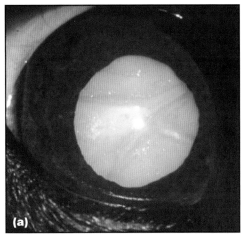

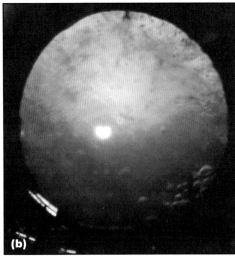

12.12 Diabetic cataracts. **(a)** Early diabetic cataract showing vacuoles, before the sudden onset of mature lens opacity. **(b)** Mature diabetic cataract – note the water clefts in the lens. The dark dull iris results from lens-induced uveitis. (Courtesy of Dr David Williams)

blindness. Although owners are often reluctant to allow a diabetic pet to undergo surgery, a great improvement in quality of life can be obtained by surgical management of cataracts, even if only one eye is treated. Other ocular complications of diabetes can include keratoconjunctivitis sicca, bacterial conjunctivitis and uveitis, with the diabetic retinopathy seen in humans being very rare.

Dermatological complications
Ulcerative skin lesions and cutaneous xanthomas have occasionally been reported in unstable canine diabetic patients. Hepatocutaneous syndrome is a rare complication of diabetes and some hepatic diseases. Severe crusting lesions of the feet and distal limbs, face and perineum are seen, and are thought to be related to an excess of glucagon. Diagnosis is confirmed by skin biopsy, but unfortunately this complication carries a poor prognosis.

Hypoglycaemia
Hypoglycaemia is rare in diabetic dogs but can be life-threatening if it occurs, so clients should be well educated about how to avoid and treat this condition. Dogs are usually protected from hypoglycaemia by

other hormones that are produced as blood glucose falls, such as glucagon, adrenaline and cortisol. Hypoglycaemia is most likely to occur when an animal does not eat their usual amount of food, exercises more than usual or receives too high a dose of insulin (sometimes accidentally). Clinical signs of mild hypoglycaemia can include lethargy, behavioural changes such as aggression or restlessness, stumbling when walking and an increased appetite. If the animal is not fed and hypoglycaemia is allowed to progress, neurological status will deteriorate to convulsions or coma, eventually resulting in cerebral damage and death. Mild hypoglycaemia can be treated by feeding any food which is not high in fibre, particularly sugar-rich food such as sweets or biscuits. If the animal cannot eat voluntarily, glucose can be applied to the dog's oral mucous membranes in the form of dextrose gel or glucose solution, where it can be directly absorbed, until the animal has recovered well enough to be fed.

In the collapsed animal, particularly following an insulin overdose, intravenous glucose must be provided immediately to limit cerebral damage. An initial intravenous bolus dose of 2 ml/kg of 25% dextrose is appropriate, followed by a 4% dextrose infusion, which can be increased if there is a poor clinical response. Glucagon has also been used to manage acute hypoglycaemia induced by insulin overdose. A 1 mg vial of glucagon can be added to 1 litre of 0.9% sodium chloride, which is then administered as a 50 ng/kg bolus, followed by constant rate infusion of 10–40 ng/kg/min, depending on response.

References and further reading

Alejandro R, Feldman EC, Shienvold FL *et al.* (1988) Advances in canine diabetes mellitus research: etiopathology and results of islet transplantation. *Journal of the American Veterinary Medical Association* **193**, 1050–1055

Atkins CE, Hill JR and Johnson RK (1979) Diabetes mellitus in the juvenile dog: a report of four cases. *Journal of the American Veterinary Medical Association* **175**, 362–368

Atkins CE and MacDonald MJ (1987) Canine diabetes mellitus has a seasonal incidence: implications relevant to human diabetes. *Diabetes Research* **5**, 83–87

Casella M, Wess G, Hassig M *et al.* (2003) Home monitoring of blood glucose concentration by owners of diabetic dogs. *Journal of Small Animal Practice* **44**, 298–305

Catchpole B, Kennedy LJ, Davison LJ *et al.* (2008) Canine diabetes mellitus: from phenotype to genotype. *Journal of Small Animal Practice* **49**, 4–10

Catchpole B, Ristic JM, Fleeman LM *et al.* (2005) Canine diabetes mellitus: can old dogs teach us new tricks? *Diabetologia* **48**, 1948–1956

Cotton RB, Cornelius LM and Theran P (1971) Diabetes mellitus in the dog: a clinicopathologic study. *Journal of the American Veterinary Medical Association* **159**, 863–870

Davison LJ, Herrtage ME and Catchpole B (2005) Study of 253 dogs in the United Kingdom with diabetes mellitus. *Veterinary Record* **156**, 467–471

Davison LJ, Herrtage ME, Steiner JM *et al.* (2003a) Evidence of anti-insulin autoreactivity and pancreatic inflammation in newly diagnosed diabetic dogs (abstract). *Journal of Veterinary Internal Medicine* **17**, 395

Davison LJ, Slater LA, Herrtage ME *et al.* (2003b) Evaluation of a continuous glucose monitoring system in diabetic dogs. *Journal of Small Animal Practice* **44**, 435–442

Davison LJ, Weenink SM, Christie MR *et al.* (2008) Autoantibodies to GAD65 and IA-2 in canine diabetes mellitus. *Veterinary Immunology and Immunopathology* **126**, 83–90

Eigenmann JE, Eigenmann RY, Rijnberk A *et al.* (1983) Progesterone-controlled growth hormone overproduction and naturally occurring canine diabetes and acromegaly. *Acta Endocrinologica (Copenhagen)* **104**, 167–176

Fall T, Hamlin HH, Hedhammar Å *et al.* (2007) Diabetes mellitus in a population of 180,000 insured dogs: incidence, survival, and breed distribution. *Journal of Veterinary Internal Medicine* **21**, 1209–1216

Fall T, Holm B, Karlsson A *et al.* (2008a) Glucagon stimulation test for estimating endogenous insulin secretion in dogs. *Veterinary Record* **163**, 266–270

Fall T, Johansson Kreuger S, Juberget A *et al.* (2008b) Gestational diabetes mellitus in 13 dogs. *Journal of Veterinary Internal Medicine* **22**, 1296–1300

Fleeman LM and Rand JS (2001) Management of canine diabetes. *Veterinary Clinics of North America: Small Animal Practice* 31, 855–880, vi

Fleeman LM and Rand JS (2003) Evaluation of day-to-day variability of serial blood glucose concentration curves in diabetic dogs. *Journal of the American Veterinary Medical Association* **222**, 317–321

Fleeman LM, Rand JS and Markwell PJ (2009) Lack of advantage of high-fibre, moderate-carbohydrate diets in dogs with stabilised diabetes. *Journal of Small Animal Practice* **50**, 604–614

Frascassi F, Boretti FS, Sieber-Ruckstuhl NS and Reusch CE (2011) Use of insulin glargine in dogs with diabetes melitus. *Veterinary Record* Oct 17 **ePub**

Graham PA (1995) Clinical and epidemiological studies on canine diabetes mellitus, *PhD Thesis*, University of Glasgow, Scotland

Graham PA and Nash AS (1995) How long will my diabetic dog live? *Proceedings of BSAVA Annual Congress*, Birmingham UK, p. 217. Cheltenham

Guptill L, Glickman L and Glickman N (2003) Time trends and risk factors for diabetes mellitus in dogs: analysis of veterinary medical data base records (1970–1999). *Veterinary Journal* **165**, 240–247

Haines DM and Penhale WJ (1985) Autoantibodies to pancreatic islet cells in canine diabetes mellitus. *Veterinary Immunology and Immunopathology* **8**, 149–156

Hess RS, Kass PH and Van Winkle TJ (2003) Association between diabetes mellitus, hypothyroidism or hyperadrenocorticism, and atherosclerosis in dogs. *Journal of Veterinary Internal Medicine* **17**, 489–494

Hess RS, Kass PH and Ward CR (2000a) Breed distribution of dogs with diabetes mellitus admitted to a tertiary care facility. *Journal of the American Veterinary Medical Association* **216**, 1414–1417

Hess RS, Saunders HM, Van Winkle TJ *et al.* (2000b) Concurrent disorders in dogs with diabetes mellitus: 221 cases (1993–1998). *Journal of the American Veterinary Medical Association* **217**, 1166–1173

Hess RS and Ward CR (2000) Effect of insulin dosage on glycemic response in dogs with diabetes mellitus: 221 cases (1993–1998). *Journal of the American Veterinary Medical Association* **216**, 217–221

Hoenig M (2002) Comparative aspects of diabetes mellitus in dogs and cats. *Molecular and Cellular Endocrinology* **197**, 221–229

Jensen AL (1995) Glycated blood proteins in canine diabetes mellitus. *Veterinary Record* **137**, 401–405

Kennedy LJ, Davison LJ, Barnes A *et al.* (2006) Identification of susceptibility and protective major histocompatibility complex haplotypes in canine diabetes mellitus. *Tissue Antigens* **68**, 467–476

Kramer JW, Klaassen JK, Baskin DG *et al.* (1988) Inheritance of diabetes mellitus in Keeshond dogs. *American Journal of Veterinary Research* **49**, 428–431

Krook L, Larsson S and Rooney JR (1960) The interrelationship of diabetes mellitus, obesity, and pyometra in the dog. *American Journal of Veterinary Research* **21**, 120–127

Ling GV, Lowenstine LJ, Pulley LT *et al.* (1977) Diabetes mellitus in dogs: a review of initial evaluation, immediate and long-term management, and outcome. *Journal of the American Veterinary Medical Association* **170**, 521–530

Mansfield CS, Jones BR and Spillman T (2003) Assessing the severity of canine pancreatitis. *Research in Veterinary Science* **74**, 137–144

Marmor M, Willeberg P, Glickman LT *et al.* (1982) Epizootiologic patterns of diabetes mellitus in dogs. *American Journal of Veterinary Research* **43**, 465–470

Mattheeuws D, Rottiers R, Kaneko JJ *et al.* (1984) Diabetes mellitus in dogs: relationship of obesity to glucose tolerance and insulin response. *American Journal of Veterinary Research* **45**, 98–103

Minkus G, Breuer W, Arun S *et al.* (1997) Ductuloendocrine cell proliferation in the pancreas of two young dogs with diabetes mellitus. *Veterinary Pathology* **34**, 164–167

Montgomery TM, Nelson RW, Feldman EC *et al.* (1996) Basal and glucagon-stimulated plasma C-peptide concentrations in healthy dogs, dogs with diabetes mellitus, and dogs with hyperadrenocorticism. *Journal of Veterinary Internal Medicine* **10**, 116–122

Peterson ME, Altszuler N and Nichols CE (1984) Decreased insulin sensitivity and glucose tolerance in spontaneous canine hyperadrenocorticism. *Research in Veterinary Science* **36**(2), 177–182

Rand JS, Fleeman LM, Farrow HA, Appleton DJ and Lederer R (2004) Canine and feline diabetes mellitus: nature or nurture? *Journal of Nutrition* 134(8 Suppl), 2072S–2080S

Redondo MJ and Eisenbarth GS (2002) Genetic control of autoimmunity in Type I diabetes and associated disorders. *Diabetologia* **45**, 605–622

Richter M, Guscett F and Spiess B (2002) Aldose reductase activity and glucose-related opacities in incubated lenses from dogs and cats. *American Journal of Veterinary Research* **63**, 1591–1597

Rijnberk A, van Herpen H, Mol JA *et al.* (1993) Disturbed release of growth hormone in mature dogs: a comparison with congenital growth hormone deficiency. *Veterinary Record* **133**, 542–545

Short AD, Catchpole B, Kennedy LJ *et al.* (2009) T cell cytokine gene polymorphisms in canine diabetes mellitus. *Veterinary Immunology and Immunopathology* **128**, 137–146

Steiner JM, Newman S, Xenoulis P *et al.* (2008) Sensitivity of serum markers for pancreatitis in dogs with macroscopic evidence of pancreatitis. *Veterinary Therapeutics* **9**, 263–273

Taplin CE and Barker JM (2008) Autoantibodies in type 1 diabetes. *Autoimmunity* **41**, 11–18

Todd JA, Bell JI and McDevitt HO (1987) HLA-DQ beta gene contributes to susceptibility and resistance to insulin-dependent diabetes mellitus. *Nature* **329**, 599–604

Watson PJ (2003) Exocrine pancreatic insufficiency as an end stage of pancreatitis in four dogs. *Journal of Small Animal Practice* **44**, 306–312

Watson PJ and Herrtage ME (2004) Use of glucagon stimulation tests to assess beta-cell function in dogs with chronic pancreatitis. *Journal of Nutrition* **134**, 2081–2083

Watson PJ, Roulois AJ, Scase T *et al.* (2007) Prevalence and breed distribution of chronic pancreatitis at post-mortem examination in first-opinion dogs. *Journal of Small Animal Practice* **48**, 609–618

13

Feline diabetes mellitus

Jacquie Rand

Introduction

Diabetes mellitus is defined as a disorder of persistent hyperglycaemia regardless of underlying cause. The typical clinical signs are polydipsia/polyuria and weight loss. It is one of the most common endocrine disorders in cats, although the prevalence varies depending on the population studied, from approximately 1 in 200 observed in a first-opinion feline-only practice (Baral *et al.*, 2003) to 1 in 100 when data from a veterinary laboratory were evaluated and 1 in 400 using data from referral institutions (Panciera *et al.*, 1990; Rand *et al.*, 1997).

The majority of cats have a disorder similar to type 2 diabetes mellitus in humans. Risk factors include obesity, physical inactivity, confinement indoors and prior administration of glucocorticoids or progestogens. Most of these risk factors decrease insulin sensitivity, leading to increased demand on beta cells to produce insulin. The incidence of feline diabetes mellitus observed in private practice is increasing (Prahl *et al.*, 2007), presumably because of a greater occurrence of predisposing factors, particularly obesity and physical inactivity.

Treatment of diabetes is aimed at normalizing circulating blood glucose concentrations, typically by administration of insulin, feeding a low carbohydrate diet and appropriate adjustment of insulin dose based on diligent monitoring of glycaemic response. In most cats, adequate glycaemic control is readily achieved, whilst in other cats consistent glycaemic control is difficult.

Cats are prone to stress hyperglycaemia, which complicates the interpretation of blood glucose concentration, and may lead to inappropriate insulin dosage changes. Home monitoring of blood glucose concentrations helps to overcome this confounding effect. Although the majority of cats are initially insulin-dependent, a substantial proportion of newly diagnosed cats undergo remission if good glycaemic control is achieved using insulin therapy and there is diligent monitoring of glycaemic response.

Aetiopathogenesis

The causes of feline diabetes mellitus are varied. In primary accession practices in Western countries the majority of cats have type 2 (previously called adult-onset or non-insulin-dependent) diabetes mellitus.

The remainder have diabetes mellitus classified as 'other specific types of diabetes' (O'Brien *et al.*, 1985; Goossens *et al.*, 1998), which typically results from insulin resistance due to acromegaly or hyperadrenocorticism, or from conditions that destroy pancreatic beta cells (pancreatitis or neoplasia) (Nelson, 2000; Rand and Marshall, 2005). Type 1 (previously called insulin-dependent or juvenile-onset diabetes) disease resulting from immune-mediated destruction of beta cells appears to be rare in cats.

Type 2 diabetes mellitus

Based on clinical characteristics and islet pathology, approximately 85–95% of diabetic cats appear to have type 2 diabetes mellitus, which results from a combination of impaired insulin secretion, insulin resistance and amyloid deposition in the pancreatic islets (O'Brien *et al.*, 1985; Panciera *et al.*, 1990; Marshall *et al.*, 2009; Roomp and Rand, 2009b). Contributory factors are outlined in Figure 13.1.

Condition	Environmental causes	Genetic causes
Insulin resistance	Obesity Physical inactivity Drugs Concurrent illness Stress Hyperglycaemia	Genetic factors Obesity Gender
Impaired insulin secretion	Islet amyloid deposition Pancreatitis Glucose toxicity Lipid toxicity	Islet amyloid deposition

13.1 Potential causes of insulin resistance and impaired insulin secretion.

Insulin resistance

Insulin resistance is a hallmark of type 2 diabetes mellitus. Diabetic cats are, on average, six times less sensitive to insulin than are healthy cats (Feldhahn *et al.*, 1999). This is of a similar magnitude to the insulin resistance in humans with type 2 diabetes mellitus. In humans, insulin resistance is predominantly the result of the sum of the underlying insulin resistance (insulin sensitivity), which is genetically determined, coupled with acquired insulin resistance, which is largely the result of obesity and physical inactivity.

Genetic and acquired factors contributing to insulin resistance are also present in cats. Risk factors of acquired insulin resistance associated with feline diabetes mellitus include obesity, physical inactivity and previous drug therapies (glucocorticoids and progestogens). Burmese cats are reported at increased risk of diabetes in Australia, New Zealand and the UK. Higher insulin concentrations in non-diabetic Burmese compared with non-diabetic domestic cats suggest that genetically determined insulin resistance is a factor. A range of insulin sensitivities are present in healthy, ideal-weight cats, and insulin sensitivity is likely genetically determined in cats, as in humans. Cats with insulin sensitivities below the population median have three times the risk of developing impaired glucose tolerance with weight gain (Appleton *et al.*, 2001).

Weight gain has a particularly profound effect on insulin resistance. In one study, insulin sensitivity was decreased by approximately 50% in cats that had increased their bodyweight by 44% over 10 months (Appleton *et al.*, 2001). In humans and dogs, physical inactivity leads to insulin resistance independent of bodyweight. Although insulin sensitivity has not been compared in inactive and active cats, indoor cats and cats rated as less active by their owners are at increased risk of developing diabetes mellitus (Lederer *et al.*, 2009; Slingerland *et al.,* 2009).

Drugs, especially long-acting or repeated glucocorticoid administration, induce insulin resistance and are a frequent precipitator of clinical signs of diabetes mellitus in cats.

Hyperglycaemia also induces insulin resistance and is reversible with improved glycaemic control.

Decreased insulin secretion

Loss of beta cell function is another hallmark of type 2 diabetes mellitus. A major cause of beta cell loss is thought to be apoptosis triggered by beta cell damage (Porte, 1991). Beta cell damage is associated with chronic hyperfunction that occurs secondary to chronic insulin resistance. Other causes of loss of beta cells include pancreatitis and islet amyloid deposition (O'Brien *et al.,* 1985; Goossens *et al.,* 1998). Some loss of function is reversible, as occurs in the early stages of glucose toxicity. Loss of beta cells occurs in the later stages of glucose toxicity, resulting in irreversible loss of beta cell insulin secretion.

Other specific types of diabetes

Other specific types of diabetes account for approximately 5–15% of cases. These types are more commonly seen in referral practice, especially tertiary referral practice, where most referred diabetic cats have disease that is difficult to control and are atypical of the majority of diabetic cats seen in first-opinion practice (O'Brien *et al.,* 1985; Goossens *et al.,* 1998). These other types also appear to account for a greater percentage of cases in developing countries where obesity is rare.

Other specific types of diabetes mellitus result from an underlying condition causing either decreased insulin secretion or impaired insulin action (insulin resistance). After type 2 diabetes, acromegaly, linked to insulin resistance, is the most commonly diagnosed underlying cause of diabetes mellitus, reported in up to 30% of cases in referral institutions in the UK and USA (Berg *et al.*, 2007; Niessen *et al.*, 2007). In cats referred with poor diabetic control and insulin doses exceeding 2 IU/kg per injection, the prevalence may be even higher. Diabetes is also linked to hyperadrenocorticism, chronic end-stage pancreatitis and pancreatic adenocarcinoma (reported to account for 9–18% of cases in referral practice), although the reported frequencies are lower than for acromegaly (O'Brien *et al.,* 1985). Pancreatitis might be underestimated as a cause of diabetes.

Glucose toxicity

Regardless of the cause of diabetes mellitus, endogenous insulin secretion at diagnosis is usually low because of the interaction between glucose toxicity and beta cell failure. Glucose toxicity describes the suppression of insulin secretion from beta cells secondary to prolonged hyperglycaemia (Unger and Grundy, 1995; Link, 2001). Insulin secretion in healthy cats is suppressed to concentrations found in insulin-dependent diabetic cats within 3–7 days of maintenance of blood glucose concentrations in the range of 30 mmol/l (Link, 2001). Glucose toxicity is dose-dependent, and less suppression occurs at lower circulating glucose concentrations.

Glucose toxicity is particularly important when superimposed on hyperfunctioning beta cells that are already compromised because of loss of beta cell mass from amyloid deposition or pancreatitis (Imamura *et al.,* 1988). With hyperfunctioning beta cells, even mild hyperglycaemia can cause a further rapid deterioration of beta cell function and worsening hyperglycaemia eventually contributes to signs of overt diabetes mellitus (Imamura *et al.,* 1988).

Suppression of insulin secretion by glucose toxicity is initially functional and reversible but later on results in structural changes of beta cells. Over weeks and months such changes become irreversible and beta cells are lost. This largely explains why cats with poorly controlled diabetes for more than 6 months have significantly reduced probability of remission, even after good glycaemic control is achieved.

Clinical features

The typical diabetic cat is 10–13 years of age and male (ratio of 2:1 male:female). Domestic Shorthair cats are the most commonly diagnosed breed. In the USA Maine Coon, Domestic Longhair, Russian Blue and Siamese are over-represented. In the UK and Australasia, Burmese cats are at increased risk; their frequency in the diabetic population is approximately three times that in the overall clinic population. One in 10 Burmese cats over the age of 8 years has diabetes mellitus in Australasia.

Clinical signs

The classical clinical signs of diabetes mellitus are:

- Polyuria, polydipsia (80% of cats)
- Weight loss (70% of cats)
- Increased appetite (reported by only 20% of owners).

At the time of diagnosis, many cats have a reduced rather than increased appetite. This is probably the result of one or more factors, including dehydration, electrolyte disturbances, ketonaemia and precipitating conditions such as infection or pancreatitis.

Clinical signs are usually present for weeks to months but may be missed by some owners. Cats are more often overweight (40%) than of normal weight or underweight. Muscle wasting and diffuse peripheral neuropathy are commonly reported (50% of cats) and result in weakness, difficulty in jumping and unsteadiness of gait. A plantigrade stance is less common and is probably indicative of more longstanding diabetes mellitus. Depression, anorexia and dehydration are present in approximately 50% of diabetic cats, but others are otherwise apparently healthy at initial presentation. In those cats that present with other specific types of diabetes mellitus, clinical signs indicative of the underlying disorder may be present.

Because diabetic cats are typically >8 years old, other concurrent diseases that may be masked by diabetes should be considered, including renal disease and hyperthyroidism.

Diagnosis

A diagnosis of uncomplicated diabetes mellitus is made based on the presence of appropriate clinical signs, persistent fasting hyperglycaemia and glucosuria. Other changes on routine clinicopathological analysis include mild anaemia, stress leucogram, hypercholesterolaemia, hypertriglyceridaemia and increased liver enzyme activities. Sick dehydrated diabetic cats may also have evidence of ketonaemia, acidosis, prerenal azotaemia and electrolyte disturbances including increased or decreased potassium and phosphorus concentrations.

Additional diagnostic tests to identify other specific types of diabetes, such as acromegaly, hyperadrenocorticism, pancreatitis and pancreatic neoplasia, are not usually performed unless pre-existing clinical signs are suggestive or there is poor response to treatment and/or evidence of significant insulin resistance. Measurement of feline pancreatic lipase immunoreactivity (fPLI) at the time of diagnosis is recommended if there are any signs consistent with pancreatitis.

Blood glucose concentration

Feline diabetes mellitus is typically diagnosed when blood glucose concentration exceeds the renal threshold, causing glucosuria and obligatory water loss and hence the signs of polyuria and polydipsia. These signs are associated with a blood glucose concentration of >14–16 mmol/l (Kruth and Cowgill, 1982).

No epidemiological studies have been performed in cats to demonstrate whether there are adverse health effects associated with persistent mild to moderate hyperglycaemia (8–14 mmol/l). In human patients, however, the cut-off blood glucose concentration for diabetes mellitus has been consistently lowered as more information has become available on the adverse effects of mild hyperglycaemia, including microvascular damage and retinopathy. It is likely that if cats were similarly classified as diabetic with a persistent fasting blood glucose concentration of 10–14 mmol/l, most would be non-insulin-dependent and a much greater proportion could be controlled with weight loss and diet alone.

Stress hyperglycaemia

Acute stress, particularly if associated with struggling, can increase blood glucose concentration by up to approximately 10 mmol/l, but often resolves within 3–4 hours. Transient illness-associated hyperglycaemia may persist for several days. Stress hyperglycaemia rarely results in blood glucose concentrations that exceed 16 mmol/l. More often glucose concentrations are in the 7–12 mmol/l range.

If a blood glucose concentration is <20 mmol/l with no, or minimal, glucosuria and typical clinical signs are absent, repeat blood glucose concentration should be measured 4 or more hours later. If the stress has largely resolved, blood glucose concentration should be within the reference interval. If the cat remains hyperglycaemic, it may be prudent to hospitalize it overnight and repeat blood glucose measurement the following morning to determine whether the hyperglycaemia persists.

If hyperglycaemia is marked (>20 mmol/l), treatment with insulin should be instituted within 24 hours if glucose concentration has not normalized, because high blood glucose concentrations can rapidly (within 24 hours) suppress insulin secretion.

Fructosamine concentration

Measurement of circulating fructosamine concentration is useful in some situations where the history is unreliable or unclear and stress hyperglycaemia cannot be ruled out as indicated above. However, over-reliance on fructosamine concentration should be avoided as there are significant problems associated with its use as a diagnostic test.

In general, measuring serum fructosamine concentration is not a sensitive indicator of persistent mild to moderate hyperglycaemia (Link and Rand, 2008). In cats with blood glucose concentrations <20 mmol/l, fructosamine concentration does not reliably differentiate cats with stress hyperglycaemia from those with diabetes mellitus. In healthy cats infused with glucose to maintain blood glucose concentrations of 17 mmol/l for 6 weeks, serum fructosamine concentration was not consistently above the upper limit of the reference interval (Link and Rand, 2008). Therefore, fructosamine measurement may significantly underdiagnose diabetes mellitus in cats with persistent hyperglycaemia of <20 mmol/l.

Ketones and lipids

Ketosis and hyperlipidaemia are likely to occur in diabetic cats with plasma glucose concentrations of >20 mmol/l, especially if present for 2 or more weeks. Experimentally, as few as 14 days of marked hyperglycaemia (at approximately 30 mmol/l) is required for plasma beta-hydroxybutyrate concentrations to exceed the reference interval in healthy cats infused with glucose (Link, 2001).

Although 60–80% of diabetic cats are ketonaemic based on plasma beta-hydroxybutyrate measurements, ketonuria is present in a smaller percentage of cats. Urine microchemistry test strips only detect acetoacetate and acetone, while beta-hydroxybutyrate is the major ketone present in diabetic ketoacidosis. Awaiting a positive stick test result can delay the diagnosis of ketonuria by approximately 5 days (Link, 2001). For an accurate diagnosis of ketosis and ketonuria, it is preferable to measure plasma or urine beta-hydroxybutyrate concentration. Although its measurement is only offered as a routine test by some veterinary laboratories, portable meters are available for use with whole blood.

Diabetic cats with mild to moderate hyperglycaemia (<20 mmol/l) do not typically develop ketonaemia and ketonuria. As a consequence, measurement of plasma beta-hydroxybutyrate is not useful for differentiating such cases from stress hyperglycaemia (Link, 2001). Healthy cats fasted for 24 hours and those on a low carbohydrate energy restricted diet for weight loss may also have mildly increased plasma beta-hydroxybutyrate concentrations (approximately 0.7 mmol/l and 1.4 mmol/l, respectively; upper limit of reference interval 0.6 mmo/l).

A diabetic ketoacidosis crisis can occur within days of demonstrating increased plasma beta-hydroxybutyrate concentrations and prompt insulin therapy should be considered in all such cases.

Urinalysis

Glucosuria in the presence of persistent hyperglycaemia is considered to be diagnostic of diabetes. Many cats also have secondary urinary tract infections. The sediment should therefore be examined for evidence of bacteria. However, there may not be an active sediment in all cases and consequently urine culture is recommended.

Treatment

Goals of therapy

The principal goal for treatment of feline diabetes mellitus has changed over the last 5 years from ameliorating clinical signs to achieving euglycaemia without the need for insulin or other hypoglycaemic therapy, commonly called 'diabetic remission'. Remission has enormous health and quality-of-life benefits for diabetic cats, and cost and lifestyle benefits for their owners. Because remission is so advantageous, in general the treatment protocol selected should maximize its probability if at all possible.

Knowledge of the likely aetiology of diabetes mellitus for each individual cat is important in determining the treatment goals for individual patients. In all newly diagnosed cats with type 2 diabetes mellitus, and in cats with correctable or reversible causes of other specific types of diabetes, including some cats with acromegaly, hyperadrenocorticism and pancreatitis, treatment should be primarily directed at achieving remission.

The primary goal of therapy in cats with long-term diabetes (>12–24 months) and uncorrectable causes of other specific types of diabetes (e.g. end-stage pancreatitis, pancreatic adenocarcinoma and many cats with acromegaly) is control of clinical signs and avoidance of clinical hypoglycaemia. Attempts should be made to identify such cases if possible. However, these cats are not typically identified until months after diagnosis, when poor control associated with a high insulin dose becomes evident, or remission does not occur despite excellent glycaemic control.

Diabetic remission

Diabetic remission is only possible if there are functional beta cells remaining. Timely resolution of glucose toxicity is critically important for its achievement.

Three factors are crucial in achieving optimal remission rates in newly diagnosed diabetic cats (Bennett *et al.*, 2006; Roomp and Rand, 2009b):

- Early initiation of appropriate insulin therapy
- Diligent and frequent monitoring of blood glucose concentrations with appropriate adjustment of insulin dose
- Feeding a suitable diet.

Several variables linked to a higher probability of remission have emerged from one study performed in 55 glargine insulin-treated cats (Roomp and Rand, 2009b). The findings of this study highlight the imperative that excellent glycaemic control be achieved as early as possible. Remission rates were 84% for cats that started intensive glycaemic control within 6 (median 4) months of diagnosis of diabetes mellitus. The rate of remission significantly decreased to 35% for cats in which the same protocol was instituted >6 months after diagnosis, even if they subsequently achieved excellent glycaemic control. Other variables associated with increased probability of remission included prior glucocorticoid treatment and absence of clinical signs of peripheral neuropathy. Gender, weight at diagnosis, age at diagnosis, presence of diabetic ketoacidosis at diagnosis, existence of chronic kidney disease or hyperthyroidism, and frequency of asymptomatic hypoglycaemia were not predictors of remission. Obesity was not shown to be negatively linked with achieving remission.

Treatment with glucocorticoids in the 6 months prior to diagnosis of diabetes mellitus was associated with an increased likelihood of diabetic remission. Sudden acquired marked insulin resistance associated with glucocorticoid treatment likely triggers a more acute onset of clinical signs, which presumably results in treatment being sought earlier than it otherwise would. Consequently there is earlier resolution of glucose toxicity.

A plantigrade stance or other milder signs of peripheral neuropathy, such as difficulty in climbing stairs, were associated with a significantly reduced probability of diabetic remission. It is likely that cats with signs of neuropathy had uncontrolled hyperglycaemia for longer periods than those without neuropathy, and therefore sustained greater destruction of beta cells arising from prolonged glucose toxicity, consequently resulting in lower remission rates.

Although 'diabetic remission' is the term commonly used to describe previously diabetic cats that maintain normoglycaemia without insulin or oral hypoglycaemic therapy, most cats in remission do not have normal glucose tolerance. The majority (80%) have a mildly impaired capacity to normalize blood glucose concentrations after a glucose challenge. A few have normal glucose tolerance and some (20–30%) have impaired fasting glucose concentrations as well as glucose intolerance. Impaired fasting glucose implies a blood glucose concentration above normal but less than that considered diabetic (6.5–11 mmol/l). Cats with impaired fasting glucose and impaired glucose tolerance should be considered pre-diabetic, and should continue to be managed with a low carbohydrate diet and normalization of bodyweight. Cats with impaired fasting glucose concentrations should be very closely monitored for relapse of their diabetes (glucose concentrations ≥11 mmol/l).

Treatment protocols for 'healthy' diabetic cats

The following relates to treatment of 'healthy' diabetic cats with minimal dehydration and no, or only mild, ketoacidosis. Cats with marked depression and dehydration, with or without ketoacidosis, should initially be treated in the same way as cats with diabetic ketoacidosis until they are stable (see Chapter 24). The protocols described below can be instituted for healthy diabetic cats and sick diabetic cats once they are stable. Because achieving diabetic remission has enormous benefits for diabetic cats and their owners, protocols that provide the greatest probability of achieving remission should initially be implemented and such protocols require insulin administration.

The aim of insulin therapy is to ensure blood glucose concentrations between 4 and 11 mmol/l throughout the day, thus maximizing the chance of diabetic remission. The type of insulin used plays a major role in achieving such rigorous glycaemic control. However, it is also dependent on the intensity of monitoring and dietary control. Although remission is achievable with most regimes commonly used, the remission rates can vary from 25% to 90% depending on the protocol implemented (Marshall and Rand, 2009; Roomp and Rand, 2009a,b).

Insulin choice

Within Europe, veterinary surgeons are legally required to use insulins registered for veterinary use as the first line of therapy. The only such insulin available is porcine lente 40 IU/ml. The previously authorized bovine lente 100 IU/ml and bovine protamine zinc insulin (PZI) (100 IU/ml) are no longer readily available. Human recombinant PZI insulin (40 IU/ml) is authorized in some countries but not yet in the UK. Recombinant human PZI has a similar action profile to the previously available 40 IU/ml beef/pork PZI (Nelson *et al.*, 2009; Norsworthy *et al.*, 2009). A wide variety of other insulins, including isophane (neutral protamine Hagedorn, NPH) are also authorized for human use.

More recently, longer-acting human-use insulin analogues have been used in cats; these include glargine and detemir.

Published data so far indicate that the use of insulin analogues such as glargine may result in higher remission rates in newly diagnosed diabetic cats than PZI, and PZI remission rates may be higher than for lente insulin, although large controlled studies are lacking. A small study of recently diagnosed diabetic cats demonstrated that 2 out of 8 cats (25%) achieved remission with porcine lente insulin, 3 of 8 (37.5%) with PZI, and 8 out of 8 with glargine (100%) (Marshall *et al.*, 2009). Remission rates for detemir are similar to those for glargine (Roomp and Rand, 2009a). Further support for higher remission rates using long-acting insulins such as glargine compared to lente insulin emanate from a recent study of 55 diabetic cats (Roomp and Rand, 2009b). These cats had previously been treated for a median of 16 weeks with other insulins, principally porcine lente insulin, but failed to achieve remission. After changing to a protocol of intensive glucose monitoring together with the use of glargine, remission rates of 84% were attained, provided the intensive protocol was initiated within 6 months of diagnosis. Similar results were obtained with detemir (Roomp and Rand, 2009b).

Given these results, PZI and porcine lente should be considered as second choice insulins. However, they may have to be used initially because of legal obligation or availability issues. Remission rates for cats are appreciably lower if intensive glucose control is not introduced early. Consequently, if these insulins are used and diabetic remission is not achieved within 4–8 weeks, it is recommended that consideration be given to changing to glargine or detemir to assist remission.

Lente and isophane insulin: When given twice daily, intermediate-acting insulins such as lente insulin have too short a duration of action for effective glycaemic control in a high proportion of cats. Because of this short duration of activity, there is usually suboptimal exogenous circulating insulin for several hours before each insulin injection, resulting in minimal glucose-lowering effect for approximately 4–8 of every 24 hours (Martin *et al.*, 2007b). Therefore, pre-insulin blood glucose concentrations are usually high (up to 20 mmol/l or higher) and the goal of achieving glucose concentrations between 4 and 11 mmol/l, which is so important for diabetic remission, is not achieved throughout the day. Although clinical signs may be relatively well controlled, the potential marked hyperglycaemia twice daily will continue to suppress and cause beta cell destruction, contributing to the lower remission rates in comparison with results obtained with longer-acting insulins (Marshall *et al.*, 2009; Roomp and Rand, 2009b).

Isophane insulin tends to have an even shorter duration of action than porcine lente insulin and is not recommended for use in cats unless no other insulin is available. Similarly, the premixed insulin analogues consisting of rapid-acting and intermediate-acting insulin analogues (e.g. 75% insulin lispro protamine suspension and 25% insulin lispro) are not recommended. There are no published data concerning their use in cats but they would not be expected to confer any advantages over lente insulin, which is also a mix of 30% short- and 70% long-acting insulin.

Protamine zinc insulin: PZI has a longer duration of action compared to lente insulin, and because of this is often preferred for use in cats. However, it is shown to be linked with lower remission rates in comparison to the new long-acting insulin analogues, detemir and glargine (Marshall *et al.*, 2009; Roomp and Rand, 2009b).

Glargine: Glargine is a synthetic insulin analogue. It is produced using recombinant DNA technology utilizing *Escherichia coli*. The insulin molecule is modified by replacing asparagine at position 21 with glycine, and by adding two arginines at the terminal portion of the insulin B chain. The glycine–arginine substitution is reflected in the name glargine. The modification shifts the isoelectric point, producing a molecule that is totally soluble at a pH of 4. In subcutaneous tissues where the pH is 7.4, the acidic solution is neutralized, allowing formation of microprecipitates, which steadily break down. This slow release of glargine into the systemic circulation produces its sustained action. The formation of microprecipitates is dependent on the interaction of the acidic insulin (pH = 4) and the relatively neutral subcutaneous tissues (pH = 7); it is therefore imperative that glargine is not mixed with other insulin or diluted before administration.

Glargine is designed for once-daily administration in humans and is marketed as a 'peakless' insulin with respect to its glucose-lowering effect. This lack of peak relates to the glucose utilization rate of glargine, a factor determined by the amount of intravenous glucose necessary to maintain a constant plasma glucose concentration after insulin is injected subcutaneously. However, when viewing the glucose and insulin concentration curves in diabetic and healthy cats, there are definite glucose nadirs and insulin peaks associated with glargine use. The blood glucose-lowering effect and the duration of insulin action in cats are comparable to those in diabetic humans (Marshall *et al.*, 2008).

In cats, clinical experience demonstrates that glargine has a long duration of action and, in stabilized cats, is not usually associated with marked hyperglycaemia at the time of the next insulin injection as occurs with lente insulin.

Detemir: The synthetic insulin analogue detemir has an extended duration of action, which is achieved via a different mechanism from glargine. Detemir is produced using recombinant DNA technology in yeast (*Saccharomyces cerevisiae*), and the insulin molecule is modified by addition of an acylated fatty acid chain. This modification facilitates reversible binding to plasma proteins, particularly albumin, from where it is released slowly into plasma. The modification also prolongs self-association in the injection depot, which delays absorption from subcutaneous tissue at the injection site and contributes to the long duration of action (Kurtzhals, 2004).

Glargine versus detemir: No clinical differences were detected between cats treated with glargine (*n* = 55) and with detemir (*n* = 18), except that a 30% lower maximal dose was required in the detemir-treated cats (median maximum glargine dose was 2.5 IU (range = 1.0–9.0 IU) compared with a median detemir dose of 1.75 IU (range = 0.5–4.0 IU)) (Roomp and Rand, 2009a,b). Because glargine has been used more widely in cats and its pharmacokinetics and dynamics are better known in comparison with detemir, glargine is currently the insulin of choice in diabetic cats. However, data from healthy cats and humans suggest that detemir has a longer duration of action and less variability between and within individuals compared to glargine, and it might yet become the insulin of choice in diabetic cats (Gilor *et al.*, 2008). Experimentally, in healthy cats detemir had a longer duration of action (median 800 minutes; range 525–915 minutes) than glargine (median 470 minutes; range 295–950 minutes) and showed less variation in duration of action between cats (Gilor *et al.*, 2008). In human patients detemir has also been shown to be more consistent in its duration of action in comparison with glargine. Therefore detemir is particularly indicated in those cats where glargine appears to have too short a duration of action with twice-daily administration.

Storage of glargine and detemir: Many questions arise because of the manufacturers' instructions regarding shelf-life for glargine and detemir, and the subsequent cost implications for owners managing their diabetic pet. Glargine is marketed for human use with a shelf-life at room temperature of 28 days after opening. It is fairly fragile but is chemically stable in solution for 6 months if kept refrigerated. Detemir is marketed with a 6-week shelf-life at room temperature after opening. Longer expiration periods are not usually recommended on multiple-use injectable medication vials for humans, even if a preservative is present, because of the risk of bacterial contamination. Glargine and detemir preparations contain the antimicrobial preservative meta-cresol, which is thought to be bacteriostatic rather than bactericidal. Authorization bodies believe that there is a reasonable probability of becoming contaminated with microbes through multiple daily punctures to withdraw medication past the arbitrary expiration date. However, in veterinary practice, owners of diabetic cats routinely use refrigerated glargine or detemir for up to 6 months or more with no evidence of problems. Owners should be instructed to immediately dispose of any insulin appearing cloudy or discoloured, because this may represent bacterial contamination or precipitation.

Frequency of insulin administration

It is important to reduce the daily exposure of beta cells to marked hyperglycaemia to aid recovery of beta cell function and maximize the likelihood of successful diabetic remission (Robertson *et al.*, 2000; Link, 2001) This is more likely if insulin is administered twice daily rather than once daily in diabetic cats.

Intermediate-acting insulin such as lente and NPH must be given twice daily in cats. However, in many cats, glycaemic control would be improved if administration were three times daily, because the duration of action is typically <8 hours. In dogs, once-daily insulin administration is associated with an increased risk of clinical hypoglycaemia, and this is also likely in cats (Hess and Ward, 2000).

Although PZI is a long-acting insulin, improved glycaemic control occurs with twice-daily administration. Glargine and detemir are also considered to be long-acting. The mean duration of action after 0.25 IU/kg of glargine in healthy cats was at least 20 hours, although in some cats it was as short as 14 hours (Marshall *et al.*, 2009). Another study measuring glucose utilization rate in healthy cats found the median duration of glargine action was 8 hours, but could be as short as 5 hours after administration of 0.5 IU/kg (Gilor *et al.*, 2008). It is clear that the duration of action of glargine, and probably detemir, varies substantially in healthy and diabetic cats, and within the same cat from day to day. Despite the lack of well controlled pharmacodynamic studies and variability within cats, clinical observations suggest that remission rates in recently diagnosed diabetic cats are higher when glargine or detemir are administered twice-daily in comparison with once-daily dosing (Weaver *et al.*, 2006; Marshall *at al.*, 2009; Roomp and Rand, 2009a,b).

Insulin dose

Dosing protocols can be successfully used for adjusting insulin dose with a range of insulins. However, it needs to be recognized that the dosing rules differ depending on whether the insulin used is intermediate-acting and unlikely to have a carry-over effect at the next insulin injection, or is long-acting with a high probability of carry-over effects.

For long-acting insulin, both the nadir (lowest) and the pre-insulin blood glucose concentration (just prior to next insulin injection) are used as a basis for increasing the dose. In contrast, with intermediate-acting insulin only the nadir blood glucose concentration is used for increasing the insulin dose.

Regardless of the type of insulin used, an initial dose of 0.25–0.5 IU/kg of the cat's ideal bodyweight is recommended for newly diagnosed cats, at 12-hourly intervals depending on blood glucose concentrations. During the first 3 days of therapy, blood glucose concentrations should be carefully monitored every 2–4 hours during the day and the insulin dose reduced if the blood glucose concentration at any one time is low.

When changing cats on to glargine from other types of insulin, they can typically be changed to the same dose, with the exception of high doses (>3 IU) of insulin. Care should be exercised in these cats until it is known how they will respond, and a smaller dose should be used initially. For detemir, a 30% lower dose than previously used is recommended as a starting dose.

Because glucose concentrations should ideally be measured every 2 hours (lente, isophane) or every 3–4 hours (glargine, detemir and PZI), portable glucose meters provide a useful tool for obtaining such results, provided they are interpreted correctly (see below). The protocols illustrated (Figures 13.2, 13.3 and 13.4) have been developed for use with intermediate (lente, NPH) and long-acting insulins (glargine, detemir and PZI).

Dose adjustments: After the initial 3 days of treatment there are two or three phases of treatment for

Blood glucose variable	Recommendation
Use an initial dose 0.5 IU/kg of lean body weight q12h if blood glucose is >20 mmol/l and 0.25 IU/Kg q12h if blood glucose <20 mmol/l; do not increase in first week but decrease if necessary	
If nadir blood glucose concentration is <3 mmol/l	Dose should be reduced by 50%
If nadir blood glucose concentration is 3–5 mmol/l	Dose should be reduced by 1 IU if poor control of clinical signs of diabetes; dose should remain the same if exemplary control of clinical signs
If nadir blood glucose concentration is 5–9 mmol/l	Dose should remain the same
If nadir blood glucose concentration is >10 mmol/l	Dose should be increased by 1 IU
If nadir blood glucose concentration occurs within 3 hours of insulin administration or blood glucose returns to baseline within 8 hours	Change to longer-acting insulin (i.e. glargine, detemir or PZI)
If the nadir blood glucose concentration occurs at 8 hours or later	Once-daily administration may be used, although twice-daily administration at a reduced dose is preferred

13.2 Dosing protocol for cats on intermediate-acting insulins (lente or isophane). Parameters for changing insulin dosage and frequency based on blood glucose measurements when using lente or isophane insulin in diabetic cats. Insulin dosage adjustments are based on monitoring blood glucose concentration every 2 weeks with serial measurements every 2 hours over 12 hours. The protocol was tested in >25 diabetic cats using lente insulin (Martin and Rand, 2007). Blood glucose values are based on measurements obtained using a portable glucose meter calibrated for human whole blood. If using a serum chemistry analyser or a portable glucose meter calibrated for feline blood, blood glucose concentrations should be adjusted by adding approximately 1.0 mmol/l to the values listed.

Parameter used for dosage adjustment	Change in dose
Begin with 0.5 IU/kg q12h if blood glucose >20 mmol/l or 0.25 IU/kg of *ideal weight* if blood glucose is lower. Do not increase in first week unless minimum response to insulin occurs, but decrease if necessary. Monitor response to therapy for first 3 days. If no monitoring is occurring in first week, begin with 1 IU/cat q12h	
If pre-insulin blood glucose concentration >12 mmol/l provided nadir is not in hypoglycaemic range *or* If nadir blood glucose concentration >10 mmol/l	Increase by 0.25 IU, depending on the severity of the hyperglycaemia and the total insulin dose
If pre-insulin blood glucose concentration 10 –12 mmol/l *or* Nadir blood glucose concentration is 5–9 mmol/l	Same dose
If pre-insulin blood glucose concentration is 11–14 mmol/l *or* If nadir glucose concentration is 3–4 mmol/l	Use nadir glucose, water intake, urine glucose and next pre-insulin glucose concentration to determine whether insulin dose is decreased or maintained
If pre-insulin blood glucose concentration <10 mmol/l *or* If nadir blood glucose concentration <3 mmol/l	Reduce by 0.5–1.0 IU or if total dose is 0.5–1.0 IU q24h, stop insulin and check for diabetic remission
If clinical signs of hypoglycaemia are observed	Reduce by 50%
If blood glucose measurements are not available	
If water intake is ≤20 ml/kg on wet food or ≤60 ml/kg on dry food	Same dose
If water intake is >20 ml/kg on wet food or >60 ml/kg on dry food	Increase dose by 0.5–1.0 IU
If urine glucose is >3+ (scale 0–4+)	Increase dose by 0.5–1.0 IU
If urine glucose is negative	Decrease dose until 0.5–1.0 IU q24h and then check for diabetic remission

13.3 Dosing protocol for cats on glargine, PZI or detemir and glucose monitoring every 1–2 weeks. Parameters for changing insulin dosage when using insulin glargine, PZI or detemir in diabetic cats being assessed with serial blood glucose measurement every 3–4 hours over 12 hours once a week (preferred) or once every 2 weeks in the first 4 months of therapy. Blood glucose values are based on measurements obtained using a portable glucose meter calibrated for human whole blood. If using a serum chemistry analyser or a portable glucose meter calibrated for feline blood, blood glucose concentrations should be adjusted by adding approximately 1.0 mmol/l to the values listed.

Parameter used for dosage adjustment	Change in dose
Phase 1: Initial dose and first 3 days on glargine or detemir	
Begin with 0.25 IU/kg of ideal weight q12h *or* If the cat has previously received another insulin, increase or reduce the starting dose taking this information into account. Glargine has a lower potency than lente insulin and PZI in most cats	
Cats with a history of developing ketosis that maintain blood glucose concentration >17 mmol/l after 24–48 hours	Increase by 0.5 IU
If blood glucose concentration is <2.8 mmol/l	Reduce dose by 0.25–0.5 IU depending on whether the cat is on low (<3 IU/cat) or high (≥3 IU/cat) dose of insulin
Phase 2: Increasing the dose	
If nadir blood glucose concentration >17 mmol/l	Increase every 3 days by 0.5 IU
If nadir blood glucose concentration 11–17 mmol/l	Increase every 3 days by 0.25-0.5 IU depending on whether cat on low or high dose of insulin

13.4 Dosing protocol for cats on glargine or detemir using daily home monitoring of blood glucose concentrations to adjust insulin dose. Reproduced with permission from Roomp and Rand (2009a). Parameters for changing insulin dosage when using insulin glargine or detemir together with home monitoring of blood glucose concentrations in a protocol aimed at achieving intensive blood glucose control. Blood glucose should be measured at least three times daily with a glucometer. Blood glucose values are based on measurements obtained using a portable glucose meter calibrated for human whole blood. If using a serum chemistry analyser or a portable glucose meter calibrated for feline blood, blood glucose concentrations should be adjusted by adding approximately 1.0 mmol/l to the values listed. (continues) ▶

Parameter used for dosage adjustment	Change in dose
Phase 2: Increasing the dose	
If nadir blood glucose concentration <11 mmol/l but peak is >11 mmol/l	Increase every 5–7 days by 0.25–0.5 IU depending on whether cat on low or high dose of insulin
If blood glucose concentration is < 2.8 mmol/l	Reduce dose by 0.25–0.5 IU depending on whether cat on low or high dose of insulin
If blood glucose concentration at the time of the next insulin injection is 2.8–5.6 mmol/l	Initially test which of the alternate methods is best suited to the individual cat: 1. Feed cat and reduce the dose by 0.25–0.5 IU depending on whether cat on low or high dose of insulin. 2. Feed the cat, wait 1–2 hours and when the glucose concentration increases to >5.6 mmol/l give the normal dose. If the glucose concentration does not increase within 1–2 hours, reduce the dose by 0.25 IU or 0.5 IU (as above). 3. Split the dose: feed cat and give most of dose immediately, and then give the remainder 1–2 hours later, when the glucose concentration has increased to >5.6 mmol/l. If all these methods lead to increased blood glucose concentrations, give the full dose if pre-insulin blood glucose concentration is 2.8–5.6 mmol/l and observe closely for signs of hypoglycaemia. In general, for most cats the best results in phase 2 occur when insulin dose is as consistent as possible, giving the full normal dose at the regular injection time
Phase 3: Holding the dose. Aim to keep blood glucose concentration between 2.8 and 11 mmol/l throughout the day	
If blood glucose concentration is <2.8 mmol/l	Reduce dose by 0.25–0.5 IU depending on whether cat on low or high dose of insulin
If nadir or peak blood glucose concentration is >11 mmol/l	Increase dose by 0.25–0.5 IU depending on whether cat on low or high dose of insulin and the degree of hyperglycaemia
Phase 4: Reducing the dose. Phase out insulin slowly by 0.25–0.5 IU depending on dose	
When the cat regularly (every day for at least one week) has its lowest blood glucose concentration in the normal range of a healthy cat and stays under 5.6 mmol/l overall	Reduce dose by 0.25–0.5 IU depending on whether the cat is on a low or high dose of insulin
If nadir glucose concentration is 2.2–<2.8 mmol/l at least three times on separate days	Reduce dose by 0.25–0.5 IU depending on whether cat on low or high dose of insulin
If nadir blood glucose concentration drops below 2.2 mmol/l	Reduce dose immediately by 0.25–0.5 IU depending on whether cat on low or high dose of insulin
If peak blood glucose concentration >11 mmol/l	Immediately increase insulin dose to last effective dose
Phase 5: Remission. Euglycaemia for a minimum of 14 days without insulin	

13.4 (continued) Dosing protocol for cats on glargine or detemir using daily home monitoring of blood glucose concentrations to adjust insulin dose. Reproduced with permission from Roomp and Rand (2009a). Parameters for changing insulin dosage when using insulin glargine or detemir together with home monitoring of blood glucose concentrations in a protocol aimed at achieving intensive blood glucose control. Blood glucose should be measured at least three times daily with a glucometer. Blood glucose values are based on measurements obtained using a portable glucose meter calibrated for human whole blood. If using a serum chemistry analyser or a portable glucose meter calibrated for feline blood, blood glucose concentrations should be adjusted by adding approximately 1.0 mmol/l to the values listed.

diabetic cats. Initially there is a phase of increasing dose, followed by a phase of consistent dosing, and finally, for cats going into remission, a phase of decreasing dose.

In the phase of increasing dose, depending on the insulin being used, either nadir or nadir and pre-insulin glucose concentrations are used as a basis for increasing the dose. If close monitoring is occurring, doses can be increased every 3 to 7 days by 0.25–1.00 IU/injection depending on whether a low (<3 IU) or high (≥ 3 IU) dose of insulin is being used and the degree of hyperglycaemia (see Figures 13.2 to 13.4). For glargine and detemir, the aim is to increase the dose until the blood glucose concentration is between 4 and 11 mmol/l; that is, consistently within or just above the reference interval throughout the day. In lente- and NPH-treated cats, this is not achievable, but the aim is for the nadir blood glucose concentration to be in the high end of the reference interval (5–9 mmol/l). Approximately 25% of cats will show an increase in glucose concentration in the first 2 to 3 days after a dose increase, which generally lasts for <24 hours. The dose should be maintained and the fluctuations disregarded.

In the phase of consistent dosing, the dose is held once the blood glucose concentrations throughout the day are between 4 and 11 mmol/l (detemir, glargine and PZI) or the nadir is between 5 and 9 mmol/l (lente, NPH). This phase of consistent dosing may last several months, although in some cats it lasts only weeks.

The final phase involves a reduction in the dose once the pre-insulin blood glucose is <10 mmol/l or if the nadir glucose concentration is <4–5 mmol/l (see Figures 13.2, 13.3 and 13.4). To determine whether remission has occurred, the insulin is stopped if the above criteria are met and the cat is on a minimal dose (e.g. 0.5 IU once or twice a day). The cat is then reassessed 12 hours later and, if at that time the blood glucose concentration has not increased to >10 mmol/l, the cat is re-checked again in one week. Insulin is immediately reinstituted if a blood glucose concentration increases to 10 mmol/l or higher within 12 hours of withholding insulin. Although remission will not be achieved in all cats, for cats that remain insulin dependent a dose reduction may be required after the phase of consistent dosing, once the insulin resistance associated with glucose toxicity resolves.

During the first weeks of insulin therapy, a frequent error is to cease insulin administration prematurely. This is often done when a pre-insulin blood glucose concentration is in the reference interval. Decreasing the dose too rapidly may reduce the chance of remission by withdrawing insulin before beta cells have fully recovered from glucose toxicity. Instead, insulin should be reduced but not withheld until the total insulin dose is 0.5 IU once or twice a day. In this phase of decreasing dose, it is critical that the rate of decrease is slow and conservative, ideally adjusting only every 7–14 days. Insulin is phased out gradually in a step-by-step manner (in 0.25 IU or 0.5 IU decrements), which is dependent on the overall dose administered. Subjectively, cats that are very slowly weaned off insulin are less likely to relapse soon after insulin is withdrawn. If the blood glucose concentration fails to remain within the reference interval after a dose reduction, the insulin dose is immediately increased to the last effective dose.

For a small number of cats, a small dose (e.g. 1 IU) of insulin administered every 48 hours is necessary when there is insufficient beta cell function to maintain euglycaemia; daily dosing would result in hypoglycaemia. In a further few cats, blood glucose concentrations remain in the reference interval for a few days following a dose reduction but then begin to increase again, and the dose will need to be increased.

The average dose for cats that remain stable on glargine, detemir, lente or PZI insulin is 0.4–0.6 IU/kg. Occasionally, cats need high total doses of insulin (5–10 IU/cat) to control blood glucose concentrations. In many of these cats the dose can be decreased once control is achieved. However, cats with acromegaly often require high (>10 IU/cat) and on occasion extreme doses (>50 IU/cat) to control blood glucose concentration. Any cat on a dose of >5 IU/cat q12h should have insulin-like growth factor (IGF-α) measured and brain imaging performed to rule out acromegaly. It is recommended that owners of cats with acromegaly measure blood glucose concentration at home before administering insulin, as growth hormone and subsequent blood glucose concentrations can vary widely from day to day.

Dose variations: There is a large variation in the glucose-lowering effect of a given dose of insulin between cats and within the same cat from day to day. This is also reported in humans and dogs. There are a variety of factors that contribute to this, including differences in rates and percentage of insulin absorbed from the subcutaneous injection site, variation in insulin sensitivity between cats and variation in the actual dose received per kg of metabolic weight (Marshall *et al.*, 2008).

The very small volume of insulin used in cats makes dosage errors likely. Many cats are receiving <2 IU at each injection. One study demonstrated that even trained paediatric nurses using 100 IU 0.3 ml syringes were unable to dose any amount under 2 IU accurately (Casella *et al.*, 1993).

Dilution is often recommended when small doses are required. However, glargine should not be diluted because of its mechanism of action; accurate dosing is therefore difficult in the majority of cats when using 100 IU/ml insulin. These errors are likely to be reduced by using 0.3 ml insulin syringes designed for 100 IU/ml insulin with 0.5 unit (and if available 0.25 unit) gradations. A magnifying glass can help more accurately dose small volumes. Many clients find the 40 IU/ml syringes assist in measuring small volumes, but care should be taken to avoid using 100 IU/ml insulin with these syringes as inappropriate calculation of differences can lead to serious dosing errors. Insulin pens more accurately dose IU increments but do not deliver a total dose smaller than 1 IU. An insulin syringe is best used for the final stages when weaning a cat off insulin. Detemir can be diluted using a solution supplied by the manufacturer.

Adverse effects of insulin

Hypoglycaemia

Biochemical hypoglycaemia is common in insulin-treated cats. Clinical hypoglycaemia is infrequent in cats treated with glargine or detemir but appears to be more common in cats treated with lente insulin (Marshall *et al.*, 2009; Roomp and Rand, 2009a,b). In human type 1 and 2 diabetics treated with glargine, the prevalence of clinical hypoglycaemia is also considerably reduced compared with shorter-acting insulins such as NPH (Fonseca *et al.*, 2004; Fulcher *et al.*, 2005). In one study of 55 cats treated with glargine using an intensive protocol designed to achieve euglycaemia, asymptomatic or biochemical hypoglycaemia was common, occurring at some point in up to 94% of cases (Roomp and Rand, 2009b). However, there was only one associated mild episode of clinical hypoglycaemia. Detemir is associated with a similar low rate of clinical hypoglycaemia.

Signs of clinical hypoglycaemia in cats can be severe and life-threatening, and are why some owners elect to euthanase diabetic cats.

Somogyi effect (overswing)

Marked hyperglycaemia following an episode of hypoglycaemia is referred to as the Somogyi effect or overswing, and insulin resistance is often mentioned as a consequence. Several studies have shown that the Somogyi effect is uncommon in human diabetic patients. In the veterinary literature to date, there are few studies describing the Somogyi effect, yet it is frequently mentioned in texts on feline diabetes mellitus. Anecdotally, the Somogyi effect followed by insulin resistance appears to be more frequent with lente and other intermediate-acting insulins, which are more potent and lead to a more rapid reduction in blood glucose following insulin injection, triggering counter-regulation. In one study of glargine-treated cats with intense home monitoring, the Somogyi effect was rarely documented despite regular occurrence of biochemical hypoglycaemia (Roomp and Rand, 2009b). Recognition of a Somogyi effect requires frequent blood glucose measurements and may be missed even with intensive monitoring protocols. The availability of continuous glucose monitoring provides the technology required to more accurately document the true incidence of the Somogyi effect associated with use of intermediate and long-acting insulins.

Oral hypoglycaemic agents

Oral hypoglycaemic drugs stimulate beta cells to secrete insulin (e.g. glipizide), or decrease insulin absorption from the gastrointestinal tract (e.g. acarbose) or increase insulin sensitivity (e.g. metformin, roziglitazone). Sole use of oral hypoglycaemic agents that stimulate insulin secretion are associated with a reduced probability of remission (remission rate <20%) compared to treatment with a long-acting insulin (remission rate >80%) and is not recommended (Feldman and Nelson, 1997; Roomp and Rand, 2009b). Remission rates associated with most other oral hypoglycaemic drugs are likely similar and so use of these drugs is also not recommended. However, the use of oral hypoglycaemic agents can be life-saving for cats when the owner elects euthanasia rather than the injection of insulin.

The alpha-glucosidase inhibitors (e.g. acarbose) reduce intestinal glucose absorption and need to be administered orally twice daily with food. Cats with a high carbohydrate diet eaten in one daily meal had significantly reduced blood glucose concentrations when given acarbose, although the same effect is achieved using a low carbohydrate diet. Acarbose may be more useful in cats on a high carbohydrate diet which are eating all their food in one or two daily meals, a typical feeding pattern for cats on a weight loss programme. Acarbose is minimally effective in cats that have multiple small meals or graze throughout the day and, as a consequence, it may not be of any real benefit in cats with a reduced appetite that are fed a high-carbohydrate and low-protein diet (e.g. for chronic kidney disease), where it might otherwise have a reasonable therapeutic indication.

Dietary management

Dietary management of feline diabetes mellitus using a low-carbohydrate diet (<15% metabolizable energy (ME)) is one of the three key strategies for increasing the probability of remission. A complete and balanced low-carbohydrate diet should be fed, including in those diabetic cats requiring weight loss. Low carbohydrate diets are associated with increased remission rates and minimize the need for beta cells to secrete insulin. Importantly, in a study comparing remission rates between a moderate-carbohydrate (26% ME) and low-carbohydrate (12% ME) diet with similar protein content (37% ME *versus* 40% ME), the low-carbohydrate diet was associated with significantly higher remission rates (68% *versus* 41%) (Bennett *et al.*, 2006). In addition, decreasing the carbohydrate content (from 50% to 25% ME) significantly reduces blood glucose concentrations in healthy cats by 20% to 25% for 3–18 hours after eating, if fed once or twice daily and throughout the day if fed *ad libitum*. For diabetic cats with reduced or no endogenous insulin secretion, the increase in blood glucose after eating is likely to be more pronounced than in healthy cats.

A restricted-carbohydrate diet should be started at the time of initiation of insulin therapy, and it is critical that the diet be continued after remission to minimize the demand on beta cells to secrete insulin. For cats already on insulin therapy, when changing from a moderate- or high-carbohydrate diet to a low-carbohydrate diet, it is recommended that the insulin dose be initially reduced by 30–50%, because hypoglycaemia can result secondary to the reduction in glucose load associated with the low-carbohydrate diet.

Ultra-low-carbohydrate diets (<5% ME) are also occasionally recommended. These diets are essentially nearly all meat or fish diets, but are often neither complete nor balanced and are high in phosphorus, which is of concern given the frequency of renal disease in diabetic cats. Although restricted carbohydrate diets are recommended if remission is a goal of therapy, there are currently no studies available that compare diets of varying carbohydrate content (2, 6 or 15% ME), to determine which is most appropriate for use in feline diabetic patients. If remission is not a realistic goal of therapy, for example if the cat has been diabetic for several years, dietary management of other health issues takes precedence.

Feeding frequency

In healthy cats, similar blood glucose concentration curves are obtained for those that are either fed the same diet once or twice daily or fed *ad libitum*. However, it is generally recommended that cats be fed twice daily at the same time as the insulin injection.

Weight management

Obesity in cats has a profound effect on insulin sensitivity, decreasing it by approximately 50% (Appleton et al., 2001). This means that more insulin is required to maintain glucose concentrations in the reference interval compared to when body condition is lean. Although many cats achieve remission in the first 4–6 weeks of insulin therapy, before substantial weight loss has occurred, obesity continues to put a high demand on beta cells to secrete insulin and likely increases the probability of relapse in the same way as it predisposes to the development of diabetes mellitus. Thus it is critically important to continue to address overweight, even if remission has been obtained. Obese cats should be energy-restricted to lose 1 to <2% of bodyweight per week (e.g. approximately 0.5 kg/month for an 8 kg cat). Because high-carbohydrate diets result in a further demand on beta cells to secrete insulin, it is recommended that obese cats are fed a low-carbohydrate balanced and complete diet designed for management of feline obesity and diabetes mellitus, even though these diets are more energy-dense and have higher fat content than traditional weight loss diets. Feeding canned food seems to increase satiety in many cats, which can facilitate owner compliance with feeding restricted amounts of food (Hoenig and Rand, 2006).

In long-term diabetic and obese cats, if a low-carbohydrate diet has not been associated with successful weight loss, a lower-energy-density diet could be used as remission is then less likely. These diets are typically high-fibre, moderate- to high-carbohydrate diets (>25% ME), which are not recommended when remission is a realistic goal. In such cases the reduction in insulin resistance associated with weight loss is unlikely to seriously affect diabetic management but it has other substantial health benefits that make it an important goal.

Monitoring response to therapy

Good glycaemic control is dependent upon close monitoring and appropriate adjustment of insulin dose. Initially, communication with the owner regarding their cat plays a large part in this process. Crucial considerations include water drunk, urine output (e.g. amount of clumping in cat litter) and bodyweight, and are evaluated along with possible signs of hypoglycaemia and developing or worsening neuropathy.

Home monitoring

Home monitoring of blood glucose concentrations provides a more accurate reflection of glycaemic control because two confounding effects often associated with a visit to a veterinary clinic are avoided.

- As eating increases blood glucose concentration, diabetic cats need to eat their normal diet and amount for an accurate blood glucose curve. This may not occur in a veterinary clinic.
- Stress increases blood glucose concentration, and struggling to resist blood sampling can increase blood glucose by up to 10 mmol/l.

Additionally, daily home monitoring provides more data and therefore facilitates more frequent insulin adjustments. This is advantageous because early optimization of blood glucose concentration increases the probability of remission. Home monitoring also allows immediate blood glucose assessment by the owner for confirming hypoglycaemia when vague but suggestive signs are present. Home monitoring may also be less expensive and more convenient for owners than having blood glucose curves obtained in the veterinary clinic.

Clients still require frequent clinic visits in the initial stabilization phase to review their home log of blood glucose concentrations and insulin dose, but do not need to leave their cat for serial blood glucose monitoring. At each visit, blood collection and glucose measurement techniques should be reviewed and the cat examined and weighed. As owners become more competent, many can confidently follow a protocol for dose adjustment. Home monitoring in combination with glargine treatment is associated with higher remission rates compared to those previously treated with other insulins, predominantly lente and PZI (Roomp and Rand, 2009b).

For home-monitored cats treated with long-acting insulins, such as glargine, detemir or PZI, it is important to obtain measurements of blood glucose concentration before each insulin injection and at the nadir point (see above). A pre-insulin glucose measurement depicts the potential carry-over effect of long-acting insulins. The time of the nadir blood glucose concentration is variable in cats, and within the same cat from day to day but can be assessed by several blood glucose measurements throughout the day.

For intermediate-acting insulins, only a nadir blood glucose measurement is required and usually occurs 2–6 hours after insulin administration. The pre-insulin glucose measurement is only useful for indicating a dose reduction when there is impending remission, or when blood glucose concentration is very high (>28 mmol/l), suggesting rebound hyperglycaemia.

Glucose meters

Portable glucose meters are frequently used for measuring blood glucose concentrations, particularly when home monitoring is being undertaken. When choosing a portable glucose meter, accuracy and precision are important considerations. A number of reputable companies manufacture glucose meters calibrated specifically for human blood, providing a whole blood or plasma equivalent value. These meters are reasonably precise. However, accuracy decreases substantially when these meters are used with feline blood. This is assumed to be a result of the different distribution of glucose between plasma and red blood cells in feline compared to human blood.

Whole blood glucose meters calibrated for human use typically report feline blood glucose concentrations approximately 20–40% or 1–2 mmol/l lower than the actual plasma glucose concentration when concentrations are within the euglycaemic range (Wess and Reusch, 2000; Reusch *et al.,* 2001). This may partly explain why some cats show no or only mild signs with moderate levels of hypoglycaemia when measured with a portable human blood glucose meter.

Glucose meters calibrated for feline blood that provide a plasma equivalent value are now available (e.g. AlphaTRAK) and more accurately reflect actual glucose concentration. If such a glucose meter or a serum chemistry analyser is used, approximately 1.0 mmol/l is added to the target blood glucose concentrations recommended when using a glucose meter for human whole blood. For example, the protocol designed for home monitoring aims for a blood glucose concentration between 2.8 and 5.6 mmol/l if measured with a whole blood meter calibrated for human use. If a plasma-equivalent meter calibrated for feline blood or a chemistry analyser is being used, the target blood glucose concentration is approximately 4.0–6.6 mmol/l. The newer feline glucose meters are also advantageous because they require substantially smaller volumes of blood (≤0.6 μl versus 1.6 μl) and have a higher upper limit for glucose concentration. It is critical that staff and clients understand the difference between meters calibrated for human and for cat blood, especially for interpreting readings within and below the reference interval.

Typically, blood is taken from the ear or a paw pad using a lancing device (Figures 13.5 to 13.7). Paw pad sampling appears to be particularly well tolerated by many cats. Either the main pad or the pisiform (carpal) pad can be used (see http://www.uq.edu.au/ccah/ppt/homemngmntslides.pdf Warming the area, for example by placing a moist cotton-wool ball in the microwave until warm and holding it on the paw for 20 seconds prior to sampling, enhances blood flow and increases success in the early stages. Likewise, rubbing the area or using other forms of heat increase blood flow. Later, with multiple use of an area, and particularly in ears, vascularization appears to increase, making sampling easier. A few owners prefer to draw blood 'free-hand' using only a lancet needle or syringe needle, but this method is more likely

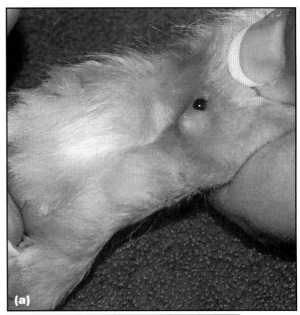
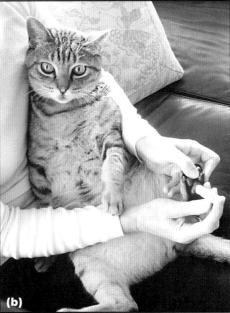

13.6 **(a)** Taking a blood sample from the carpal (pisiform) pad. (Courtesy of S. Ford)
(b) Sampling the main paw pad is well tolerated in many cats. (Courtesy of W. Milledge)

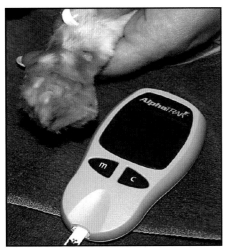

13.5 The Abbott AlphaTRAK meter is calibrated for feline blood, and only requires a 0.3 μl sample, making it ideal for measuring blood glucose in paw pad or ear samples. (Courtesy of S. Ford)

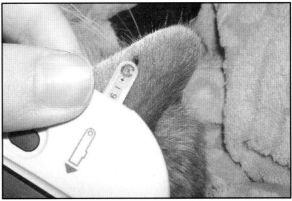

13.7 Measuring blood glucose from an ear sample. Best results occur if the area is rubbed or warmed first to increase blood supply. (Courtesy of S. Ford)

to be painful and is not recommended initially until experience is gained.

Certain lancets work better in certain sites, in certain cats and with certain owners; a successful approach is to test various areas and lancets in the consulting room in order to determine the best device and site that will maximize the likelihood of obtaining an adequate sample.

Water intake and urine glucose output

Water intake and urine glucose estimations are useful indicators of glycaemic control, but are inferior to daily home blood glucose measurements. Water intake measured at home was shown to be a better indicator of recent mean blood glucose concentration than measurement of fructosamine concentration (Martin *et al.*, 2007a). This is probably because fructosamine concentration reflects mean blood glucose concentration over the preceding 1–3 weeks, and during the phase of increasing dose when managing diabetic cats, mean blood glucose concentration can change substantially. Observant owners may become aware of a sudden marked increase in glucose concentrations over several hours because the cat drinks substantially more.

Estimation of urine glucose is useful and can be achieved using special 'chips' added to cat litter. Specially designed litter boxes are also available, with trays to catch urine beneath the litter. In fractious cats in which blood glucose measurements cannot be obtained, or where the owner is unwilling to measure blood glucose concentration, urine glucose and water intake can be used as crude indicators for adjusting insulin dose with glargine and detemir. However, with intermediate-acting insulins more commonly than with long-acting insulin, marked glucosuria occurs with both under- and overdosing because of rebound hyperglycaemia and the short duration of insulin action. Therefore, using urine glucose to increase the dose of intermediate-acting insulin is often problematic.

Urine glucose measurements are less useful for detecting remission in glargine- and detemir-treated cats because once cats are on the correct dose of glargine or detemir, they should have negative or trace glucosuria. Conversely, repeated negative urine glucose is more often an indicator of remission in cats treated with lente or NPH insulin.

Fructosamine

In general, measurement of serum fructosamine concentration is of much less value than serial blood glucose measurements for dose adjustment. However, fructosamine measurement is sometimes useful for monitoring glycaemic control, especially when reliable owner observations of clinical signs are unavailable or when clinical signs and blood glucose concentrations are conflicting (e.g. when blood glucose concentrations measured in the veterinary clinic are high, but the owner reports signs of good control at home). Because changes in fructosamine lag behind glucose concentrations by 1–3 weeks, it is considerably inferior to home monitoring in the early stages of therapy before the insulin dose has stabilized or when aiming for remission. It is more useful once the patient is stable and clinic revisits are only scheduled every 3–6 months.

Outcome and prognosis

Approximately 25–30% of cats in remission will relapse and, of those, 25% can achieve a second remission and some may achieve a third (Roomp and Rand, 2009b). Although there have been no studies published of factors associated with relapse, anecdotal observations and knowledge of pathophysiology indicate that conditions associated with increasing demand on the remaining beta cells to secrete insulin are involved. Therefore, important aspects of management of cats in remission include:

- Continuing to feed a low carbohydrate diet
- Avoiding glucocorticoid administration if possible
- Normalizing body condition
- Managing underlying chronic conditions such as dental disease.

If glucocorticoids must be administered, concurrent low-dose long-acting insulin therapy, for example glargine 0.5–1.0 IU administered once daily, may help maintain euglycaemia.

Glucose concentrations should be checked weekly for cats in remission; if this is not possible, urine glucose and water intake should be monitored closely. A second remission is more likely to be obtained if beta cell loss from glucose toxicity is minimized. If insulin therapy can be instituted early before blood glucose concentration chronically rises above the renal threshold, toxic glucose damage is reduced. If hyperglycaemia occurs e.g. >10 mmol/l, insulin should be reinstituted immediately to prevent further damage to beta cells.

In the absence of remission, prognosis depends on the underlying cause of the diabetes and the degree of glycaemic control that can be achieved. One study from a tertiary referral institution reported a mean survival of 17 months (Goossens *et al.*, 1998). Survival times in first-opinion practice are longer because of the lower percentage of cats with significant underlying disease and the higher percentage that achieve remission.

Whilst high remission rates (>80%) can be achieved in first-opinion practice using long-acting (glargine or detemir) insulin, low carbohydrate diets and intense home monitoring of blood glucose concentrations, these are not always possible to achieve. Where there is a legal requirement to use a veterinary-registered insulin initially, if remission has not occurred within 4–8 weeks of initiating therapy, the insulin may be changed to glargine or detemir to increase the probability of remission. Cats with obvious insulin resistance should be tested for other specific types of diabetes (see Chapter 23).

References and further reading

Appleton DJ, Rand JS and Sunvold GD (2001) Insulin sensitivity decreases with obesity, and lean cats with low insulin sensitivity are at greatest risk of glucose intolerance with weight gain. *Journal of Feline Medicine and Surgery* **3**, 211–228

Bantle JP and Laine DC (1988) Day-to-day variation in glycaemic control in type I and type II diabetes mellitus. *Diabetes Resource* **8**, 147–149

Baral RM, Rand JS, Catt MJ *et al.* (2003) Prevalence of feline diabetes mellitus in a feline private practice. *Journal of Veterinary Internal Medicine* **17**, 433–434

Bennett N, Greco DS, Peterson ME *et al.* (2006) Comparison of a low carbohydrate–low fiber diet and a moderate carbohydrate–high fiber diet in the management of feline diabetes mellitus. *Journal of Feline Medicine and Surgery* **8**(2), 73–84

Berg RI, Nelson RW, Feldman EC *et al.* (2007) Serum insulin-like growth factor-I concentration in cats with diabetes mellitus and acromegaly. *Journal of Veterinary Internal Medicine* **21**, 892–898

Casella SJ, Mongilio MK, Plotnick LP *et al.* (1993) Accuracy and precision of low-dose insulin administration. *Pediatrics* **91**, 1155–1157

DiBartola S and Panciera DL (2006) Fluid therapy in endocrine and metabolic disorders. In: *Fluid, electrolyte, and acid–base disorders in small animal practice, 3rd Edition*, ed. A Winkel and S Stringer, pp. 478–489 Saunders Elsevier, St Louis.

D'Orazio P, Burnett RW, Fogh-Andersen N *et al.* (2005) Approved IFCC recommendation on reporting results for blood glucose (abbreviated). *Clinical Chemistry* **51**, 1573–1576

Elliott DA, Feldman EC, Koblik PD *et al.* (2000) Prevalence of pituitary tumors among diabetic cats with insulin resistance. *Journal of the American Veterinary Medical Association* **216**, 1765–1768

Feldman EC and Nelson RW (2004) *Diabetic ketoacidosis*. In: *Canine and Feline Endocrinology and Reproduction, 3rd edn*, ed. Feldman EC and Nelson RW, pp. 580–615. Elsevier Science, USA

Feldman EC, Nelson RW and Feldman MS (1997) Intensive 50-week evaluation of glipizide administration in 50 cats with previously untreated diabetes mellitus. *Journal of the American Veterinary Medical Association* **210**, 772–777.

Feldhahn JR, Rand JS and Martin GJ (1999) Insulin sensitivity in normal and diabetic cats. *Journal of Feline Medicine and Surgery* **1**, 107–115

Fonseca V, Bell DS, Berger S *et al.* (2004) A comparison of bedtime insulin glargine with bedtime Neutral protamine Hagedorn in patients with type 2 diabetes: subgroup analysis of patients taking once-daily insulin in a multicenter, randomized, parallel group study. *American Journal of Medical Science* **328**, 274–280

Fulcher GR, Gilbert RE and Yue DK (2005) Glargine is superior to NPH for improving glycated hemoglobin and fasting blood glucose levels during intensive insulin therapy. *Internal Medicine Journal* **35**, 536–542

Gilor C, Keel T, Attermeier KJ *et al.* (2008) Hyperinsulinemic-euglycemic clamps using insulin detemir and insulin glargine in healthy cats. *Journal of Veterinary Internal Medicine* **22**, 728 [abstract]

Goossens MMC, Nelson RW, Feldman EC *et al.* (1998) Response to treatment and survival in 104 cats with diabetes mellitus (1985–1995). *Journal of Veterinary Internal Medicine* **12**, 1–6

Hess RS and Ward CR (2000) Effect of insulin dosage on glycemic response in dogs with diabetes mellitus: 221 cases (1993–1998). *Journal of the American Veterinary Medical Association* **216**(2), 217–221

Hoenig M and Rand JS (2006) Pathogenesis and management of feline obesity. In: *Consultations in Feline Internal Medicine, Volume 5*, ed. A Winkel and S Stringer, pp. 175–182. Saunders Elsevier, St. Louis

Imamura T, Koffler M, Helderman JH *et al.* (1988) Severe diabetes induced in subtotally depancreatized dogs by sustained hyperglycaemia. *Diabetes* **37**, 600–609

Koenig A, Drobatz KJ, Beale AB *et al.* (2004) Hyperglycemic, hyperosmolar syndrome in feline diabetics: 17 cases (1995–2001). *Journal of Veterinary Emergency Medicine and Critical Care* **14**, 30–40

Kruth SA and Cowgill LD (1982) Renal glucose transport in the cat. *Proceedings, American College of Veterinary Internal Medicine Forum* **78** [abstract]

Kurtzhals P (2004) Engineering predictability and protraction in a basal insulin analogue: the pharmacology of insulin detemir. *International Journal of Obesity Related Metabolic Disorders* **28**, 23–28

Lederer R, Rand JS, Jonsson NN, Hughes IP and Morton JM (2009) Frequency of feline diabetes mellitus and breed predisposition in domestic cats in Australia. *The Veterinary Journal* **179**, 254–258

Link KRJ (2001) *Feline Diabetes: Diagnostics and Experimental Modelling.* Doctoral thesis, University of Queensland

Link KRJ and Rand JS (2008) Changes in blood glucose concentration are associated with relatively rapid changes in circulating fructosamine concentrations in cats. *Journal of Feline Medicine and Surgery* **10**, 583–592

Marshall RD and Rand JS (2010) Glargine administered intramuscularly is effective for treatment of feline diabetic ketoacidosis. *Proceedings, American College of Veterinary Internal Medicine Forum* pp. 686–687

Marshall RD, Rand JS and Morton JM (2008) Insulin glargine has a long duration of effect following administration either once daily or twice daily in divided doses in healthy cats. *Journal of Feline Medicine Surgery* **10**, 488–494

Marshall R, Rand JR and Morton JM (2009) Treatment with glargine insulin improves glycemic control and results in a higher rate of non-insulin dependence than protamine zinc or lente insulins in newly diagnosed diabetic cats. *Journal of Feline Medicine and Surgery* **11**, 683–691

Martin GJ and Rand JS (2007a) Comparisons of different measurements for monitoring diabetic cats treated with porcine insulin zinc suspension. *Veterinary Record* **161**, 52–58

Martin GJ and Rand JS (2007b) Control of diabetes mellitus in cats with porcine insulin zinc suspension. *Veterinary Record* **161**, 88–94

Moberg E, Kollind M, Lins PE *et al.* (1995) Day-to-day variation of insulin sensitivity in patients with type 1 diabetes: role of gender and menstrual cycle. *Diabetes Medicine* **12**, 224–228

Nelson RW (2000) Diabetes mellitus. In: *Textbook of Veterinary Internal Medicine, 5th edn*, ed. EC Feldman and S Ettinger, p. 1438. WB Saunders, Philadelphia

Nelson RW, Henley K, Cole C [PZIR Clinical Study Group] (2009) Field safety and efficacy of protamine zinc recombinant human insulin for treatment of diabetes mellitus in cats. *Journal of Veterinary Internal Medicine* **23**, 787–793

Niessen SJM, Petrie G, Gaudiano F *et al.* (2007) Feline acromegaly: an underdiagnosed endocrinopathy? *Journal of Veterinary Internal Medicine* **21**, 899–905

Norsworthy G, Lynn R and Cole C (2009) Preliminary study of protamine zinc recombinant insulin for the treatment of diabetes mellitus in cats. *Veterinary Therapeutics* **10**, 24–8

O'Brien TD, Hayden DW, Johnson KH *et al.* (1985) High dose intravenous tolerance test and serum insulin and glucagon levels in diabetic and non-diabetic cats: relationships to insular amyloidosis. *Veterinary Pathology* **22**, 250–261

Panciera DL, Thomas CB, Eicker SW *et al.* (1990) Epizootiological patterns of diabetes mellitus in cats: 333 cases (1980–1986). *Journal of American Veterinary Medicine Association* **197**, 1504–1508

Porte DJ (1991) Beta-cells in type 2 diabetes mellitus. *Diabetes* **40**, 166–180

Prahl A, Guptill L, Glickman NW, Tetrick M and Glickman LT (2007) Time trends and risk factors for diabetes mellitus in cats presented to veterinary teaching hospitals. *Journal of Feline Medicine and Surgery* **9**, 351–358

Rand JS, Bobbermein LM and Hendrik JK (1997) Over-representation of Burmese in cats with diabetes mellitus in Queensland. *Australian Veterinary Journal* **75**, 402–405

Rand J, Fleeman L, Farrow H, Appleton D and Lederer R (2004) Canine and feline diabetes mellitus: Nature or nurture? *Journal of Nutrition* **134**, 2072–2080

Rand JS and Marshall R (2005) Diabetes mellitus in cats. *Veterinary Clinics of North America: Small Animal Practice* **35**, 211

Reusch CE, Wess G and Casella M (2001) Home monitoring of blood glucose concentration in the management of diabetes mellitus. *Compendium on Continuing Education for the Practicing Veterinarian* **23**, 544–556

Robertson RP, Tanaka Y, Sacchi G *et al.* (2000) Glucose toxicity of the β-cell: cellular and molecular mechanisms. In: *Diabetes Mellitus*, ed. D LeRoith and JM Olefsky, p. 125. Lippincott Williams & Wilkins, New York

Roomp K and Rand J (2009a) Detemir results in similar glycaemic control to glargine in diabetic cats. *Journal of Veterinary Internal Medicine* **23** [abstract]

Roomp K and Rand J (2009b) Intensive blood glucose control is safe and effective in diabetic cats using home monitoring and treatment with glargine. *Journal of Feline Medicine and Surgery* **11**, 668–682

Slingerland LI, Fazilova VV, Plantinga EA *et al.* (2009) Indoor confinement and physical inactivity rather than the proportion of dry food are risk factors in the development of feline type 2 diabetes mellitus. *The Veterinary Journal* **179**, 247–253

Steffes MW and Sacks DB (2005) Measurement of circulating glucose concentrations: the time is now for consistency among methods and types of samples. *Clinical Chemistry* **51**, 1569–1570

Unger RH and Grundy S (1995) Hyperglycaemia as an inducer as well as a consequence of impaired islet cell function and insulin resistance: implications for the management of diabetes. *Diabetologia* **28**, 119–121

Weaver KE, Rozanski EA, Mahony OM *et al.* (2006) Use of glargine and lente insulins in cats with diabetes mellitus. *Journal of Veterinary Internal Medicine* **20**, 234–238

Wess G and Reusch C (2000) Assessment of five portable blood glucose meters for use in cats. *American Journal of Veterinary Research* **61**, 1587–1592

Selected articles and updated protocols are available on: www.uq.edu.au/ccah

14

Insulinoma and other gastrointestinal tract tumours

Peter P. Kintzer

Insulinoma

Insulinomas are tumours that arise from the beta cells of the pancreatic islets and secrete excessive amounts of insulin, resulting in clinical signs of hypoglycaemia. As the secretion of insulin is usually episodic, so also are the resulting clinical signs. Insulinomas in dogs are typically malignant and almost always metastasize; even those appearing benign on histopathological evaluation usually behave in an aggressive manner (Leifer, 1986). Metastasis to the liver, local lymph nodes and omentum is common, and is found in approximately 50% of dogs at the time of diagnosis.

Due to the small number of reported cases in cats, the expected behaviour of insulinoma in this species is unclear.

Clinical features

Signalment
Insulinomas are rare in dogs. They are typically seen in middle-aged to older dogs but have been reported in dogs ranging from 3.5 to 15 years of age. There is no apparent sex predilection. Breeds reported as being at increased risk of developing an insulinoma include German Shepherd Dogs, Boxers, Standard Poodles, Irish Setters, collies and Fox Terriers (Caywood *et al.*, 1988; Nelson and Salisbury, 2000).

Insulinomas are extremely rare in cats, with only four cases, ranging in age from 12–17 years, reported. Three of these cats were Siamese (Hawks *et al.*, 1992).

Clinical signs
Most animals with insulinoma present with clinical signs related to hyperinsulinism and resulting episodes of hypoglycaemia. Clinical signs result from neuroglycopenia or the increased adrenergic tone induced by hypoglycaemia.

Seizures are the most common presenting complaint. The brain is dependent on a steady supply of glucose, as it has limited energy reserves and limited ability to utilize other fuels. Other reported clinical signs of hypoglycaemia are listed in Figure 14.1.

Clinical signs are typically episodic and may be related to fasting, exercise or, counterintuitively, to feeding in some cases. The duration of clinical signs before diagnosis is variable (usually 1–6 months),

- Seizures
- Weakness
- Paresis
- Collapse
- Tremors
- Lethargy
- Dullness
- Ataxia
- Behaviour changes
- Nervousness
- Muscle fasciculation
- Exercise intolerance
- Polyphagia
- Tachycardia (occasionally bradycardia)
- Tachypnoea
- Pupillary dilation
- Polyneuropathy
- Decerebrate posture
- Coma

14.1 Clinical signs of hypoglycaemia.

and most patients exhibit multiple signs that increase in severity and frequency as the disease progresses. The severity of a hypoglycaemic crisis is dependent on three factors:

- The glucose nadir
- The rate of decrease in the blood glucose concentration
- The duration of the hypoglycaemia.

Differential diagnosis of hypoglycaemia
The major causes of hypoglycaemia are listed in Figure 14.2 and its investigation is described in greater detail in Chapter 25. Evaluation of the signalment, history, physical examination and routine clinicopathological data will allow the clinician to exclude many of these disorders in a given patient.

- The primary differential diagnosis is a paraneoplastic hypoglycaemia, secondary to extrapancreatic neoplasia.
- Hepatocellular carcinoma, hepatoma, leiomyosarcoma, leiomyoma, haemangiosarcoma, melanoma and leukaemia have been implicated in extrapancreatic hypoglycaemia in dogs (Leifer, 1986).
- Mechanisms of extrapancreatic tumour hypoglycaemia include:
  - Secretion of an insulin-like substance

- Insulinoma
- Extrapancreatic neoplasia
- Sepsis
- Infections – *Babesia*, parvovirus
- Neonatal hypoglycaemia
- Toy-breed hypoglycaemia
- Hunting dog hypoglycaemia
- Prolonged starvation
- Hepatic insufficiency
- Hypoadrenocorticism (primary and secondary)
- Renal failure
- Panhypopituitarism
- Iatrogenic – oral hypoglycaemic drugs, propranolol, exogenous insulin excess
- Toxins – xylitol, ethylene glycol
- Severe polycythaemia

14.2 Causes of hypoglycaemia.

- Excess glucose utilization by the tumour
- Inhibition of hepatic glycogenolysis and gluconeogenesis.

Such extrapancreatic tumours are usually large malignant lesions readily demonstrable on diagnostic imaging studies.

Diagnosis

The diagnosis of insulinoma is made when a patient with hypoglycaemia (glucose <3.5 mmol/l) has a high serum insulin concentration.

- Simultaneous serum glucose and insulin concentrations are evaluated in animals suspected of having an insulinoma.
- Use of the insulin:glucose and amended insulin:glucose ratios as diagnostic tests for insulinoma is controversial. They probably provide no more information than evaluation of insulin and glucose measured simultaneously and are no longer recommended.

If hypoglycaemia is not present on initial presentation, the animal is fasted under observation (in case signs of hypoglycaemia occur), and blood glucose concentrations determined every 1–2 hours until hypoglycaemia is documented. Point-of-care glucose analysers are usually adequate for this purpose (Steiner and Bruyette, 1996; Nelson and Salisbury, 2000). Such analysers should be calibrated against standard laboratory results, as some machines tend to give falsely low concentration, particularly in the hypoglycaemic range.

Although 12 hours of fasting is usually sufficient to demonstrate hypoglycaemia, some patients require prolonged fasting (>24 hours). Once hypoglycaemia is documented, a blood sample for determination of simultaneous insulin and glucose concentrations is submitted to the diagnostic laboratory. Serum samples for determination of insulin concentration must be handled appropriately (see Chapter 1).

- An elevated insulin concentration (>140 pmol/l) in a hypoglycaemic patient (absolute hyperinsulinaemia) is consistent with insulinoma.

- If the insulin concentration is within the mid to high (70–140 pmol/l) portion of the reference interval (relative hyperinsulinaemia), insulinoma is still likely because insulin concentration should be low to undetectable once blood glucose concentrations fall below 2 mmol/l.
- Serum insulin concentrations in the low (35–70 pmol/l) end of the reference interval are equivocal and considered non-diagnostic. An insulinoma remains a possibility.
- An insulin concentration below the reference interval (<35 pmol/l) in a hypoglycaemic animal is the normal physiological response and is therefore not consistent with the diagnosis of insulinoma.

In cases where equivocal results are found (i.e. hypoglycaemia with serum insulin concentrations in the low end of the reference range), additional simultaneous insulin and glucose determinations may be necessary. Demonstration of a low circulating fructosamine concentration is useful in diagnosing chronic hypoglycaemia when blood glucose concentrations remain within the reference interval at the time of investigation (Mellanby and Herrtage, 2002). Haematology, serum biochemistry, urinalysis and survey radiographs are typically unremarkable.

A pancreatic mass or evidence of metastasis may be detected using ultrasonography, although in many cases the lesion is too small to image. The sensitivity of this modality is highly dependent on the resolution of the equipment and the experience of the ultrasonographer. Other imaging modalities such as computed tomography (CT) or magnetic resonance imaging (MRI) may be helpful (Robben *et al.*, 2005; Mai and Caceres 2008) but are not commonly utilized. Scintigraphy using a radiolabelled somatostatin analogue, [111]Indium pentetreotide, has been described in a few cases, and may detect the insulinoma as well as metastatic lesions. A false negative study would result if the tumour cells do not express somatostatin receptors. A positive scan may also predict whether the tumour will be responsive to treatment with somatostatin analogues (Simpson and Dykes, 1997; Garden *et al.*, 2005).

Treatment

Emergency treatment of symptomatic hypoglycaemia

Symptomatic hypoglycaemia is treated with the intravenous injection of dextrose as a bolus (1 ml/kg 50% dextrose injection diluted to 25% in normal saline and administered slowly over 5–10 minutes) and subsequently glucose (2.5% or 5% dextrose solution) as an intravenous infusion as necessitated by the patient's condition. The goal is to ameliorate the clinical signs of hypoglycaemia, but not necessarily return the blood glucose concentration to normal.

Overzealous administration of intravenous dextrose should be avoided to prevent the potential stimulation of insulin release from the tumour and worsening of the hypoglycaemia. Such rebound hypoglycaemia may result in a vicious cycle that is difficult to break and potentially fatal. Frequent feeding of small meals should be instituted as soon as the animal is stable.

Persistence of seizures following resolution of hypoglycaemia may be an indication of an underlying neurological problem, such as cerebral oedema. Mannitol and/or a rapid-acting glucocorticoid preparation may be indicated and diazepam or other anticonvulsants may be necessary to control the seizures. Although uncommon, cerebral lesions (laminar and pseudo-laminar necrosis) can cause continued intermittent acquired seizure activity as a result of prolonged or recurrent episodes of hypoglycaemia. Such cases may need long-term therapy with phenobarbital or other anticonvulsant medications.

Surgery for insulinoma

The initial treatment of choice for dogs and cats with insulinoma is surgery. Symptomatic hypoglycaemia must be adequately controlled prior to anaesthesia and surgery. This may involve: frequent feedings; dextrose-containing intravenous fluids; prednisolone/prednisone; or more aggressive medical therapy (discussed later) as dictated by the patient's response.

Laparotomy provides histological confirmation of the diagnosis and allows resection of the neoplastic tissue and staging of the disease. A ventral midline approach is used. A balanced intravenous electrolyte solution containing dextrose is administered intraoperatively at approximately 10 ml/kg/h aiming to maintain blood glucose concentrations around 2.5 mmol/l. Appropriate preoperative and intraoperative fluid therapy is important to maintain systemic blood pressure and splanchnic perfusion and to decrease the incidence of postoperative pancreatitis.

The pancreas should be carefully inspected both visually and by palpation. Insulinomas are typically firmer than the normal parenchyma and may be small and obscured by the normal pancreatic tissue, thus difficult to visualize. Insulinomas occur with approximately equal frequency in the right and left lobes of the pancreas. In addition, multiple nodules are seen in approximately 15% of dogs. Diffuse infiltration by neoplastic beta cells without identifiable nodules has also been reported. Intraoperative ultrasonography may be useful in identifying nodules that cannot be seen or palpated.

If no tumour can be identified definitively, some authorities recommend removing 50% or more of the pancreas in the hope of excising the tumour (Matthiesen and Mullen, 1990). Any identifiable pancreatic nodules should be removed by partial pancreatectomy if possible, as this has been reported to result in longer survival times than simple excision of the tumour.

Surgical technique: Surgical technique is similar in both the dog and cat (see *BSAVA Manual of Canine and Feline Abdominal Surgery* for more details). The pancreas must be handled gently during palpation and surgery to minimize the incidence of postoperative pancreatitis. Tumours in the left lobe or distal right lobe should be removed by partial pancreatectomy as follows.

1. Resect the portion of the lobe containing the tumour 1–2 cm proximal to the insulinoma.
2. Divide the mesentery around the lobe. Ligate and transect the vessels.
3. After incising through the surface, bluntly dissect the pancreatic tissue from both sides to isolate the pancreatic duct. Ligate the duct with non-absorbable suture and transect.
4. Thoroughly lavage, and close the abdomen routinely.

Tumours in the body of the pancreas or proximal right lobe should be removed by local excision, along with 1–2 cm of surrounding normal pancreas by the following technique:

1. Separate the pancreatic tissue by blunt dissection.
2. Take care to avoid trauma to the pancreaticoduodenal vessels, the main and accessory pancreatic ducts and the common bile duct.
3. Attend to haemostasis as needed.
4. Thoroughly lavage, and close the abdomen routinely.

Special considerations: Cytoreduction of any visible metastatic lesions should be attempted, as this may result in longer hypoglycaemia-free survival periods or make subsequent medical management easier. Even if gross metastatic disease is not evident, biopsy of the liver and appropriate lymph nodes must be done, as occult metastatic disease is common.

Close intraoperative monitoring of the serum glucose concentration is imperative, as manipulation of the pancreas during surgery can stimulate insulin release from the tumour and result in hypoglycaemia – signs of which may not be evident in an anaesthetized patient. The intravenous administration of dextrose is adjusted as needed, based on serial blood glucose determinations.

In the immediate postoperative period, blood glucose concentrations are monitored every hour for the first 4–6 hours and then every 2–4 hours, with the administration of dextrose boluses or dextrose-containing solutions being adjusted accordingly. Some dogs may be normoglycaemic or hyperglycaemic after surgery and do not require dextrose-containing fluids.

Complications: Potential complications include hyperglycaemia, persistent hypoglycaemia and pancreatitis.

In some dogs, transient hyperglycaemia develops after surgical removal of the islet cell tumour. In most cases the diabetic state resolves in a few days, although on rare occasions, persistent hyperglycaemia can result in dogs requiring exogenous insulin therapy. Such cases must be closely monitored by home urine glucose determinations and periodic serial blood glucose curves, as in almost all cases the diabetic state will resolve eventually and the patient will need to be evaluated for recurrence of the insulinoma. Transient hyperglycaemia does occur in cats, but there have been few reported cases.

Persistence of hypoglycaemia postoperatively or recurrence of hypoglycaemia any time postoperatively should prompt consideration of symptomatic medical management or the use of chemotherapy. In patients who have had a significant hypoglycaemia-free period after surgery, a second operation may result in several months of normoglycaemia unless gross metastatic disease is present. In these cases medical management is indicated, as discussed below.

Pancreatitis is a potential complication in animals undergoing surgery for insulinoma and can be severe or even life-threatening. Appropriate preoperative, intraoperative and postoperative intravenous fluid administration is important in decreasing the risk of this complication.

Postoperative care: Following surgery, food and water should be withheld for 24–48 hours, or longer if signs of pancreatitis are evident. Thereafter, water and then a bland diet are offered. If there are no problems, normal diet can be resumed within a few days.

Long-term medical management of hypoglycaemia

Frequent feedings
In some cases of insulinoma, frequent feedings may control clinical hypoglycaemia. Diets high in protein, fats and complex carbohydrates are recommended. These are the type of diets typically recommended as adjunctive management of diabetes mellitus. In animals with insulinoma, they are useful in decreasing postprandial hyperglycaemia, potentially resulting in a marked insulin surge.

Prednisolone/prednisone
Prednisolone or prednisone (0.2–0.5 mg/kg orally q12h) can be given if dietary management alone is not effective. Higher doses can be administered if necessary, but the development of iatrogenic hyperadrenocorticism is ultimately dose limiting.

Diazoxide
Although infrequently used, the non-diuretic benzothiadiazide antihypertensive agent diazoxide can be successful in controlling hypoglycaemia in patients not responding to diet and judicious glucocorticoid administration. Diazoxide inhibits pancreatic beta cell insulin secretion, enhances hepatic glycogenolysis and gluconeogenesis, and inhibits glucose uptake by peripheral tissues (Meleo and Caplan, 2000). The initial dosage is 10 mg/kg orally q24h, which can be increased as needed to control hypoglycaemia. The recommended maximum dose is 60 mg/kg orally q24h.

Common adverse effects include vomiting and anorexia. Other potential adverse effects include: bone marrow suppression; sodium retention; diarrhoea; tachycardia; aplastic anaemia; hyperglycaemia; and cataracts. The other major drawbacks of diazoxide are its limited availability and considerable expense.

Somatostatin analogues
The long-acting somatostatin analogue octreotide has been successfully used as palliative therapy to control hypoglycaemia in a few dogs with insulinoma, refractory to usual symptomatic medical therapy (Nelson and Couto, 2003; Robben et al., 2006). Somatostatin inhibits the release of insulin from pancreatic beta cells. The initial dosage is 10–40 µg/dog s.c. q 8–12h (Nelson and Couto, 2003). The dosage is increased as needed to control hypoglycaemia.

The responsiveness of insulinomas to octreotide is dependent on the presence of somatostatin receptors on the cell membranes of the tumour cells, hence not all patients will respond to this therapy. In addition, some patients become refractory to the medication. Octreotide is expensive but appears to be well tolerated. Longer-acting slow-release somatostatin analogues have not been adequately studied in dogs and cats with insulinoma, but may be useful as well as more convenient.

Miscellaneous medications
Other medications, such as propranolol and diphenylhydantoin, have been used in human patients with insulinoma and discussed as adjunctive therapy for beta cell tumours in dogs. These agents have not been sufficiently evaluated in dogs with insulinoma for therapeutic recommendations to be given.

Chemotherapy of insulinoma

Streptozotocin
Streptozotocin is a nitrosourea alkylating agent that is cytotoxic to pancreatic beta cells and has been used to treat humans with non-resectable or metastatic insulinomas. In initial reports in two dogs, bolus injection of streptozotocin caused acute fatal renal failure. However, a recent study (Moore et al., 2002) has shown that multiple doses of streptozotocin can be safely given to dogs with insulinoma if an aggressive saline diuresis protocol is used prior to and following the infusion of the chemotherapeutic agent (Figure 14.3).

Pretreatment diuresis
• Administer 0.9% saline at a rate of 18.3 ml/kg/h i.v. for 3 hours
Streptozotocin infusion
• Administer streptozotocin (500 mg/m²) diluted in the appropriate volume of 0.9% saline at a rate of 18.3 ml/kg/h i.v. over the next 2 hours
Antiemetic treatment
• Give butorphanol at a dose of 0.4 mg/kg i.m. during or after the streptozotocin infusion
Post-treatment diuresis
• Administer 0.9% saline at a rate of 18.3 ml/kg/h i.v. for 2 hours

14.3 Protocol for use of streptozotocin as chemotherapeutic treatment of insulinoma in dogs.

The current recommended dose is 500 mg/m^2 per treatment. Five treatments are given at 3-week intervals, unless side effects dictate otherwise, progressive disease is detected or hyperglycaemia occurs. If metastatic disease is present, imaging studies should also be used to monitor treatment. Butorphanol is administered during the streptozotocin infusion for its antiemetic effects (see Figure 14.3). The use of other antiemetic agents can also be considered.

The incidence of nephrotoxicity in the study was low and acute renal failure was not reported. Other reported adverse effects included: bone marrow suppression, which was generally mild; vomiting, which was occasionally severe; anorexia; diarrhoea; elevated alanine aminotransferase activity; transient hypoglycaemia; and insulin-dependent diabetes mellitus. Streptozotocin is efficacious in some dogs with insulinoma and its use should be considered in dogs with non-resectable or metastatic disease (particularly those that are hypoglycaemic), dogs remaining hypoglycaemic after surgery (indicating residual disease) and dogs in which hypoglycaemia recurs.

Doxorubicin

The use of doxorubicin (commonly used in veterinary oncology) has been reported in a few human patients with insulinoma, but its efficacy in veterinary patients with insulinoma is not known. Use of doxorubicin could be contemplated in certain cases and its activity against canine and feline insulinoma needs further investigation.

Other potential chemotherapies

Other reported chemotherapeutic protocols used for non-resectable and metastatic insulinomas in humans include crisantaspase (L-asparaginase) and combinations of streptozotocin with doxorubicin and streptozotocin with fluorouracil (**NB fluorouracil cannot be used in cats**). Use of these agents in veterinary patients with insulinoma warrants further evaluation.

Prognosis

The long-term prognosis for dogs and cats with insulinoma is guarded. Tumour burden, presence of metastatic disease and owner willingness to treat aggressively all appear to impact upon survival time. Approximately two-thirds to three-quarters of dogs survive 6 months or longer after surgery (often over a year) before intractable hypoglycaemia recurs. Reported survival time is longer in dogs initially treated with surgery (median survival time (MST) 381 days, range 20–1758 days) compared to medical therapy alone (MST 74 days, range 8–508 days). Another study reported an MST of 547 days overall, 785 days for dogs undergoing surgery, and 1316 days for those dogs that were placed on prednisolone when hypoglycaemia eventually recurred after surgery (Nelson and Couto, 2003; Polton *et al.*, 2007). Individualization of therapy with the use of combinations of medical and surgical therapy based on the stage and extent of disease may improve prognosis and survival time in a given patient. Cats have been reported to have MST of approximately 6.5 months with a range of 0–18 months (Bennett, 2007).

Gastrinoma

Gastrinomas are rare gastrin-secreting neuroendocrine non-beta cell tumours of the pancreas, with <50 cases reported. The excessive production of gastrin results in parietal cell growth and hypersecretion of hydrochloric acid in the stomach. Metastasis involving regional lymph nodes, omentum and/or liver is identified in approximately three-quarters of patients.

Clinical features

Signalment
The age range of dogs and cats affected by gastrinomas is 3–12 years. The median age of canine patients is reported to be 8 years. No breed or sex predilection is apparent (Simpson and Dykes, 1997).

Clinical signs
Clinical signs seen in dogs and cats with gastrinoma result from the effects of the excessive gastrin secretion, gastric mucosal hypertrophy and subsequent overproduction of gastric acid, which can lead to ulceration of the oesophagus, stomach and duodenum, and disruption of intestinal function. Additional clinical signs may be caused by the physical effects of large tumours or metastatic lesions. Common clinical signs are listed in Figure 14.4. Severity of clinical signs varies from mild in early disease to life-threatening in patients with perforated ulcers and peritonitis.

Clinical sign	Approximate percentage
Vomiting	95
Weight loss	90
Anorexia	70
Lethargy	65
Diarrhoea	65
Polyuria/polydipsia	25
Melaena	25
Fever	20
Abdominal pain	15
Haematemesis	15
Haematochezia	10
Tachycardia	7
Polyphagia	4

14.4 Approximate percentages of dogs and cats affected by the clinical signs associated with gastrinoma.

Diagnosis

Routine clinicopathological features

Complete blood counts may reveal leucocytosis, neutrophilia, regenerative anaemia and decreased total protein. Serum chemistry abnormalities may include hypoproteinaemia, hypoalbuminaemia, hypocalcaemia, hypokalaemia, hypochloraemia and metabolic alkalosis. Vomiting and gastrointestinal blood loss would account for these abnormalities.

Circulating gastrin concentration

Demonstration of an elevated fasting serum gastrin concentration is an important component in establishing the diagnosis. The assay is available at a few veterinary diagnostic laboratories and the laboratory should be contacted for specific sample handling instructions (see Chapter 1). Differential diagnosis for hypergastrinaemia includes administration of proton pump inhibitor, H2 blocker or antacid drugs, liver disease, chronic renal failure, gastric outflow obstruction, atrophic gastritis, intestinal resection, gastric dilatation and volvulus, and immunoproliferative enteropathy of Basenjis. In humans, a tentative diagnosis of gastrinoma (pending histopathological confirmation) is made when the serum gastrin concentration is 10-fold higher than the upper end of the reference interval. A similar approach has been used in veterinary patients and almost all cases tested have had a fasting serum gastrin concentration at least three times higher than the upper end of the reference interval. In cases where the elevation is less pronounced or borderline, stimulation tests can be performed. The secretin response test and the calcium response test have been described (Simpson and Dykes, 1997; Steiner, 2004). Secretin and calcium both stimulate gastrin secretion in patients with gastrinoma; a significant increase in the serum gastrin concentration following the administration of either secretagogue is consistent with the presence of a gastrinoma. These tests are rarely performed in practice. They could be considered in the unusual case that has a borderline fasting serum gastrin concentration and in which a gastrinoma is still suspected. Definitive diagnosis of a gastrinoma requires histopathological examination.

Diagnostic imaging

Abdominal radiography is typically unrewarding. Ultrasonography of the abdomen may reveal evidence of a pancreatic tumour or metastatic disease, but is unremarkable in many cases. The sensitivity of ultrasonography is highly dependent on the resolution of the equipment and the experience of the operator. Advanced imaging (CT and MRI) may be more sensitive, but these modalities also often fail to find the pancreatic lesion. Nuclear medicine scans for somatostatin receptors and endoscopic ultrasonography appear to be the most sensitive techniques for identifying the primary lesion in people, but are rarely employed in veterinary patients (Altschul *et al.*, 1997; Steiner, 2004).

Treatment

Exploratory laparotomy should be considered in most patients with gastrinoma. Preoperative evaluation for metastatic disease is indicated, as patients with extensive metastatic disease may not be ideal surgical candidates. The surgeon should find (or confirm) and remove the primary pancreatic lesion, repair any perforated or severe gastrointestinal ulcers, evaluate for metastatic disease and debulk metastatic lesions. Surgical technique, complications, special considerations and postoperative management are similar to that described for insulinomas above.

The proton pump inhibitor omeprazole is administered at an initial dose of 0.5–1.5 mg/kg q24h to decrease gastric acid production and control clinical signs. Long-term therapy and subsequent dose increases may be necessary. Sucralfate (0.5–1 g/dog q8h) may be added to bind to and protect the gastric mucosal surface while active ulceration is present. The use of the prostaglandin E_1 analogue misoprostol (2–5 μg/kg q8h) may be indicated in patients whose ulcer disease is not adequately controlled with omeprazole and sucralfate.

The somatostatin analogue octreotide (5–20 μg/dog s.c. q8–12h) may be effective in decreasing gastrin secretion and controlling clinical signs, and its use has been reported in a few patients (Altschul *et al.*, 1997; Simpson and Dykes, 1997). Octreotide may also impair tumour growth. The response to octreotide is dependent on the presence of somatostatin receptors on the cell membranes of the tumour cells, hence not all patients may respond to this therapy. In addition, some patients may become less responsive to the medication over time. Octreotide is expensive but appears to be well tolerated. Longer-acting slow-release somatostatin analogues may become available in the future.

Chemotherapy for gastrinoma has not been adequately evaluated in dogs and cats. Use of streptozotocin or doxorubicin could be considered in selected patients, such as those with metastatic disease, or those whose owners have refused surgery. The use of radiation therapy and interferon has been reported to palliate a significant portion of human patients with gastrinoma, but has not yet been evaluated in veterinary patients.

Prognosis

The long-term prognosis for dogs and cats with gastrinoma is poor. MST is reported to be 5.5 months, with a reported range of 1 week to 2.8 years. Two dogs treated with octreotide lived 10 and 14 months, respectively (Simpson and Dykes, 1997; Hughes, 2006). Nonetheless, with appropriate surgical and medical therapy many patients enjoy a good quality of life until the disease becomes widespread. With aggressive medical management, even some patients with extensive metastasis can have their disease adequately palliated for a period of time. Earlier diagnosis, individualized combinations of surgical and medical therapy and application of newer therapeutic modalities are expected to improve MSTs in the future.

Glucagonoma

Glucagonomas are rare glucagon-secreting neuro-endocrine non-beta cell tumours of the pancreas. They originate from the alpha cells of the pancreatic islets and have been diagnosed in a small number of dogs (<20 reported cases). Metastasis to lymph nodes and liver often occurs.

Clinical features

Signalment
The small number of reported cases precludes definitive conclusions regarding signalment, but it would appear that glucagonomas are more prevalent in middle-aged to older dogs.

Clinical signs
Findings reported in dogs with glucagonoma include decreased appetite, lethargy, lymphadenopathy and diarrhoea. Patients typically have skin lesions termed superficial necrolytic dermatitis, characterized by erythema, scaling, crusting and ulceration of the footpads, mucocutaneous junctions, face, elbows, hocks and ventral abdomen (Gross *et al.*, 1990). The footpads may be significantly hyperkeratotic. Secondary skin infections are not uncommon. Superficial necrolytic dermatitis can also be seen more commonly in dogs with severe liver disease.

Diagnosis
Most dogs with glucagonoma have hyperglycaemia or overt diabetes mellitus, which may be present when skin lesions are noted or develop months after they are first observed. Hypoaminoacidaemia has been reported in dogs with glucagonoma and is felt to contribute to the pathogenesis of the superficial necrolytic dermatitis. Diagnosis is based on the exclusion of other causes of superficial necrolytic dermatitis and on finding significantly increased circulating glucagon concentrations in a dog with a pancreatic tumour positive for glucagon on immuno-histochemistry. Glucagon assays may not be readily available at veterinary diagnostic laboratories. If a human laboratory is used, the laboratory should be contacted for specific shipping and handling instructions. Other disorders reportedly resulting in elevated glucagon levels in people include chronic renal failure, pancreatitis, sepsis, hyperadrenocorticism and diabetic ketoacidosis (Steiner, 2004).

Diagnostic imaging
Abdominal radiographs are typically unrewarding. Advanced imaging (CT and MRI) may be more sensitive, but these modalities also often fail to find the pancreatic lesion. Abdominal ultrasonography may be unremarkable or it may reveal a pancreatic tumour or evidence of metastasis to lymph nodes or liver. The sensitivity of ultrasonography is highly dependent on the resolution of the equipment and the experience of the operator.

Treatment
Surgery is recommended in most dogs with glucagonoma. Recommendations for surgical technique, exploratory evaluation, complications and postoperative management are similar to those described for insulinomas and gastrinomas (see above).

Medical management may include intravenous or oral amino acid supplementation, insulin therapy, octreotide injections, hydrotherapy, and antibiotics for secondary infections. Medical therapy should be considered to hasten resolution of skin lesions after surgery in patients with residual or recurrent tumour or if surgery is not performed. Chemotherapy with streptozotocin or dacarbazine has been used in human patients with glucagonoma.

Prognosis
The long-term prognosis for dogs with glucagonoma is usually poor, as metastatic disease and recurrence are not unusual. Appropriate surgical and medical therapy may help some patients enjoy a good quality of life and short-term prognosis. Individualization of therapy, with the use of combinations of medical and surgical therapy based on the extent of disease, may improve prognosis and survival time in a given patient.

Carcinoid

Carcinoids are neuroendocrine tumours that arise from APUD (amine precursor uptake and decarboxylation) tissue, usually involving gastrointestinal enterochromaffin cells. They are rare, with <30 canine and <5 feline cases reported. Carcinoids have been found in the gastrointestinal tract, lung and liver of dogs and in the gastrointestinal tract, liver and heart of cats. These tumours can produce serotonin, histamine, bradykinins, tachykinins, prostaglandins and substance P. In humans, release of these substances into the systemic circulation results in flushing, diarrhoea, abdominal cramping and hyperventilation. This constellation of signs, termed the carcinoid syndrome, has not been reported in dogs and cats with carcinoid tumours.

Clinical features

Signalment
The small number of reported cases precludes definitive conclusions regarding signalment, except that carcinoids are more prevalent in older animals.

Clinical signs
Clinical signs of carcinoids in dogs and cats have been associated with a mass effect of the tumour, including intestinal and common bile duct obstruction, or the presence of metastatic disease. Metastasis to lymph nodes, liver, lung, pancreas, omentum and peritoneal cavity has been described (Patnaik *et al.*, 1980; Steiner, 2004). Reported clinical signs in animals have included anorexia, weight loss, lethargy, vomiting, diarrhoea, abdominal pain, gastrointestinal bleeding, liver failure and cardiac abnormalities.

Diagnosis

In humans, diagnosis is based on the clinical signs (carcinoid syndrome), demonstration of elevated urinary concentrations of tumour products, and histopathology. In dogs and cats, definitive diagnosis has been achieved using histopathology, although significantly elevated serum serotonin concentrations were described in one dog with metastatic intestinal carcinoid (Sako *et al.*, 2003).

Routine clinicopathological features

A complete blood count may reveal leucocytosis, neutrophilia and mild anaemia, which is usually non-regenerative. Serum biochemistry abnormalities may include liver enzyme elevations and electrolyte disturbances.

Diagnostic imaging

Abdominal and thoracic radiographs may show evidence of a mass lesion. Abdominal ultrasonography may be unremarkable or may reveal a primary tumour or evidence of metastasis. Advanced imaging (CT and MRI) are more sensitive, but these modalities may also fail to identify a primary lesion. Scintigraphy with radiolabelled somatostatin analogues is often successful for identification and localization of carcinoids in humans, but has not been described in dogs and cats.

Treatment

Surgery is recommended in most cases. Preoperative evaluation for metastatic disease is indicated, as patients with extensive metastatic spread may not be ideal surgical candidates. The surgeon should excise or debulk the primary tumour, correct any obstructions and evaluate for metastatic disease. Cytoreduction of any visible metastatic lesions should be attempted. Streptozotocin, fluorouracil, imatinib, carboplatin, etoposide and interferon chemotherapy and radiotherapy have all been employed in human patients. Adjuvant carboplatin chemotherapy following surgical excision of a jejunal carcinoid has been reported in one dog (Spugnini *et al.*, 2008).

Prognosis

The prognosis is generally considered guarded to poor and depends on the size and location of the primary tumour as well as the presence and extent of metastatic disease.

Other islet cell tumours

Rare cases of syndromes resulting from the excessive secretion of somatostatin, pancreatic polypeptide or vasoactive polypeptide by islet cell tumours have been reported in humans. Although the presence of some of these hormones has been demonstrated in canine islet cell tumours with immunohistochemistry (Hawkins, 1987; Boosinger *et al.*, 1988), clinical syndromes associated with oversecretion of these hormones have not been conclusively identified in dogs and cats.

References and further reading

Altschul M, Simpson KW, Dykes NL *et al.* (1997) Evaluation of somatostatin analogues for the detection and treatment of gastrinoma in a dog. *Journal of Small Animal Practice* **38**, 286–291

Bennett N (2007) Insulinoma. In: *Blackwell's Five-Minute Veterinary Consult, 4th edn,* ed. LP Tilley and FWK Smith, pp.758–759. Blackwell Publishing, Ames

Birchard SJ (2005) The pancreas. In: *BSAVA Manual of Canine and Feline Abdominal Surgery,* ed. JM Williams and JD Niles, pp. 210–219. BSAVA Publications, Gloucester

Boosinger TR, Zerbe CA, Grabau JH and Pletcher JM (1988) Multihormonal pancreatic endocrine tumor in a dog with duodenal ulcers and hypertrophic gastropathy. *Veterinary Pathology* **25**, 237–239

Caywood DD, Klausner JS, O'Leary TP and Withrow SJ (1988) Pancreatic insulin secreting neoplasms: clinical, diagnostic and prognostic features in 73 dogs. *Journal of the American Animal Hospital Association* **24**, 577–586

Garden OA, Reubi JC, Dykes NL *et al.* (2005) Somatostatin receptor imaging in vivo by planar scintigraphy facilitates the diagnosis of canine insulinomas. *Journal of Veterinary Internal Medicine* **19**, 168–176

Gross TL, O'Brien TD, Davies AP and Long RE (1990) Glucagon-producing pancreatic endocrine tumors in two dogs with superficial necrolytic dermatitis. *Journal of the American Veterinary Medical Association* **197**, 1619–1622

Hawkins KL (1987) Immunocytochemistry of normal pancreatic islets and spontaneous islet cell tumors in dogs. *Veterinary Pathology* **24**, 170–179

Hawks D, Peterson ME, Hawkins KL and Rosebury WS (1992) Insulin-secreting pancreatic (islet cell) carcinoma in a cat. *Journal of Veterinary Internal Medicine* **6**, 193–199

Hughes SM (2006) Canine gastrinoma: a case study and literature review of therapeutic options. *New Zealand Veterinary Journal,* **54**, 242–247

Leifer CE (1986) Hypoglycemia. In: *Current Veterinary Therapy IX,* ed. RW Kirk, pp. 982–987. WB Saunders, Philadelphia

Mai W and Caceres AV (2008) Dual-phase computed tomographic angiography in three dogs with pancreatic insulinoma. *Veterinary Radiology and Ultrasound* **49**, 141–148

Matthiesen DT and Mullen HS (1990) Problems and complications associated with endocrine surgery in the dog and cat. *Problems in Veterinary Medicine,* **2**, 627–667

Meleo KA and Caplan ER (2000) Treatment of insulinoma in the dog, cat, and ferret. In: *Kirk's Current Veterinary Therapy XIII,* ed. JD Bonagura, pp. 357–361. WB Saunders, Philadelphia

Mellanby RJ and Herrtage ME (2002) Insulinoma in a normoglycaemic dog with low serum fructosamine. *Journal of Small Animal Practice* **43**, 506–508

Moore AS, Nelson RW, Henry CJ *et al.* (2002) Streptozocin for treatment of pancreatic islet cell tumours in dogs: 17 cases (1989–1999). *Journal of the American Veterinary Medical Association* **221**, 811–818

Nelson RW and Couto CG (2003) Disorders of the endocrine pancreas. In: *Small Animal Internal Medicine, 3rd edn,* ed. RW Nelson and CG Couto, pp. 729–777. Mosby, St. Louis

Nelson RW and Salisbury SK (2000) Pancreatic beta cell neoplasia. In: *Saunders' Manual of Small Animal Practice, 2nd edn,* ed. SJ Birchard and RG Sherding, pp. 288–294. WB Saunders, Philadelphia

Patnaik AK, Hurvitz AI and Johnson GF (1980) Canine intestinal adenocarcinoma and carcinoid. *Veterinary Pathology* **17**, 149–163

Polton GA, White RN, Brearley MJ and Eastwood JM (2007) Improved survival in a retrospective cohort of 28 dogs with insulinoma. *Journal of Small Animal Practice* **48**, 151–156

Robben JH, Pollak YW, Kirpensteijn J *et al.* (2005) Comparison of ultrasonography, computed tomography and single-photon emission computed tomography for the detection and localization of canine insulinoma. *Journal of Veterinary Internal Medicine* **19**, 15–22

Robben JH, van den Brom WE, Mol JA, van Haeften TW and Rijnberk A (2006) Effect of octreotide on plasma concentrations of glucose, insulin, glucagon, growth hormone and cortisol in healthy dogs and dogs with insulinoma. *Research in Veterinary Science* **80**, 25–32

Sako T, Uchida E, Okamoto M *et al.* (2003) Immunohistochemical evaluation of a malignant intestinal carcinoid in a dog. *Veterinary Pathology* **40**, 212–215

Simpson KW and Dykes NL (1997) Diagnosis and treatment of gastrinomas. *Seminars in Veterinary Medicine and Surgery (Small Animal)* **12**, 274–281

Spugnini EP, Gargiulo M, Assin R *et al.* (2008) Adjuvant carboplatin for the treatment of intestinal carcinoid in a dog. *In Vivo* **22**, 759–761

Steiner JM (2004) Unusual gastrointestinal endocrine disorders. In: *BSAVA Manual of Canine and Feline Endocrinology, 3rd edn,* ed. CT Mooney and ME Peterson, pp. 222–228. BSAVA Publications, Gloucester

Steiner JM and Bruyette DS (1996) Canine insulinoma. *Compendium on Continuing Education for the Practicing Veterinarian* **8**, 13–25

15

Canine hypoadrenocorticism

David B. Church

Introduction

Canine hypoadrenocorticism is the clinical syndrome caused by a significant reduction in the principal biologically active glucocorticoid, cortisol, usually in association with a significant reduction in the principal biologically active mineralocorticoid, aldosterone. While once thought of as a relatively rare disorder, the prevalence appears to have increased over the last 5 years. This may be due to an increasing awareness of the variety of signs with which affected dogs may present. As a result, veterinary surgeons have a higher index of suspicion for hypoadrenocorticism and are testing for the disease, probably justifiably, earlier and with less classical supporting evidence, often in dogs with only vague or non-specific signs of 'not doing well'.

The vast majority of dogs with clinically significant hypoadrenocorticism have primary hypoadrenocorticism. In a proportion of these dogs there is selective loss of glucocorticoid secreting capacity only; this disorder is referred to as 'atypical' Addison's disease. Additionally, selective glucocorticoid deficiency can occur as a result of secondary hypoadrenocorticism associated with reduced adrenocorticotropic hormone (ACTH) secretion, although this is an extremely rare occurrence.

Physiology of the adrenal cortex

The major adrenocortical hormones are synthesized in different areas of the adrenal cortex. The adrenal cortex comprises approximately 75% of the adrenal gland and is divided into three morphologically distinct regions: the inner zona reticularis; the zona fasciculata; and the outer zona glomerulosa. These three zones of the adrenal cortex are responsible for producing a range of endogenous steroid hormones or corticosteroids. All corticosteroids are produced by sequential hydrolysis, oxidation and methylation of cholesterol. These reactions are catalysed by a variety of enzymes and produce a range of intermediate steroids.

Cells of the zona reticularis and fasciculata produce cortisol, the principal endogenous glucocorticoid. Androgens and oestrogens are also produced in these zones. In common with other glucocorticoids, cortisol has a wide range of actions that help maintain general body homeostasis. Cortisol acts both through non-gene-regulated intracellular pathways and by binding to specific glucocorticoid receptors within the nucleus to alter gene expression. In summary, through these actions cortisol alters the regulation of many processes, including enzyme synthesis and activity, cell and lysosomal membrane permeability, numerous intracellular and transcellular transport processes and a range of genetic expressions that relate to alteration and management of cell structure. Cortisol also plays a seminal role in glucose homeostasis through its capacity to modify glycogen metabolism.

The zona glomerulosa has a less clearly defined structure and its cells tend to be scattered in the regions directly beneath the capsule. Aldosterone, the principal endogenous mineralocorticoid, is synthesized in the zona glomerulosa.

The differences in steroid synthesis are related to variations in the concentrations of specific steroid synthesizing enzymes in each region of the adrenal cortex. Compared to the zona fasciculata, the zona glomerulosa has a low concentration of 17α-hydroxylase, the enzyme that converts pregnenolone and progesterone to substrates for glucocorticoid/androgen/oestrogen production. The zona glomerulosa also has high concentrations of aldosterone synthase, the cytochrome P450 enzyme that converts corticosterone to aldosterone.

Aldosterone secretion is stimulated via activation of the renin–angiotensin system and through elevations in plasma potassium concentration acting directly on the zona glomerulosa (Figure 15.1).

Renin catalyses the conversion of angiotensinogen to angiotensin I, which is itself converted to angiotensin II. Angiotensin II is both a potent vasoconstrictor and an aldosterone secretagogue. Renin release is stimulated by the activation of various effectors that include:

- Baroreceptors in the walls of the afferent arterioles of the glomeruli
- Cardiac and arterial baroreceptors that regulate sympathetic neural activity
- Concentration of circulating catecholamines which enhance renin secretion via β-1 adrenergic receptors
- Cells of the macula densa in the early distal tubule, which appear to be stimulated by a reduction in chloride delivery.

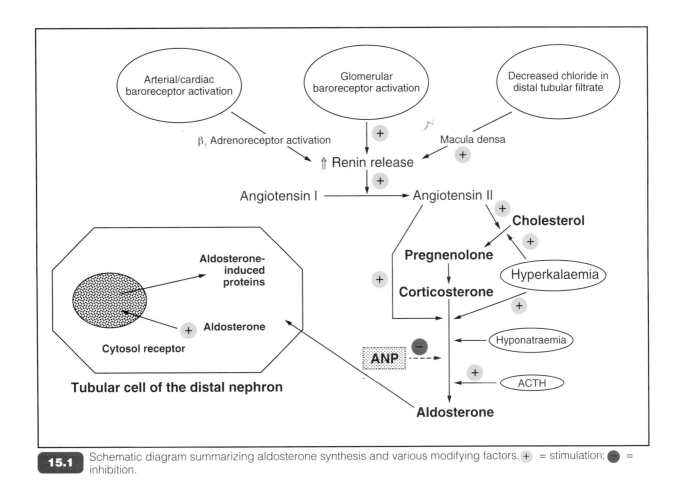

15.1 Schematic diagram summarizing aldosterone synthesis and various modifying factors. + = stimulation; − = inhibition.

Angiotensin II and hyperkalaemia act on the zona glomerulosa, promoting the conversion of cholesterol to pregnenolone and, more importantly, of corticosterone to aldosterone via stimulation of aldosterone synthase. Aldosterone release can also be stimulated by other factors, including ACTH and hyponatraemia, and is suppressed by atrial natriuretic peptide.

The primary sites of action of aldosterone are the connecting segment and collecting tubules of the distal nephron where sodium and chloride resorption and potassium and hydrogen ion secretion are stimulated.

Aldosterone acts through specific cytosolic receptors contained within its major target cells of the distal nephron. Once aldosterone binds to these receptors, the hormone–receptor complex migrates to the nucleus, where it modifies nuclear chromatin transcription to produce so-called aldosterone-induced proteins (AIPs). These AIPs modify transcellular ionic transport in the aldosterone-sensitive cells of the distal nephron. Cortisol has similar affinity for the aldosterone receptor and has approximately 1000 times the plasma concentration of aldosterone. However, cortisol does not act as a major mineralocorticoid due to intracellular pre-receptor enzymatic modification by the enzyme 11β-hydroxysteroid dehydrogenase. This enzyme exists in at least two isoforms: 11β-hydroxysteroid dehydrogenase type 1 and type 2. Type 1 11β-hydroxysteroid dehydrogenase converts biologically inactive cortisone to its

active form, cortisol, while type 2 converts cortisol (but not aldosterone) to its inactive form cortisone. The major target cells for aldosterone possess significant amounts of 11β-hydroxysteroid dehydrogenase type 2, thus ensuring aldosterone and not cortisol has the major mineralocorticoid activity in these distal nephron tubular target cells.

Aldosterone stimulates ionic transport in these cells by increasing the number of open sodium and potassium channels in the luminal membrane as well as the activity of the sodium–potassium–ATPase pump in the basolateral membrane. The aldosterone-induced elevation in luminal sodium permeability promotes sodium diffusion into the tubular cell which is returned to the systemic circulation by the sodium–potassium–ATPase pump. The movement of sodium through its luminal channel creates a negative potential. Electroneutrality is maintained either by passive chloride resorption or by potassium secretion from the cell into the tubule lumen. Aldosterone further enhances intraluminal potassium secretion as the extracellular transport of sodium via the sodium–potassium–ATPase pump increases intracellular movement of potassium and ensures a continued intracellular supply of potassium for its ongoing excretion.

Aldosterone-stimulated hydrogen ion secretion occurs in different collecting tubular cells and is mediated through an H^+–ATPase pump in the luminal membrane. Aldosterone also indirectly stimulates tubular hydrogen ion secretion via its effect on sodium resorption. The associated generation of a luminal negative electrical potential through sodium resorption creates a favourable electrical gradient for hydrogen ion accumulation in the tubular lumen.

Primary hypoadrenocorticism

Aetiology

Impaired adrenocortical function may develop as a result of disease of any part of the hypothalamic–pituitary–adrenal axis. However, in dogs and cats hypoadrenocorticism is generally a result of substantial destruction of adrenocortical tissue. Although any destruction of adrenocortical tissue may impair adrenocortical reserve, in non-stressful situations approximately 90% of the adrenal cortex needs to be non-functional before this impairment becomes clinically significant (Herrtage, 2005).

In most cases the underlying reason for adrenal destruction appears to be idiopathic or immune-mediated. Several investigators have described bilateral adrenocortical atrophy with mononuclear infiltrates (Schaer et al., 1986; Boujon et al., 1994). In addition, anti-adrenal antibodies have been detected in variable proportions of dogs with primary hypoadrenocorticism (Schaer et al., 1986; Weller et al., 1996). In humans, immune-mediated adrenocortical destruction has been associated with two heritable conditions resulting in immune-mediated polyendocrinopathies. Interestingly, a marked genetic predisposition for hypoadrenocorticism has been demonstrated in a number of different breeds of dogs (see below).

Both temporary and permanent hypoadrenocorticism develops not uncommonly in dogs with hyperadrenocorticism treated with either mitotane or trilostane (Braddock et al., 2003; Chapman et al., 2004). In an as yet undetermined proportion of dogs with pituitary-dependent hyperadrenocorticism treated with trilostane, permanent adrenocortical destruction appears to result from generalized bilateral adrenocortical infarction (see Chapter 16). This bilateral adrenal haemorrhage and subsequent necrosis may be a consequence of chronic hyperstimulation by markedly elevated plasma ACTH concentrations, as has been reported in humans and more recently in rats with experimentally induced pituitary-dependent hyperadrenocorticism (Rao, 1995; Burkhardt et al., 2009).

A variety of different drugs can inhibit adrenocortical steroid production both specifically and non-specifically. These include etomidate, most members of the imidazole drug group and various agents such as metyrapone, aminoglutethimide and mifepristone. However, as their effects are generally relatively short-acting, they rarely result in clinically significant hypoadrenocorticism.

Less well documented causes of adrenal destruction in dogs include infectious and infiltrative diseases as well as possible adrenocortical destruction secondary to haemorrhage induced by coagulopathies.

Clinical features

Signalment

Primary hypoadrenocorticism has been reported in dogs ranging from 2 months to 14 years of age, although most affected animals present in young to middle age. The disease is most over-represented in Standard Poodles and Bearded Collies. Other breeds such as Nova Scotia Duck Tolling Retrievers, Leonbergers, Portuguese Water Spaniels, Great Danes, Rottweilers, Wheaten Terriers and West Highland White Terriers also appear predisposed (Smallwood and Barsanti, 1995; Peterson et al., 1996; Burton et al., 1997). A genetic predilection has been confirmed in a number of these breeds.

In Standard Poodles the heritability appears to be influenced by a single recessive locus (Famula et al., 2003), while in Bearded Collies the mechanism of inheritance, although studied remains undetermined (Oberbauer et al., 2002). A recent evaluation of the mode of heritability of hypoadrenocorticism in the Portuguese Water Dog, using complex segregation analysis, suggested the mode of inheritance was under the control of a single autosomal recessive locus and that the risk was no different in males and females (Oberbauer et al., 2006). Another study investigated hypoadrenocorticism in 25 Nova Scotia Duck Tolling Retrievers, where the disorder appeared to have an autosomal recessive mode of inheritance (Hughes et al., 2007). In these dogs, hypoadrenocorticism was diagnosed at an earlier age (median, 2.6 years) compared with published reports of a median age at diagnosis of 4.0 years among the general affected population (Peterson et al., 1996). Interestingly up to one-third of these diseased retrievers had no serum electrolyte abnormalities at the time of diagnosis.

In those breeds in which a marked breed predilection has not been reported, female dogs are more commonly affected with a ratio of approximately 2.3:1.

Clinical signs

The clinical features of hypoadrenocorticism vary from a variety of vague and non-specific signs to acute collapse with generalized underperfusion (Figure 15.2). The more subacute clinical scenarios often suggest that the animal is unwell but do not indicate any particular body system or disease. It is not uncommon for dogs with primary hypoadrenocorticism to have a waxing and waning history characterized by vague illness with variable gastrointestinal signs and depression/weakness interspersed with periods of apparent normality. The clinician's index of suspicion for hypoadrenocorticism is heightened by such a history, particularly if the animal has shown a dramatic clinical response to symptomatic fluid therapy.

Patients presenting with acute collapse usually have evidence of generalized, marked hypovolaemia and dehydration, together with vomiting, diarrhoea, abdominal pain and hypothermia. Some may have severe gastrointestinal haemorrhage with melaena and occasional haematemesis (Medinger et al.,

Presenting complaints
• Inappetence [a]
• Lethargy [a]
• Weakness [b]
• Vomiting [b]
• Diarrhoea
• Weight loss
• Shivering and/or muscle stiffness
• Polyuria
• Polydipsia

Physical examination findings
• Depression [a]
• Weakness [a]
• Dehydration [b]
• Inappropriately slow heart rate
• Hypothermia

15.2 Clinical signs encountered in dogs with hypoadrenocorticism. [a] Present in almost all cases. [b] Common.

1993). The expected compensatory tachycardia may not be apparent. Mineralocorticoid deficiency results in hyperkalaemia, which with increasing severity tends to decrease the heart rate. The lack of a compensatory tachycardia in a patient that is clearly hypovolaemic is surprising, and this finding should further increase the index of suspicion for hypoadrenocorticism (or any other cause of marked hyperkalaemia in a hypovolaemic patient). However, many dogs with hypoadrenocorticism present with normal or increased heart rates.

Dogs with acute hypoadrenocorticism are unstable and represent a true medical emergency that requires rapid stabilization with parenteral fluid therapy, at least initially. As such the diagnosis of primary hypoadrenocorticism needs to be considered relatively early in the investigation of these patients.

While the acute hypoadrenocorticoid patient is a dramatic medical emergency, the majority of patients with primary hypoadrenocorticism present with vague and non-specific clinical features, usually attributable to variable impairment of the gastrointestinal, renal and neurological systems. These may include any combination of lethargy, weakness, depression, inappetence, vomiting and diarrhoea. These signs may vary in severity in individual dogs. Polydipsia and polyuria are rarely primary complaints, although their presence may be revealed during questioning of the owners. Additionally a small proportion of hypoadrenocorticoid patients will present with a reversible megaoesophagus (where regurgitation is the primary presenting complaint), or other signs of neuromuscular dysfunction such as generalized muscle cramping (Burrows, 1987; Lifton *et al.*, 1996; Saito *et al.*, 2002). The most consistent findings on physical examination in these dogs include depression, lethargy or weakness and variable degrees of dehydration or hypovolaemia. Like those presenting with acute illness described above, these animals may be bradycardic or have evidence of gastrointestinal haemorrhage.

It is important to remember that all dogs with primary hypoadrenocorticism are potentially unstable as they are variably hypovolaemic and are prone to marked hypotension. This hypotensive potential is due to a lack of aldosterone secretion and is possibly further exacerbated by concurrent decreased vascular responsiveness to normal pressor effects, mediated through the overproduction of nitric oxide (Orbach *et al.*, 2001). Consequently, if primary hypoadrenocorticism is being considered in any patient, they should be treated as a potentially critical case until their adrenocortical function has been clarified.

Diagnosis

Haematology
In the presence of appropriate clinical signs, suspicion for hypoadrenocorticism is dramatically increased by the presence of lymphocytosis and/or eosinophilia or simply the absence of a stress leucogram (lymphopenia and eosinopenia) in a clearly unwell or 'stressed' patient (Figure 15.3).

Haematology
• Non-regenerative anaemia
• Absence of lymphopenia and eosinopenia in a 'stressed' animal
• Lymphocytosis
• Eosinophilia
• Neutrophilic leucocytosis
• Mild neutropenia

Serum biochemistry
• Hyperkalaemia
• Hyponatraemia
• Hypochloraemia
• Prerenal azotaemia
• Hyperphosphataemia
• ± Hypercalcaemia
• ± Hypoglycaemia
• Metabolic acidosis (low total CO_2 and HCO_3^-)

Urinalysis
• Urine SG varies from inappropriately dilute to concentrated

15.3 Clinicopathological abnormalities in dogs with hypoadrenocorticism.

Hypoadrenocorticism commonly results in a non-regenerative anaemia of chronic illness although often the severity of this anaemia is masked by concurrent hypovolaemia and/or dehydration. Occasionally, gastrointestinal haemorrhage can result in profound anaemia (Peterson *et al.*, 1996). Again the magnitude of the reduction in packed cell volume underestimates the severity of the true anaemia because of the concurrent hypovolaemia/dehydration. If severe enough, gastrointestinal haemorrhage on occasions may result in a regenerative anaemia.

Biochemistry
The most consistent biochemical abnormalities found in dogs with primary hypoadrenocorticism include azotaemia, hyponatraemia, hyperkalaemia, hypochloraemia and less commonly hypoglycaemia and hypercalcaemia (see Figure 15.3).

Electrolyte abnormalities: Hyponatraemia and hyperkalaemia with a sodium:potassium ratio of <23:1 are considered characteristic features of primary hypoadrenocorticism. In various studies evaluating diseases associated with these electrolyte abnormalities, hypoadrenocorticism was the most common explanation for the presence of concurrent hyponatraemia and hyperkalaemia (Roth and Tyler, 1999; Neiger and Gundersen, 2003; Adler *et al.*, 2007).

In patients with hypoadrenocorticism, circulating sodium concentrations are usually <135 mmol/l and potassium concentrations are usually >5.5 mmol/l. However, because of the variation in the magnitude of these changes, the ratio of sodium to potassium concentration is frequently recommended as a more reliable indicator of hypoadrenocorticism. In one study evaluating dogs with subnormal plasma Na:K ratios, 28% of dogs with a ratio <25:1 had primary hypoadrenocorticism and this proportion increased to 64% of cases when the Na:K ratio was <20:1 (Neiger and Gunderson, 2003).

Circulating chloride concentration is also reduced in patients with hypoadrenocorticism and concentrations of <100 mmol/l are frequently encountered.

Although the presence of hyponatraemia, hyperkalaemia, hypochloraemia and a significantly reduced Na:K ratio support a diagnosis of hypoadrenocorticism, these changes can occur in a variety of other conditions (Roth and Tyler, 1999; Neiger and Gunderson, 2003; Nielsen *et al.*, 2008). Non-adrenal diseases associated with moderate to marked hyponatraemia and hyperkalaemia include acute and chronic urinary tract disease, various gastrointestinal disorders including pancreatitis, secretory enteropathies and diffuse small bowel disease, chronic end stage heart or liver failure, pleural and peritoneal effusions, neoplasia, and on occasions uncomplicated pregnancy (Roth and Tyler, 1999; Schaer *et al.*, 2001; Neiger and Gunderson, 2003; Nielsen *et al.*, 2008). In addition, artefactual hyperkalaemia may be a confusing consequence of post-collection haemolysis, particularly in Japanese Akitas (Degen, 1987) or of marked leucocytosis or thrombocytosis (Reimann *et al.*, 1989). Consequently, many non-adrenal illnesses may result in a subnormal Na:K ratio. Indeed, any disease that results in significant metabolic acidosis or in marked tissue destruction with release of intracellular contents may produce marked hyperkalaemia.

Approximately 10–30% of dogs with primary hypoadrenocorticism have serum or plasma electrolyte concentrations within their respective reference intervals or have only mild hyponatraemia without hyperkalaemia at the time of diagnosis. While it is clear that these animals have primary hypoadrenocorticism, the explanation for relatively mild or absent electrolyte derangements remains a topic of some debate. In some animals, prior therapy may mask previously abnormal electrolyte concentrations. Some animals may be detected earlier in the course of their disease and electrolyte changes are potentially less apparent if the dog is fed a diet that is relatively high in sodium. It has been suggested that these animals represent a subset of patients with primary selective glucocorticoid deficiency or 'atypical' Addison's disease (Lifton *et al.*, 1996; Sadek and Schaer, 1996; Thompson *et al.*, 2007). However, this remains a hypothesis as large studies evaluating aldosterone production in such affected patients have not yet been carried out. Regardless of the underlying explanation, it is important to emphasize that the diagnosis of primary and typical hypoadrenocorticism is ***not*** precluded in animals with normal or only mildly abnormal electrolyte concentrations.

Azotaemia: As with all hypovolaemic conditions, animals with primary hypoadrenocorticism develop azotaemia secondary to renal underperfusion. However, unlike many other hypovolaemic conditions, where renal concentrating ability is maintained, dogs with primary hypoadrenocorticism are generally unable to concentrate their urine effectively. Impaired urine concentrating ability is due to mineralocorticoid deficiency and resultant chronic renal sodium loss, depletion of normal renal medullary sodium concentration gradient and impaired water resorption from the renal collecting ducts. As a consequence, azotaemia is usually accompanied by inappropriately dilute urine increasing the potential for affected animals to be mistakenly diagnosed with severe primary renal disease.

Other abnormalities: Dogs with hypoadrenocorticism tend to have increased circulating calcium concentrations and this increase has been reported in both the total and ionized fractions (Adamantos and Boag, 2008; Gow *et al.*, 2009). Although it has been hypothesized that hypercalcaemia is due to volume depletion, this does not explain the ionized hypercalcaemia (Adamantos and Boag, 2008). Any tendency towards metabolic acidosis increases the ionized calcium fraction by altering the affinity of the serum- binding proteins and thus may play a role in some dogs. Equally, the impairment of renal function secondary to hypovolaemia may also contribute to an increased total serum calcium concentration. From one small study of eight cases, the hypercalcaemia did not appear to be related to any increase in parathyroid hormone or Vitamin D concentrations (Gow *et al.*, 2009). Currently, the mechanism is poorly understood. It is likely to be multifactorial, and glucocorticoid deficiency itself may play a role. Regardless of the underlying mechanism, the hypercalcaemia is generally mild, clinically insignificant and does not appear to be associated with the degree of alteration in the sodium:potassium ratio. Hypoadrenocorticism remains, however, an important differential of hypercalcaemia in dogs (see Chapter 21).

Other biochemical abnormalities occasionally encountered in dogs and cats with hypoadrenocorticism include hypoglycaemia and varying degrees of hypoalbuminaemia or hypoproteinaemia. As with anaemia, the severity of the hypoproteinaemia may be masked by the hypovolaemia/dehydration. Hypoproteinaemia can be a result of gastrointestinal haemorrhage.

Supplementary diagnostic aids

Other diagnostic aids that may provide supporting evidence for hypoadrenocorticism include electrocardiography, thoracic radiography and abdominal ultrasonography.

Electrocardiography: Electrocardiography may be helpful, as animals with hyperkalaemia tend to have specific changes in electrocardiographic complex morphology. These include peaking of the T-wave, shortening of the Q–T interval, prolongation of the P–R interval and reduction in P-wave amplitude. Unfortunately, these changes occur in any condition that induces hyperkalaemia. They are therefore not particularly suggestive of reduced adrenocortical function. Electrocardiographic changes are notoriously unreliable indicators of the existence or degree of hyperkalaemia. Some animals with substantial electrolyte derangements do not have dramatic electrocardiographic changes.

Diagnostic imaging: Thoracic radiography of affected animals may reveal a reduction in the size of the cardiac silhouette, the prominence of the pulmonary vasculature and the diameter of the caudal vena cava. Although these signs are invariably present in dogs with hypoadrenocorticism they are simply a reflection of hypovolaemia (Melian *et al.,* 1999). Additionally, when present, the megaoesophagus that may be associated with hypoadrenocorticism is likely to be noticeable on plain thoracic radiography.

It has been suggested that ultrasonographic imaging of both adrenal glands may facilitate the diagnosis of primary hypoadrenocorticism. In one study, objective evaluation of adrenal gland size using abdominal ultrasonography confirmed a significant reduction in the size of both adrenal glands with minimal overlap between normal and affected dogs (Hoerauf and Reusch, 1999). It is possible that in the hands of a skilled ultrasonographer with appropriate equipment this may provide further support to increase the index of suspicion for a diagnosis of hypoadrenocorticism.

Adrenal function tests

It is important to note that none of the above potential abnormalities, either alone or in combination, can be considered sufficient evidence to confirm a diagnosis of hypoadrenocorticism. Many other conditions potentially produce such clinical signs and abnormalities in the various diagnostic aids described. Consequently, documenting impaired adrenal steroid production is necessary to confirm a diagnosis of hypoadrenocorticism. For diagnosing hypoadrenocorticism, the recommended tests are safe, easy to perform, relatively inexpensive and have excellent specificity and sensitivity.

ACTH response test: Dogs with primary hypoadrenocorticism are likely to have both hypocortisolaemia and hypoaldosteronaemia. However, a proportion of patients may only be afflicted with hypocortisolaemia. It appears poorly documented and probably exceptionally rare to have isolated aldosterone deficiency without hypocortisolaemia.

Estimating basal concentrations of adrenal hormones can be supportive of a deficiency, but the degree of overlap between affected and non-affected patients limits their diagnostic value. Equally, measurement of a decreased urinary corticoid:creatinine ratio may provide some indication of hypoadrenocorticism in a patient with supporting clinical signs, but this does not assess adrenal reserve and consequently true hypofunction may not be detected. A definitive diagnosis is therefore more commonly made by measuring circulating cortisol concentration before and after stimulation with exogenous ACTH. This provides no information on mineralocorticoid deficiency but this is not required in the vast majority of dogs with impaired adrenocortical function.

A diagnosis of hypoadrenocorticism is confirmed by demonstration of subnormal basal and post-ACTH circulating cortisol concentrations in an animal that has not recently received exogenous glucocorticoid therapy. The ACTH response test is best performed by sampling before and 30–60 minutes after the intravenous or intramuscular administration of 250 μg (or the intravenous administration of 5 μg/kg) of the synthetic ACTH analogue tetracosactrin (cosyntropin).

As hydrocortisone, prednisolone and prednisone all cross-react in cortisol assays, it is essential that the ACTH response test is performed *before* these agents are administered to the dog. By contrast, dexamethasone does not cross-react in cortisol assays and consequently can be used to provide glucocorticoid support to critically ill patients if deemed necessary. Although dexamethasone directly inhibits endogenous cortisol production, this effect usually takes at least 4–6 hours to be expressed. Consequently, any artefactual lowering of post-ACTH cortisol concentrations can be avoided by ensuring that the ACTH response test is completed within 2–3 hours of dexamethasone administration. Delaying glucocorticoid therapy until the ACTH response test is completed is rarely problematic, provided that adequate intravenous fluid therapy has been instituted.

The administration of a supraphysiological dose of ACTH should result in a predictable increase in circulating cortisol values in healthy animals and often an enhanced post-ACTH cortisol concentration in dogs with clinically significant non-adrenal illness (Figure 15.4). An abnormally poor response to this test defined as minimal stimulation with a post-ACTH cortisol concentration of less than approximately 50 nmol/l confirms a diagnosis of hypoadrenocorticism. In the majority of affected dogs, both pre and post ACTH cortisol concentrations are generally undetectable in standard commercial cortisol assays.

Although the 'gold standard' for confirming a diagnosis of hypoadrenocorticism is the ACTH response test, it does not differentiate between animals with naturally occurring primary and atypical hypoadrenocorticism. In addition, similar results occur in animals with secondary adrenal insufficiency as a result of chronic pituitary dysfunction or previous but recently

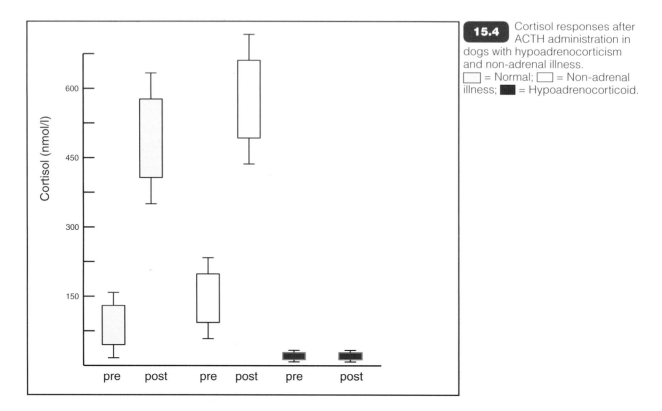

15.4 Cortisol responses after ACTH administration in dogs with hypoadrenocorticism and non-adrenal illness. ☐ = Normal; ☐ = Non-adrenal illness; ■ = Hypoadrenocorticoid.

discontinued chronic glucocorticoid administration. Differentiation of these explanations for diminished adrenocortical function requires estimation of the endogenous circulating ACTH concentration or circulating aldosterone concentrations.

Endogenous ACTH: Estimating a basal circulating ACTH concentration in an animal with clearly demonstrable subnormal adrenocortical function (as described above) is a reliable means of differentiating primary from secondary hypoadrenocorticism. Dogs with primary hypoadrenocorticism have markedly elevated plasma ACTH concentrations (usually >66 pmol/l; reference interval 15–45 pmol/l) whereas those patients with secondary hypoadrenocorticism have subnormal or undetectable values (usually <7 pmol/l).

Sample processing needs to be meticulous, as the measurable ACTH is readily decreased because of post-collection proteolysis and/or haemolysis. Consequently there must be sufficient evidence that the sample arrived at the laboratory in appropriate order prior to ACTH measurement. In addition, the ACTH assay must be validated for use in dogs (see Chapter 2).

Endogenous ACTH concentrations can be rapidly and dramatically suppressed by any exogenous glucocorticoid. Consequently, estimation of endogenous ACTH should only be performed on samples collected before glucocorticoid supplementation has begun. Modern ACTH assays can be reliably performed on EDTA plasma separated and frozen within 30 minutes of collection. However, in a busy clinical setting the practicalities of preparing these samples at the same time as administering supportive therapy to a critical patient often results in the ACTH estimation not being performed.

Circulating aldosterone concentration: Estimation of circulating aldosterone concentrations, before and after ACTH administration, is theoretically helpful in differentiating primary typical from secondary hypoadrenocorticism. In addition, and more importantly, it helps to confirm dogs with selective glucocorticoid deficiency or 'atypical' Addison's disease. Although assays for measurement of aldosterone concentrations are not widely available, aldosterone is well preserved across species and hence most assays used for estimation of human aldosterone can be adapted for use in dogs. The absolute values will differ between laboratories but usually reference basal values range between 5.5 and 270 pmol/l (mean 135 pmol/l) with post-ACTH concentrations between 404 and 1437 pmol/l (mean 848 pmol/l) (Golden and Lothrop, 1988; Feldman and Nelson, 2004).

Dogs with primary hypoadrenocorticism will have reduced circulating cortisol and aldosterone concentrations before and after ACTH administration. Dogs with primary disease but reference range electrolyte concentrations (because of previous therapy) will have a similar response. By contrast, those with secondary hypoadrenocorticism have relatively normal aldosterone concentrations. Dogs with selective glucocorticoid deficiency or 'atypical' disease may have a cortisol and aldosterone response indistinguishable from that of patients with secondary hypoadrenocorticism. However, the aldosterone response may be blunted and it is as yet unclear whether all such animals develop aldosterone deficiency and true Addison's disease in time.

ACTH:cortisol ratio and/or renin:aldosterone ratio: An alternative method of measuring an animal's capacity to produce adequate amounts of glucocorticoid and mineralocorticoid is to measure paired variables, such as the ratio of circulating concentrations of cortisol to ACTH (CAR) or the ratio of circulating concentrations of aldosterone to renin (ARR). Reference ranges for both ratios were established in 60 healthy dogs (CAR: 1.1–26.1 and ARR: 0.1–1.5; numbers based on SI units). Using such a range, the CAR and ARR clearly discriminated between healthy dogs and those with hypoadrenocorticism (Javadi *et al.,* 2006). Although animals with non-adrenal illness have not been studied, it does suggest that basal concentrations of cortisol and aldosterone, when interpreted with basal concentrations of ACTH and renin respectively, can provide a sensitive and possibly specific indicator of primary hypocortisolism and hypoaldosteronism. However, the same practical limitations to measuring ACTH as discussed above apply. In addition, assays for renin are not widely available, limiting the diagnostic utility of such ratios.

Treatment

Because of the combination of a potentially critical patient and the inability to rapidly confirm a diagnosis by cortisol estimation, there are times when hypoadrenocorticism requires treatment before a diagnosis has been reliably confirmed. Initially most affected animals require intravenous fluid therapy and concurrent parenteral glucocorticoid/mineralocorticoid replacement therapy (Figure 15.5). Dogs with atypical primary hypoadrenocorticism, at least initially, require only glucocorticoid supplementation.

Fluid therapy
Type: 0.9% saline solution Rate: 10–30 ml/kg/h i.v. initially for first 2–3 hours then reduced to no >5–7.5 ml/kg/h. Monitor circulating sodium concentration and ensure it does not increase by more than 10–12 mmol/l in the first 24 hours Potassium supplementation: Contraindicated until plasma potassium concentration normalizes Dextrose: Rarely required unless hypoglycaemic. Use 2.5% dextrose infusion (add 50 ml of 50% dextrose to each litre of i.v. fluids) and monitor glycaemic response
Mineralo/glucocorticoid therapy
Parenteral therapy should continue until the animal is rehydrated, gastrointestinal tract function has normalized, food and water are being consumed normally and oral maintenance therapy can be started. Recommended options include: • HSS at 1 mg/ml administered as a continuous infusion of 0.5 mg/kg/h • HSS as a bolus of 4–10 mg/kg i.v. every 6 hours • Prednisolone sodium succinate [a] at 4–20 mg/kg i.v., then dexamethasone sodium phosphate at 0.05–0.1 mg/kg in i.v. fluids infused over 12 hours • Dexamethasone sodium phosphate [a] at 0.1–2 mg/kg i.v., then 0.05–0.1 mg/kg in i.v. fluids infused over 12 hours

15.5 Initial treatment required to manage dogs with acute, critical hypoadrenocorticism. HSS, hydrocortisone sodium succinate; [a] Prednisolone/prednisone and dexamethasone lack mineralcortocoid activity necessitating the concurrent use of a parenteral mineralocorticoid. The only agent currently available (USA only) is desoxycorticosterone pivalate (DOCP) given as a single intramuscular injection at 2.2 mg/kg.

Initial stabilization or acute therapy

Intravenous fluid therapy should be started as soon as possible in the acutely unwell patient. Patients with hypoadrenocorticism are susceptible to fluid overload and, additionally, rapid correction of any hyponatraemia may result in structural neurological disease and myelinolysis, characterized by a variety of variably reversible neurological signs (Brady *et al.,* 1999; MacMillan, 2003). There is therefore a conflict between the need to correct the severe hypovolaemia quickly whilst ensuring the sodium concentration does not increase too rapidly.

Consequently the fluid of choice is normal saline (0.9%), and most endocrinologists and criticalists recommend an initial rate of 10–30 ml/kg/h with a subsequent reduction to around two to three times maintenance levels (5–7.5 ml/kg/h) after 2–3 hours. Because of the potential for excessively rapid correction of the hyponatraemia, circulating sodium concentration should be monitored closely. Experimental and clinical observations suggest that the degree of correction over the first 24 hours is most important and problems are unlikely if the sodium does not increase by more than 10–12 mmol/l in the first 24 hours.

Although fluid therapy alone generally results in a marked reduction in circulating potassium concentration (because of restoration of renal perfusion and correction of acidosis) it should be complemented by treatment with a parenteral agent possessing both glucocorticoid and mineralocorticoid activity. Currently, hydrocortisone sodium succinate (HSS) is the only commercially available parenteral steroid with both glucocorticoid and mineralocorticoid activity. Although soluble dexamethasone or prednisolone preparations can be used, their lack of mineralocorticoid activity makes them less attractive alternatives to HSS. Using HSS, additional treatment for hyperkalaemia (e.g. intravenous dextrose, insulin, calcium or bicarbonate) is virtually never required.

HSS is an ester of hydrocortisone or cortisol, the principal steroid produced by the adrenal cortex in dogs. It has equipotent glucocorticoid and mineralocorticoid activity. However, it has only 25% of the glucocorticoid potency of prednisolone and <1% of the mineralocorticoid potency of fludrocortisone. At the recommended doses it provides sufficient glucocorticoid and mineralocorticoid activity to treat the clinical consequences of primary hypoadrenocorticism and can be effectively used in the short-term management of these patients (Church *et al.,* 1999).

HSS is administered as an intravenous infusion at a dose of 0.5 mg/kg/h until normal gastrointestinal function has returned, the dog is eating and drinking and can be switched to oral steroid supplementation. In a dog with clinically significant hypoadrenocorticism this dose is likely to produce plasma cortisol concentrations of approximately 1000 nmol/l within 2–3 hours. Such a cortisol concentration is likely to provide adequate glucocorticoid and mineralocorticoid replacement in stressed dogs with impaired adrenocortical function (Church *et al.,* 1994; Church *et al.,* 1999).

As there is potential for HSS to adhere to plastic or glass at low concentrations, it is best to administer it in its own fluid bag or in a syringe driver diluted to a concentration of no less than 1mg/ml. It is incompatible with a variety of different solutions, including ampicillin sodium, and it is therefore best to dilute the HSS in normal saline.

If fluid therapy is adequate and an HSS infusion has been used, the response to therapy is usually dramatic, with most patients showing a good to excellent response within hours. It is recommended that circulating sodium and potassium concentrations are monitored at least hourly initially and that care is taken to ensure that there is an adequate clinical response, a decrease in the degree of azotaemia and appropriate urine production. Close monitoring is essential because in many cases a definitive diagnosis will not yet have been made and there is a possibility of inducing neurological damage with inappropriate changes in circulating sodium concentrations.

Maintenance therapy

Once the patient is stabilized, glucocorticoid and mineralocorticoid replacement therapy is almost always required for the remainder of the animal's life. Traditionally, a semi-selective mineralocorticoid, fludrocortisone acetate and a semi-selective glucocorticoid (cortisone acetate or prednisolone) are initially used together.

Patients can also be maintained on a combination of a selective mineralocorticoid, desoxycorticosterone pivalate (DOCP) and a semi-selective glucocorticoid (cortisone acetate or prednisolone). Because DOCP has no glucocorticoid activity it must always be used with a glucocorticoid. Currently, DOCP is not available in the UK or Europe.

Fludrocortisone acetate: Fludrocortisone acetate is a synthetic adrenocortical steroid with a fluoride ion substituted at the 9α position and an 11β-hydroxyl group, giving it both glucocorticoid and mineralocorticoid potency.

Because of the 9α fluoride substitution, fludrocortisone acetate has potent mineralocorticoid activity while the 11β-hydroxylation confers significant glucocorticoid activity. As a result, fludrocortisone has 10 times the glucocorticoid activity and 125 times the mineralocorticoid activity of cortisol.

The dose of fludrocortisone acetate is 10–30 µg/kg orally q24h. Typically a lower dose is used initially, with subsequent titration based on clinical response and circulating electrolyte concentrations. Dose adjustments are usually made after weekly electrolyte evaluations. Once these are stable and within or close to their reference intervals for healthy dogs, adjustments can be made every 4–6 months.

Although fludrocortisone acetate is primarily used for its mineralocorticoid activity, as stated above it also has inherent glucocorticoid activity. Based on daily cortisol production in healthy dogs, the theoretical glucocorticoid activity required for maintenance is approximately 0.2 mg/kg/day. Given the inherent glucocorticoid activity of fludrocortisone

acetate (10 times that of cortisol) it is possible for patients to be well controlled on this drug alone. However, because of differences in individual requirements, steroid metabolism and bioavailability, not all animals can be stabilized effectively on fludrocortisone acetate alone. In these individuals specific glucocorticoid supplementation is also required. Whether or not glucocorticoid supplementation is required in normal circumstances, if the animal is stressed through non-adrenal factors (e.g. illness, trauma, environmental change) then the inherent requirement for glucocorticoids should be accommodated by introducing glucocorticoid supplementation or increasing the daily dose.

In patients receiving concurrent long-term fludrocortisone acetate and prednisolone, it is not uncommon for the dose of fludrocortisone acetate to be increased gradually, as there appears to be a reduction in its efficacy over time (Kintzer and Peterson, 1997). Although many possible mechanisms for this exist, it is tempting to speculate that this represents accelerated metabolism of both steroids in response to the chronic 'supraphysiological' state created by long-term daily prednisolone administration and the well described steroid-induced tachyphylaxis. In the author's opinion, this 'fludrocortisone creep' is not as common a feature in patients treated with concurrent cortisone acetate and fludrocortisone acetate or the latter alone. In such treated patients, the fludrocortisone acetate dose required to maintain normal electrolyte concentrations is generally at the lower end of the suggested dose range.

Desoxycorticosterone pivalate: DOCP is a long-acting mineralocorticoid. As it has neither 11β- nor 17α-hydroxylation, it theoretically has little if any glucocorticoid activity.

The recommended dose of DOCP is 2.2 mg/kg by deep intramuscular injection every 25 days, although subcutaneous injection has been shown to be an effective alternative (McCabe et al., 1995). Plasma electrolyte, urea and creatinine concentrations are monitored every 2 weeks to determine the duration of action and help individualize the dose. Once stabilized it is prudent to check electrolytes every 3–6 months. Most dogs are well controlled on 1.1–2.2 mg/kg q3–4wk, although it has been suggested that occasional individuals will require more frequent dosing. As DOCP has no glucocorticoid activity, it is essential that patients receive concurrent glucocorticoid supplementation with either cortisone acetate or prednisolone.

Cortisone acetate: Cortisone is a synthetic steroid with an 11-keto substitution. Once absorbed, it is rapidly activated to hydrocortisone by a distinct 11β-hydroxysteroid dehydrogenase operating in a reductive mode. As cortisone is rapidly hydroxylated to cortisol, it provides a complete replacement for any form of cortisol deficiency. As it has equipotent glucocorticoid and mineralocorticoid activity it will also provide more mineralocorticoid activity than other synthetic glucocorticoids such as prednisolone. In addition, its shorter half-life and lower overall activity means it is less likely to create iatrogenic hyperadrenocorticism with long-term administration.

In patients with hypoadrenocorticism, orally administered cortisone acetate can be used as an effective long-term cortisol replacement. The dose of cortisone acetate must be individualized according to the severity of the condition, the response obtained and the other glucocorticoid or mineralocorticoid that is concurrently administered. As animals recover from an acute crisis, start eating and drinking normally and are changed from parenteral to oral medication, most patients are started on a dose of 0.5–1.0 mg/kg either once or divided twice daily. However once stable, generally a dose of 0.5 mg/kg either once or divided twice daily provides adequate additional glucocorticoid supplementation.

Prednisolone: Prednisolone is a synthetic adrenal steroid with moderately potentiated glucocorticoid activity (approximately 5 times that of hydrocortisone) and <10% of hydrocortisone's mineralocorticoid activity. Some clinicians advocate its use as a glucocorticoid supplement in the long-term management of hypoadrenocorticism at a dose rate of between 0.2 and 0.5 mg/kg once daily.

If the only formulation of prednisolone available is 5 mg tablets, then cortisone acetate may be a more effective alternative for glucocorticoid maintenance treatment in any dog that weighs <30 kg. In this situation, using prednisolone as the agent to provide maintenance glucocorticoid therapy makes it difficult to avoid overdosing in dogs under this weight.

Monitoring response to therapy

Regardless of the formulation(s) chosen for hormone replacement, monitoring the success of therapy is best achieved by concentrating on the clinical picture whilst being guided by the 'natural biomarkers' of glucocorticoid and mineralocorticoid function.

The natural biomarkers for glucocorticoid activity that are readily available to clinicians are all contained within the leucogram. Specifically, well managed hypoadrenocorticoid patients should ideally have a normal white cell count with mid-normal range absolute counts for lymphocytes, eosinophils and neutrophils and a normal neutrophil:lymphocyte ratio. The easily obtainable natural biomarkers for mineralocorticoid activity are not surprisingly the plasma concentrations of sodium and potassium together with the Na:K ratio.

There is no value in measuring circulating cortisol concentrations, basal or otherwise in hypoadrenocorticoid patients receiving glucocorticoids and/or mineralocorticoids. While determining basal endogenous circulating ACTH concentrations can provide some insight into the current level of glucocorticoid activity, various practical difficulties with sample collection and processing as well as cost make this an unattractive option.

However, it is important to stress that whenever there is some disagreement it is generally advisable to follow the old adage 'we should treat the patient not the numbers'. A happy, bright dog that appears well controlled in every other way should not be subjected to repeated testing and dose changes simply because it has a mild hyperkalaemia.

Secondary hypoadrenocorticism

Although canine adrenocortical insufficiency secondary to impaired hypothalamic–pituitary activity may occur as a result of a specific destructive lesion (Herrtage, 2005; Platt *et al.*, 1999), it is most commonly secondary to excessive, exogenous glucocorticoid supplementation.

Depending on the dose, preparation and duration of therapy, suppression of the hypothalamic–pituitary–adrenal axis can persist for weeks or months after cessation of exogenous therapy.

As aldosterone secretion is principally controlled by plasma concentrations of renin and potassium rather than ACTH, secondary hypoadrenocorticism is not characterized by signs referable to mineralocorticoid deficiency. Consequently although these patients may be clinically indistinguishable from animals with primary hypoadrenocorticism, they will not have hyponatraemia and hyperkalaemia.

Demonstration of suppression of the hypothalamic–pituitary–adrenal axis is best elucidated with an ACTH response test. As stated above suppression of the pituitary adrenal axis will persist for a variable period depending upon both the dose and duration of administration and also the preparation. In terms of recovery from the suppressive effects of glucocorticoid supplementation, basal circulating endogenous ACTH concentration is the first parameter to normalize, followed by basal cortisol and finally post-ACTH plasma cortisol concentration.

If treatment is required, secondary hypoadrenocorticism can usually be managed by replacement glucocorticoid therapy alone.

Prognosis

Hypoadrenocorticism is a readily treatable disease with an excellent prognosis, provided that treatment is maintained for life. Patients on adequate maintenance therapy should expect to lead relatively healthy lives, with no obvious impairment to exercise or other usual activities. However, it is vitally important to stress to owners that affected dogs only remain well while they continue to receive adequate glucocorticoid and mineralocorticoid supplementation. Additionally, as these dogs have no adrenocortical reserve, any non-adrenal illness or stressful event needs to be matched with an appropriate increase in the amount of glucocorticoid administered. Dogs with atypical disease should be carefully monitored for subsequent mineralocorticoid deficiency.

References

Adamantos S and Boag A (2008) Total and ionised calcium concentrations in dogs with hypoadrenocorticism. *The Veterinary Record* **163**, 25–26

Adler JA, Drobatz KJ and Hess RS (2007) Abnormalities of serum electrolyte concentrations in dogs with hypoadrenocorticism. *Journal of Veterinary Internal Medicine* **21**, 1168–1173

Boujon CE, Bornand-Jaunin V, Scharer V *et al.* (1994) Pituitary gland changes in canine hypoadrenocorticism: a functional and immunocytochemical study. *Journal of Comparative Pathology* **111**, 287–295

Braddock JA, Church DB, Roberston ID *et al.* (2003) Trilostane treatment in dogs with pituitary-dependent hyperadrenocorticism. *Australian Veterinary Journal* **81**, 600–607

Brady CA, Vite CH and Drobatz KJ (1999) Severe neurologic sequelae in a dog after treatment of hypoadrenal crisis. *Journal of the American Veterinary Medical Association* **215**, 222–225

Burkhardt WA, Boretti FS, Guscetti F *et al.* (2009) Severe adrenal vacuolization and haemorrhage caused by adrenocorticotropic hormone. *Proceedings, 19th ECVIM–CA Congress*, p. 269

Burrows CF (1987) Reversible mega-oesophagus in a dog with hypoadrenocorticism. *Journal of Small Animal Practice* **28**, 1073–1078

Burton S, DeLay J, Holmes A *et al.* (1997) Hypoadrenocorticism in young related Nova Scotia duck tolling retrievers. *Canadian Veterinary Journal* **38**, 231–234

Chapman PS, Kelly DF, Archer J *et al.* (2004) Adrenal necrosis in a dog receiving trilostane for the treatment of hyperadrenocorticism. *Journal of Small Animal Practice* **45**, 307–310

Church DB, Lamb WA and Emslie DR (1999) Plasma cortisol concentrations in normal dogs given hydrocortisone sodium succinate. *Australian Veterinary Journal* **77**, 316–317

Church DB, Nicholson AL, Ilkiw JE and Emslie DR (1994) Effect of non-adrenal illness anaesthesia and surgery on plasma cortisol concentrations in dogs. *Research in Veterinary Science* **56**, 129–131

Degen M (1987) Pseudohyperkalemia in Akitas. *Journal of the American Veterinary Medical Association* **190**, 541–543

Dunn KJ, Herrtage ME and Dunn JK (1995) Use of ACTH stimulation tests to monitor the treatment of canine hyperadrenocorticism. *The Veterinary Record* **137**, 161–165

Famula TR, Belanger JM and Oberbauer AM (2003) Heritability and complex segregation analysis of hypoadrenocorticism in the standard poodle. *Journal of Small Animal Practice* **44**, 8–12

Feldman EC and Nelson RW (2004) Hypoadrenocorticism. In: *Canine and Feline Endocrinology and Reproduction, 3rd edn*, ed. EC Feldman and RW Nelson, pp. 394–439. WB Saunders, Philadelphia

Golden DL and Lowthrop CD (1988) A retrospective study of aldosterone secretion in normal and adrenopathic dogs. *Journal of Veterinary Internal Medicine* **2**, 121–125

Gow AG, Gow DJ, Bell R *et al.* (2009) Calcium metabolism in eight dogs with hypoadrenocorticism. *Journal of Small Animal Practice* **50**, 426–430

Herrtage ME (2005) Hypoadrenocorticism. In: *Textbook of Veterinary Internal Medicine, 6th edn*, ed. SJ Ettinger and EC Feldman, pp. 1612–1622. WB Saunders, Philadelphia

Hoerauf A and Reusch C (1999) Ultrasonographic evaluation of the adrenal glands in six dogs with hypoadrenocorticism. *Journal of American Animal Hospital Association* **35**, 214–218

Hughes AM, Nelson RW, Famula TR and Bannasch DL (2007) Clinical features and heritability of hypoadrenocorticism in Nova Scotia Duck Tolling Retrievers: 25 cases (1994–2006). *Journal of the American Veterinary Medical Association* **231**, 407–412

Javadi S, Galac S, Boer P *et al.* (2006) Aldosterone-to-renin and cortisol-to-adrenocorticotropic hormone ratios in healthy dogs and dogs with primary hypoadrenocorticism. *Journal of Veterinary Internal Medicine* **20**, 556–551

Kintzer PP and Peterson ME (1997) Treatment and long-term follow-up of 205 dogs with hypoadrenocorticism. *Journal of Veterinary Internal Medicine* **11**, 43–49

Lifton SJ, King LG and Zerbe CA (1996) Glucocorticoid deficient hypoadrenocorticism in dogs: 18 cases (1986–1995). *Journal of the American Veterinary Medical Association* **209**, 2076–2081

MacMillan KL (2003) Neurologic complications following treatment of canine hypoadrenocorticism. *Canadian Veterinary Journal*, **44**, 490–492

McCabe MD, Feldman EC, Lynn RC and Kass PH (1995) Subcutaneous administration of desoxycorticosterone pivalate for the treatment of canine hypoadrenocorticism. *Journal of the American Animal Hospital Association* **31**, 151–155

Medinger TL, Williams DA and Bruyette DS (1993) Severe gastrointestinal tract haemorrhage in three dogs with hypoadrenocorticism. *Journal of the American Veterinary Medical Association* **202**, 1869–1872

Melian C, Stefanacci J, Peterson ME and Kintzer PP (1999) Radiographic findings in dogs with naturally-occurring primary hypoadrenocorticism. *Journal of the American Animal Hospital Association* **35**, 208–212

Neiger R and Gunderson HC (2003) Decreased sodium:potassium ratio in dogs: 50 cases. *BSAVA Congress Scientific Proceedings, Veterinary Programme*, p. 600 [abstract]

Nielsen L, Bell R, Zoia A *et al.* (2008) Low ratios of sodium to potassium in the serum of 238 dogs. *The Veterinary Record* **162**, 431–435

Oberbauer AM, Bell JS, Belanger JM and Famula TR (2006) Genetic evaluation of Addison's disease in the Portuguese Water Dog. *BMC Veterinary Research* **2**, 2–15

Oberbauer AM, Benemann KS, Belanger JM *et al.* (2002) Inheritance of hypoadrenocorticism in bearded collies. *American Journal of Veterinary Research* **63**, 643–647

Orbach P, Wood CE and Keller-Wood M (2001) Nitric oxide reduces pressor responsiveness during ovine hypoadrenocorticism. *Clinical Experimental Pharmacology and Physiology* **28**, 459–462

Peterson ME, Kintzer PP and Kass PH (1996) Pretreatment clinical and laboratory findings in dogs with hypoadrenocorticism: 225 cases (1979–1993). *Journal of the American Veterinary Medical Association* **208**, 85–91

Platt SR, Chrisman CL, Graham J and Clemmons RM (1999) Secondary hypoadrenocorticism associated with craniocerebral trauma in a dog. *Journal of the American Animal Hospital Association* **35**, 117–122

Rao RH (1995) Bilateral massive adrenal haemorrhage. *Medical Clinics of North America* **79**, 107–129

Reimann KA, Knowlen GG and Tvedten HW (1989) Factitious hyperkalemia in dogs with thrombocytosis. *Journal of Veterinary Internal Medicine* **3**, 47–52

Roth L and Tyler RD (1999) Evaluation of low sodium:potassium ratios in dogs. *Journal of Veterinary Diagnostic Investigations* **11**, 60–64

Sadek D and Schaer M (1996) Atypical Addison's disease in the dog: a retrospective survey of 14 cases. *Journal of the American Animal Hospital Association* **32**, 159–63

Saito M, Olby NJ, Obledo L and Goodkin JL (2002) Muscle cramps in two standard poodles with hypoadrenocorticism. *Journal of the American Animal Hospital Association* **38**, 437–443

Schaer M, Riley WJ, Buergelt CD *et al.* (1986) Autoimmunity and Addison's disease in the dog. *Journal of the American Animal Hospital Association* **22**, 789–794

Schaer M, Halling KB, Collins KE and Grant DC (2001) Combined hyponatremia and hyperkalemia mimicking acute hypoadrenocorticism in three pregnant dogs. *Journal of the American Veterinary Medical Association* **218**, 897–899

Smallwood LJ and Barsanti JA (1995) Hypoadrenocorticism in a family of Leonbergers. *Journal of the American Animal Hospital Association* **31**, 301–305

Thompson AL, Scott-Moncrieff JC and Anderson JD (2007) Comparison of classic hypoadrenocorticism with glucocorticoid-deficient hypoadrenocorticism in dogs: 46 cases (1985–2005). *Journal of the American Veterinary Medical Association* **230**, 1190–1194

Weller RE, Buschbom RL, Dagle GE *et al.* (1996) Hypoadrenocorticism in beagles exposed to aerosols of plutonium-238 dioxide by inhalation. *Radiation Research* **146**, 688–693

16

Canine hyperadrenocorticism

Michael E. Herrtage and Ian K. Ramsey

Introduction

Adrenal glands are each composed of a cortex and a medulla; these are embryologically and functionally separate endocrine glands. The adrenal cortex produces three groups of hormones: mineralocorticoids, which are important in electrolyte and water homeostasis; glucocorticoids, which promote gluconeogenesis; and small quantities of sex hormones, particularly male hormones that have weak androgenic activity. The cortex is essential for life, whereas the medulla is not. Hyperadrenocorticism describes the excessive production or administration of glucocorticoids and is one of the most commonly diagnosed endocrinopathies in the dog. Hyperadrenocorticism is rare in the cat and is described in Chapter 17.

Physiology of the adrenal gland

Control of glucocorticoid release

Glucocorticoid release is controlled almost entirely by adrenocorticotropic hormone (ACTH) secreted by the anterior pituitary, which in turn is regulated by corticotropin-releasing hormone (CRH) from the hypothalamus (Figure 16.1). Cortisol has direct negative feedback effects on the hypothalamus, to decrease formation of CRH, and the anterior pituitary gland, to decrease the formation of ACTH. These feedback mechanisms help regulate the plasma concentration of cortisol.

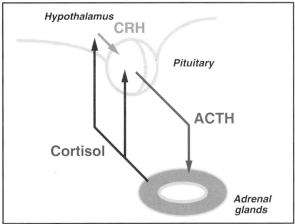

16.1 Regulation of glucocorticoid release. ACTH = adrenocorticotropic hormone; CRH = corticotropin-releasing hormone.

Secretion of CRH and ACTH is normally episodic and pulsatile, which results in fluctuating cortisol concentrations throughout the day. Diurnal variation is superimposed on this type of release. Anecdotally, in the dog CRH, ACTH and thus cortisol concentrations are highest in the early hours of the morning, whereas in the cat they are greatest in the evening. However, a true circadian rhythm of cortisol concentrations has been difficult to confirm in the dog (Kemppainen and Sartin, 1984).

Functions of glucocorticoids

Cortisol has more diverse effects on the body than any other hormone (Figure 16.2). It is best regarded as a hormone that has evolved to play a pivotal role in the body's response to long-term stresses such as starvation, chronic inflammation and infection. During periods of stress, both ACTH and cortisol are maintained at high concentrations, because the effects of stress tend to override the normal negative feedback control. Challenges to the immune system also activate the hypothalamic–pituitary–adrenal axis as cytokines, principally interleukin-1, stimulate the release of CRH from the hypothalamus.

In response to such stresses, cortisol acts to maintain blood glucose concentrations by increasing the production of glucose from non-carbohydrate sources (gluconeogenesis). Protein and fat catabolism are stimulated to provide amino and fatty acids for this process. In these respects, and in many others, cortisol counteracts the effects of insulin (which conversely may be viewed as having evolved to store the products of recent feeding). As a result, when cortisol is present in excessive quantities, this brings about a reduction in protein and fat stores in all tissues of the body except the liver. The catabolic actions of glucocorticoids on protein result in muscle wastage and weakness. They also result in the increased formation of hepatic gluconeogenic enzymes, which act on amino acids to produce glucose.

The catabolic effects on fat stores are countered by insulin, which inhibits lipolysis and stimulates lipogenesis. As a result, adipose tissue tends to be redistributed to the abdomen and back of the neck in dogs with excess concentrations of glucocorticoids and an adequate nutritional supply. Ketogenesis occurs if the effects of insulin are exceeded.

In response to chronic immunological and inflammatory stresses, cortisol has multiple and profound

Liver
• Increased gluconeogenesis • Increased glycogen stores • Induction of certain enzymes

Muscle
• Increased protein catabolism – muscle wasting and weakness

Bone
• Osteopenia associated with increased protein catabolism and negative calcium balance

Skin
• Increased protein catabolism – thin skin, poor wound healing and poor scar formation

Blood
• Erythrocytosis • Decrease in circulating lymphocytes • Decrease in circulating eosinophils • Increase in circulating neutrophils

Kidney
• Increased glomerular filtration rate and interference with vasopressin release or action (polyuria) • Increased calcium excretion

Immune system
• Diminished inflammatory response • Reduced immune response

Adipose tissue
• Increased lipolysis • Redistribution of fat deposits

Pituitary and hypothalamus
• Suppression of ACTH and CRH secretion

16.2 Effects of glucocorticoids on different body systems. ACTH = adrenocorticotropic hormone; CRH = corticotropin-releasing hormone.

effects that tend to prevent the body's pro-inflammatory reactions from becoming excessive or harmful. As a result, when cortisol is present in excess, it is anti-inflammatory and immunosuppressive.

Causes of hyperadrenocorticism

Hyperadrenocorticism can be spontaneous or iatrogenic. Spontaneously occurring hyperadrenocorticism may be associated with inappropriate secretion of ACTH by the pituitary (pituitary-dependent hyperadrenocorticism) or associated with a primary adrenal disorder (adrenal-dependent hyperadrenocorticism) (Figure 16.3).

Pituitary-dependent hyperadrenocorticism
Pituitary-dependent hyperadrenocorticism accounts for over 80% of dogs with naturally occurring hyperadrenocorticism. Excessive ACTH secretion results in bilateral adrenocortical hyperplasia and excess

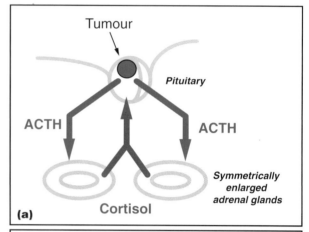

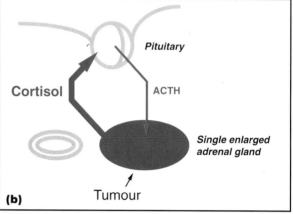

16.3 **(a)** The pituitary–adrenal axis in pituitary-dependent hyperadrenocorticism. **(b)** The pituitary–adrenal axis in adrenal-dependent hyperadrenocorticism. ACTH = adrenocorticotropic hormone; CRH = corticotropin-releasing hormone.

cortisol secretion. There is a failure of the negative feedback mechanism of cortisol on ACTH. However, ACTH secretion may remain episodic, resulting in fluctuating cortisol concentrations, which may at times fall within the reference interval.

More than 90% of dogs with pituitary-dependent hyperadrenocorticism have a pituitary tumour. Adenomas of the corticotropic cells of the pars distalis and pars intermedia are the most common type of canine pituitary tumour reported. Most of these pituitary tumours are microadenomas (<10 mm in diameter). Detection of such small tumours requires careful microdissection, experience and special stains. In one study using immunocytochemical staining, more than 80% of dogs with pituitary-dependent hyperadrenocorticism were positive for pituitary adenomas (Peterson *et al*, 1982). Macroadenomas (>10 mm diameter) are seen in about 10–15% of dogs (Duesberg *et al.*, 1995). These may compress the remaining pituitary gland and extend dorsally into the hypothalamus (Figure 16.4). However, they are generally slow growing and may not produce neurological signs. Corticotropic adenocarcinomas have been reported but are rare.

Hypersecretion of ACTH in the absence of pituitary neoplasia has also been suggested as a cause of pituitary-dependent hyperadrenocorticism. The cause is unknown, but suggestions include:

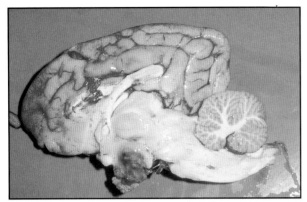

16.4 Pituitary macroadenoma found on post-mortem examination of a 13-year-old Golden Retriever that had been successfully treated with mitotane for hyperadrenocorticism for 5 years. There were no neurological signs associated with this tumour.

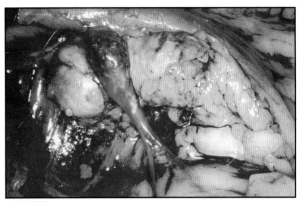

16.5 An adrenocortical carcinoma of the right adrenal gland invading the phrenicoabdominal vein. The caudal vena cava can be seen at the top of the photograph.

- An excessive stimulation of pituitary corticotropic cells secondary to an, as yet unknown, hypothalamic disorder
- A primary failure of the negative feedback response by cortisol
- An overproduction of CRH from the hypothalamus causing diffuse hyperplasia of the corticotropic cells in the anterior pituitary.

From a clinical point of view, the precise pituitary pathology is not of great importance unless neurological signs are present at the time of diagnosis or if they become apparent during the initial treatment.

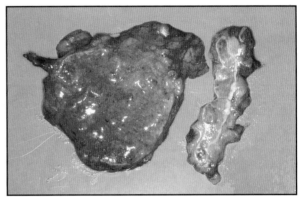

16.6 The cut surface of both adrenal glands from the same case as Figure 16.4. Note the severe cortical atrophy (pale rim) in the contralateral adrenal gland.

Adrenal-dependent hyperadrenocorticism

The remaining 15–20% of spontaneous cases of hyperadrenocorticism are caused by unilateral adrenal tumours. Bilateral adrenal tumours have also been reported, but appear to be rare (Ford *et al.*, 1993). Adrenocortical tumours may be benign or malignant, although it can be difficult, histologically, to distinguish between an adrenocortical adenoma and a carcinoma unless there is evidence of invasion or metastasis. Benign tumours are usually small and well circumscribed, and are commonly partly calcified (Reusch and Feldman, 1991). In contrast, adrenocortical carcinomas are usually larger, locally invasive, haemorrhagic and necrotic. They are also often calcified. Carcinomas, especially of the right adrenal gland, frequently invade the phrenicoabdominal vein and caudal vena cava and metastasize to the liver, lung and kidney (Figure 16.5).

In dogs, adrenocortical adenomas and carcinomas occur with approximately equal frequency. The cortex contiguous to the tumour, and that of the contralateral gland, atrophy in the presence of functional adenomas and carcinomas (Figure 16.6).

Other causes of hyperadrenocorticism

A few reports exist in which dogs with pituitary-dependent hyperadrenocorticism have concurrent adrenal tumours (Greco *et al.*, 1999). Ectopic ACTH production would appear to be a very rare cause of hyperadrenocorticism in the dog, with only one suspected case reported (Galac *et al.*, 2005). In humans, however, a number of tumours are capable of synthesizing and secreting excessive quantities of ACTH; for example oat cell carcinomas of the lung. Moreover, hypercortisolism independent of ACTH or tumours is also recognized in humans, and there is one report of food-associated hypercortisolaemia in a dog (Galac *et al.*, 2008). These reports have led to the suggestion that hyperadrenocorticism in the dog be classified as ACTH-dependent (including pituitary and other tumours producing ACTH) and ACTH-independent (including adrenal tumours and food-associated hypercortisolaemia).

Clinical features

Signalment

Age

Pituitary-dependent hyperadrenocorticism is usually a disease of the middle-aged to older dog, with an age range of 2–16 years and reported median age of 7–9 years. Dogs with adrenal-dependent hyperadrenocorticism tend to be older, ranging from 6 to 16 years, with mean age reported as 11.3 years (Reusch and Feldman, 1991).

Breed

Any breed can develop hyperadrenocorticism; however, Poodles, Dachshunds and small terriers (e.g. Yorkshire, Jack Russell, Staffordshire Bull Terriers) appear at greater risk of developing pituitary-dependent hyperadrenocorticism. Adrenocortical tumours occur more frequently in larger breeds, with approximately 50% of affected dogs weighing >20 kg (Reusch and Feldman, 1991).

Sex

There is no significant difference in sex distribution in pituitary-dependent hyperadrenocorticism; however, bitches are more likely to develop adrenal tumours. In one study, 60–65% of dogs with functional adrenocortical tumours were female (Reusch and Feldman, 1991).

Clinical signs

Affected dogs usually develop a classic combination of clinical signs associated with increased glucocorticoid concentrations and these are listed in Figure 16.7 in approximate decreasing order of frequency. Larger breeds of dogs and those with recent onset of disease, however, may only show a few characteristic signs, rather than the classic array of clinical signs usually observed in smaller breeds.

- Polydipsia and polyuria
- Polyphagia
- Abdominal distension
- Liver enlargement
- Muscle wasting/weakness
- Lethargy, poor exercise tolerance
- Skin changes
- Alopecia
- Persistent anoestrus or testicular atrophy
- Calcinosis cutis
- Myotonia
- Neurological signs
- Hypertensive retinopathy

16.7 Clinical signs of canine hyperadrenocorticism in approximate order of frequency.

Hyperadrenocorticism has an insidious onset and is slowly progressive over many months or even years. Many owners consider the early signs (e.g. alopecia, lethargy) as part of the normal ageing process of their dog, or misinterpret the signs (e.g. increased appetite) as indicating good health. In a few cases, clinical signs may be intermittent, with periods of remission and relapse; in others there may be an apparent rapid onset and progression of clinical signs.

Polydipsia and polyuria

Polydipsia and polyuria are noted in nearly all cases of hyperadrenocorticism. Polydipsia is nearly always noticeable in dogs when water consumption exceeds 100 ml/kg/day. However, some astute owners may note polydipsia even if water consumption does not exceed this figure. Excessive thirst, nocturia, incontinence and/or urination in the house are usually reported by owners. The polydipsia occurs secondary to the polyuria. However, the precise cause

of the polyuria remains obscure, but may be due to increased glomerular filtration rate, inhibition of the release of arginine vasopressin (antidiuretic hormone (ADH)), inhibition of the action of ADH on the renal tubules or possibly accelerated inactivation of ADH. The end result is a partial secondary diabetes insipidus. Dogs with macroadenomas may show signs of concurrent central diabetes insipidus due to compression of the posterior lobe of the pituitary and hypothalamus.

Polyphagia and weight gain

Increased appetite is common and, although many owners dismiss it as a sign of good health, a voracious appetite or scavenging/stealing of food may give rise to concern, especially if the dog previously had a poor appetite. Polyphagia is assumed to be a direct effect of glucocorticoids centrally, but there is little real evidence to support this theory.

Hyperadrenocorticism is also associated with an increase in weight in many cases, despite a concurrent loss of muscle mass. The weight gain is partly due to polyphagia, but even dogs fed normal maintenance rations may gain weight if they develop hyperadrenocorticism. This may be because cortisol decreases maintenance energy requirement and overall metabolic rate or because of its effect on exercise tolerance. Cortisol also has effects on fat distribution, such that increased fat deposits tend to occur over the dorsum and within the abdomen. This gives affected dogs the typical 'table top' appearance when viewed from above.

Abdominal distension

A pot-bellied appearance (Figure 16.8) is very common in hyperadrenocorticism, but may be so insidious that owners fail to recognize its significance. Abdominal distension is associated with the redistribution of fat to the abdomen, liver en-largement and weakness of the abdominal muscles. The weakness of the abdominal muscles makes palpation of the pendulous abdomen easier and more rewarding.

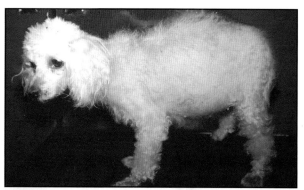

16.8 A 6-year-old Poodle bitch with pituitary-dependent hyperadrenocorticism. Note the abdominal distension, muscle wasting, alopecia and thin skin.

Muscle wasting/weakness

The gradual onset of lethargy and poor exercise tolerance is initially considered by many owners as compatible with ageing. Owners may only become concerned when muscle weakness leads to an inability to climb stairs or jump into a car. Lethargy, excessive panting and poor exercise tolerance are probably an expression of muscle wasting and weakness. Apart from the development of a pendulous abdomen, decreased muscle mass may be noted around the limbs, over the spine or over the temporal region. Muscle weakness is the result of muscle wasting caused by protein catabolism and a direct effect of cortisol on cell membrane excitability.

Occasionally, dogs with hyperadrenocorticism develop myotonia, characterized by persistent active muscle contractions that continue after voluntary or involuntary stimuli. The condition appears to be especially prevalent in the Miniature Poodle but has been noted in other breeds (Siliart et al., 2002). All limbs may be affected, but the signs are usually more severe in the hindlegs. Animals with myotonia walk with a stiff, stilted gait or rabbit hop. The affected limbs are rigid and rapidly return to extension after being passively flexed. In some cases, passive flexion may be difficult or impossible to achieve because of the persistent muscle tone. Spinal reflexes are difficult to elicit because of the rigidity, but pain sensation is normal. The muscles are usually slightly hypertrophied rather than being atrophied and a myotonic dimple can be elicited by percussion of the affected muscle. Bizarre high-frequency discharges are noted on electromyography (Duncan et al., 1977). These bizarre myotonic and pseudomyotonic discharges may be found in some dogs with hyperadrenocorticism that do not show obvious clinical manifestations of myotonia.

Dermatological features

The skin, particularly over the ventral abdomen, becomes thin and inelastic because of atrophy of the dermal connective tissues. Elasticity can be assessed clinically by tenting the skin between the thumb and forefinger (Figure 16.9). In the normal dog, the skin will flow back to a smooth contour, whereas in hyperadrenocorticism it remains tented. Striae (stretch marks) can form as a result of this inelasticity. The abdominal veins are prominent and easily visible through the thin skin (Figure 16.10).

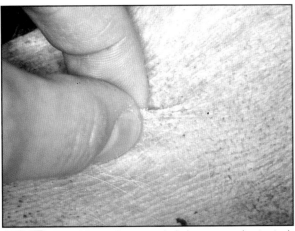

16.9 The skin on the ventral abdomen can be tented to assess elasticity.

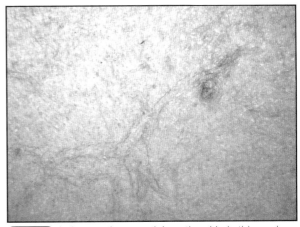

16.10 In hyperadrenocorticism, the skin is thin and inelastic and remains tented. The abdominal veins are visible through the skin.

There is often excessive surface scale, and comedones caused by follicular plugging are seen, especially around the nipples (Figure 16.11). Hyperpigmentation of the skin is rare in canine hyperadrenocorticism.

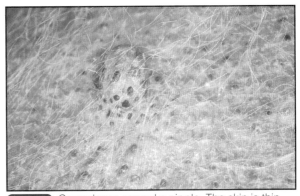

16.11 Comedones around a nipple. The skin is thin and abdominal veins are visible.

Protein catabolism, causing atrophic skin collagen, also leads to excessive bruising following venepuncture or other minor trauma (Figure 16.12). Wound healing is extraordinarily slow, presumably because of inhibition of fibroblast proliferation and collagen synthesis. Healing wounds often undergo dehiscence and even old scars may start to break down (Figure 16.13).

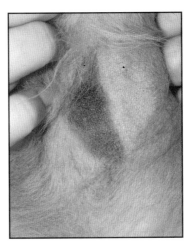

16.12 Extensive bruising on the neck of a Pomeranian with hyperadrenocorticism. This resulted from a single needle insertion with minimal restraint and pressure being applied for a minute or so afterwards.

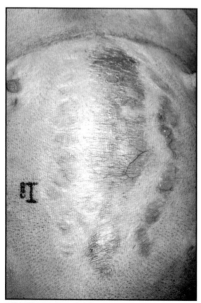

16.13 Partial breakdown of an abdominal incision in a Boxer with hyperadrenocorticism.

Calcinosis cutis is a frequent finding in biopsy material from the skin but clinical evidence of calcinosis cutis is less common. The gross appearance can vary but the predilection sites are the neck, axilla, ventral abdomen and inguinal areas (Figure 16.14). Calcinosis cutis usually appears as a firm, slightly elevated, white or cream plaque surrounded by a rim of erythema. Large plaques tend to crack, become secondarily infected and develop a crust containing white powdery material. The exact pathogenesis is unclear, but circulating calcium and phosphate concentrations are usually normal.

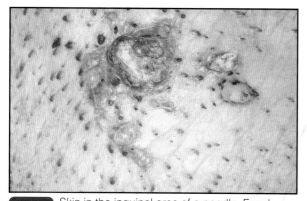

16.14 Skin in the inguinal area of a poodle. Focal areas of calcinosis cutis can be seen eroding through the epidermis. Comedones are also present.

Thinning of the haircoat leading to bilaterally symmetrical alopecia is frequently seen with hyperadrenocorticism and occurs because of the inhibitory effect of cortisol on the anagen (growth) phase of the hair cycle. The remaining hair is dull and dry because it is in the telogen (resting) phase of the hair cycle. The alopecia is non-pruritic and affects mainly the flanks, ventral abdomen and chest, perineum and neck. The head, feet and in some cases the tail are usually the last areas to be affected (see Figure 16.8). The coat colour is often lighter than normal. Occasionally, affected dogs do not lose

their haircoat but retain it, becoming hypertrichotic. When hair has been clipped in dogs with hyperadrenocorticism, it will frequently fail to regrow or the regrowth will be poor or sparse.

Occasionally, these skin and hair coat changes may be the owner's main reason for presentation (Zur and White, 2011).

Anoestrus/testicular atrophy
Entire bitches with hyperadrenocorticism usually cease to have regular oestrous cycles. The length of anoestrus, which is often years, indicates the duration of the disease process. In the intact male, both testes become soft and spongy. Anoestrus or testicular atrophy occurs due to the negative feedback effect of high concentrations of cortisol on the pituitary, which also suppress secretion of gonadotropic hormones.

Neurological signs
Although uncommon at the time of presentation, a few cases will develop neurological signs associated with a large functional pituitary tumour. The size of the tumour is less important than its rate of growth in determining such effects. The most common clinical signs are dullness, depression, disorientation, loss of learned behaviour, anorexia, aimless wandering or pacing, head pressing, circling, ataxia, blindness, anisocoria and seizures. More often, however, neurological signs develop during initial treatment of pituitary-dependent hyperadrenocorticism with trilostane or mitotane. This is thought to involve removal of the negative feedback inhibition of cortisol on the pituitary and hypothalamus, which then allows some pituitary tumours to enlarge rapidly, resulting in oedema and increased intracranial pressure.

Intracranial haemorrhage from the pituitary tumour may lead to pituitary apoplexy, which is characterized by an acute severe depression and diabetes insipidus that is often, though not universally, fatal (Long *et al.*, 2003; Bertolini *et al.*, 2007). Trigger factors for pituitary apoplexy are not known in dogs, but in humans there is an association with recent endocrine testing (including ACTH response tests). The reason for this is not known.

Hypertension
Systemic hypertension occurs in >50% of dogs with untreated hyperadrenocorticism. The mechanisms underlying the hypertension potentially include excessive secretion of renin, activation of the renin–angiotensin system, enhanced vascular sensitivity to catecholamines and a reduction of vasodilator prostaglandins (Goy-Thollot *et al.*, 2002). In the majority of cases, the moderate degree of hypertension is not associated with clinical signs, but hypertension-induced blindness due to intraocular haemorrhage and retinal detachment has been reported, albeit rarely. Hypertension may also exacerbate left ventricular hypertrophy and congestive heart failure and cause glomerular damage and proteinuria. In general, hypertension does not resolve following treatment of hyperadrenocorticism. The explanation for this is currently not known.

Respiratory signs

The most frequent respiratory abnormality noted is excessive panting (see above). However, pulmonary thromboembolism is a potential but rare complication of hyperadrenocorticism. Pulmonary thromboembolism may be related to glomerular protein loss, resulting in decreased antithrombin III concentrations. Clinical signs of hyperpnoea progressing to overt dyspnoea are consistent with this condition.

Routine clinicopathological features

The main haematological, biochemical and urinalysis findings are listed in Figure 16.15.

Haematology

- Lymphopenia (<1.5 x 10⁹/l)
- Eosinopenia (<0.2 x 10⁹/l)
- Neutrophilia
- Monocytosis
- Erythrocytosis
- Thrombocytosis

Biochemistry

- Increased alkaline phosphatase (often markedly elevated)
- Increased alanine aminotransferase
- High normal fasting blood glucose; rarely diabetic
- Decreased blood urea
- Increased cholesterol (>8 mmol/l)
- Increased triglycerides (lipaemic plasma/serum)
- Increased bile salts

Urinalysis

- Urine specific gravity <1.015 and often <1.008
- Urinary tract infection
- Urine protein
- Urine glucose (<10% of cases)

Other findings

- Low total thyroxine concentrations
- Subnormal response to thyroid-stimulating hormone stimulation
- Increased parathyroid hormone concentrations

16.15 Clinicopathological and other hormonal features of canine hyperadrenocorticism.

Haematology

The most consistent haematological finding is a stress leucogram with a relative and absolute lymphopenia (<1.5 x 10⁹/l) and eosinopenia (<0.2 x 10⁹/l). Lymphopenia is most likely the result of steroid lymphocytolysis, and eosinopenia results from bone marrow sequestration of eosinophils. A mild to moderate neutrophilia and monocytosis may be found and is thought to result from decreased capillary margination and diapedesis associated with excess glucocorticoids.

The red cell count is usually normal, although mild polycythaemia may occasionally be noted. Platelet counts may also be increased. These findings are thought to result from stimulatory effects of glucocorticoids on the bone marrow.

Biochemistry

Alkaline phosphatase

Alkaline phosphatase (ALP) activity is increased in >90% of cases of canine hyperadrenocorticism. The increase is commonly 5–40 times the upper end of the reference interval and is perhaps the most sensitive biochemical screening test for hyperadrenocorticism. However, it is also the least specific. The increased activity occurs because glucocorticoids, both endogenous or exogenous, induce a specific hepatic isoenzyme of ALP, an effect unique to the dog. A reference interval serum ALP activity does not exclude a diagnosis of hyperadrenocorticism. Equally, increases in ALP activity may be due to other conditions.

Measurement of the glucocorticoid-induced isoenzyme of ALP is as sensitive for hyperadrenocorticism as is measuring total ALP, but is no more specific. This is because the glucocorticoid-induced isoenzyme can be increased in other disorders, including primary hepatopathies, diabetes mellitus, and in dogs treated with anticonvulsants and glucocorticoids (Teske et al., 1989).

Alanine aminotransferase

Alanine aminotransferase (ALT) activity is commonly increased in hyperadrenocorticism, but the increase is usually only mild. Any increase is believed to result from liver damage caused by glycogen accumulation in hepatocytes.

Glucose

Blood glucose concentration is usually in the high end of the reference interval. Approximately 10% of cases develop overt diabetes mellitus, caused by antagonism to the action of insulin by the gluconeogenic effects of excess glucocorticoids.

Urea and creatinine

Blood urea concentration is usually normal to decreased due to the continual urinary loss associated with glucocorticoid-induced diuresis. Serum creatinine concentration also tends to be at the low end of the reference interval. Urea and creatinine concentrations at the high end of the reference interval are therefore of some concern, as affected animals may become overtly azotaemic when treatment for the hyperadrenocorticism is instituted.

Cholesterol and triglyceride

Cholesterol and triglyceride concentrations are increased because of glucocorticoid stimulation of lipolysis. Cholesterol concentration is usually >8 mmol/l. This is not a specific finding, as cholesterol is also increased in hypothyroidism, diabetes mellitus, cholestatic liver disease and protein-losing nephropathy, all of which may be differential diagnoses. Hypertriglyceridaemia can also occur, although less frequently. Lipaemia can interfere with the accurate assessment of a number of other laboratory parameters.

Electrolytes

Sodium, potassium, calcium and phosphate concentrations are usually within their respective reference intervals. However, phosphate concentrations may be increased when compared to age-matched controls (Ramsey *et al.*, 2005).

Bile acids

Resting and postprandial serum bile acid concentrations may show a mild to moderate increase in some cases of hyperadrenocorticism due to steroid hepatopathy. When abnormal results are obtained, it may prove difficult to differentiate hyperadrenocorticism from primary liver disorders. The patient's appetite, thirst, weight change and other clinical signs may be useful in making this distinction, but if not hepatic biopsy may be required.

Urinalysis

Specific gravity

The specific gravity of urine is usually <1.015 and the urine is often hyposthenuric (<1.008) provided water has not been withheld. Dogs with hyperadrenocorticism can usually concentrate their urine if water is deprived, but their concentrating ability is frequently reduced. However, in some cases of pituitary-dependent hyperadrenocorticism with a macroadenoma, compression of the posterior lobe of the pituitary and suprasellar extension into the hypothalamus may cause disruption to ADH production and release and subsequently signs of central diabetes insipidus.

Culture

Urinary tract infection (UTI) occurs in approximately 50% of cases of hyperadrenocorticism. There is an increased risk of UTI because urine is retained in an over-distended bladder due to incomplete voiding resulting from muscle weakness. There is often little evidence of blood or inflammatory cells in the sediment of the urine, and indeed few clinical signs of UTI due to the immunosuppressive action of excess glucocorticoids. Therefore, culture of urine samples obtained by cystocentesis is required to demonstrate infection. UTIs can also ascend to the kidneys to cause pyelonephritis.

Protein

Up to 45% of dogs with untreated hyperadrenocorticism have proteinuria, defined as a urine protein:creatinine ratio >1.0, in the absence of UTI (Hurley and Vaden, 1998). The proteinuria is usually mild and may be associated with systemic hypertension.

Glucose

Glucosuria is present in the 10% of cases with overt diabetes mellitus.

Effects on other endocrine test results

Thyroid function tests

Serum total thyroxine (T4) and/or triiodothyronine (T3) concentrations are decreased in approximately 70% of dogs with hyperadrenocorticism (Peterson *et al.*, 1984). In addition, >60% of dogs with decreased serum total T4 concentrations also have decreased free T4 concentrations (Ferguson and Peterson, 1992). The total T4 response to thyrotropin-releasing hormone (TRH) or thyroid-stimulating hormone (TSH; thyrotropin) administration usually parallels a normal response, but actual values both pre- and post-TRH or TSH are subnormal. These effects are thought to be due to inhibition of pituitary secretion of TSH and a blunted TSH response to TRH stimulation (Ramsey and Herrtage, 1998). However, the situation is complex, as in some cases of spontaneous hyperadrenocorticism canine TSH concentrations may be increased. Other potential causes include cortisol-induced alteration in thyroid hormone binding to plasma proteins or enhancement of thyroid hormone metabolism. In one study, an increased free T4 fraction indicative of reduced serum T4 binding was identified in nearly 40% of dogs with hyperadrenocorticism (Ferguson and Peterson, 1992). Treatment of the hyperadrenocorticism (with trilostane) results in an expected increase in both total T4 and TSH (Kenefick and Neiger, 2008). Treatment has also been associated with a decrease in free T4 concentration, although most remained within the reference interval (Kenefick and Neiger, 2008). The explanation for this observation is not clear.

Parathyroid hormone

Glucocorticoids are known to increase urinary calcium excretion in canine hyperadrenocorticism. In order to maintain normal circulating concentrations of calcium, parathyroid hormone (PTH; parathormone) concentrations are increased in >80% of cases of hyperadrenocorticism (Ramsey *et al.*, 2005). PTH concentrations increase early in the course of the disease in both pituitary- and adrenal-dependent hyperadrenocorticism. Trilostane results in a reduction in PTH concentrations; however, many values do not return to the reference interval (Tebb *et al.*, 2005).

Growth hormone and insulin-like growth factor 1

Chronic glucocorticoid excess reduces spontaneous and stimulated growth hormone (GH) secretion by enhancing release of somatostatin from the hypothalamus. Reduced GH secretion from the pituitary may result in reduced serum insulin-like growth factor 1 (IGF-1) concentrations.

Insulin and C-peptide

It has been shown that both insulin and C-peptide (released in equimolar concentrations to insulin) concentrations are increased in dogs with hyperadrenocorticism and that their response to glucagon is exaggerated when compared to healthy dogs (Montgomery *et al.*, 1996). This observation is explained by cortisol inducing peripheral insulin resistance, which may ultimately result in overt diabetes mellitus.

Diagnostic imaging

Advances in diagnostic imaging have improved the ability of clinicians to identify the cause of spontaneous hyperadrenocorticism and the extent of the underlying pathology so that treatment can be directed more specifically to the individual patient. However, finding a pituitary or adrenal mass does not necessarily mean that a functional tumour is present. Therefore, diagnostic imaging should always be interpreted in association with the clinical signs and endocrine test results.

Radiography

Radiographic examination of the thorax and abdomen is advisable in all cases of suspected or proven hyperadrenocorticism. Although positive diagnostic information is only obtained in the small number of cases in which adrenal enlargement or mineralization can be detected, survey radiographs may reveal significant concurrent disease, which might alter the prognosis. In addition, there are a number of common radiological changes consistent with hyperadrenocorticism that provide a useful aid to diagnosis: these are listed in Figure 16.16.

Abdominal radiographs
• Liver enlargement • Good radiographic contrast • Pot-bellied appearance • Calcinosis cutis/soft tissue mineralization • Distended bladder • Cystic calculi • Adrenal enlargement/mineralization • ± Osteopenia
Thoracic radiographs
• Tracheal and bronchial wall mineralization • Pulmonary metastasis from adrenocortical carcinoma • Osteopenia • Congestive heart failure (rare) • Pulmonary thromboembolism (rare)

16.16 Radiological signs compatible with hyperadrenocorticism.

Liver enlargement

Hepatomegaly is the most consistent radiographic finding in hyperadrenocorticism. There is good radiographic contrast to permit easy identification of the abdominal structures because of the large deposits of intra-abdominal fat. The pot-bellied appearance is usually obvious on the recumbent lateral projection (Figure 16.17).

Adrenal enlargement/mineralization

Normal adrenal glands are not visible on abdominal radiographs. Adrenomegaly is a rare finding but if present it suggests gross enlargement, typical though not diagnostic of an adrenocortical carcinoma. Unilateral mineralization in the region of an adrenal gland also suggests the possibility of an adrenal tumour, although the presence of mineralization cannot be used to distinguish benign from malignant tumours as both may become mineralized (Figure 16.18).

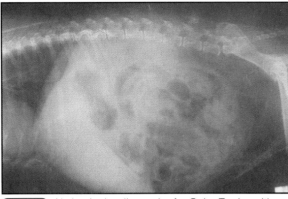

16.17 Abdominal radiograph of a Cairn Terrier with pituitary-dependent hyperadrenocorticism. The radiographic signs include hepatomegaly, abdominal distension, calcinosis cutis, dystrophic calcification in the soft tissues along the spine, an enlarged bladder and osteopenia.

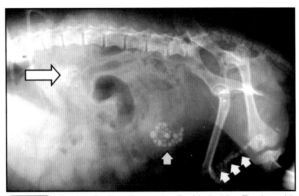

16.18 Abdominal radiograph of a Yorkshire Terrier with an adrenal tumour. The calcified mass can be seen in the dorsocranial area of the abdomen (open arrow). In addition, cystic (blue arrow) and urethral (yellow arrows) calculi are present. Despite this extensive urolithiasis, the dog was able to urinate normally. The anti-inflammatory effects of the excessive glucocorticoids may have contributed to this.

Soft tissue mineralization

Calcinosis cutis tends to have a nodular mineralization pattern, whereas calcification in the fascial planes, for example just dorsal to the thoracolumbar spine, tends to be linear (see Figure 16.17). Mineralization may also be seen in the lung, renal pelvis, liver, gastric mucosa and abdominal aorta. Tracheal and bronchial wall mineralization is frequently seen radiographically in cases of hyperadrenocorticism. Calcification of these structures, however, can be seen in normally ageing animals and is not considered to be significant.

Urinary bladder

A grossly distended urinary bladder may be seen radiographically, even when the animal has been allowed to urinate prior to the radiographic examination. Cystic calculi may also be present (see Figure 16.18) and are usually associated with UTI.

Osteopenia

Although glucocorticoids cause histopathological changes of osteopenia in dogs, objective evaluation of skeletal demineralization is notoriously difficult (Schwarz *et al.*, 2000). However, occasionally the impression of osteopenia is gained from a distinct reduction in radiographic density of the lumbar vertebral bodies relative to the vertebral end plates (see Figures 16.17 and 16.18).

Other changes
Thoracic radiographs should also be examined for evidence of lung metastasis from an adrenocortical carcinoma, congestive heart failure, and pulmonary thromboembolism (although in many cases of pulmonary thromboembolism, the radiographs may reveal no abnormalities).

Abdominal ultrasonography
With high-resolution ultrasound equipment, it is possible for an experienced ultrasonographer to image both adrenal glands of most dogs. The best images of the adrenals are obtained by scanning from the right and left lateral intercostal and abdominal approaches.

Location
The right adrenal gland is more difficult to image than the left because of its deeper and more cranial location under the ribs. The right adrenal gland is located craniomedial to the right kidney, lying between the cranial pole of the kidney and dorsal or dorsolateral to the caudal vena cava and just cranial to the cranial mesenteric artery. The left adrenal gland is more variable in location. It may be found anywhere from craniomedial to the left kidney to a more midline position ventrolateral to the aorta adjacent to the first or second lumbar vertebra. The left adrenal gland is located between the origin of the cranial mesenteric artery and the left renal artery.

Appearance
The normal adrenal gland is somewhat flattened, bilobed and hypoechoic compared to the surrounding tissues. The medulla of the normal adrenal is slightly hyperechoic compared to the cortex. The maximum dimensions (length x thickness) of normal canine adrenal glands are in the range of 10–52 mm x 2–12 mm (Grooters *et al.*, 1995; Douglass *et al.*, 1997). There is poor correlation between these dimensions and bodyweight and there are no published adrenal measurements for different breeds of dog.

The challenge for the ultrasonographer is to distinguish consistently between normal, hyperplastic and neoplastic glands. Although the adrenal glands of dogs with pituitary-dependent hyperadrenocorticism have been characterized as being symmetrically enlarged and of normal conformation, the diagnosis of adrenal hyperplasia is a somewhat subjective evaluation. Hyperplastic adrenal glands should be larger and easier to image than normal glands, but should still have a normal, homogeneous hypoechoic pattern (Figure 16.19a). Some studies have shown that adrenal gland thickness (ventrodorsal dimension) and width are significantly greater in dogs with pituitary-dependent hyperadrenocorticism

when compared with weight- and age-matched controls (Bartez *et al.*, 1995; Grooters *et al.*, 1996). However, although a thickness of >7.5 mm for the left adrenal gland is considered to provide the best sensitivity and specificity as a diagnostic test for pituitary-dependent hyperadrenocorticism (Bartez *et al.*, 1995), increases in adrenal thickness are not specific enough to warrant the use of adrenal ultrasonography as a screening test for hyperadrenocorticism, as there is considerable overlap between normal and hyperplastic adrenal gland measurements (Gould *et al.*, 2001). However, ultrasonographic identification of both adrenal glands of similar size with normal architecture in a dog with clinical signs of hyperadrenocorticism and a positive endocrine screening test confirms pituitary-dependent hyperadrenocorticism.

Tumour detection
Abdominal ultrasonography can also detect adrenocortical tumours (Kantrowitz *et al.*, 1986) (Figure 16.19b). There is a propensity for malignant adrenal tumours to invade nearby vessels and surrounding tissues; therefore a thorough ultrasonographic examination of adjacent vessels and tissues should be performed (Figure 16.19c). Mineralization is frequently associated with both benign and malignant

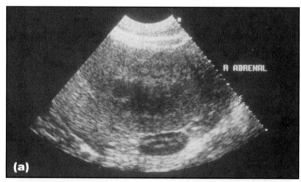
(a)

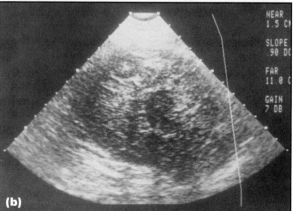
(b)

16.19 Ultrasonography of the canine adrenal gland. **(a)** Ultrasonograph of the right adrenal of an 8-year-old crossbreed dog with pituitary-dependent hyperadrenocorticism showing the thickened hypoechoic cortex surrounding a normal echogenic medulla. **(b)** Ultrasonograph of the right adrenal of an 8-year-old German Shepherd bitch with adrenal-dependent hyperadrenocorticism. The adrenal tumour is the large mixed echogenic mass in the centre of the scan that has completely replaced the normal architecture of the adrenal gland. (continues) ▶

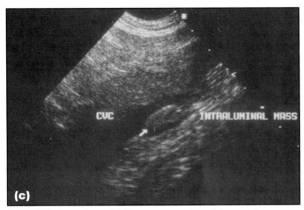

16.19 (continued) Ultrasonography of the canine adrenal gland. **(c)** Ultrasonograph of the cranial abdomen of a 10-year-old Labrador Retriever bitch with an adrenocortical carcinoma which has invaded the caudal vena cava (CVC).

adrenocortical tumours in the dog, and acoustic shadowing may aid in localizing the adrenal tumour. Ultrasonography cannot, however, differentiate a functional adrenocortical tumour from a non-functional tumour, a phaeochromocytoma, a metastatic lesion or a granuloma.

If an adrenal mass is identified, the liver, spleen and kidneys should also be examined ultrasonographically for evidence of metastases.

Whilst ultrasonography has been shown to be a reasonably reliable and practical method of determining the cause of hyperadrenocorticism, there are some cases of pituitary-dependent hyperadrenocorticism where the adrenal glands are not similar in size. The degree of asymmetry, as measured by the thickness of each gland, can vary and it has been shown that a difference of up to 5 mm makes the diagnosis of adrenal-dependent hyperadrenocorticism unlikely (Benchekroun *et al.*, 2010).

Computed tomography and magnetic resonance imaging

CT and MRI have proved useful in the diagnosis of adrenal tumours, adrenal hyperplasia and large pituitary tumours (Voorhout *et al.*, 1988; Bertoy *et al.*, 1995; Duesberg *et al.*, 1995) but both techniques are expensive and not always available. In a study comparing abdominal survey radiography with CT for the detection of adrenocortical tumours, CT accurately localized all tumours, whereas abdominal radiography accurately localized only 55% of the cases (Voorhout *et al.*, 1990). This was due to the fact that tumours <20 mm in diameter could not be detected on abdominal radiographs. CT can also identify invasion of the caudal vena cava by the tumour and adhesions between the adrenal gland and the caudal vena cava.

MRI has been found to be superior to CT in detecting ACTH-secreting tumours of the pituitary gland in humans, where it is considered to be the modality of choice for the evaluation. A comparison of CT and low-field MRI has been performed in a small series of dogs with pituitary-dependent hyperadrenocorticism (Auriemma *et al.*, 2009). Although both techniques provided comparable information

on the presence of pituitary adenomas, MRI produced better image quality with both increased signal-to-noise ratio and contrast-to-noise ratio.

MRI is extremely sensitive and can detect pituitary tumours as small as 3 mm at their greatest height (Bertoy *et al.*, 1995). About 50% of dogs with pituitary-dependent hyperadrenocorticism have a detectable pituitary mass on MRI (Figure 16.20). These masses usually continue to grow despite treatment with mitotane or trilostane (Bertoy *et al.*,

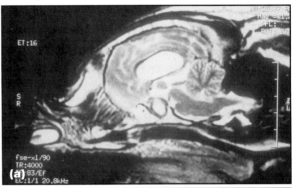

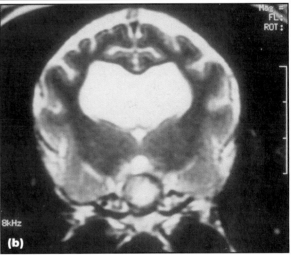

16.20 MRI: **(a)** T2-weighted midline sagittal image, and **(b)** T2-weighted transverse image showing a pituitary macroadenoma in a 10-year-old Bulldog with pituitary-dependent hyperadrenocorticism and central diabetes insipidus.

1996). Correlation between pituitary tumour size and the presence or development of neurological signs is not clear cut. Large pituitary tumours (up to 12 mm in diameter) have been shown to be present without causing neurological signs, whereas pituitary masses ranging in size from 8 to 24 mm may be associated with neurological signs (Duesberg *et al.*, 1995). In those cases with neurological signs, MRI or CT examination of the brain is essential for accurately planning therapy if pituitary irradiation is to be considered.

Diagnostic endocrine tests

A presumptive diagnosis of hyperadrenocorticism can be made from clinical signs, routine clinico-pathological features and diagnostic imaging findings, but the diagnosis must be confirmed by hormone assay (Figure 16.21). A single resting or basal plasma or serum cortisol determination is of limited diagnostic value because of the overlap in cortisol concentrations obtained from normal and abnormal disease states. The most commonly used screening tests are the ACTH response test or the low-dose dexamethasone suppression (LDDS) test; however, the urinary corticoid:creatinine ratio has also proved useful. None of these tests is perfect and all are capable of giving false positive and false negative results. If a dog with clinical signs compatible with hyperadrenocorticism produces a negative result with one screening test, an alternative screening test should be used. False positive results can be obtained in dogs suffering from non-adrenal disease (Kaplan *et al.*, 1995). A definitive diagnosis of hyperadrenocorticism should never be made purely on the basis of results of any screening tests, especially in dogs without classic signs of hyperadrenocorticism or in dogs with known non-adrenal disease.

The protocols for these tests are given in Figure 16.22. The relative merits of each test and interpretation are discussed below. The authors' preference is to use the ACTH response test as the first screening test and the LDDS test if the ACTH response test gives a result within the reference interval in a dog with clinical signs suspicious for hyperadrenocorticism.

ACTH response test

The ACTH response test is the best screening test for distinguishing spontaneous from iatrogenic hyperadrenocorticism. In spontaneous hyperadrenocorticism, the ACTH response test reliably identifies >50% of dogs with adrenal dependent hyperadrenocorticism and about 85% of dogs with pituitary-dependent hyperadrenocorticism. Occasional false positive results do occur; false negative results are more common.

The test is simple, robust and quick to perform and documents excessive production of glucocorticoids

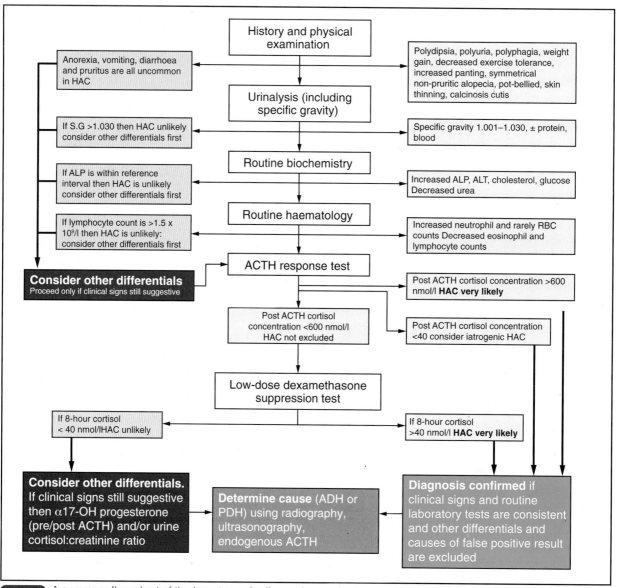

16.21 A summary flow chart of the key stages in diagnosing canine hyperadrenocorticism. ADH = adrenal-dependent hyperadrenocorticism; PDH = pituitary-dependent hyperadrenocorticism.

ACTH response test
1. Collect a blood sample for basal cortisol concentration[a]
2. Inject 250 μg of synthetic ACTH (tetracosactide, cosyntropin) i.v. or i.m. to dogs >5 kg. Use only 125 μg in dogs <5 kg[b]
3. Collect a second sample for cortisol concentration 30–60 minutes later

Low-dose dexamethasone suppression screening test
1. Collect a blood sample for cortisol determination
2. Inject 0.01–0.015 mg/kg of dexamethasone i.v.
3. Collect a second sample for cortisol concentration 3–4 hours later and a third sample 8 hours after dexamethasone administration

Urine corticoid:creatinine ratio
1. Collect a urine sample in the morning for corticoid and creatinine measurements. It is preferable for the dog to be at home for this test so that it is minimally stressed
2. Determine the urine corticoid:creatinine ratio by dividing the urine corticoid concentration (μmol/l) by the urine creatinine concentration (μmol/l)

16.22 Protocols for screening tests for hyperadrenocorticism. [a] The recent administration of glucocorticoids such as hydrocortisone, prednisolone or prednisone may result in elevated cortisol concentrations due to cross-reactivity in many cortisol assays. For this reason glucocorticoids should be withheld for at least 24 hours before testing. There is no cross-reactivity with dexamethasone, but like other glucocorticoids, dexamethasone will suppress cortisol concentrations in patients with an intact hypothalamic–pituitary adrenal axis. [b] Doses as low as 5 μg/kg administered intravenously have also been shown to maximally stimulate cortisol production in healthy dogs and those with hyperadrenocorticism but care must be taken to time the post-ACTH sample correctly (Kerl *et al.*, 1999).

by the adrenal cortex in cases of hyperadrenocorticism. The information gained is also useful in providing baseline information for monitoring subsequent trilostane or mitotane therapy, although different criteria are used to interpret cortisol results during treatment. The cost of ACTH varies considerably in different countries and, when expensive, can limit the widespread use of this test. Doses as low as 0.5 μg/kg have been tested and, at least in healthy dogs, appear adequate (Martin *et al.*, 2007).

The ACTH response test does not, however, reliably differentiate adrenal-dependent from pituitary-dependent hyperadrenocorticism. A diagnosis of hyperadrenocorticism should not be excluded on

the basis of a normal ACTH response if the clinical signs are compatible with the disease. Occasionally, an animal under chronic stress may develop some degree of adrenal hyperplasia, which produces an abnormal ACTH response. This may be seen for example with diabetes mellitus or pyometra and in these cases a normal cortisol response to ACTH stimulation will be obtained after treatment of the underlying disease.

It is essential to use absolute values for pre- and post-ACTH plasma cortisol concentrations rather than a ratio or percentage increase over baseline. In healthy dogs, pre-ACTH cortisol concentrations are usually between 20 and 250 nmol/l, with post-ACTH cortisol concentrations between 200 and 450 nmol/l. Regardless of the pre-ACTH cortisol value, a diagnosis of hyperadrenocorticism can be confirmed by demonstrating a post-ACTH cortisol concentration >600 nmol/l in dogs with compatible clinical signs and without evidence of concurrent non-adrenal disease (Figure 16. 23).

Concurrent measurement of 17α-hydroxyprogesterone

Some dogs with classic clinical signs of hyperadrenocorticism and typical haematological and biochemical findings have a normal cortisol response to both ACTH stimulation and low-dose dexamethasone suppression. These cases have been termed 'atypical hyperadrenocorticism'. It has been suggested that cases of atypical hyperadrenocorticism may have a derangement of the steroid production pathway and that some of the precursors of cortisol, such as 17α-hydroxyprogesterone, may be abnormally increased. Circulating 17α-hydroxyprogesterone concentrations exhibit an exaggerated response to ACTH stimulation in both typical and atypical hyperadrenocorticism, with 17α-hydroxyprogresterone concentrations increasing to between 6.5 and 38 nmol/l after stimulation (Ristic *et al.,* 2002). Both pituitary-dependent and adrenal-dependent atypical hyperadrenocorticism cases have been reported (Norman *et al.,* 1999; Syme *et al.,* 2001; Ristic *et al.*, 2002).

In healthy dogs, pre-ACTH 17α-hydroxyprogesterone concentrations range from <1–1.9 nmol/l and stimulate to between 1.0 and 5.5 mmol/l after ACTH administration. As with cortisol measurements on ACTH stimulation testing, abnormal 17α-hydroxyprogesterone responses can be found

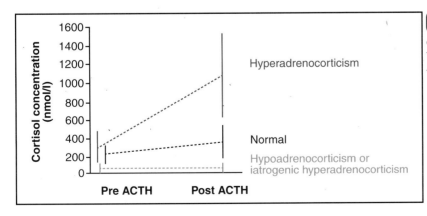

16.23 Interpretation of measurements of plasma cortisol concentrations before and after the administration of synthetic ACTH. ACTH = adrenocorticotropic hormone

in cases of non-adrenal illnesses (Chapman *et al.,* 2003; Sieber-Ruckstuhl *et al.,* 2008). Measurement of plasma 17α-hydroxyprogesterone concentration is probably most useful in distinguishing mild cases of hyperadrenocorticism from other mild diseases (Benitah *et al.,* 2005).

Plasma 17α-hydroxyprogesterone concentrations can be used to monitor treatment of atypical cases treated with mitotane. However, the measurement of 17α-hydroxyprogesterone is not helpful in monitoring cases treated with trilostane as the concentrations can remain the same or become further increased as treatment is instituted.

Low-dose dexamethasone suppression test

The LDDS test is more reliable than the ACTH response test in confirming hyperadrenocorticism, as the results are diagnostic in the majority of adrenal-dependent cases and in 90–95% of dogs with pituitary-dependent hyperadrenocorticism. Occasional false negative results do occur; false positive results are more common.

The LDDS test is not as accurate as the ACTH response test for the detection of iatrogenic hyperadrenocorticism. It is also affected by more variables than the ACTH response test, takes 8 hours to complete and does not provide pre-treatment information that may be used in monitoring the effects of mitotane or trilostane therapy.

Interpretation of the results of the LDDS test must be based on the laboratory's reference interval for the dose and preparation of dexamethasone administered. If the dose of dexamethasone fails to suppress circulating cortisol concentrations adequately in a dog with compatible clinical signs, a diagnosis of hyperadrenocorticism is confirmed. Whilst basal and 8-hour post-dexamethasone samples are most important for interpretation of the test (Figure 16.24), one or more samples taken at intermediate times (for example, 2, 3 or 4 hours) during the test period may also prove helpful in distinguishing the cause of the hyperadrenocorticism. If a plasma cortisol concentration determined 2–6 hours after dexamethasone injection is suppressed normally (to below approximately 40 mmol/l), while the 8-hour sample shows escape from cortisol suppression, or there is >50% suppression compared to baseline value, then a

diagnosis of pituitary-dependent hyperadrenocorticism is supported. If the cortisol is not suppressed by the dexamethasone then the cause of the hyperadrenocorticism cannot be determined. A few dogs with pituitary-dependent hyperadrenocorticism confirmed by other methods may show an 'inverse' pattern of results, i.e. a failure of suppression at 4 hours but suppression at 8 hours (Mueller *et al.,* 2006). As the 4-hour result is not normal, these dogs cannot be described as false negatives. The importance, reliability and specificity of this pattern of test result have yet to be determined.

Urinary corticoid:creatinine ratio

Evaluation of urinary corticoid:creatinine ratio, rather than the more laborious 24-hour urinary corticoid excretion, has been shown to be a simple and valuable screening test for hyperadrenocorticism (Rijnberk *et al.,* 1988).

Cortisol and its metabolites are excreted in urine. By measuring urinary corticoids in the morning sample, the concentration will reflect cortisol release over a period of several hours, thereby adjusting for fluctuations in plasma cortisol concentrations. Relating the urine corticoid concentration to urine creatinine concentration provides a correction for any differences in urine concentration.

Urine is collected in the morning for cortisol and creatinine estimations. It is preferable for the dog to be at home for this test so that the dog is subjected to as little stress as possible otherwise abnormal cortisol concentrations will be found in the urine. The urine cortisol:creatinine ratio is determined by dividing the urine cortisol concentration (in μmol/l) by the urine creatinine concentration (in μmol/l).

Although differences between labortories exist, the reference ratio for normal dogs is <10 x10⁻⁶. The urine corticoid:creatinine ratio is increased to >10 x 10⁻⁶ in dogs with hyperadrenocorticism. However, the ratio is also increased in many dogs with non-adrenal illness (Smiley and Peterson, 1993). Therefore, while this simple test appears highly sensitive in detecting hyperadrenocorticism in dogs, it is not specific. The test does provide a good screening test for hyperadrenocorticism, in that values within the reference interval make a diagnosis of hyperadrenocorticism highly unlikely. The urine corticoid:creatinine ratio does not

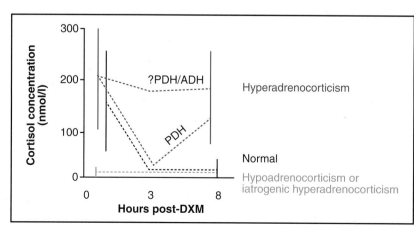

16.24 Interpretation of measurements of plasma cortisol concentrations before and after the administration of a low dose of dexamethasone (DXM). ?PDH/ADH represents the type of response seen in cases of pituitary-dependent or adrenal-dependent hyperadrenocorticism. PDH represents the response in pituitary-dependent cases where suppression occurs.

reliably differentiate pituitary-dependent from adrenal-dependent hyperadrenocorticism unless the ratio exceeds 100 x 10^{-6}, when it is likely that the dog is suffering from pituitary-dependent hyperadrenocorticism (Galac *et al.,* 1997). The test can be combined with dexamethasone suppression, but this does not increase the diagnostic yield when compared to the more conventional protocols that measure circulating cortisol concentration. The test is of little value in monitoring the response to mitotane or trilostane therapy in dogs with hyperadrenocorticism (Guptill *et al.,* 1997; Galac *et al.,* 2009).

Tests to differentiate the cause of hyperadrenocorticism

The ability to differentiate between pituitary- and adrenal-dependent hyperadrenocorticism can have important implications for provision of the most effective method of management. The high-dose dexamethasone suppression test used to be the most commonly used test for differentiating the cause of hyperadrenocorticism, but its accuracy has recently been brought into question. Canine ACTH assays are now readily available and the determination of plasma ACTH concentration has been shown to provide reliable discrimination between pituitary and adrenal causes (Gould *et al.,* 2001). Diagnostic imaging techniques, particularly abdominal ultrasonography, have also proved sensitive in distinguishing dogs with pituitary-dependent hyperadrenocorticism from dogs with adrenocortical tumours.

Plasma endogenous ACTH concentration

Stringent and meticulous sample handling is crucial, as ACTH activity in the plasma will reduce rapidly, resulting in falsely low values and incorrect interpretation (Chapter 1). The endogenous ACTH assay used must be validated for dogs.

Measurement of basal endogenous ACTH concentration is of no value in the diagnosis of hyperadrenocorticism because of the episodic secretion of ACTH in healthy dogs and the overlap of values in dogs with hyperadrenocorticism.

Endogenous ACTH concentrations in healthy dogs range from 2.91 to 11 pmol/l. Dogs with adrenal tumours have very low endogenous ACTH concentrations (<1.1 pmol/l), whereas those with pituitary-dependent hyperadrenocorticism tend to have high reference interval to increased concentrations of endogenous ACTH (>6 pmol/l), which discriminates the cause with a high sensitivity and specificity (Rodríguez Piñero *et al.,* 2009). It has also been recognized that there is a positive correlation between the plasma ACTH concentration and the size of the pituitary mass in pituitary-dependent hyperadrenocorticism (Théon and Feldman, 1998).

Diagnostic imaging

Abdominal radiography, abdominal ultrasonography and abdominal and cranial CT/MR imaging can be used to differentiate between pituitary-dependent hyperadrenocorticism and adrenal-dependent

hyperadrenocorticism. Recognition of metastatic lesions with radiography and/or ultrasonography, however, is the only method that can reliably distinguish dogs with adenomas from dogs with carcinomas in the absence of histopathology (Reusch and Feldman, 1991).

Treatment of pituitary-dependent hyperadrenocorticism

Trilostane

Trilostane is a synthetic steroid with no inherent hormonal activity. The clinical use of trilostane in canine hyperadrenocorticism, and in particular pituitary-dependent disease, has now been evaluated in several published clinical studies from centres across the world (Neiger *et al.,* 2002; Ruckstuhl *et al.,* 2002; Braddock *et al.,* 2003; Galac *et al.,* 2008).

Mode of action

Trilostane primarily acts as a competitive, and therefore reversible, inhibitor of the 3β-hydroxysteroid dehydrogenase enzyme system, which blocks adrenal synthesis of glucocorticoids, mineralocorticoids and sex hormones. However, 17α-hydroxyprogesterone concentrations do not change or may increase in dogs treated with trilostane. In addition, trilostane appears to have a more marked suppressive effect on cortisol compared with cortisone. This has been suggested as evidence of an effect on 11β-hydroxylase and possibly on the interconversion of cortisol and cortisone by 11β-hydroxysteroid dehydrogenase (11β-HSD) (Sieber-Ruckstuhl *et al.,* 2006; Sieber-Ruckstuhl *et al.,* 2008).

Safety

Handling trilostane does not require any special safety precautions; although, as a drug with anti-progesterone effects, it should be avoided by women who are pregnant or intending to become pregnant.

Starting dose

The starting dose recommended by the manufacturer is in the range 3–6 mg/kg orally q24h. A range of capsule sizes (10, 30, 60 and 120 mg) is available in the UK, but in other countries reformulation may be necessary for the lower doses. The tablets are more effective if administered with food. There are no studies that directly compare different frequencies of administration of trilostane. However, it is known that the suppressive effect of trilostane on cortisol lasts <24 hours and in some cases switching from once- to twice-daily dosing is beneficial (Bell *et al.,* 2006). Some studies have looked at starting treatment with twice-daily dosing. Initial results suggested a higher frequency of adverse effects when using trilostane twice daily (Alenza *et al.,* 2006). However, later studies using lower starting doses demonstrated a lower rate of adverse events and lower total daily doses (Vaughan *et al.,* 2008; Feldman, 2011). Given that treatment is long term, many owners will opt for once-daily treatment, at least initially.

Monitoring

Dogs on trilostane should be monitored every 3–6 months. Most clinical studies to date have used the clinical signs and ACTH stimulation test results as the primary methods of assessing control. It is important to interpret all monitoring tests in the light of clinical findings. Trilostane causes significant reductions in both the mean basal and post-ACTH stimulation cortisol concentrations in dogs with hyperadrenocorticism in the first month of treatment. The manufacturer currently recommends that blood samples are taken for biochemistry (including electrolytes) and an ACTH stimulation test is done after 10 days, 4 weeks, 12 weeks and thereafter every 3 months following initial diagnosis and after each dose adjustment. Dose adjustments should be small and, if increasing the dose, should not be more than 50% higher than the current dose. Most animals will stabilize within the range of 2–7 mg/kg/day. However, a small number of animals may require doses significantly in excess of 10 mg/kg/day.

As the effects of trilostane are relatively short lived, the results obtained by an ACTH response test vary considerably with the time of testing relative to dosing (Bell *et al.*, 2006). The manufacturer recommends that ACTH response tests are performed 4–6 hours after dosing to enable accurate interpretation of results. However, many endocrinologists currently prefer to start the ACTH response test 2–4 hours after dosing, as this is more likely to be the nadir of cortisol production following trilostane administration.

Various cortisol target concentrations for the ACTH response test have been used to monitor trilostane therapy. The lower the target range, the greater the possibility of the animal developing signs of hypoadrenocorticism. A commonly recommended target range for the post-ACTH cortisol concentration is 40–120 nmol/l for ACTH response tests started 2–4 hours after dosing. However, if dogs have a post-ACTH cortisol concentration of 120–200 nmol/l and are responding well to treatment then an increase in monitoring rather than dose may be more acceptable to the owners. It should be noted that, despite its widespread use, the ACTH response test has never been validated for trilostane therapy. Other methods of monitoring trilostane are still under active investigation.

The short duration of action of trilostane has a protective effect against the development of hypoadrenocorticism. Many dogs with minimal serum cortisol response to ACTH stimulation 2–4 hours after trilostane dosing do not develop signs of hypoadrenocorticism. In contrast, some dogs that have a target post-ACTH stimulation test serum cortisol concentration will maintain signs of hyperadrenocorticism (Braddock *et al.*, 2003; Bell *et al.*, 2006). In this situation, switching to twice-daily administration of trilostane will help at least some of these cases. Anecdotal evidence suggests that about 20% of dogs with hyperadrenocorticism in first-opinion practice are more stable if trilostane is given twice daily.

Efficacy and survival

Trilostane has been found to be between 67% and 90% effective in resolving the various signs of hyperadrenocorticism over 3–6 months.

The reported median survival times of dogs treated with trilostane range from 662 to 900 days; this is comparable to or better than the median survival times of dogs treated with mitotane (which ranged from 708 to 720 days in the same studies) (Barker *et al.*, 2005; Clemente *et al.*, 2007). However, one study compared twice-daily trilostane with a non-selective adrenocorticolytic protocol (Clemente *et al.*, 2007). In those countries that do not currently regard either routine twice-daily dosing with trilostane or non-selective adrenocorticolysis with mitotane as first-choice protocols this study has more relevance to animals that have failed a conventional first-choice protocol.

Side effects

The prevalence of side effects from trilostane is generally considered to be lower than from mitotane. If the various clinical studies are combined, then only approximately 15% of dogs treated with trilostane developed adverse effects that are directly attributable to the drug. This figure compares favourably to those reported with mitotane (25–42%).

If failure to respond is regarded as an adverse effect, then this is probably the most common adverse effect of trilostane administration. In these cases, an increase in the dose (and/or frequency) or a change to an alternative medication (such as mitotane) is indicated. Other side effects are summarized in Figure 16.25.

Other common side effects include an increase in the size of the adrenal glands and a change in their echotexture (Mantis *et al.*, 2003).

Adrenal necrosis: Acute adrenal necrosis is the most serious side effect of trilostane identified to date (Chapman *et al.*, 2004; Ramsey *et al.*, 2008). Although deaths are rare, histopathological evidence of adrenal necrosis is more common (Reusch *et al.*, 2007). Necrosis of the adrenal cortex cannot be directly explained by the competitive inhibition of steroidogenesis. The development of adrenal necrosis could be due to the hypersecretion of ACTH, which, together with increasing the size of the adrenal glands, may also, paradoxically, result in necrosis and haemorrhage of the adrenal glands.

Hypoadrenocorticism: Overdosing with trilostane will result in hypoadrenocorticism. Most cases of hypoadrenocorticism associated with trilostane recover rapidly following temporary cessation of the drug, but will continue to require the drug to control the clinical signs of hyperadrenocorticism. Most cases that develop hypoadrenocorticism have typical electrolyte changes (hyponatraemia, hyperkalaemia).

Hyperkalaemia: Some clinical studies of trilostane have recorded a mild increase in serum potassium concentrations. Dogs that develop hyperkalaemia but whose cortisol concentrations are adequate do

Problem	Management
Profound weakness, depression and anorexia	Discontinue trilostane and re-assess patient. Check sodium and potassium concentrations and institute prednisolone (0.2 mg/kg orally q24h). Reassess ACTH stimulation test
Acute onset of neurological signs	Reassess patient. Continue trilostane unless dog is anorexic, vomiting or depressed. Give prednisolone 2.0 mg/kg orally q24h or dexamethasone 0.1 mg/kg orally q24h and decrease dose slowly once neurological signs have resolved. If no response, consider radiotherapy
Failure to resume normal water intake	Recheck urinalysis and blood urea. Re-assess ACTH stimulation test. Increase trilostane by 50% if post-ACTH cortisol >200 nmol/l. If post-ACTH cortisol <120 nmol/l, consider increasing frequency of medication. Consider central diabetes insipidus in association with a macroadenoma
Failure of hair to regrow	Re-assess ACTH response test. Increase trilostane by 50% if post-ACTH cortisol >200 nmol/l. If post-ACTH cortisol <120 nmol/l, consider increasing frequency of medication. Consider concurrent hypothyroidism (determine baseline total T4 and cTSH)
Failure to respond despite ACTH response test results that suggest adequate dose of trilostane	Consider switching to mitotane after 2 weeks of treatment.

16.25 Possible problems that may be encountered during trilostane therapy, and their management.

not appear to have low aldosterone concentrations (Ramsey and Neiger, unpublished observations). The mechanism of action of this hyperkalaemia has not been identified. Any trilostane-treated dog with a mild increase in potassium should have an ACTH response test performed, rather than empirically reducing the dose. Trilostane can then be safely withheld whilst waiting for the results of the test.

Other side effects: Trilostane is associated with vomiting and diarrhoea in some dogs, independently of any effects on cortisol concentration. The best treatment is to administer the tablets with food or to change to an alternative medication.

Successful treatment with trilostane might also lead to the development of previously suppressed immune-mediated, inflammatory or neoplastic diseases. However, there have been no reports of these side effects. There is also a theoretical risk that trilostane-induced adrenal hyperplasia could undergo neoplastic transformation or that it could cause an increase in the size of pituitary tumours. However no evidence for this has been published.

Other uses of trilostane in dogs
Trilostane has been demonstrated as effective in the treatment of Alopecia X in Pomeranians, Poodles and Alaskan Malamutes; many authorities consider Alopecia X to be a mild, slowly progressive form of pituitary-dependent hyperadrenocorticism (Cerundolo *et al.*, 2004; Leone *et al.*, 2005) (see Chapter 26). The doses used in these separate studies were different (9–11 mg/kg orally q24h for the Pomeranians and Miniature Poodles; 3.0–3.6 mg/kg orally q24h for the Alaskan Malamutes). As the condition does not usually progress rapidly or cause other significant effects (such as polyuria or polyphagia), the need for, and risks of, therapy should be carefully discussed with owners before commencing trilostane therapy.

Mitotane therapy
Mitotane (o,p'-DDD) is an adrenocorticolytic drug. It selectively destroys the zona fasciculata and zona reticularis, whilst tending to preserve the zona glomerulosa. Mitotane requires a Special Treatment Authorization from the Veterinary Medicines Directorate for its use in the UK. It should therefore only be used in the treatment of pituitary-dependent hyperadrenocorticism when trilostane has been shown to be ineffective, when adverse effects have meant that trilostane cannot be used, or when pre-existing disorders preclude the use of trilostane.

Pre-treatment assessment
Mitotane therapy should only be considered once the diagnosis of hyperadrenocorticism has been confirmed. Because of its powerful effects, it should never be used empirically. Before treatment is instigated, the dog's daily water consumption should be measured over at least two consecutive 24-hour periods. If the water intake and appetite are not increased then pre-treatment cortisol concentrations, both before and after ACTH stimulation, are required in order for the effects of treatment to be monitored.

Initial treatment
It is preferable to have patients hospitalized for the initial course of treatment, although many clinicians have dogs treated by their owners at home, with the owners doing the necessary monitoring.

Mitotane is given orally at a dose rate of 50 mg/kg/day. It should be administered with food, as it is a fat-soluble drug and its absorption is poor when administered orally to fasted animals. Daily mitotane therapy should be continued until any of the following changes are noted:

- The water intake of a polydipsic dog drops to ≤60 ml/kg/day
- The dog takes longer to consume its meal than before treatment or stops eating completely
- The dog develops vomiting or has diarrhoea
- The dog becomes listless and depressed.

The initial mitotane course is then stopped and the dog put on maintenance therapy (see below).

The importance of close monitoring of the patient during this period cannot be over-emphasized.

The majority of dogs with pituitary-dependent hyperadrenocorticism require between 7 and 14 days, treatment, with an average of 10 days before water consumption reduces to ≤60 ml/kg/day. If the dog is not polydipsic or polyphagic, treatment should continue until the serum cortisol concentrations, both before and after ACTH stimulation, are <120 mmol/l. Some dogs respond in 2–3 days, but this is rare; others require >60 consecutive days of treatment. It is important to emphasize that each dog must be treated as an individual if the therapy is to be successful and that an ACTH response test should be performed to check that the induction course of therapy has adequately suppressed adrenal function before maintenance therapy is introduced. If serum cortisol concentrations are undetectable and do not respond to ACTH stimulation then the introduction of maintenance therapy should be delayed until the cortisol concentrations are between 20 and 120 nmol/l after ACTH stimulation.

Maintenance therapy
Having produced sufficient adrenocortical damage with daily mitotane treatment, it is important to continue therapy, albeit at a lower dose, otherwise the adrenal cortex will regenerate a hyperplastic zona fasciculata and zona reticularis and the clinical signs will recur.

Mitotane is given at a dose of 50 mg/kg/week with food. Dogs whose conditions are well controlled may sleep for a few hours after the weekly dose and for that reason it is often recommended that the treatment is given in the evening. More profound depression or weakness requires re-evaluation using the ACTH response test and possibly a reduction or splitting of the maintenance dose. Failure to control the polydipsia may require an increased dose of mitotane.

Re-examination
Treated dogs should be re-examined 4–8 weeks after initiation of maintenance therapy, unless problems are encountered. Marked improvement should be noted at this time. The most obvious and rapid response is a reduction in water intake, urine output and appetite and this is usually obvious at the end of the initial course of therapy. Muscle strength and exercise tolerance improve over the first 3–4 weeks. Skin and haircoat changes take longer and their progress is variable. Alopecia may get markedly worse before improving. Although improvement should be noted at 8 weeks, the skin and haircoat may not return to normal for 3–6 months (Figure 16.26).

Re-evaluation every 3–6 months is recommended for the remainder of the animal's life. The dosage of mitotane should be adjusted according to the results of ACTH response testing. The goal of therapy is to achieve an ACTH test result with serum cortisol concentrations between 20 and 120 nmol/l. Relapses (serum cortisol >200 nmol/l) do occur in up to 55% of cases (Kintzer and Peterson, 1991). These should be treated with a short course of daily

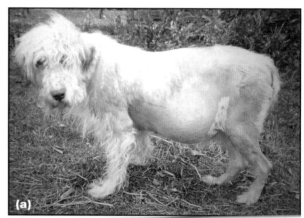

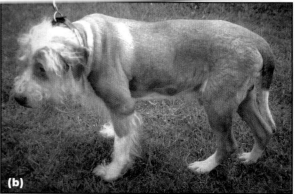

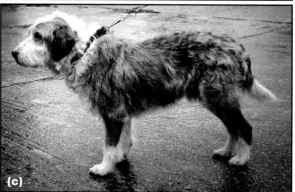

16.26 A 10-year-old crossbred dog with pituitary-dependent hyperadrenocorticism. **(a)** Before treatment; **(b)** after commencing treatment with mitotane; **(c)** 6 months later.

mitotane therapy or an increase in the maintenance dosage. Overdose (serum cortisol <20 nmol/l) is less frequent (5–10%) and requires a reduction in the frequency or dose of maintenance therapy (Kintzer and Peterson, 1991; Dunn *et al.,* 1995).

Side effects
Mitotane therapy is comparatively safe and the most frequent adverse effects (anorexia, vomiting or diarrhoea) are rarely serious provided they are noticed early on, so that mitotane therapy can be withheld. Some of the problems that can be encountered during treatment are summarized in Figure 16.27, together with their suggested management.

The use of prednisolone and other glucocorticoids is not necessary; although they are often recommended during induction to prevent signs of

Problem	Management
Vomiting or anorexia within first 3 days of treatment (gastric irritation)	Discontinue mitotane and re-assess patient. Divide dose and give 2–4 times a day
Profound weakness, depression and anorexia usually around fourth or fifth day of treatment with mitotane	Discontinue mitotane and re-assess patient. Check sodium and potassium concentrations and institute prednisolone (0.2 mg/kg orally q24h). Reassess ACTH response test. Start maintenance therapy with mitotane
Acute onset of neurological signs	Reassess patient. Continue mitotane unless dog is anorexic, vomiting or depressed. Give prednisolone 2.0 mg/kg orally q24h or dexamethasone 0.1 mg/kg orally q24h and decrease dose slowly once neurological signs have resolved. If no response, consider radiotherapy
Failure to resume normal water intake	Recheck urinalysis and blood urea. Re-assess ACTH stimulation test. Increase mitotane by 50% if post-ACTH cortisol >200 nmol/l. Consider central diabetes insipidus in association with a macroadenoma
Failure of hair to regrow	Re-assess ACTH stimulation test. Determine baseline total T4 and cTSH. Increase mitotane by 50% if post-ACTH cortisol >200 nmol/l. Consider concurrent hypothyroidism
Excessive depression or weakness related to weekly maintenance therapy on mitotane	Re-assess patient. Check sodium and potassium concentrations. Repeat ACTH stimulation test. If post-ACTH cortisol <20 nmol/l reduce maintenance dose or give every other week

16.27 Possible problems that may be encountered during mitotane therapy and their management.

hypocortisolaemia, there is limited evidence of a true reduction in the incidence of adverse effects and they may mask the indicators of the endpoint of daily induction. In addition, at least for prednisolone, the interpretation of subsequent ACTH response test results is difficult, due to the cross-reactivity of prednisolone in most cortisol assays (Dunn *et al.*, 1995). However, if the dog is being treated at home, the owner should be given a small supply of prednisolone tablets to be used in an emergency.

Successful treatment with mitotane might also lead to the development of previously suppressed immune-mediated, inflammatory or neoplastic diseases.

Neurological signs: Rarely, dogs will develop neurological signs during the induction course of treatment with mitotane as a result of enlargement of a pituitary tumour. Most of these cases will respond favourably to treatment with glucocorticoids. If the glucocorticoid therapy is slowly withdrawn over several weeks, the brain can often adapt to the enlargement of the pituitary tumour. If there is no response to glucocorticoid therapy, radiotherapy should be considered.

Hypoadrenocorticism: Primary hypoadrenocorticism (Addison's disease) with both glucocorticoid and mineralocorticoid insufficiency occurs in 5–17% of treated dogs during maintenance therapy (see Chapter 15). Although Addison's disease can develop at any time during treatment, most cases of primary hypoadrenocorticism occur during the first year of treatment. There is, unfortunately, no way to predict which dogs will develop complete adrenocortical insufficiency, but if hypoadrenocorticism does develop, maintenance mitotane therapy should be stopped and the dog treated with mineralocorticoid and glucocorticoid supplementation, as for primary hypoadrenocorticism.

Survival data

The mean survival time of treated dogs was 30 months in one study, with a range of a few days to over 7 years (Dunn *et al.*, 1995). The highest mortality was seen in the first 16 weeks of treatment, and dogs that survived this period had a longer mean survival time. Other studies have shown similar survival times (Kintzer and Peterson, 1991).

Other treatments

Selegiline

Selegiline (L-deprenyl) is a monoamine oxidase inhibitor (MAOI) and as such it should inhibit ACTH secretion by increasing dopaminergic tone to the hypothalamic–pituitary axis. Depletion of dopamine and a consequent increase in ACTH secretion is considered to be a possible aetiology for pituitary-dependent hyperadrenocorticism in the dog. Selegeline is not authorized for use in pituitary-dependent hyperadrenocorticism in the UK, but is authorized for behavioural disorders in dogs.

The recommended dose of selegiline for canine hyperadrenocorticism is 1 mg/kg orally q24h. If there is an inadequate response after 2 months, the dosage is increased to 2 mg/kg q24h. If this dosage also proves ineffective, alternative treatment should be employed. Selegiline is not recommended for pituitary-dependent hyperadrenocorticism in dogs with concurrent diabetes mellitus, pancreatitis, heart failure, renal disease or other severe illnesses. It should not be used in cases of adrenal-dependent hyperadrenocorticism as it is largely ineffective. The drug should not be administered with other MAOIs, opioids or tricyclic antidepressants.

Preliminary trials with selegiline have shown that the efficacy is poor, with about 80% of dogs failing to show improvement of clinical signs. However, an advantage of selegiline is that there are no severe adverse effects with this treatment. Monitoring therapy with endocrine testing is difficult, since there are only minor reductions in serum cortisol concentrations during LDDS or ACTH response tests (Reusch et al., 1999).

Selegiline may be considered for treatment of cases in which clinical signs of pituitary-dependent hyperadrenocorticism are very mild and the risk of trilostane or mitotane considered too great, or for treatment of cases that have obvious signs of hyperadrenocorticism and a positive diagnosis, but where the owner does not consider these to be causing the dog any major problems, and thus any adverse effect from another treatment would not be tolerated.

Ketoconazole

Ketoconazole is an imidazole antifungal drug, which has a similar mode of action to trilostane. Ketoconazole has been used effectively in the management of canine hyperadrenocorticism, but has more side effects than trilostane (Feldman et al., 1992; Lien and Huang 2008). Adverse effects include anorexia, vomiting, diarrhoea, hepatopathy and jaundice. Higher doses are associated with a higher incidence of adverse effects. Ketoconazole should not be used unless trilostane and mitotane have failed or are not available.

The initial dose of ketoconazole is 5 mg/kg orally q12h for 7 days to assess drug tolerance. If there are no adverse reactions, the dose is increased to 10 mg/kg q12h for 14 days. The efficacy of the treatment is determined by an ACTH response test using the same criteria as for monitoring mitotane therapy. If sufficient suppression of cortisol is not achieved (i.e. serum cortisol >120 nmol/l), then the dose should be increased to 15 mg/kg q12h. Occasionally, doses of 20 mg/kg q12h are required to control the disease.

The treatment is expensive and not always effective. About 25% of dogs treated with ketoconazole fail to respond adequately.

Others

Various other drugs have been suggested for the treatment of hyperadrenocorticism, including phosphatidylserine, retinoic acid, cyproheptadine, cabergoline, metyrapone and aminoglutethimide (Perez et al., 2002; Castillo et al., 2008). Some of these drugs have been found to be ineffective, others associated with unacceptable side effects and others have not yet been properly investigated. None is currently regarded as a useful treatment for canine hyperadrenocorticism.

Pituitary irradiation

Pituitary irradiation is indicated for dogs with neurological signs associated with pituitary tumours. CT or MRI of the brain is required to plan the treatment protocol. Radiotherapy using megavoltage irradiation from a linear accelerator or cobalt 60 source is required to penetrate to the depth of the pituitary gland without seriously injuring overlying soft tissues. Most treatment protocols involve the administration of 40–50 Gy in 3–4 Gy fractions (Goosens et al., 1998; Théon and Feldman, 1998). There is

often a dramatic response, although in some cases improvement takes several weeks. The resolution of neurological signs parallels the reduction in size of the tumour, which can continue to decrease for a year or more after the completion of the radiotherapy. Reduction in ACTH secretion by the tumour is less predictable, occurring in only about 20% of cases and, if it does occur, may not be evident for 6–12 months after therapy. Therefore, medical management of hyperadrenocorticism with trilostane or mitotane is indicated, at least initially.

Hypophysectomy

Hypophysectomy has been successfully performed in the dog for the treatment of pituitary-dependent hyperadrenocorticism using the trans-sphenoidal approach (Meij et al., 1998). The operation is technically difficult and should only be carried out by a surgeon with considerable skill and experience of the technique, otherwise it is associated with high morbidity and mortality. In experienced hands, perioperative mortality is 8% and the surgical failure rate (i.e. the condition recurs) is 6% (Hanson et al., 2005). Haemorrhage and incomplete visualization and removal of larger lesions are common complications. Diabetes insipidus, which may be transient, develops in about 50% of cases and requires treatment, and all dogs will require lifelong thyroid and glucocorticoid replacement therapy.

Bilateral adrenalectomy

Bilateral adrenalectomy has been employed successfully but involves the risk of putting an ill animal with a compromised immune system and poor wound healing, through a difficult surgery procedure. With other more effective treatments available, there is little to recommend this technique. Dogs treated by this approach will require lifelong treatment for hypoadrenocorticism.

Treatment of adrenal-dependent hyperadrenocorticism

There are three main treatment options for adrenal-dependent hyperadrenocorticism.

Surgical adrenalectomy

Dogs with adrenal-dependent hyperadrenocorticism carry the best prognosis if the tumour can be completely removed surgically. However, animals with untreated adrenal-dependent hyperadrenocorticism represent difficult surgical candidates because of the increased anaesthetic risk (due to poor respiratory and hepatic function), hypercoagulability (leading to an increased risk of pulmonary thromboembolism) and the poor vascular tone (leading to poor haemostasis). Primary wound healing is delayed, but wound breakdown is rare. The anatomical location and surrounding blood vessels make surgical exposure and removal difficult. Furthermore, many adrenal tumours are quite friable and haemorrhagic. Unilateral adrenalectomy, therefore, requires considerable experience and expertise. Acute postoperative hypoadrenocorticism due to pre-existing contralateral adrenal atrophy is common. Postoperative intensive care facilities are, therefore, essential.

Inexperienced surgeons or those without adequate facilities, including assistance in anaesthesia, should not attempt adrenalectomy. Even in referral institutes, perioperative mortality rates are often in the range of 20–30% (van Sluijs *et al.*, 1995; Schwartz *et al.*, 2008). Almost all animals that undergo adrenalectomy suffer some sort of complication.

If surgery is an option then preoperative staging of the adrenal tumour should include thoracic radiographs and abdominal ultrasonography to assess the presence of vascular invasion and metastatic spread. Administration of trilostane or mitotane is recommended by some authors in order to attempt to control the hyperadrenocorticism before surgery. Preoperative stabilization probably improves survival, but this has not been clearly demonstrated. Mitotane may be less useful than trilostane or ketoconazole in this respect, because it may make the tumour more friable, but objective data are not available.

Adrenalectomy is best performed by a ventral midline laparotomy (Scavelli *et al.*, 1986; Anderson *et al.*, 2001). The paracostal approach that has been advocated by some authors provides inadequate exposure. The contralateral adrenal gland should be checked for the presence of bilateral tumours, and other abdominal organs should be checked for metastases. The renal vessels and caudal vena cava should be carefully examined for the presence of tumour. If there is local invasion, debulking surgery is still worthwhile, providing this can be accomplished safely; if not, a small biopsy should be taken. The abdomen should be closed with suture materials that are slowly absorbed.

During and following surgery, glucocorticoid (and sometimes mineralocorticoid) supplementation is required. For this purpose, intravenous hydrocortisone (5–10 mg/kg q6h or 0.5 mg/kg/h constant rate infusion) would be a logical choice but dexamethasone (0.1–2.0 mg/kg i.v. q6h) or oral prednisolone with fludrocortisone, if needed, can also be used. Therapy should be slowly discontinued over a period of weeks to months, depending on the results of electrolyte monitoring, assessment of appetite and results of ACTH response tests.

If surgery is successful and the patient survives the perioperative period then the prognosis is good. In one study, the median survival time was just less than 2 years, although some dogs survived >4 years (van Sluijs *et al.*, 1995).

Mitotane

Mitotane is effective and relatively safe in dogs with adrenal-dependent hyperadrenocorticism. Dogs with adrenal tumours, however, tend to be more resistant to mitotane than dogs with pituitary-dependent hyperadrenocorticism (Feldman *et al.*, 1992). Generally, dogs with adrenal-dependent hyperadrenocorticism require higher daily induction doses (50–75 mg/kg orally q24h) and a longer period of induction (>14 days) than dogs with pituitary-dependent hyperadrenocorticism (Kintzer and Peterson, 1994). However, approximately 20% of cases respond successfully to the recommended protocol for pituitary-dependent hyperadrenocorticism. Frequent monitoring of treatment by ACTH response testing is important to ensure adequate control of the hyperadrenocorticism.

Maintenance doses are also generally higher (75–100 mg/kg/week) and again frequent monitoring of the cortisol response to ACTH stimulation is required to maintain optimal control of the disease. Adverse effects of treatment are similar to those described for pituitary-dependent hyperadrenocorticism. Those dogs requiring higher dose rates tend to be more prone to adverse effects. The adrenal tumour and metastatic mass will often reduce in size, due the cytotoxic effects of mitotane, but in other cases the tumour will continue to grow, despite increasing doses of mitotane. In one study of adrenocortical tumours treated using mitotane therapy, the median survival time was 11 months, with a range of a few weeks to >5 years (Kintzer and Peterson, 1994).

Trilostane

Trilostane has also been used to control the clinical signs in adrenal-dependent hyperadrenocorticism with some success (Eastwood *et al.*, 2003; Benchekroun *et al.*, 2008; Helm *et al.*, 2011). Comparisons of mitotane- and trilostane-treated dogs suggest survival times are not significantly different (Helm *et al.*, 2011). There is currently limited evidence that increased trilostane doses are required than for pituitary-dependent hyperadrenocorticism. As an enzyme inhibitor, however, trilostane only provides control of the clinical signs without treating the underlying neoplastic disease process.

References and further reading

Anderson CR, Birchard SJ, Powers BE *et al.* (2001) Surgical treatment of adrenocortical tumors: 21 cases (1990–1996). *Journal of the American Animal Hospital Association* **37**, 93–97

Auriemma E, Barthez PY, van der Vlugt-Meijer RH, Voorhout G and Meij BP (2009) Computed tomography and low-field magnetic imaging of the pituitary gland of dogs with pituitary-dependent hyperadrenocorticism: 11 cases (2001–2003). *Journal of the American Veterinary Medical Association* **235**, 409–414

Barker E, Campbell S, Tebb A *et al.* (2005) A comparison of the survival times of dogs treated for hyperadrenocorticism with trilostane or mitotane. *Journal of Veterinary Internal Medicine* **19**, 810–815

Bartez PY, Nyland TG and Feldman EC (1995) Ultrasonographic evaluation of the adrenal glands in dogs. *Journal of the American Veterinary Medical Association* **207**, 1180–1183

Bell R, Neiger R, McGrotty Y and Ramsey IK (2006) Effects of once daily trilostane administration on cortisol concentrations and ACTH responsiveness in hyperadrenocorticoid dogs. *Veterinary Record* **159**, 277–281

Benchekroun G, de Fornel-Thibaud P, Lafarge S *et al.* (2008) Trilostane therapy for hyperadrenocorticism in three dogs with adrenocortical metastasis. *Veterinary Record* **163**, 190–192

Benchekroun G, de Fornel-Thibaud P, Rodríguez Piñero MI *et al.* (2010) Ultrasonography criteria for differentiating ACTH dependency and ACTH independency in 47 dogs with hyperadrenocorticism and equivocal asymmetry. *Journal of Veterinary Internal Medicine* **24**, 1077–1085

Benitah N, Feldman EC, Kass PH and Nelson RW (2005) Evaluation of serum 17-hydroxyprogesterone concentration after administration of ACTH in dogs with hyperadrenocorticism.

Journal of the American Veterinary Medical Association **227**, 1095–1101

Bertolini G, Rossetti E and Caldin M (2007) Pituitary apoplexy-like disease in 4 dogs. *Journal of Veterinary Internal Medicine* 21, 1251–1257

Bertoy EH, Feldman EC, Nelson RW *et al.* (1995) Magnetic resonance imaging of the brain in dogs with recently diagnosed but untreated pituitary-dependent hyperadrenocorticism. *Journal of the American Veterinary Medical Association* **206**, 651–656

Bertoy EH, Feldman EC, Nelson RW *et al.* (1996) One-year follow-up evaluation of magnetic resonance imaging of the brain of dogs with pituitary-dependent hyperadrenocorticism. *Journal of the American Veterinary Medical Association* **208**, 1268–1273

Braddock JA, Church DB, Robertson ID, and Watson AD. (2003) Trilostane treatment in dogs with pituitary-dependent hyperadrenocorticism. *Australian Veterinary Journal* **81**, 600–607

Castillo VA, Gómez NV, Lalia JC, Cabrera Blatter MF and García JD (2008) Cushing's disease in dogs: cabergoline treatment. *Research in Veterinary Science* **85**, 26–34

Cerundolo R, Lloyd DH, Persechino A, Evans H and Cauvin A (2004) Treatment of canine Alopecia X with trilostane. *Veterinary Dermatology* **15**, 285–293

Chapman PS, Kelly DF, Archer J, Brockman DJ and Neiger R (2004) Adrenal necrosis in two dogs receiving trilostane for the treatment of hyperadrenocorticism. *Journal of Small Animal Practice* **45**, 307–310

Chapman PS, Mooney CT, Ede J *et al.* (2003) Evaluation of the basal and post-adrenocorticotrophic hormone serum concentrations of 17-hydroxyprogesterone for the diagnosis of hyperadrenocorticism in dogs. *Veterinary Record* **153**, 771–775

Clemente M, De Andrés PJ, Arenas C *et al.* (2007) Comparison of non-selective adrenocorticolysis with mitotane or trilostane for the treatment of dogs with pituitary-dependent hyperadrenocorticism. *Veterinary Record* **161**, 805–809

Douglass JP, Berry CR and James S (1997) Ultrasonographic adrenal gland measurements in dogs without evidence of adrenal disease. *Veterinary Radiology and Ultrasound* **38**, 124–130

Duesberg CA, Feldman EC, Nelson RW *et al.* (1995) Magnetic resonance imaging for the diagnosis of pituitary macrotumors in dogs. *Journal of the American Veterinary Medical Association* **206**, 657–662

Duncan ID, Griffiths IR and Nash AS (1977) Myotonia in canine Cushing's disease. *Veterinary Record* **100**, 30–31

Dunn KJ, Herrtage ME and Dunn JK (1995) Use of ACTH stimulation tests to monitor the treatment of canine hyperadrenocorticism. *Veterinary Record* **137**, 161–165

Eastwood JM, Elwood CM and Hurley KJ (2003) Trilostane treatment of a dog with functional adrenocortical neoplasia. *Journal of Small Animal Practice* **44**, 126–131

Feldman EC (2011) Evaluation of twice-daily lower-dose trilostane treatment administered orally in dogs with naturally occurring hyperadrenocorticism. *Journal of the American Veterinary Medical Association* **238**, 1441–1451

Feldman EC, Nelson RW, Feldman MS and Farver TB (1992) Comparison of mitotane treatment for adrenal tumor versus pituitary-dependent hyperadrenocorticism in dogs. *Journal of the American Veterinary Medical Association* **200**, 1642–1647

Ferguson DC and Peterson ME (1992) Serum free and total iodothyronine concentrations in dogs with hyperadrenocorticism. *American Journal of Veterinary Research* **53**, 1636–1640

Ford SL, Feldman EC and Nelson RW (1993) Hyperadrenocorticism caused by bilateral adrenocortical neoplasia in dogs: four cases (1983–1988). *Journal of the American Veterinary Medical Association* **202**, 789–792

Galac S, Buijtels JJ and Kooistra HS (2009) Urinary corticoid : creatinine ratios in dogs with pituitary-dependent hypercortisolism during trilostane treatment. *Journal of Veterinary Internal Medicine* **23**, 1214–1219

Galac S, Buijtels JJ, Mol JA and Kooistra HS (2010) Effects of trilostane on the pituitary-adrenocortical and renin-aldosterone axis in dogs with pituitary-dependent hypercortisolism. *Veterinary Journal* **183**, 75–80

Galac S, Kars VJ, Voorhout G, Mol JA and Kooistra HS (2008) ACTH-independent hyperadrenocorticism due to food-dependent hypercortisolemia in a dog: a case report. *Veterinary Journal* **177**, 141–3

Galac S, Kooistra HS, Kirpensteijn J *et al.* (2005) Hyperadrenocorticism in a dog due to ectopic ACTH secretion. *Domestic Animal Endocrinology* **28**, 338–348

Galac S, Kooistra HS, Teske E and Rijnberk A (1997) Urinary corticoid/creatinine ratios in the differentiation between pituitary-dependent hyperadrenocorticism and hyperadrenocorticism due to adrenocortical tumour in the dog. *Veterinary Quarterly* **19**, 17–20

Goossens MMC, Feldman EC, Theon AP and Koblik PD (1998) Efficacy of cobalt 60 radiotherapy in dogs with pituitary-dependent hyperadrenocorticism. *Journal of American Veterinary Medical Association* **212**, 374–376

Gould SM, Baines EA, Mannion PA, Evans H and Herrtage ME (2001) Use of endogenous ACTH concentration and adrenal ultrasonography to distinguish the cause of canine hyperadrenocorticism. *Journal of Small Animal Practice* **42**, 113–121

Goy-Thollot I, Péchereau D, Kéroack S, Dezempte JC and Bonnet JM (2002) Investigation of the role of aldosterone in hypertension associated with spontaneous pituitary-dependent hyperadrenocorticism in dogs. *Journal of Small Animal Practice* **43**, 489–492

Greco DS, Peterson ME, Davidson AP, Feldman EC and Komurek K (1999) Concurrent pituitary and adrenal tumors in dogs with hyperadrenocorticism: 17 cases (1978–1995). *Journal of the American Veterinary Medical Association* **214**, 1349–1353.

Grooters AM, Biller DS and Merryman J (1995) Ultrasonographic parameters of normal canine adrenal glands: comparison to necropsy findings. *Veterinary Radiology and Ultrasound* **36**, 126–130

Grooters AM, Biller DS, Theisen SK and Miyabayashi T (1996) Ultrasonographic characteristics of adrenal glands in dogs with pituitary-dependent hyperadrenocorticism: comparison with normal dogs. *Journal of Veterinary Internal Medicine* **10**, 110–115

Guptill L, Scott-Moncrieff JC, Bottoms G *et al.* (1997) Use of urine cortisol : creatinine ratio to monitor treatment response in dogs with pituitary-dependent hyperadrenocorticism. *Journal of the American Veterinary Medical Association* **210**, 1158–1161

Hanson JM, van't HM, Voorhout G *et al.* (2005) Efficacy of transsphenoidal hypophysectomy in treatment of dogs with pituitary-dependent hyperadrenocorticism. *Journal of Veterinary Internal Medicine* **19**, 687–694

Helm JR, Mclauchlan G, Frowde P *et al.* (2011) A comparison of factors that influence survival in dogs treated with mitotane or trilostane with adrenal-dependent hyperadrenocorticism. *Journal of Veterinary Internal Medicine* **25** , 251–260

Hurley KJ and Vaden SL (1998) Evaluation of urine protein content in dogs with pituitary-dependent hyperadrenocorticism. *Journal of the American Veterinary Medical Association* **212**, 369–373

Kantrowitz CM, Nyland TG and Feldman EC (1986) Adrenal ultrasonography in the dog: detection of tumours and hyperplasia in hyperadrenocorticism. *Veterinary Radiology* **27**, 91–96

Kaplan AJ, Peterson ME and Kemppainen RJ (1995) Effects of disease on the results of diagnostic tests for use in detecting hyperadrenocorticism in dogs. *Journal of the American Veterinary Medical Association* **207**, 445–451

Kemppainen RJ and Sartin JL (1984) Evidence for episodic but not circadian activity in plasma concentrations of adrenocorticotropin, cortisol and thyroxine in dogs. *Journal of Endocrinology* **103**, 219–226

Kenefick SJ and Neiger R (2008) The effect of trilostane treatment on circulating thyroid hormone concentrations in dogs with pituitary-dependent hyperadrenocorticism. *Journal of Small Animal Practice* **49**, 139–143

Kerl ME, Peterson ME, Wallace MS, Meliàn C and Kemppainen RJ (1999) Evaluation of a low-dose synthetic adrenocorticotropic hormone stimulation test in clinically normal dogs and dogs with naturally developing hyperadrenocorticism. *Journal of the American Veterinary Medical Association* **214**, 1497–1501

Kintzer PP and Peterson ME (1991) Mitotane (o,p'-DDD) treatment of 200 dogs with pituitary-dependent hyperadrenocorticism. *Journal of Veterinary Internal Medicine* **5**, 182–190

Kintzer PP and Peterson ME (1994) Mitotane treatment of 32 dogs with cortisol-secreting adrenocortical neoplasms. *Journal of the American Veterinary Medical Association* **205**, 54–60

Leone F, Cerundolo R, Vercelli A and Lloyd DH (2005) The use of trilostane for the treatment of alopecia X in Alaskan malamutes. *Journal of the American Animal Hospital Association* **41**, 336–342

Lien YH and Huang HP (2008) Use of ketoconazole to treat dogs with pituitary-dependent hyperadrenocorticism: 48 cases (1994–2007). *Journal of the American Veterinary Medical Association* **233**, 1896–1901

Long S, Michieletto A, Anderson TJ, Williams A and Knottenbelt CM (2003) Suspected pituitary apoplexy in a German short-haired pointer. *Journal of Small Animal Practice* **44**, 497–502

Mantis P, Lamb CR, Witt AL and Neiger R (2003) Changes in ultrasonographic appearance of adrenal glands in dogs with pituitary-dependent hyperadrenocorticism treated with trilostane. *Veterinary Radiology and Ultrasound* **44,** 682–685

Martin LG, Behrend EN, Mealey KL, Carpenter DM and Hickey KC (2007) Effect of low doses of cosyntropin on serum cortisol concentrations in clinically normal dogs. *American Journal of Veterinary Research* **68**, 555–560

Meij BP, Voorhout G, van den Ingh TSGAM *et al.* (1998) Results of transsphenoidal hypophysectomy in 52 dogs with pituitary-dependent hyperadrenocorticism. *Veterinary Surgery* **27**, 246–261

Montgomery TM, Nelson RW, Feldman EC, Robertson K and Polonsky KS (1996) Basal and glucagon-stimulated plasma C-peptide concentrations in healthy dogs, dogs with diabetes mellitus, and dogs with hyperadrenocorticism. *Journal of Veterinary Internal Medicine* **10**, 116–122

Mueller C, Sieber-Ruckstuhl N, Wenger M, Kaser-Hotz B and Reusch CE (2006) Low-dose dexamethasone test with 'inverse' results a possible new pattern of cortisol response. *Veterinary Record* **159**, 489–491

Neiger R, Ramsey I, O'Connor J, Hurley KJ and Mooney CT (2002) Trilostane treatment of 78 dogs with pituitary-dependent hyperadrenocorticism. *Veterinary Record* **150**, 799–804

Norman EJ, Thompson H and Mooney CT (1999) Dynamic adrenal function testing in eight dogs with hyperadrenocorticism associated with adrenocortical neoplasia. *Veterinary Record* **144**, 551–554

Pérez AM, Guerrero B, Melián C, Ynaraja E and Peña L (2002) Use of aminoglutethimide in the treatment of pituitary-dependent hyperadrenocorticism in the dog. *Journal of Small Animal Practice* **43**, 104–108

Perez Alenza D, Arenas C, Lopez ML and Melian C (2006) Long-term efficacy of trilostane administered twice daily in dogs with pituitary-dependent hyperadrenocorticism. *Journal of the American Animal Hospital Association* **42**, 269–276

Peterson ME, Ferguson DC, Kintzer PP and Drucker WD (1984) Effects of spontaneous hyperadrenocorticism on serum thyroid hormone concentrations in the dog. *American Journal of Veterinary Research* **45**, 2034–2038

Peterson ME, Krieger DT, Drucker WD and Halmi NS (1982) Immunocytochemical study of the hypophysis in 25 dogs with pituitary-dependent hyperadrenocorticism. *Acta Endocrinologica* **101**, 15–24

Ramsey IK and Herrtage ME (1998) The effect of thyrotropin releasing hormone on thyrotropin concentrations in euthyroid, hypothyroid and hyperadrenocorticoid dogs. *Journal of Veterinary Internal Medicine* **12**, 235.

Ramsey IK, Richardson J, Lenard Z, Tebb AJ and Irwin PJ (2008) Persistent isolated hypocortisolism following brief treatment with trilostane. *Australian Veterinary Journal* **86**, 491–495

Ramsey IK, Tebb A, Harris E, Evans H and Herrtage ME (2005) Hyperparathyroidism in dogs with hyperadrenocorticism. *Journal of Small Animal Practice* **46**, 531–536

Reusch CE and Feldman EC (1991) Canine hyperadrenocorticism due to adrenocortical neoplasia: pretreatment evaluation in 41 dogs. *Journal of Veterinary Internal Medicine* **13**, 291–301

Reusch CE, Sieber-Ruckstuhl N, Wenger M, Lutz H, Perren A and Pospischil A (2007) Histological evaluation of the adrenal glands of seven dogs with hyperadrenocorticism treated with trilostane. *Veterinary Record* **160**, 219–224

Reusch CE, Steffen T and Hoerauf A (1999) The efficacy of L-deprenyl in dogs with pituitary-dependent hyperadrenocorticism. *Journal of Veterinary Internal Medicine* **5**, 3–10

Rijnberk A, Van Wees A and Mol JA (1988) Assessment of two tests for the diagnosis of canine hyperadrenocorticism. *Veterinary Record* **122**, 178–180

Ristic JME, Ramsey IK, Heath FM, Evans HJ and Herrtage ME (2002) The use of 17-hydroxyprogesterone in the diagnosis of canine hyperadrenocorticism. *Journal of Veterinary Internal Medicine* **16**, 433–439

Rodríguez Piñero MI, Benchekroun G, de Fornel-Thibaud P *et al.* (2009) Accuracy of an adrenocorticotropic hormone (ACTH) immunoluminometric assay for differentiating ACTH-dependent from ACTH-independent hyperadrenocorticism in dogs. *Journal of Veterinary Internal Medicine* **23**, 850–855

Ruckstuhl NS, Nett CS and Reusch CE (2002) Results of clinical examinations, laboratory tests, and ultrasonography in dogs with pituitary-dependent hyperadrenocorticism treated with trilostane. *American Journal of Veterinary Research* **63**, 506–512

Scavelli TD, Peterson ME and Matthiesen DT (1986) Results of surgical treatment for hyperadrenocorticism caused by adrenocortical neoplasia in the dog: 25 cases (1980-1984). *Journal of the American Veterinary Medical Association* **189**, 1360–1364

Schwartz P, Kovak JR, Koprowski A *et al.* (2008) Evaluation of prognostic factors in the surgical treatment of adrenal gland tumors in dogs: 41 cases (1999–2005). *Journal of the American Veterinary Medical Association* **232**, 77–84

Schwarz T, Störk CK, Mellor D and Sullivan M (2000) Osteopenia and other radiographic signs in canine hyperadrenocorticism. *Journal of Small Animal Practice* **41**, 491–495

Semple CG, Thomson JA, Stark AN, McDonald M and Beastall GH (1982) Trilostane and the normal hypothalamic-pituitary-adrenocortical axis. *Clinical Endocrinology (Oxford)* **17**, 569–575

Sieber-Ruckstuhl NS, Boretti FS, Wenger M, Maser-Gluth C and Reusch CE (2006) Cortisol, aldosterone, cortisol precursor, androgen and endogenous ACTH concentrations in dogs with pituitary-dependant hyperadrenocorticism treated with trilostane. *Domestic Animal Endocrinology* **31**, 63–75

Sieber-Ruckstuhl NS, Boretti FS, Wenger M, Maser-Gluth C and Reusch CE (2008) Serum concentrations of cortisol and cortisone in healthy dogs and dogs with pituitary-dependent hyperadrenocorticism treated with trilostane. *Veterinary Record* **163**, 477–481

Siliart B, Marouze C, Martin L and Gayet C (2002) Pseudomyotonia associated with hyperadrenocorticism in the French Poodle: 151 clinical cases (1993–2000). *Proceedings of 12th ECVIM-CA/ESVIM Congress*

Smiley LE and Peterson ME (1993) Evaluation of a urine cortisol:creatinine ratio as a screening test for hyperadrenocorticism in dogs. *Journal of Veterinary Internal Medicine* **7**, 163–168

Syme HM, Scott-Moncrieff J, Treadwell NG *et al.* (2001) Hyperadrenocorticism associated with excessive sex hormone production by an adrenocortical tumor in two dogs. *Journal of the American Veterinary Medical Association* **219**, 1725–1728

Tebb AJ, Arteaga A, Evans H and Ramsey IK (2005) Canine hyperadrenocorticism: effects of trilostane on parathyroid hormone, calcium and phosphate concentrations. *Journal of Small Animal Practice* **46**, 537–542

Teske E, Rothuizen J, de Bruijne JJ and Rijnberk A (1989) Corticosteroid-induced alkaline phosphatase isoenzyme in the diagnosis of canine hypercorticism. *Veterinary Record* **125**, 12–14

Théon AP and Feldman EC (1998) Megavoltage irradiation of pituitary macrotumours in dogs with neurological signs. *Journal of the American Veterinary Medical Association* **213**, 225–231

van Sluijs FJ, Sjollema BE, Voorhout G, van den Ingh TSGAM and Rijnberk A (1995) Results of adrenalectomy in 36 dogs with hyperadrenocorticism caused by adrenocortical tumour. *Veterinary Quarterly* **17**, 113–116

Vaughan MA, Feldman EC, Hoar BR and Nelson RW (2008) Evaluation of twice-daily, low-dose trilostane treatment administered orally in dogs with naturally occurring hyperadrenocorticism. *Journal of the American Veterinary Medical Association* **232**, 1321–1328

Voorhout G, Stolp R, Lubberink AAME and van Waes PFGM (1988) Computed tomography in the diagnosis of canine hyperadrenocorticism not suppressible by dexamethasone. *Journal of the American Veterinary Medical Association* **192**, 641–646

Voorhout G, Stolp R, Rijnberk A and van Waes PFGM (1990) Assessment of survey radiography and comparison with X-ray computed tomography for detection of hyperfunctioning adrenocortical tumors in dogs. *Journal of the American Veterinary Medical Association* **196**, 1799–1803

Zur G and White SD (2011) Hyperadrenocorticism in 10 dogs with skin lesions as the only presenting clinical sign. *Journal of the American Animal Hospital Association* **47**, 419–427

17

Feline hyperadrenocorticism

Mark E. Peterson

Introduction

In cats, as in other species, hyperadrenocorticism (Cushing's syndrome) is the constellation of clinical signs resulting from chronic glucocorticoid excess. Naturally occurring hyperadrenocorticism is caused by primary hyperfunction of either the pituitary or adrenal gland, whereas iatrogenic hyperadrenocorticism is caused by administration of synthetic glucocorticoids. Of the two causes of the naturally occurring disease, pituitary-dependent hyperadrenocorticism results from excessive secretion of adrenocorticotropic hormone (ACTH) from an adenoma arising in the pars distalis or pars intermedia of the pituitary gland, which induces bilateral adrenocortical hyperplasia. Unilateral adenoma or carcinoma of the adrenal cortex secretes excessive cortisol autonomously, resulting in suppression of pituitary ACTH secretion and atrophy of the contralateral adrenal cortex.

Whilst naturally occurring hyperadrenocorticism is rare in cats, both pituitary-dependent hyperadrenocorticism and cortisol-secreting adrenal tumours are well recognized. Approximately 75–80% of cats with hyperadrenocorticism have the pituitary-dependent form of the disorder; the remaining 20–25% have unilateral adrenal tumours. Of the cats with functional adrenocortical tumours, approximately two-thirds have unilateral adenoma; the remainder have adrenal carcinoma.

Although cats tend to be more resistant than dogs to the effects of exogenous glucocorticoid excess, iatrogenic hyperadrenocorticism is a well recognized disorder in cats (Lien *et al.*, 2006; Lowe *et al.*, 2008).

Progesterone-secreting adrenal tumours have also been recognized in cats, albeit rarely. Clinical signs are similar to those in cats with cortisol-secreting tumours but, as in the dog, measurement of cortisol precursors is necessary for diagnosis (see Chapter 16).

Clinical features

Hyperadrenocorticism is a disease of middle-aged to older cats, with a median age of 10–11 years. Whilst a slight female sex predilection was once suggested, most case series of cats with hyperadrenocorticism have shown no sex predilection. There is no reported breed predilection in cats that develop hyperadrenocorticism.

Clinical signs and abnormal laboratory findings in cats with hyperadrenocorticism are listed in Figure 17.1. The most common clinical signs are:

- Polyuria/polydipsia
- Polyphagia
- Pendulous abdomen
- Cutaneous changes.

Cats with advanced or long-term untreated hyperadrenocorticism also show other signs typical for the disease in dogs, such as bilaterally symmetrical hair loss, weight gain and muscle atrophy.

Clinical signs	Approximate percentage of hyperadrenocorticoid cats with these features
Polyuria and polydipsia	85–90
Pot-bellied appearance	70–85
Increased appetite	65–75
Unkempt, seborrhoeic hair coat	60–70
Muscle wasting	60–65
Bilateral symmetrical hair thinning or alopecia	40–60
Lethargy	40–60
Insulin resistance (high daily insulin dose)	45–55
Weight loss	50–60
Fragile, tearing skin	30–50
Infection or sepsis	30–40
Obesity/weight gain	20–40
Hepatomegaly	25–35
Calcinosis cutis	0

17.1 Clinical signs in cats with hyperadrenocorticism. (Data from Duesberg *et al.*, 1995; Goossens *et al.*, 1995; Watson and Herrtage, 1998; Feldman and Nelson, 2004)

Differences in clinical presentation between cats and dogs
Despite the apparent similarity between cats and dogs with hyperadrenocorticism, there are major differences in clinical presentation.

Polyuria and polydipsia
Polyuria and polydipsia are usually the earliest signs of hyperadrenocorticism in dogs and develop in >80% of cases. In dogs, it appears that glucocorticoids inhibit the secretion or action of vasopressin (antidiuretic hormone, ADH) resulting in polyuria with secondary polydipsia. Although hyperglycaemic osmotic diuresis might also contribute to these signs, most dogs with hyperadrenocorticism have a normal or only mildly increased blood glucose concentration and are not overtly diabetic.

In contrast to dogs with hyperadrenocorticism, the onset of polyuria and polydipsia in cats that are treated with large doses of glucocorticoids, as well as those that develop naturally occurring hyperadrenocorticism, is often delayed. Polyuria usually coincides with the development of moderate to severe hyperglycaemia and glucosuria, with subsequent osmotic diuresis. Therefore, polyuria and polydipsia are not typically present in cats during the early stages of hyperadrenocorticism when glucose tolerance is still normal (i.e. before development of diabetes mellitus).

Although rare in cats with hyperadrenocorticism, polyuria and polydipsia can develop either without concurrent diabetes or prior to the progression to overt diabetes mellitus (Watson and Herrtage, 1998; Feldman and Nelson, 2004). The mechanism for the development of polyuria and polydipsia in non-diabetic cats is unclear, but may be related to concurrent renal disease.

Skin fragility
Extreme fragility of the skin is one of the major cutaneous manifestations of hyperadrenocorticism seen in cats, although rare in dogs with the disorder. Skin fragility somewhat resembling that seen in cats with cutaneous asthenia (Ehlers–Danlos syndrome) develops in approximately half of all cats with hyperadrenocorticism. In affected cats, the skin tends to tear with routine handling or whilst playing with other cats, leaving large denuded areas (Figure 17.2).

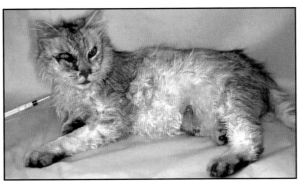

17.2 Cat with hyperadrenocorticism caused by a unilateral adrenal adenoma. Note the unkempt hair coat, chronic eye infection and open non-healing wound on the ventral abdomen. The non-healing wound is secondary to severe thinning of the skin.

Although many of the other cutaneous features of hyperadrenocorticism in cats are similar to those reported in dogs (e.g. unkempt hair coat, bilaterally symmetric hair loss, atrophic thin skin and bruising of the skin), skin fragility appears to be a unique but serious manifestation of the disease in cats (see Figure 17.1).

Weight loss
In contrast to the canine disease, many cats with hyperadrenocorticism have a history of weight loss rather than weight gain or obesity (see Figure 17.1). In most of these cats, the weight loss occurs secondary to poorly controlled diabetes mellitus (present in up to 90% of cats with hyperadrenocorticism). Insulin resistance may be a feature of the diabetes in some cats, but most do not require extremely high doses of insulin for adequate glycaemic control. Insulin resistance, when present, is not as severe as in cats with acromegaly, where extremely high insulin doses may be required for any glycaemic control (see Chapter 5).

Diagnosis

Routine clinicopathological analyses
The results of routine clinicopathological tests are variable and are often not specific for the disease (Figure 17.3). The classic haematological changes of mature leucocytosis, eosinopenia, lymphopenia

Abnormal laboratory findings	Approximate percentage of hyperadrenocorticoid cats with these features
Complete blood count	
Lymphopenia	60–65
Eosinopenia	55–60
Mature leucocytosis	45–55
Monocytosis	20–25
Serum biochemical analysis	
Hyperglycaemia	80–90
Hypercholesterolaemia	30–45
High alanine aminotransferase activity	35–40
High alkaline phosphatase activity	10–20
Urinalysis	
Glucosuria	85–90
Urine specific gravity <1.015	5–10
Ketonuria	5–10

17.3 Abnormal laboratory findings in cats with hyperadrenocorticism. (Data from Duesberg *et al.*, 1995; Goossens *et al.*, 1995; Watson and Herrtage, 1998; Feldman and Nelson, 2004)

and monocytosis may be reported, but these findings are inconsistent.

By far the most striking serum biochemical abnormality reported is severe hyperglycaemia and glucosuria. Hypercholesterolaemia develops in approximately one-third to one-half of affected cats and is probably caused, at least in part, by a poorly controlled diabetic state. High activity of serum alanine aminotransferase (ALT) also develops in approximately a third of affected cats, probably related to the hepatic lipidosis associated with diabetes mellitus. In dogs with hyperadrenocorticism, steroid induction of a specific hepatic isoenzyme of alkaline phosphatase (ALP) causes increases in the serum activity of this enzyme in 85–90% of cases; whereas only 10–20% of cats with hyperadrenocorticism have high ALP activity. The mild increase in serum ALP activity found in some cats probably results from the poorly regulated diabetic state rather than from a direct effect of glucocorticoid excess, as it may normalize with insulin treatment alone, despite progression of the hyperadrenocorticism.

Despite clinical polyuria and polydipsia, cats with hyperadrenocorticism usually maintain urine specific gravity of >1.020. Cats rarely exhibit the dilute urine commonly noted in dogs with hyperadrenocorticism. Again, this difference in urine concentration probably reflects the fact that polyuria in most cats is the result of hyperglycaemia and glucosuria, rather than being a direct inhibitory effect on secretion or action of ADH as in dogs.

Pituitary–adrenal function tests

Endocrinological evaluation of cats with suspected hyperadrenocorticism is a two-step process, in which screening tests to confirm the diagnosis are first used, followed by discriminatory tests to distinguish pituitary-dependent disease from functional adrenal tumours. Test results can be difficult to interpret because clinical signs are often less dramatic in cats than in dogs, and results of individual tests may be inconsistent with poor sensitivity or specificity. In many cases, it is necessary to use a combination of tests to determine whether hyperadrenocorticism is present as well as to establish the underlying cause of the disorder.

Screening tests

The three tests used for diagnosis of cats suspected of having hyperadrenocorticism include the ACTH response test, urine cortisol:creatinine ratio (UCCR), and low-dose dexamethasone suppression (LDDS) test. Test protocols are summarized in Figure 17.4. It is important to realize that none of the tests is perfect and that each has advantages and disadvantages. Therefore, it is recommended that the diagnosis of hyperadrenocorticism be reserved for cats with clinical signs of the disease together with endocrine test results consistent with that diagnosis.

ACTH response test: The ACTH response test is commonly used as a screening test for hyperadrenocorticism in dogs and has also been recommended for cats. The advantages of this test are that it

Test	Test protocol
Screening tests	
ACTH response test	Collect baseline blood sample for serum cortisol measurement. Administer synthetic ACTH (tetracosactrin or cosyntropin at 125 µg/cat i.v.). Collect blood sample for post-ACTH cortisol determination 1 hour later
Urine cortisol:creatinine ratio (UCCR)	Owner collects urine specimen from cat at home. Owner drops off urine sample to veterinary clinic. Submit urine to laboratory.
Low-dose dexamethasone suppression (LDDS) test	Collect baseline blood sample for serum cortisol measurement. Administer dexamethasone (0.1 mg/kg i.v.). Collect blood samples for post-dexamethasone cortisol determination 4 and 8 hours later
Combined dexamethasone suppression/ACTH response test	Collect baseline blood sample for serum cortisol determination. Administer dexamethasone (0.1 mg/kg i.v.). Collect blood sample for post-dexamethasone cortisol determination 4 hours later. Immediately after collecting this sample, administer synthetic ACTH (tetracosactrin or cosyntropin at 125 µg/cat i.v.). Collect blood sample for post-ACTH cortisol determination 1 hour later
Discrimination tests	
High-dose dexamethasone suppression (HDDS) test	Collect baseline blood sample for serum cortisol measurement. Administer dexamethasone (1.0 mg/kg i.v.). Collect blood samples for cortisol determination 4 and 8 hours later
HDDS test plus UCCR	Owner collects urine from cat at home on two consecutive mornings for determination of the baseline UCCR. On the second day, owner then administers three doses of dexamethasone (0.1 mg/kg q8h orally) at 8pm, 4pm and midnight. On the third day, the owner collects a third urine sample at 8am for the post-dexamethasone UCCR determination
Plasma endogenous ACTH concentration	Collect plasma in chilled tube with protease inhibitor added if available. Immediately separate and freeze plasma until assayed
Abdominal ultrasonography	Need equipment and skilled operator to perform procedure

17.4 A summary of diagnostic test protocols used in cats with suspected hyperadrenocorticism.

requires little time (1 hour) and only two venepunctures (see Figure 17.4), and is the only test that can be used to distinguish iatrogenic from naturally occurring hyperadrenocorticism. Regardless of the basal cortisol concentration, diagnosis of naturally occurring hyperadrenocorticism depends on demonstration of a post-ACTH cortisol concentration that is higher than the reference interval. By contrast, cats with iatrogenic hyperadrenocorticism are expected to have a subnormal response to exogenous ACTH administration.

In cats, the main problem with the ACTH response test is its poor sensitivity for hyperadrenocorticism. Only 35–50% of cats with naturally occurring disease exhibit an exaggerated serum cortisol response, whereas up to two-thirds of cats with the disease have reference interval test results. Therefore, the ACTH response test is not as useful for detecting naturally occurring hyperadrenocorticism in cats as in dogs, where the test sensitivity is approximately 0.85. However, if iatrogenic hyperadrenocorticism is suspected, the ACTH response test remains the screening test of choice to document secondary adrenocortical suppression (Peterson *et al.*, 1994; Duesberg and Peterson, 1997; Hoenig, 2002; Feldman and Nelson, 2004).

Studies have reported that a variety of chronic illnesses (not associated with hyperadrenocorticism) can also influence ACTH-stimulated cortisol secretion in cats (Zerbe *et al.*, 1987). It is likely that the 'stress' associated with chronic illness results in some degree of bilateral adrenocortical hyperplasia in sick cats, which could account for an exaggerated cortisol response to ACTH. Therefore, the diagnosis of hyperadrenocorticism should be based on the cat's history, clinical signs and routine clinicopathological findings, and not solely on the results of basal or ACTH-stimulated serum cortisol concentrations.

Sex hormone-secreting adrenal tumours have been recognized rarely in cats (Boord and Griffin, 1999; Rossmeisl *et al.*, 2000; Declue *et al.*, 2005; Briscoe *et al.* 2009; Millard *et al.*, 2009; Quante *et al.* 2009). Clinical signs are similar to those of cats with cortisol-secreting tumours but, as in the dog, measurement of cortisol precursors is necessary for diagnosis (see Chapter 16). Measurement of serum or plasma sex hormones (e.g. progesterone, 17α-hydroxyprogesterone, androstenedione, testosterone or oestradiol) before and after ACTH stimulation is often recommended. However, ACTH stimulation testing is of limited value in these cats, as most are found to have high basal serum concentrations of these steroids, making stimulation tests unnecessary.

A commonly employed protocol for testing is shown in Figure 17.4. In cats, intravenous administration of ACTH (125 μg/cat) induces greater and more prolonged adrenocortical stimulation than the intramuscular route and is therefore preferred (Peterson and Kemppainen, 1992). Lower doses of synthetic ACTH (1.25 and 12.5 μg/cat) produce comparable cortisol stimulation (Peterson and Kemppainen, 1993) but more prolonged stimulation is attained after administration of the higher dose (125 μg/cat). For obese cats, doses as high as 250 μg/cat have been recommended, particularly if sampling is delayed for any reason (Schoeman *et al.*, 2000).

Overall, the ACTH response test is *not* recommended as the initial screening test for hyperadrenocorticism in cats because it lacks sensitivity; most cats with hyperadrenocorticism will have reference interval results. Two alternative screening tests, which have increased sensitivity, are available (see below) and are clearly superior.

Urine cortisol: creatinine ratio: UCCR is a valuable, highly sensitive measure that can be used to help diagnose hyperadrenocorticism in cats (Goosens *et al.*, 1995; Feldman and Nelson, 2004). The test sensitivity for diagnosing hyperadrenocorticism ranges from 0.8–0.9, higher than the sensitivity of the ACTH response test. However, the finding of a high (false positive) UCCR is common in cats with moderate to severe non-adrenal illness (Henry *et al.*, 1996; de Lange *et al.*, 2004).

To avoid the stress of travel or hospitalization (which could falsely increase the UCCR), it is best to have the owner collect the urine specimen from the cat at home and bring the sample to the veterinary clinic for submission to the laboratory. Although it can be difficult for many owners to collect a urine sample from their cat, use of non-absorbent cat litter or replacement of the cat litter with non-absorbent aquarium gravel may be helpful.

Overall, UCCR is a sensitive measure for distinguishing cats with hyperadrenocorticism from those that do not have the disease. However, since the specificity of this test appears to be low, the cat's history and physical examination must be carefully evaluated when interpreting the test results. If the UCCR values are suggestive of hyperadrenocorticism, the diagnosis is best confirmed with another more specific test, such as the LDDS test.

Low-dose dexamethasone suppression test: The LDDS test is performed differently in cats than in dogs. For cats, a 10-fold higher dose of dexamethasone is required (Peterson *et al.*, 1994; Duesberg and Peterson, 1997; Hoenig, 2002; Feldman and Nelson, 2004; Kley *et al.*, 2007). The protocol for cats is described in Figure 17.4. Dexamethasone at 0.1 mg/kg i.v. will consistently suppress serum cortisol concentrations to approximately <40 nmol/l at 4 and 8 hours in healthy cats and in those with non-adrenal illness. Inadequate serum cortisol suppression at both 4 and 8 hours, diagnostic for hyperadrenocorticism, is found in all cats with cortisol-secreting adrenal tumours. The vast majority of cats with pituitary-dependent hyperadrenocorticism will also fail to suppress serum cortisol concentration at 4 or 8 hours.

Overall, the LDDS test is an excellent screening test, with a sensitivity close to 1 and acceptable specificity. As this test is clearly better than the ACTH response test and has better test specificity than the UCCR, it is the test of choice for evaluating a cat with suspected hyperadrenocorticism.

***Combined ACTH response/dexamethasone
suppression test:*** The ACTH response test and
LDDS test (0.1 mg/kg) are both useful screening
tests for hyperadrenocorticism in cats. It is possible
to combine the two and perform them in a single
day so that only three blood samples need to be
collected over a 5-hour period (see Figure 17.4).

Almost all cats with hyperadrenocorticism fail to
demonstrate adequate serum cortisol suppression
after dexamethasone administration, and approximately half have an exaggerated cortisol response
after ACTH administration. By contrast, healthy cats
and almost all diabetic cats without hyperadrenocorticism exhibit marked serum cortisol suppression after
dexamethasone and have a reference range cortisol
response after ACTH stimulation (Peterson *et al.*,
1994; Duesberg and Peterson, 1997; Hoenig, 2002).

Overall, because of the low sensitivity of the
ACTH response test, the combined ACTH response/
dexamethasone suppression test is *not* recommended as a screening test for hyperadrenocorticism. Use of the 8-hour LDDS test, as outlined
above, is a better diagnostic test for cats with suspected hyperadrenocorticism.

Discriminatory tests

Once a diagnosis of hyperadrenocorticism has been
confirmed, pituitary-dependent disease must be dis-
tinguished from adrenal-dependent hyperadrenocorticism, as this has important implications for
treatment. Tests include the high-dose dexamethasone suppression (HDDS) test and endogenous
plasma ACTH measurement. Imaging techniques
such as abdominal radiography, ultrasonography,
computed tomography and magnetic resonance
imaging can also be extremely helpful in determining the cause. In addition, it is only possible to
detect metastatic lesions from an adrenal carcinoma
by use of these imaging techniques, in the absence
of adrenal biopsy and histopathology.

High-dose dexamethasone suppression test: In
cats with confirmed hyperadrenocorticism, an
HDDS test can be performed to help differentiate
pituitary-dependent hyperadrenocorticism from cortisol-secreting adrenocortical tumours. The protocol
is described in Figure 17.4.

Adequate cortisol suppression is generally
defined as a serum cortisol concentration of <30
nmol/l; or a cortisol concentration <50% of the
baseline value at 4 or 8 hours. In cats with functional
adrenocortical neoplasia, this dose of dexamethasone never adequately suppresses cortisol concentration, whereas it suppresses serum cortisol
concentration in approximately 50% of cats with
pituitary-dependent hyperadrenocorticism (Peterson
et al., 1994; Duesberg and Peterson, 1997; Feldman
and Nelson, 2004). In contrast, 85% of dogs with
pituitary-dependent hyperadrenocorticism will demonstrate adequate cortisol suppression after administration of this high dose of dexamethasone.

Overall, this in-hospital test is relatively easy to
perform. Suppression of serum cortisol concentrations, when demonstrated, is consistent with

pituitary-dependent hyperadrenocorticism. Unfortunately, the test cannot reliably determine the cause of
the disorder, as half of the cats with pituitary-
dependent hyperadrenocorticism fail to demonstrate
any suppression. In these cases, either plasma
ACTH should be measured or abdominal
ultrasonography should be performed to determine
the cause of the hyperadrenocorticism.

HDDS test (UCCR measurements): The protocol
is described in Figure 17.4: urine is collected on
three consecutive mornings, and the three oral dexamethasone doses are all administered on the second day.

If UCCR after dexamethasone administration is
suppressed by >50% of the average basal UCCR
then pituitary-dependent hyperadrenocorticism is
likely. If suppression is <50%, no discrimination is
possible, as is the case for the standard HDDS test
described above. In contrast to the standard HDDS
test, in which half of cats with pituitary-dependent
hyperadrenocorticism fail to demonstrate suppression, approximately 75% of cats with pituitary-
dependent hyperadrenocorticism will demonstrate
suppression with this test (Goosens *et al.*, 1995;
Meij *et al.*, 2001). This makes this test more reliable
for distinguishing the cause of hyperadrenocorticism
in cats.

Overall, this test is generally easier to perform
and is better at determining the cause of the disorder than the standard in-hospital test. Therefore,
for those owners who can administer dexamethasone orally, this protocol can be recommended both
as a screening test (baseline UCCR) and discrimination test (post-dexamethasone UCCR).

Endogenous ACTH: The basal endogenous ACTH
concentration is valuable for differentiating the origin of hyperadrenocorticism in cats with clinical
signs and screening test results diagnostic for the
disease (Peterson *et al.*, 1994; Duesberg and
Peterson, 1997). The endogenous ACTH concentration is high to high–normal in cats with pituitary-
dependent hyperadrenocorticism, whereas the
concentration in cats with functional adrenocortical
tumours is low to undetectable.

It is important that blood samples for determination of endogenous ACTH concentration are handled carefully, as ACTH degrades rapidly in plasma
after collection. Special handling requirements
include the addition of a protease inhibitor (e.g.
aprotinin) when blood is collected and rapid separation of plasma and proper storage temperatures
until the assay is performed. Mishandling of samples may result in a falsely low value that could erroneously suggest an adrenal tumour (see Chapter 1).

Diagnostic imaging

Abdominal radiography and abdominal ultrasonography are commonly used to help differentiate pituitary-dependent hyperadrenocorticism and
cortisol-secreting adrenal tumours. Computed
tomography (CT) and magnetic resonance imaging
(MRI) have also proven useful in the detection of

pituitary tumours (>3 mm diameter) as well as unilateral adrenal tumours, but both techniques require specialized equipment, are expensive to perform and are not widely available.

Although a large adrenocortical tumour can occasionally be visualized on abdominal radiographs, radiography is of no value in confirming bilateral adrenocortical hyperplasia in cats with pituitary-dependent hyperadrenocorticism. Bilateral calcification of the adrenal gland can occasionally be detected in older cats and this should not be interpreted as evidence of an adrenal tumour as it is in dogs (Peterson *et al.*, 1994).

Ultrasonographic evaluation of adrenal size and morphology is extremely useful in determining the cause of the hyperadrenocorticism in cats. Adrenal glands are relatively easy to identify in cats: in contrast to the dog, where the left and right adrenal glands differ in shape, in cats both the adrenal glands are oblong and oval to bean-shaped. In cats with hyperadrenocorticism, if both adrenal glands are large or of equal size, the diagnosis is pituitary-dependent hyperadrenocorticism. If, on the other hand, one adrenal gland is large or misshapen and the contralateral adrenal is small or cannot be visualized on ultrasonographic evaluation, a cortisol-secreting adrenal tumour is diagnosed (Peterson *et al.*, 1994; Duesberg and Peterson, 1997; Feldman and Nelson, 2004; Kley *et al.*, 2007).

Treatment

In cats, hyperadrenocorticism is difficult to treat successfully. Treatment options are summarized in Figure 17.5. Potential options for medical treatment include the use of the adrenocorticolytic agent mitotane (o,p'-DDD) or drugs that block one or more of the enzymes involved in cortisol synthesis (e.g. ketoconazole, metyrapone or trilostane). Surgical treatment of cats with pituitary-dependent hyperadrenocorticism includes bilateral adrenalectomy or hypophysectomy, whereas unilateral adrenalectomy is indicated in cats with an adrenocortical tumour. Finally, external radiation therapy can also be used for pituitary-dependent hyperadrenocorticism, especially when the cat has a large pituitary adenoma.

Treatment	Indication	Comments
Medical therapy		
Mitotane (o,p'-DDD)	PDH or adrenal tumour	Initial dose 25–50 mg/kg orally q24h. Drug fails to suppress adrenocortical function adequately in most cats. Adverse effects common. Not strongly recommended
Ketoconazole	PDH or adrenal tumour	Ineffective in suppressing adrenocortical function in most cats. Adverse effects common. Not recommended
Metyrapone	PDH or adrenal tumour	Initial dose, 250–500 mg/cat orally q24h. Potential adverse effects include vomiting and anorexia. Beneficial effects on suppressing adrenocortical function may be transient. Most useful as preoperative preparation for adrenalectomy. Unavailability of drug is a frequent problem
Trilostane	PDH or adrenal tumour	Initial dose 15–30 mg/cat orally q24h; increase to 60–90 mg/cat q24h if needed. Adverse effects uncommon. Effective in suppressing adrenocortical function. Useful as preoperative preparation for adrenalectomy and possibly for long-term use. Not authorized for use in cats
Radiation therapy		
Pituitary radiation treatment	PDH	Offers a potential cure for pituitary-dependent hyperadrenocorticism. May be the only treatment for cats with a large or invasive pituitary tumour. Treatment response typically delayed, so use of concurrent medical therapy or bilateral adrenalectomy recommended. Limited availability and expense disadvantages
Surgery		
Unilateral adrenalectomy	Adrenal tumour	Pre-surgical medical stabilization (e.g. metyrapone or trilostane) helpful. Postoperative complications may include pancreatitis and wound dehiscence. Clinical signs resolve by 2–4 months postoperatively. Glucocorticoid supplementation required for approximately 2 months postoperatively, until function of the atrophied remaining adrenal gland recovers. With complete removal of adrenal tumour, cure of disease accomplished
Bilateral adrenalectomy	PDH	Pre-surgical medical stabilization (e.g. metyrapone or trilostane) helpful. Postoperative complications common. Clinical signs resolve by 2–4 months postoperatively. Lifelong replacement of both mineralocorticoid and glucocorticoid hormones required. Pituitary defect (e.g. pituitary adenoma) remains; may later develop pituitary macroadenoma
Hypophysectomy	PDH	Offers potential cure for hyperadrenocorticism. Pre-surgical medical stabilization (e.g. metyrapone or trilostane) helpful. Requires highly skilled surgeon and advanced imaging facilities. Postoperative complications (diabetes insipidus) common. Recurrence of disease possible

17.5 A summary of the treatment options for cats with hyperadrenocorticism. (Data from Peterson *et al.*, 1994; Duesberg *et al.*, 1995; Duesberg and Peterson, 1997; Watson and Herrtage, 1998; Moore *et al.*, 2000; Hoenig, 2002; Feldman and Nelson, 2004)

From collected experience over the last 2 decades, adrenalectomy has proven the most successful mode of treatment in cats, whereas medical management and use of pituitary radiotherapy have yielded mixed results. With the introduction and more widespread use of the drug trilostane, however, most cats with hyperadrenocorticism can now be reasonably controlled medically, at least for a few weeks to months.

Medical therapy

Mitotane

Mitotane is an adrenocortical cytolytic agent that has been used extensively for the treatment of hyperadrenocorticism in dogs. A number of different protocols for mitotane treatment of cats with hyperadrenocorticism have been used, with limited short-term success, and long-term results have been generally discouraging (Peterson *et al.*, 1994; Duesberg and Peterson, 1997; Schwedes, 1997, Feldman and Nelson, 2004). In most cats treated with the standard dosages of mitotane used for dogs with pituitary-dependent hyperadrenocorticism (25–50 mg/kg orally q24h), the drug neither effectively suppresses adrenocortical function nor alleviates clinical signs of the disease, even after prolonged daily treatment periods. Adverse effects such as anorexia, vomiting and lethargy are relatively common, even in cats where the drug has not lowered serum cortisol concentrations. Because of mitotane's poor effectiveness and high rate of adverse effects, this drug is not recommended for cats with hyperadrenocorticism.

Ketoconazole

Ketoconazole, a drug used principally for treatment of mycotic disease, inhibits the first step in cortisol biosynthesis (cholesterol side-chain cleavage to pregnenolone) and, to a lesser extent, the conversion of 11-deoxycortisol to cortisol. Although ketoconazole has been used successfully in both humans and dogs with hyperadrenocorticism, it does not reliably suppress adrenocortical function in healthy cats, or in cats with hyperadrenocorticism, and may cause serious side effects such as thrombocytopenia (Peterson *et al.*, 1994; Duesberg and Peterson, 1997, Feldman and Nelson, 2004). Therefore, ketoconazole cannot be recommended for treatment of cats with hyperadrenocorticism.

Metyrapone

Metyrapone, a drug that inhibits the action of 11β-hydroxylase (the enzyme that converts 11-deoxycortisol to cortisol), has been used with mixed results in cats with hyperadrenocorticism. Total dosages ranging from 250–500 mg/day have been used (Daley *et al.*, 1993; Peterson *et al.*, 1994; Duesberg and Peterson, 1997; Moore *et al.,* 2000). Most cats appear to tolerate the drug reasonably well, but drug-induced vomiting and anorexia have necessitated the discontinuation of the drug in some cats. If treatment is effective, metyrapone reduces both basal and ACTH-stimulated cortisol concentrations and ameliorates the clinical signs of disease.

Overall, the effectiveness of metyrapone in cats with hyperadrenocorticism is variable and may be transient, so the drug is best used short-term to prepare for surgical adrenalectomy. However, metyrapone is difficult to obtain, precluding its widespread use for cats with hyperadrenocorticism.

Trilostane

Trilostane reversibly inhibits the 3β-hydroxysteroid dehydrogenase enzyme system in the adrenal cortex, which decreases the synthesis of both glucocorticoids and mineralocorticoids. Trilostane is an effective medical treatment for dogs with hyperadrenocorticism (see Chapter 16), and experience collected over the last few years indicates that it is also a valuable treatment for cats with the disorder.

Thus far, trilostane treatment has been reported in seven cats with hyperadrenocorticism (six with pituitary-dependent disease and one with an adrenal tumour), using a daily dose of 4.2–13.6 mg/kg orally (Skelly *et al.,* 2003; Boag *et al.,* 2004; Neiger *et al.* 2004). Clinical signs of hyperadrenocorticism resolved to varying degrees after trilostane administration.

Based on both reported studies and personal experience, the recommended starting dose in cats with hyperadrenocorticism is 20–30 mg/cat orally per day, administered once daily or divided between feeding times. The daily trilostane dose frequently needs to be adjusted in cats, based upon resolution of clinical signs, serum biochemistry results and repeat ACTH response testing.

Cats on trilostane treatment should be evaluated at 2 weeks, 1 month, 2–3 months and every 1–3 months thereafter. At each recheck (scheduled at approximately 3–4 hours after the morning trilostane dose), the owner should be questioned and the cat examined. Blood is then collected for routine clinico-pathological analyses, and an ACTH response test is performed. Although the ideal target range for the post-ACTH cortisol concentration for cats receiving trilostane has yet to be determined, a post-ACTH cortisol concentration of 50–150 nmol/l should be targeted. In cats with persistent clinical signs and serum cortisol values higher than this range, the dose of trilostane is increased to 30–60 mg/cat per day, administered once daily or divided at the time of feeding. Additional dosage adjustments are made as required, based upon subsequent recheck examinations and ACTH response testing. In some cats, daily doses as high as 90–120 mg have been required to control clinical signs and lower ACTH-stimulated cortisol concentrations into the ideal range.

If a cat on trilostane presents with clinical signs consistent with hypocortisolism, one should stop the trilostane and perform an ACTH response test to confirm whether clinical signs are due to low cortisol concentrations. If hypoadrenocorticism is confirmed but serum electrolytes are normal, trilostane should be stopped and glucocorticoids administered. If hypoadrenocorticism is associated with hyperkalaemia or hyponatraemia, trilostane should be discontinued for a month and both glucocorticoids and mineralocorticoids administered.

Overall, although further investigation is needed, trilostane appears to be a valuable option for treatment of cats with hyperadrenocorticism and provides a useful medical alternative to metyrapone. Trilostane should be extremely useful in the preoperative preparation of cats with hyperadrenocorticism, prior to unilateral or bilateral adrenalectomy, but the drug may also be useful as the sole agent in the long-term management of some cats.

Radiation therapy

Pituitary radiotherapy

Radiation therapy has been used with partial success to treat a number of cats with pituitary-dependent hyperadrenocorticism (Peterson *et al.*, 1994; Duesberg and Peterson, 1997, Feldman and Nelson, 2004, Mayer *et al.*, 2006; Sellon *et al.*, 2009). Pituitary radiotherapy may help decrease tumour size and prolong survival in cats with a large or invasive pituitary tumour, and also offers a potential cure for cats with pituitary-dependent hyperadrenocorticism. However, because the decrease in both tumour size and ACTH secretion are often delayed, many cats die of complications attributable to hyperadrenocorticism before radiotherapy can adequately control the disease. Use of medical therapy (e.g. trilostane) to help control hyperadrenocorticism is therefore recommended prior to performing radiotherapy in cats with pituitary-dependent hyperadrenocorticism.

Other disadvantages of radiotherapy for treatment of cats with hyperadrenocorticism include its limited availability and high expense, as well as the frequent anaesthesia and extended hospitalization periods required to perform the treatment. In addition, multiple radiation treatments may be required in some cats (Sellon *et al.*, 2009).

Surgery

Unilateral and bilateral adrenalectomy

Details of the surgical procedures can be found in the *BSAVA Manual of Canine and Feline Abdominal Surgery*. Adrenalectomy appears to be the most successful method of treating cats with hyperadrenocorticism. Unilateral adrenalectomy should be performed in cats with a unilateral, cortisol-secreting adrenocortical tumour. Bilateral adrenalectomy must be performed in cats with pituitary-dependent bilateral adrenocortical hyperplasia.

Unfortunately, cats debilitated by chronic hypersecretion of glucocorticoids have an increased risk of infection and delayed wound healing postoperatively. Other postoperative complications include pancreatitis, thromboembolic phenomena, wound dehiscence, and hypoadrenocorticism. Pre-surgical medical stabilization (e.g. trilostane) of cats with severe clinical signs improves the postoperative outcome. In cats with pituitary-dependent hyperadrenocorticism that undergo successful bilateral adrenalectomy, the pituitary defect (e.g. pituitary adenoma) remains; these cats may later develop neurological signs associated with a compressive pituitary tumour.

Cats undergoing unilateral adrenalectomy generally require glucocorticoid supplementation for approximately 2 months postoperatively, until the glucocorticoid secretory function of the atrophied contralateral gland recovers. In contrast, cats undergoing bilateral adrenalectomy require constant, lifelong replacement of both mineralocorticoid and glucocorticoid hormones.

Cats with hyperadrenocorticism that are successfully treated by adrenalectomy typically have resolution of clinical signs (polyuria, polydipsia, polyphagia and lethargy) and physical abnormalities (pot belly, muscle wasting, alopecia, thin skin, hepatomegaly and infection) within 2–4 months postoperatively (Duesberg *et al.*, 1995; Watson and Herrtage, 1998; Feldman and Nelson, 2004). In addition, many cats have decreased requirements for exogenous insulin therapy.

Hypophysectomy

Microsurgical trans-sphenoidal hypophysectomy has been found to be an effective method of treatment for cats with pituitary-dependent hyperadrenocorticism (Meij *et al.*, 2001). However, as it requires an experienced, highly skilled veterinary surgeon and ad-vanced CT imaging facilities, this procedure remains a highly specialized form of treatment. Although it appears highly effective, at least in cats with a small pituitary tumour, hypophysectomy is associated with significant morbidity and the procedure is not likely to be effective in cats with a large pituitary adenoma. Another disadvantage of this treatment is that hypopituitarism develops during the immediate postoperative period, resulting in hypocortisolism, hypothyroidism and transient diabetes insipidus; therefore, substitution therapy with glucocorticoids, thyroxine and desmopressin are required for at least 2–4 weeks or lifelong after hypophysectomy.

Prognosis

Hyperadrenocorticism is a serious disease with a guarded to grave prognosis. Without treatment most cats will succumb to complications of the disease within a few weeks to months of diagnosis. One common reason for death of untreated cats is the deleterious effects of glucocorticoid excess on skin fragility, which leads to tearing of skin, opening of wounds and a delay in wound healing. The immuno-suppressive effects of glucocorticoid excess also predispose cats to infection. Finally, chronic hypercortisolism may adversely affect the cardiovascular system, leading to hypertension, pulmonary thromboembolism or congestive heart failure. Thus, the deleterious consequences of chronic cortisol excess on metabolic, immune and cardiovascular function are frequently responsible for the death of untreated cats with hyperadrenocorticism.

References and further reading

Boag AK, Neiger R and Church DB (2004) Trilostane treatment of bilateral adrenal enlargement and excessive sex steroid hormone production in a cat. *Journal of Small Animal Practice* **45**, 263–266
Boord M and Griffin C (1999) Progesterone-secreting adrenal mass in a cat with clinical signs of hyperadrenocorticism. *Journal of the American Veterinary Medicine Association* **214**, 666–669

Briscoe K, Barrs VR, Foster DF and Beatty JA (2009) Hyperaldosteronism and hyperprogesteronism in a cat. *Journal of Feline Medicine and Surgery* **11**, 758–762

Daley CA, Zerbe CA, Schick RO and Powers RD (1993) Use of metyrapone to treat pituitary-dependent hyperadrenocorticism in a cat with large cutaneous wounds. *Journal of the American Veterinary Medical Association* **202**, 956–960

Declue AE, Breshears LA, Pardo ID *et al.* (2005) Hyperaldosteronism and hyperprogesteronism in a cat with an adrenal cortical carcinoma. *Journal of Veterinary Internal Medicine* **19**, 355–358

de Lange MS, Galac S, Trip MR and Kooistra HS (2004) High urinary corticoid/creatinine ratios in cats with hyperthyroidism. *Journal of Veterinary Internal Medicine* **18**, 152–155

Duesberg CA, Nelson RW, Feldman EC, Vaden SL and Scott-Moncrieff JCR (1995) Adrenalectomy for treatment of hyperadrenocorticism in cats: 10 cases (1988–1992). *Journal of the American Veterinary Medical Association* **207**, 1066–1070

Duesberg C and Peterson ME (1997) Adrenal disorders in cats. *Veterinary Clinics of North America: Small Animal Practice* **27**, 321–347

Feldman EC and Nelson RW (2004) Hyperadrenocorticism in cats (Cushing's syndrome). In: *Canine and Feline Endocrinology and Reproduction, 3rd edn*, ed. EC Feldman and RW Nelson, pp. 358–393. WB Saunders, Philadelphia

Goossens MM, Meyer HP, Voorhout G and Sprang EP (1995) Urinary excretion of glucocorticoids in the diagnosis of hyperadrenocorticism in cats. *Domestic Animal Endocrinology* **12**, 355–362

Henry CJ, Clark TP, Young DW and Spano JS (1996) Urine cortisol:creatinine ratio in healthy and sick cats. *Journal of Veterinary Internal Medicine* **10**, 123–126

Hoenig M (2002) Feline hyperadrenocorticism – where are we now? *Journal of Feline Medicine and Surgery* **4**, 171–174

Kley S, Alt M, Zimmer C, Hoerauf A and Reusch CE (2007) Evaluation of the low-dose dexamethasone suppression test and ultrasonographic measurements of the adrenal glands in cats with diabetes mellitus. *Schweizer Archiv für Tierheilkunde* **149**, 493–500

Lien YH, Huang HP and Chang PH (2006) Iatrogenic hyperadrenocorticism in 12 cats. *Journal of the American Animal Hospital Association* **42**, 414–423

Lowe AD, Campbell KL, Barger A, Schaeffer DJ and Borst L (2008) Clinical, clinicopathological and histological changes observed in 14 cats treated with glucocorticoids. *Veterinary Record* **162**, 777–783.

Mayer MN, Greco DS and LaRue SM (2006) Outcomes of pituitary tumor irradiation in cats. *Journal of Veterinary Internal Medicine* **20**, 1151–1154

Meij BP, van der Vlugt-Meijer RH, van den Ingh TS, Flik G and Rijnberk (2005) Melanotroph pituitary adenoma in a cat with diabetes mellitus. *Veterinary Pathology* **42**, 92—97

Meij BP, Voorhout G, Van Den Ingh TS and Rijnberk A (2001) Transsphenoidal hypophysectomy for treatment of pituitary-dependent hyperadrenocorticism in 7 cats. *Veterinary Surgery* **30**, 72–86

Millard RP, Pickens EH, Wells KL (2009) Excessive production of sex hormones in a cat with an adrenocortical tumor. *Journal of the American Veterinary Medical Association* **234**, 505–508

Moore LE, Biller DS and Olsen DE (2000) Hyperadrenocorticism treated with metyrapone followed by bilateral adrenalectomy in a cat. *Journal of the American Veterinary Medicine Association* **217**, 691–694

Neiger R, Witt AL, Noble A and German AJ (2004) Trilostane therapy for treatment of pituitary-dependent hyperadrenocorticism in 5 cats. *Journal of Veterinary Internal Medicine* **18**, 160–164

Peterson ME and Kemppainen RJ (1992) Comparison of intravenous and intramuscular routes of administering cosyntropin for corticotropin stimulation testing in cats. *American Journal of Veterinary Research* **53**, 1392–1395

Peterson ME and Kemppainen RJ (1993) Dose-response relation between plasma concentrations of corticotropin and cortisol after administration of incremental doses of cosyntropin for corticotropin stimulation testing in cats. *American Journal of Veterinary Research* **54**, 300–304

Peterson ME, Randolph JF and Mooney CT (1994) Endocrine diseases. In: *The Cat: Diagnosis and Clinical Management, 2nd edn*, ed. RG Sherding, pp. 1404–1506. Churchill Livingstone, New York

Quante S, Sieber-Ruckstuhl N, Wilhelm S *et al.* (2009) Hyperprogesteronism due to bilateral adrenal carcinomas in a cat with diabetes mellitus. *Schweizer Archiv für Tierheilkunde* **151**, 437–442

Rossmeisl JH Jr, Scott-Moncrieff JC, Siems J *et al.* (2000) Hyperadrenocorticism and hyperprogesteronemia in a cat with an adrenocortical adenocarcinoma. *Journal of the American Animal Hospital Association* **36**, 512–517

Schoeman JP, Evans HJ, Childs D and Herrtage ME (2000) Cortisol responses to two different doses of intravenous synthetic ACTH (tetracosactrin) in overweight cats. *Journal of Small Animal Practice* **41**, 552–557

Schwedes CS (1997) Mitotane (o,p'-DDD) treatment in a cat with hyperadrenocorticism. *Journal of Small Animal Practice* **38**, 520–524

Sellon RK, Fidel J, Houston R and Gavin PR (2009) Linear-accelerator-based modified radiosurgical treatment of pituitary tumors in cats: 11 cases (1997–2008). *Journal of Veterinary Internal Medicine* **23**, 1038–1044

Skelly BJ, Petrus D and Nicholls PK (2003) Use of trilostane for the treatment of pituitary-dependent hyperadrenocorticism in a cat. *Journal of Small Animal Practice* **44**, 269–272

Watson PJ and Herrtage ME (1998) Hyperadrenocorticism in six cats. *Journal of Small Animal Practice* **39**, 175—184

Zerbe CA, Refsal KR, Peterson ME *et al.* (1987) Effect of nonadrenal illness on adrenal function in the cat. *American Journal of Veterinary Research* **48**, 451–454

Zimmer C, Horauf A and Reusch C (2000) Ultrasonographic examination of the adrenal gland and evaluation of the hypophyseal–adrenal axis in 20 cats. *Journal of Small Animal Practice* **41**, 156–160

18

Feline hypoadrenocorticism

Mark E. Peterson

Introduction

Hypoadrenocorticism is caused by deficient adreno-cortical secretion of glucocorticoids, either alone or concurrent with reduced secretion of mineralocorti-coids, and can be either naturally occurring or iatro-genic. Hypoadrenocorticism is extremely rare in cats: in the time since the first cat with primary hypoadrenocorticism was described almost 30 years ago (Johnessee *et al.*, 1983), fewer than 20 well documented cases of naturally occurring adre-nal insufficiency have been reported.

Aetiology and pathophysiology

Hypoadrenocorticism may result from primary adrenal failure, in which the destruction of >85–90% of both adrenal cortices leads to deficient secretion of glucocorticoids and mineralocorticoids. This is known as primary hypoadrenocorticism.

Alternatively, the disorder may result from insuffi-cient pituitary adrenocorticotropic hormone (ACTH) secretion, leading to atrophy of the adrenal cortex and impaired glucocorticoid secretion. This is known as secondary hypoadrenocorticism. How-ever, because the zona glomerulosa is spared in cats with secondary hypoadrenocorticism, adequate mineralocorticoid secretion is maintained.

Primary hypoadrenocorticism

In cats with naturally occurring primary hypoadreno-corticism, the cause of the complete destruction or atrophy of both adrenal cortices is usually unknown (idiopathic atrophy). As in humans and dogs with the disease, it is likely that many of these cats have immune-mediated destruction of the adrenal corti-ces. Less commonly, cats with primary hypoadreno-corticism may have a history of abdominal trauma, and in these cases it is thought that adrenal haem-orrhage is responsible for their disease (Berger and Reed, 1993; Brain, 1997). Primary hypoadrenocorti-cism secondary to bilateral adrenal gland infiltration by multicentric lymphoma has also been described in cats (Parnell *et al.*, 1999).

Although iatrogenic primary hypoadrenocorticism is rare in cats, this disorder is a well recognized complication of surgical treatment for pituitary-dependent hyperadrenocorticism (Cushing's disease) by bilateral adrenalectomy (Duesberg *et al.*, 1995).

In all cats with primary hypoadrenocorticism, the deficiency of both glucocorticoids and mineralocorti-coids causes the clinical signs observed. As the primary insult is to the adrenal glands, pituitary pro-duction of ACTH continues unhindered. In fact, reduced cortisol production results in decreased negative feedback at the pituitary gland, which allows an increased release of ACTH. For this rea-son, circulating concentrations of ACTH are usually greatly increased in cats with primary hypoadreno-corticism (Peterson *et al.*, 1989; Berger and Reed, 1993; Stonehewer and Tasker, 2001).

Secondary hypoadrenocorticism

Secondary hypoadrenocorticism can develop be-cause of deficient ACTH production associated with an underlying hypothalamic–pituitary disorder (e.g. pituitary or hypothalamic tumour) or from administra-tion of drugs that suppress pituitary ACTH produc-tion (Middleton *et al.*, 1987; Peterson *et al.*, 1994; Duesberg and Peterson, 1997). In cats, secondary hypoadrenocorticism has not yet been recognized as a naturally occurring disorder. It is likely to develop in some cats with large pituitary tumours, but clinical signs may be masked by those caused by the pitui-tary mass itself.

Iatrogenic hypoadrenocorticism, due to chronic administration of either glucocorticoids or progesto-gens, is the most common type of secondary adreno-cortical failure encountered in cats (Middleton *et al.*, 1987; Peterson, 1987; Peterson *et al.*, 1994; Duesberg and Peterson, 1997). Although hypophy-sectomy is not commonly used as a treatment for pituitary-dependent hyperadrenocorticism in cats, iatrogenic secondary hypoadrenocorticism is a well recognized complication of this procedure (Meij *et al.*, 2001).

Deficient ACTH secretion results in atrophy of the zona fasciculata and zona reticularis and a subse-quent decrease in glucocorticoid production. As ACTH has little stimulatory effect on mineralocorti-coid production, the adrenal zona glomerulosa is preserved. The deficiency in glucocorticoid produc-tion results in clinical signs similar to those observed in cats with primary hypoadrenocorticism; except that the derangements associated with mineralocorticoid deficiency (and subsequent electrolyte disturbances) are absent. Therefore, the clinical signs observed are usually less severe than those that develop in cats with primary hypoadrenocorticism.

Clinical features

Naturally occurring primary hypoadrenocorticism has been well documented in 18 cats: of these, 14 had idiopathic atrophy of the adrenal cortex, 2 had traumatically induced hypoadrenocorticism and 2 had adrenal lymphoma. The cats with idiopathic hypoadrenocorticism were of mixed breeding, ranging in age from 1 to 14 years (median age 4 years), with no obvious sex predilection.

The clinical signs and physical examination findings in the 18 reported cats with primary hypoadrenocorticism are similar to those observed in dogs with the disease. The most common owner complaints include lethargy, anorexia and weight loss (Figure 18.1). Vomiting, polyuria and polydipsia are less commonly reported. In some cats, the clinical manifestations may wax and wane; this temporary remission usually occurs after parenteral fluid and corticosteroid administration.

On physical examination, the most common findings are depression, dehydration, weakness, hypothermia, extended capillary refill time and a weak pulse. Collapse, bradycardia and a painful abdomen are observed less frequently.

Diagnosis

Routine clinicopathological features

Haematology

Haematological abnormalities that may develop in cats with primary hypoadrenocorticism include lymphocytosis and eosinophilia, as well as mild normocytic, normochromic, non-regenerative anaemia (Figure 18.2). The finding of reference interval or high eosinophil and lymphocyte counts in a sick cat with signs suggestive of hypoadrenocorticism is clinically significant, because the expected response to stress is eosinopenia and lymphopenia.

Clinical feature	Number of cats	Percentage of cats
Historical owner complaints		
Lethargy or depression	18	100
Anorexia	17	94
Weight loss	14	78
Vomiting	10	56
Waxing–waning course	7	39
Previous response to therapy	6	33
Polyuria and polydipsia	5	28
Dysphagia	1	6
Physical examination findings		
Depression	18	100
Dehydration	16	89
Weakness	14	78
Hypothermia	12	67
Extended capillary refill time	8	44
Weak pulse	7	39
Collapse/inability to rise	5	28
Bradycardia	2	11
Painful abdomen	1	6
Constipation	1	6

18.1 Clinical features in 18 cats with primary hypoadrenocorticism. (Data from Johnessee *et al.*, 1983; Peterson *et al.*, 1989; Berger and Reed, 1993; Ballmer-Rusca, 1995; Brain, 1997; Parnell *et al.*, 1999; Tasker *et al.*, 1999; Stonehewer and Tasker, 2001; Redden, 2005)

Diagnostic feature	Number of cats	Percentage of cats
Haematology		
Anaemia	5	28
Lymphocytosis	4	22
Eosinophilia	1	6
Biochemistry		
Sodium-to-potassium ratio <27:1	18	100
Hyponatraemia	18	100
Hyperkalaemia	17	94
Azotaemia	15	83
Hyperphosphataemia	13	72
Hypochloraemia	13	72
Low total CO_2 (metabolic acidosis)	4	22
Hypercalcaemia	3	17
Urinalysis		
Specific gravity <1.030	10/15	75
Specific gravity >1.030	5/15	25
Pituitary–adrenal function tests		
Low basal serum cortisol	17	94
Subnormal ACTH-stimulated cortisol	17/17	100
High endogenous ACTH concentration	10/10	100

18.2 Diagnostic features in 18 cats with primary hypoadrenocorticism. (Data from Johnessee *et al.*, 1983; Peterson *et al.*, 1989; Berger and Reed, 1993; Ballmer-Rusca, 1995; Brain, 1997; Parnell *et al.*, 1999; Tasker *et al.*, 1999; Stonehewer and Tasker, 2001; Redden, 2005)

Biochemistry

Most cats with primary hypoadrenocorticism develop the classical electrolyte changes associated with mineralocorticoid deficiency, including hyponatraemia, hypochloraemia and hyperkalaemia (Figure 18.2). The extracellular fluid volume contraction (and subsequent decreased renal perfusion) associated with primary adrenocortical insufficiency often results in prerenal azotaemia and hyperphosphataemia.

It is important to realize, however, that most sick cats in which altered serum electrolyte changes are found on serum biochemical testing will *not* have primary hypoadrenocorticism. In one study of 49 sick cats with decreased sodium-to-potassium ratios, the final diagnoses included gastrointestinal disease, urinary disease, cardiorespiratory disease and artefactually decreased Na:K ratios (Bell, *et al.,* 2005). None of these 49 cats had a final diagnosis of hypoadrenocorticism.

Urinalysis

As in dogs with primary hypoadrenocorticism, pretreatment urine specific gravity varies but urine may be more dilute than would be expected in a cat with prerenal azotaemia. Care must be taken not to misdiagnose primary renal failure in these cases. The cause of this apparent loss of renal concentrating ability is poorly understood, but may be secondary to renal sodium loss with resultant medullary washout.

Radiography and electrocardiography

Radiography demonstrated hypoperfusion of the lungs and microcardia in approximately half of the cats with primary hypoadrenocorticism. Electrocardiography revealed sinus bradycardia in 2 of the 18 cats, and atrial premature contractions in one (Peterson *et al.,* 1989). None of the cats with primary hypoadrenocorticism showed other ECG changes commonly associated with hyperkalaemia in dogs and humans, such as peaking of the T wave, reduced or absent P wave or atrial standstill.

Pituitary–adrenal function tests

ACTH response test

The most accurate screening test for hypoadrenocorticism in cats is the ACTH response test. The finding of a low basal serum cortisol concentration with a subnormal or negligible response to ACTH is diagnostic for adrenocortical insufficiency, but does not differentiate between primary and secondary causes of hypoadrenocorticism. When interpreting the test results, it is imperative to compare them to reference interval values obtained in healthy cats; this is because cats tend to respond to ACTH with a smaller rise in peak serum cortisol concentrations than do dogs (Peterson *et al.,* 1994; Duesberg and Peterson, 1997).

One common protocol for ACTH response testing in cats is to collect blood for determination of circulating cortisol concentration before and at 60 minutes after administration of 0.125 mg synthetic ACTH (tetracosactide or cosyntropin) intravenously. Use of the intravenous route for ACTH administration is very important in cats with suspected hypoadrenocorticism, especially if the cat is dehydrated. In addition, findings in healthy cats indicate that ACTH given by the intravenous route induces a greater and more prolonged adrenocortical stimulation than intramuscular administration (Peterson and Kemppainen, 1992).

Many glucocorticoid preparations, including hydrocortisone and prednisolone/prednisone, cross-react in most cortisol assays to give a falsely elevated endogenous cortisol determination, and therefore should not be administered until the ACTH response test is completed. Dexamethasone, on the other hand, can be administered before the ACTH response test because it has little or no influence on the measurement of endogenous cortisol concentrations.

A subnormal serum cortisol response to ACTH administration accompanied by serum electrolyte findings of hyperkalaemia and hyponatraemia is consistent with primary hypoadrenocorticism. If serum electrolyte changes are not found, one of the following may be present:

- Early primary hypoadrenocorticism with at least some residual mineralocorticoid secretion
- Secondary hypoadrenocorticism resulting from pituitary or hypothalamic disease
- Most commonly, secondary hypoadrenocorticism resulting from the administration of drugs such as glucocorticoids or progestogens.

Endogenous ACTH concentration

Once steroid or progestogen administration (or any other iatrogenic cause of hypoadrenocorticism) has been excluded, circulating ACTH concentration should be determined to help distinguish between primary and secondary hypoadrenocorticism. Plasma ACTH concentrations are extremely high in cats with primary hypoadrenocorticism (Peterson *et al.,* 1989; Berger and Reed, 1993; Stonehewer and Tasker, 2001), whereas cats with secondary hypoadrenocorticism have inappropriately low plasma ACTH concentrations when compared with circulating cortisol concentrations (Peterson *et al.,* 1994; Duesberg and Peterson, 1997).

Samples for plasma ACTH determination must be collected prior to treatment with glucocorticoids, as these drugs suppress pituitary ACTH secretion and may result in 'false' reference interval or low plasma ACTH concentrations in cats with primary hypoadrenocorticism. It is also important to remember that blood samples for determination of endogenous ACTH concentration need to be handled carefully, as ACTH can degrade rapidly after collection. Special sample handling is required as outlined in Chapter 1. Mishandling of samples potentially results in falsely decreased values, which could erroneously suggest secondary rather than primary hypoadrenocorticism.

Treatment

Initial treatment

Fluid therapy

In cats with acute or life-threatening primary adrenal failure, initial therapy should be aimed at restoring the circulating blood volume, providing an immediate source of glucocorticoid, and correcting serum electrolyte disturbances (i.e. hyperkalaemia, hyponatraemia). An indwelling intravenous catheter should be placed, preferably in the jugular vein, to allow for the administration of large volumes of isotonic fluids. The intravenous fluid of choice is 0.9% saline, administered at 20–40 ml/kg/h during the first 1–3 hours. If the cat begins to improve, the rate of administration may be slowed before the total bolus has been given. The endpoint of resuscitation is an improvement in tissue perfusion, which is clinically recognized by an improvement in mucous membrane colour, better quality pulses, a decrease in the heart rate towards normal and improved mentation.

Once fluid deficits are restored, the rate of fluid administration should be decreased to maintenance rates of 2.5 ml/kg/h (60 ml/kg/day), given by continuous infusion. Fluid administration is tapered as described when azotaemia resolves, serum electrolyte abnormalities are corrected, and the cat is eating and drinking on its own.

Glucocorticoid therapy

Rapid intravenous administration of a glucocorticoid is also extremely important in the initial management of severe adrenocortical insufficiency. In most cases, dexamethasone at 0.5 mg/kg i.v. is adequate and will not interfere with concurrent ACTH response testing. Alternatively, hydrocortisone can be administered at 5–10 mg/kg i.v. q6h or as a continuous infusion (0.5–0.625 mg/kg/h) for the first 24 hours. However, these doses are based on studies in dogs (see Chapter 15) and no feline-specific dosages have been evaluated. If hydrocortisone is used as initial glucocorticoid therapy, it should not be administered until the ACTH response test has been completed.

Once the test has been completed and the cat is stable, glucocorticoid replacement should then be continued as prednisolone (0.2 mg/kg i.m. q24h). Oral administration of this daily glucocorticoid dosage can be instituted once the cat can swallow without vomiting. In cats, use of prednisolone is preferred over the pro-drug prednisone, which must be converted to prednisolone to be metabolically active. In one study of cats, only 21% of orally administered prednisone was absorbed and converted to prednisolone in the circulation (Graham-Mize *et al.*, 2005). For that reason, prednisolone is the glucocorticoid of choice for long-term treatment of hypoadrenocorticism in cats.

Mineralocorticoid therapy

Once the cat is stabilized and can swallow without vomiting, mineralocorticoid replacement therapy should also be started with fludrocortisone acetate, administered orally at 0.1 mg/cat/day (Peterson *et al.*, 1989, 1994; Duesberg and Peterson, 1997; Tasker *et al.*, 1999). Although not available in most countries other than the USA, the mineralocorticoid desoxycorticosterone pivalate (DOCP) also works well in most cats when administered intramuscularly at an initial dosage of 12.5 mg/cat/month (Peterson *et al.*, 1989, 1994; Duesberg and Peterson, 1997; Redden, 2005). The mineralocorticoid effects of either fludrocortisone acetate or DOCP enhance renal potassium excretion and sodium resorption, thereby normalizing serum electrolyte abnormalities.

In contrast to dogs, in which the major clinical signs of primary hypoadrenocorticism usually resolve rapidly within a day or two of treatment, signs of weakness, lethargy and anorexia may persist for 3–5 days in cats with acute adrenocortical insufficiency, despite appropriate management (Peterson *et al.*, 1989; Tasker *et al.*, 1999).

Long-term treatment and prognosis

Once stabilized, maintenance therapy for cats with primary adrenocortical insufficiency consists of life-long mineralocorticoid and glucocorticoid supplementation. With appropriate replacement therapy, the long-term prognosis for cats with primary (especially idiopathic) hypoadrenocorticism is excellent.

Either oral fludrocortisone acetate or intramuscular injections of DOCP can be given for chronic mineralocorticoid therapy (Peterson *et al.*, 1989; Berger and Reed, 1993; Peterson *et al.*, 1994; Duesberg and Peterson, 1997; Tasker *et al.*, 1999; Stonehewer and Tasker, 2001; Redden, 2005). The dosage of mineralocorticoid supplementation is adjusted as needed, based on serial serum electrolyte concentrations, determined every 1–2 weeks during the initial maintenance period. The goal of mineralocorticoid treatment is normalization of the serum sodium and potassium concentrations.

Glucocorticoid replacement, as needed, is usually accomplished with oral administration of prednisolone, at a total dosage of 1–1.25 mg/cat q24h. If owners find it difficult to give oral medication to their cat, glucocorticoid supplementation can be given intramuscularly as repositol methylprednisolone acetate, at a total dosage of 10 mg/cat/month. At these low replacement glucocorticoid doses, adverse effects associated with iatrogenic hyperadrenocorticism (i.e. polyuria, polydipsia, polyphagia, pendulous abdomen, hair loss) rarely, if ever, develop in cats.

References and further reading

Ballmer-Rusca E (1995) What is your diagnosis? Hypoadrenocorticism in a domestic cat. *Schweizer Archiv für Tierheilkunde* **137**, 65–67

Bell R, Mellor DJ, Ramsey I, and Knottenbert C (2005) Decreased sodium:potassium ratios in cats: 49 cases. *Veterinary Clinical Pathololology* **34**, 110–114

Berger SL and Reed JR (1993) Traumatically induced hypoadrenocorticism in a cat. *Journal of the American Animal Hospital Association* **29**, 337–339

Brain PH (1997) Trauma-induced hypoadrenocorticism in a cat. *Australian Veterinary Practitioner* **27**, 178–181

Duesberg CA, Nelson RW, Feldman EC, Vaden SL and Scott-Moncrieff JCR (1995) Adrenalectomy for treatment of hyperadrenocorticism in cats: 10 cases (1988–1992). *Journal of the American Veterinary Medical Association* **207**, 1066–1070

Duesberg C and Peterson ME (1997) Adrenal disorders in cats. *Veterinary Clinics of North America: Small Animal Practice* **27**, 321–347

Graham-Mize CA, Rosser EJ and Hauptman J (2005) Absorption, bioavailability, and activity of prednisone and prednisolone in cats. In: *Advances in Veterinary Dermatology, Vol.5*, ed. A Hiller *et al.*, pp. 152–158. Blackwell, Oxford

Johnessee JS, Peterson ME and Gilbertson SR (1983) Primary hypoadrenocorticism in a cat. *Journal of the American Veterinary Medical Association* **183**, 881–882.

Meij BP, Voorhout G, Van Den Ingh TS and Rijnberk A (2001) Transsphenoidal hypophysectomy for treatment of pituitary-dependent hyperadrenocorticism in 7 cats. *Veterinary Surgery* **30**, 72–86

Middleton DJ, Watson AD, Howe CJ and Caterson ID (1987) Suppression of cortisol responses to exogenous adrenocorticotrophic hormone, and the occurrence of side effects attributable to glucocorticoid excess, in cats during therapy with megestrol acetate and prednisolone. *Canadian Journal of Veterinary Research* **51**, 60–65

Parnell NK, Powell LL, Hohenhaus AE, Patnaik AK and Peterson ME (1999). Hypoadrenocorticism as the primary manifestation of lymphoma in two cats. *Journal of the American Veterinary Medical Association* **214**, 1208–1211

Peterson ME (1987) Effects of megestrol acetate on glucose tolerance and growth hormone secretion in the cat. *Research in Veterinary Science* **42**, 354–357

Peterson ME, Greco DS and Orth DN (1989) Primary hypoadrenocorticism in ten cats. *Journal of Veterinary Internal Medicine* **3**, 55–58

Peterson ME and Kemppainen RJ (1992) Comparison of intravenous and intramuscular routes of administering cosyntropin for corticotropin stimulation testing in cats. *American Journal of Veterinary Research* **53**, 1392–1395

Peterson ME, Randolph JF and Mooney CT (1994) Endocrine diseases. In: *The Cat: Diagnosis and Clinical Management, 2nd edn*, ed. RG Sherding, pp. 1404–1506. Churchill Livingstone, New York

Redden B (2005) Feline hypoadrenocorticism. *Compendium on Continuing Education for the Practicing Veterinarian* **27**, 697–706

Stonehewer J and Tasker S (2001) Hypoadrenocorticism in a cat. *Journal of Small Animal Practice* **42**, 186–190

Tasker S, MacKay AD and Sparkes AH (1999) A case of feline primary hypoadrenocorticism. *Journal of Feline Medicine and Surgery* **1**, 257–260

19

Feline hyperaldosteronism

Andrea M. Harvey and Kent R. Refsal

Introduction

Hyperaldosteronism results from increased secretion of aldosterone from the adrenal glands and may be primary or secondary in origin. Secondary hyperaldosteronism occurs in response to stimulation of the renin–angiotensin–aldosterone system (RAAS) and may therefore be a consequence of any disorder that stimulates the RAAS, such as dehydration, hypotension, reduced renal perfusion (most commonly secondary to renal disease) or sodium deficiency (reduced intake or increased loss). Renin-secreting tumours have been reported in humans as a cause of secondary hyperaldosteronism but have not been reported as such in cats.

Animals suffering from primary hyperaldosteronism (PHA) undergo an inappropriate increase in aldosterone secretion, independent of the RAAS. This is most commonly caused by unilateral adrenal neoplasia. Bilateral adrenal tumours and bilateral adrenal hyperplasia have also been described in cats. Until recently primary hyperaldosteronism (PHA) was considered a rare disease, but it is now increasingly recognized as a cause of hypokalaemia and/or hypertension in cats.

Primary hyperaldosteronism was first reported in an elderly Domestic Shorthair (DSH) cat presenting with hypokalaemic polymyopathy (Eger *et al.*, 1983). Since 1999, PHA has been reported in at least a further 35 cats. Adrenocortical adenoma or adenocarcinoma was identified in 24 cats, and 13 cases were included in a single case series (Ash *et al.*, 2005), allowing a more detailed description of this disease. Of the 13 cats in this series, 9 were diagnosed at a single first-opinion practice in the UK, raising the possibility that the condition is more common than previously thought. Some aldosterone-secreting adrenal neoplasms may also produce excessive progesterone and/or corticosterone.

A second case series of 11 cats described a non-tumourous form of hyperaldosteronism that shares similarities with idiopathic adrenal hyperplasia in humans (Javadi *et al.*, 2005). The authors now regularly encounter cases of primary hyperaldosteronism in cats and receive frequent advice calls from general practitioners, adding to the suspicion that this disease is more common than previously recognized.

Physiology of the RAAS

The RAAS acts to maintain the volume of extracellular fluid, circulatory pressure, and electrolyte homeostasis through the integrated effects of various enzymes and hormones, chiefly on the vasculature and kidney (Figure 19.1).

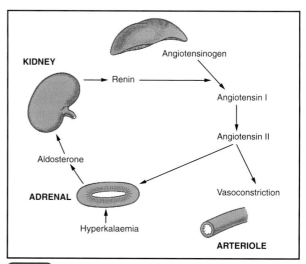

19.1 Regulation of aldosterone release.

Active release of renin is stimulated predominantly by decreased renal perfusion detected by baroreceptors in the afferent arterioles. Other stimuli include a decrease in sodium content in glomerular filtrate, as detected by the macula densa cells of the proximal tubule, and sympathetic nerve stimulation via alpha-adrenergic receptors. In the circulation, renin acts on angiotensinogen to cleave angiotensin I, which is then converted to angiotensin II by angiotensin-converting enzyme (ACE). Angiotension II has potent biological effects, principally arising from its binding to type 1 receptors to mediate vasoconstriction, promote renal tubular reabsorption of sodium, stimulate release of aldosterone from the adrenal cortex, and exert negative feedback on the release of renin.

The synthesis and effects of aldosterone

Aldosterone is synthesized from cholesterol through a series of intermediary metabolites, including progesterone, 11-deoxycorticosterone and corticosterone (Figure 19.2) in the zona glomerulosa of the

204

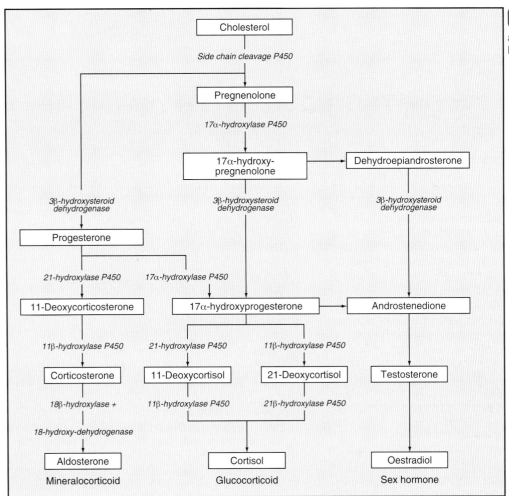

19.2 Simplified diagram of adrenal steroid biosynthesis.

adrenal cortex. In addition to the stimulus from angiotensin II, aldosterone is released as a direct response to hyperkalaemia and, to a lesser extent, after adrenocorticotropic hormone (ACTH) release from the anterior pituitary gland.

After secretion into the circulation, aldosterone enters target tissues and exerts its effects through binding to mineralocorticoid receptors. In the kidneys aldosterone acts on the distal collecting tubule and collecting ducts to stimulate activity of epithelial sodium channels, promoting sodium reabsorption with concurrent loss of potassium and hydrogen ions. Therefore, when stimulated, the classic cascade of events in the RAAS results in an increase of circulatory pressure via vasoconstriction and retention of sodium.

Aetiology

Adrenal neoplasia

Unilateral adrenocortical neoplasia is the most commonly described cause of PHA in cats, with adenomas and carcinomas appearing to occur with approximately equal frequency.

Bilateral adrenal neoplasms have been described only very rarely in cats. Bilateral adrenal adenomas were identified in two cats, although the bilateral nature of the adrenal disease was only discovered on post-mortem examination, highlighting the necessity for careful evaluation of both adrenal glands at initial investigation (Ash et al., 2005). A further patient underwent surgery for the removal of a left adrenal adenoma and went on to develop a right adrenal carcinoma within 2 years (MacKay et al., 1999).

Aldosterone-producing adrenal neoplasms have also been recognized in conjunction with other endocrinopathies, albeit very rarely. Presumed multiple endocrine neoplasia type 1 was reported in one cat with an aldosterone-producing adenoma and concurrent insulinoma and functional parathyroid adenoma (Reimer et al., 2005). Some adrenocortical tumours, especially carcinomas, secrete glucocorticoids or sex steroids in addition to mineralocorticoids. In particular, hyperprogesteronism with associated diabetes mellitus has been reported in combination with hyperaldosteronism (De Clue et al., 2005; Briscoe et al., 2009). The putative mechanism for concurrent hyperprogesteronism and hyperaldosteronism is increased production of progesterone, as an intermediate in the synthesis of aldosterone, from neoplastic cells of the zona glomerulosa alone. Alternatively, there may be increased secretion of aldosterone and progesterone from neoplastic cells of the zona glomerulosa and fasciculata/reticularis respectively, although there is no evidence for this. A recently reported laboratory survey measured progesterone, cortisol and corticosterone in feline serum samples submitted for plasma aldosterone assay and found a significant number of samples with elevated aldosterone (especially >3000 pmol/l; reference interval 110–500 pmol/l) also had marked elevations in progesterone and corticosterone (Refsal and Mazaki-Tovi, 2009).

Adrenal hyperplasia

In 2005, a series of 11 cats were described as having non-tumourous PHA (Javadi *et al.*, 2005). These cases appear similar to bilateral adrenal hyperplasia, a disorder well described in humans. Most cats have laboratory evidence of mild renal disease. At necropsy, the presence of bilateral adrenal hyperplasia with identification of nodular hyperplasia of the zona glomerulosa bilaterally is seen. Histopathological changes in the kidneys reveal hyaline arteriolar sclerosis, glomerular sclerosis, tubular atrophy and interstitial fibrosis; these are changes classically recognized in humans with the disorder.

Clinical features

Signalment

Feline PHA is a disease of middle-aged to older cats. The reported age of onset ranges from 5 to 20 years, with an average of 11 years for cases of adrenal neoplasia. The age for cases of adrenal hyperplasia appears similar, ranging from 11 to 18 years. There does not appear to be any breed predisposition; most reported cases have been DSH cats, with one case each of Domestic Longhair (DLH), Siamese, Burmese and Burmilla being diagnosed with adrenal neoplasia. No sex predisposition exists; all reported cases have been neutered, with roughly equal numbers of female and male cats.

Clinical signs

The major clinical signs are similar, whether PHA results from adrenal adenoma, carcinoma or hyperplasia. Most commonly, the major initial presenting signs relate directly to increased aldosterone concentrations and can be divided broadly into either hypokalaemic myopathy or acute onset blindness – or both.

Hypokalaemic polymyopathy

This is the most common presentation for cases with adrenal neoplasia, with most presenting with various signs consistent with muscle dysfunction, particularly cervical ventroflexion (Figure 19.3), hindlimb weakness and ataxia, or, less commonly, limb stiffness, dysphagia and collapse. In some cases the muscular features are mild and episodic, while in others they are acute and severe in onset. This presentation is less common in adrenal hyperplasia, with only a few reported cases having signs of hypokalaemic polymyopathy.

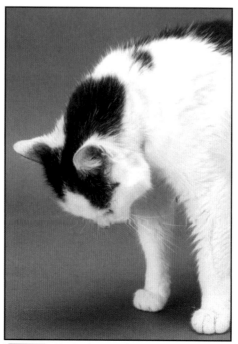

19.3 Typical ventroflexion of the neck in a hypokalaemic cat. (Courtesy of Ellie Mardell and Andy Sparkes)

Acute-onset blindness

Intraocular haemorrhage (Figure 19.4) or acute-onset blindness resulting from retinal detachment (Figure 19.5) is less commonly the main presenting sign in adrenal neoplasia. In both cats shown in Figures 19.4 and 19.5, hypertension was severe (systolic blood pressure >200 mmHg), and no other clinical signs were reported. Although not always the main presenting sign, subclinical hypertension is common. Hypertensive retinopathy (Figure 19.6) appears to be a more common major presenting sign in cases of adrenal hyperplasia, with the majority of cases presenting with retinal detachment or subretinal, intraretinal and intravitreal haemorrhages associated with systemic hypertension. Overall, hypertension was more severe in this group of cats: all systolic blood pressures were >185 mmHg, with some >200 mmHg.

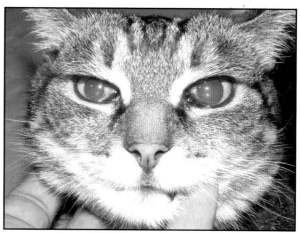

19.4 Bilateral iridal haemorrhage in a cat with systemic hypertension. (Courtesy of Tim Knott, Rowe Veterinary Group)

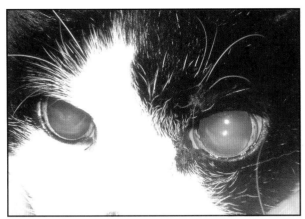

19.5 Bilateral retinal detachment in a cat with systemic hypertension. This cat presented with sudden onset blindness. (Courtesy of Tim Knott, Rowe Veterinary Group)

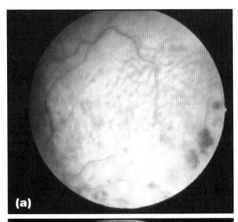

(a)

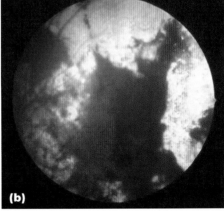

(b)

19.6 Hypertensive retinopathy can have a variable appearance, such as **(a)** retinal oedema with patchy areas of retinal haemorrhage or **(b)** more diffuse retinal haemorrhage. (Courtesy of Jim Carter, University of Bristol)

Other possible signs

Although not yet described specifically in association with hyperaldosteronism, hypertension may also result in central nervous system oedema, haemorrhage or ischaemia, which may contribute to neurological signs such as seizures, ataxia, and behavioural changes. Polyuria and polydipsia are reported in about 15% of PHA cases (due to adrenal tumours) and may arise secondary to concurrent conditions such as hyperthyroidism; this may be either as a direct consequence of hypokalaemia or as a result of vasopressin resistance and increased osmotic threshold of vasopressin release. Polyphagia is reported in 10% of cases, the cause of which is unknown. Concurrent hypercortisolaemia may be responsible, although it has not yet been clearly documented. Unrecognized hyperprogesteronism may also account for this (see below).

Clinical signs related to other steroid excess

There are two single case reports of cats with aldosterone-secreting adrenal tumours that had concurrent hyperprogesteronism. One of these had an adrenocortical carcinoma; the large adrenal mass in the other case was presumed to be a carcinoma but histopathological examination was not available. In these cases the signs of hyperprogesteronism predominated; this results in very similar clinical signs to those encountered with hypercortisolaemia, namely secondary diabetes mellitus, polyuria, polydipsia, polyphagia, poor coat condition, seborrhoea, thin fragile skin and a pot-bellied appearance (Figure 19.7). Elevated serum progesterone concentrations may also contribute to muscle weakness, which may be attributed initially to hypokalaemic polymyopathy. Clinical signs of hypertension may be present.

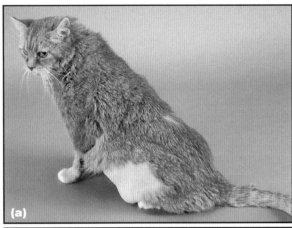

(a)

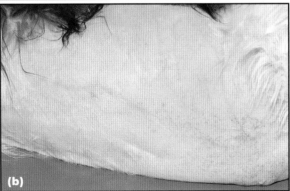

(b)

19.7 Both these cats were diagnosed with concurrent hyperaldosteronism and hyperprogesteronism, due to unilateral adrenal carcinomas. **(a)** This cat's primary presenting problems were progressive symmetrical alopecia, seborrhoea oleosa, abdominal distension and, more recently, diabetes mellitus, polyphagia, failure of hair regrowth and hindlimb weakness. **(b)** Note the very thin skin and prominent cutaneous blood vessels commonly seen in cases of hyperprogesteronism. (Courtesy of Langford Veterinary Services)

Clinical signs related to concomitant illness

Because cats affected with PHA are older, the possibility of concurrent diseases that may divert attention from hyperaldosteronism must also be considered. Concomitant illnesses such as chronic kidney disease or hyperthyroidism may be wrongly assumed to be the cause of hypokalaemia and/or hypertension. In general, hypertension associated with hyperthyroidism alone is mild; if severe hypertension is seen, the possibility of concurrent PHA should be considered. Left ventricular hypertrophy secondary to hypertension and/or concurrent disease such as hyperthyroidism may be present, resulting in typical clinical findings of cardiomyopathy, such as a systolic heart murmur, tachycardia, gallop rhythm or dysrhythmias. Development of congestive heart failure as a consequence of hypertension alone is rare. Cardiac disease associated solely with PHA has not been described in cats, and the possibility of secondary hyperaldosteronism should be considered if a patient in congestive heart failure has an elevated PAC. However, the cardiac effects of elevated aldosterone are well recognized in humans and it is therefore possible that cardiac disease could arise as a consequence of PHA.

Clinicopathological features

No specific haematological abnormalities of PHA have been identified. On serum biochemistry, hypokalaemia is most often present; however, the degree is variable. Because hypokalaemia is identified in cats for many other reasons (Figure 19.8), a mild to moderate hypokalaemia may be easily overlooked without consideration of hyperaldosteronism. Currently, most reported cases of PHA due to adrenal neoplasia are hypokalaemic; however, this could, in part, reflect the fact that hypokalaemia is often considered a prerequisite before evaluation for hyperaldosteronism is initiated. Persistence of hypokalaemia despite supplementation with potassium often prompts suspicion of hyperaldosteronism in cats. However, normokalaemia does not exclude the possibility of PHA, and PHA should certainly be considered as a differential diagnosis for unexplained hypertension (Figure 19.9), even in the absence of hypokalaemia. In fact, only approximately half of the described cases of adrenal hyperplasia were hypokalaemic (usually mild) at initial presentation. Such cases could easily be missed if hypokalaemia is considered a prerequisite for evaluation of PHA.

Serum sodium concentrations are usually within the reference interval. Hypernatraemia has only been reported in a few patients with PHA and, in all cases, was mild. The lack of significant hypernatraemia may be explained by concurrent volume expansion secondary to sodium retention. Creatine kinase is usually elevated in cats with polymyopathy, but again the degree of elevation is highly variable. A metabolic alkalosis may be observed, related to aldosterone-mediated excretion of hydrogen ions. Urea and creatinine may be elevated at the time of diagnosis, and progression of renal disease may be the cause of death in some cases. The presence of azotaemia may hinder the diagnosis in some cases, because

Reduced potassium intake
• Inappetence/anorexia
• Potassium-depleted diet
• Potassium-deficient intravenous fluid

Potassium translocation
• Alkalaemia
• Insulin administration
• Diabetic ketoacidosis
• Bicarbonate administration
• Periodic hypokalaemia (Burmese)
• Hypothermia
• Stimulation by catecholamines

Gastrointestinal loss of potassium
• Vomiting
• Diarrhoea
• Malabsorption

Renal loss of potassium
• Polyuria
• Chronic renal failure
• Acute renal failure (polyuric phase)
• Diuretic administration (loop or thiazide)
• Primary hyperaldosteronism
• Hyperadrenocorticism
• Renal tubular acidosis

Endocrine disease
• Hyperthyroidism
• Hyperadrenocorticism

Other diseases
• Hepatic failure
• Portal hypertension
• Congestive heart failure

19.8 Differential diagnosis of feline hypokalaemia.

Most common
• Renal disease (NB renal disease can also be secondary to PHA)
• Hyperthyroidism (usually mild hypertension)
• Primary hyperaldosteronism

Other possible causes (not proven in cats)
• Diabetes mellitus
• Hyperadrenocorticism
• Hyperprogesteronism (alone or with PHA)
• Obesity

19.9 Differential diagnoses for hypertension.

hypokalaemia and/or hypertension may simply be considered a consequence of the renal disease itself. In humans, progressive renal disease is a recognized sequel to PHA, with renal damage occurring because of a combination of elevated intraglomerular capillary pressure, inflammation and fibrosis, which are a direct effect of angiotensin II and chronic hypokalaemia. This is thought to also occur in cats, particularly in the adrenal hyperplasia cases where a progressively worsening azotaemia was documented in all reported cases.

Diagnostic imaging

Adrenal masses are rarely visible using radiography, and if a mass *is* seen it is more likely to be an adrenocortical carcinoma. Pulmonary metastases can occur, albeit infrequently; thoracic radiography (including right and left lateral projections) should therefore be performed prior to consideration of surgery, in order to screen for metastases.

Currently, ultrasonography is the best described imaging modality for detecting adrenal masses in cats. In all reported feline cases of PHA in which adrenal ultrasonography has been performed, unilateral adrenal enlargement with evidence of an adrenal mass has been identified, with sizes ranging from 10 to 46 mm in diameter (Figure 19.10). The contralateral adrenal gland may appear normal in appearance or may be unidentifiable. It is vital that the contralateral gland be assessed, as bilateral adenomas have been reported, albeit rarely. Bilateral adrenal carcinomas have also been reported in a cat with hyperprogesteronism (Quante *et al.*, 2009). Ultrasonography may also identify the presence and degree of invasion of the caudal vena cava by the tumour or related thrombus, and the presence of metastases to other organs. A close association of the tumour with the caudal vena cava is usually evident; however, to date imaging has not been useful in preoperative assessment of the likely ease of surgical removal of adrenal masses, or the likelihood of postoperative complications.

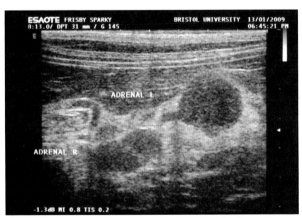

19.10 Ultrasonogram illustrating the typical hypoechoic appearance of an adrenal mass of the left adrenal gland. This mass was an adrenal adenoma. A unilateral adrenalectomy was successful in managing this case. The normal appearance of the right adrenal gland can also be seen. (Courtesy of Langford Veterinary Services)

Other imaging modalities, including magnetic resonance imaging (MRI; Figure 19.11), computed tomography (CT) and saphenous venography, have been reported in a small number of cases in an attempt to establish the extent of the adrenal mass before undertaking surgery. Results from MRI in one cat showed no evidence of extension into the caudal vena cava; however, the cat succumbed to fatal haemorrhage postoperatively. Saphenous venography was used in one cat to demonstrate lack of invasion of the caudal vena cava by an adrenal tumour, but surgery was not subsequently performed in that

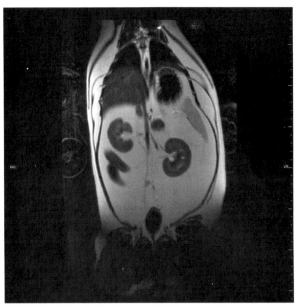

19.11 T2-weighted coronal MRI scan of the abdomen from the same case as Figure 19.10, demonstrating the significantly enlarged left adrenal gland, in comparison to the right. It can be seen that there is no evidence of invasion of the caudal vena cava in this case. (Courtesy of Langford Veterinary Services)

cat. CT, the imaging modality of choice in human patients, has been used successfully in a cat, but further data are needed to define its diagnostic utility compared to ultrasonography. Radionuclide scintigraphy has not been reported in assessment of feline PHA.

In the reported cases of non-tumourous PHA, ultrasonography and/or CT examination showed subtle abnormalities, such as an increase in adrenal echogenicity or areas of calcification and thickening and/or rounding of one pole of one or both adrenal glands, without evidence of adrenal neoplasia. Some cats had no visible adrenal changes.

Diagnosis

Plasma aldosterone concentration and other corticosteroids

The possibility of PHA should be considered in any case with hypokalaemia and/or hypertension, or when there is identification of an adrenal mass. Confirmation of diagnosis relies mainly on demonstrating an elevated plasma aldosterone concentration (PAC). The assay is widely available at commercial endocrine laboratories and requirements for collection and handling of serum or plasma are routine. There is no clear evidence for improved diagnostic performance by undertaking an ACTH stimulation test for aldosterone measurement. Baseline PAC has been elevated with respect to laboratory reference values in all reported cases of feline PHA related to an adrenocortical tumour. However, there may be wide variation in PAC in healthy cats and those with secondary hyperaldosteronism, and therefore results must be assessed relative to clinical signs.

Demonstration of an elevated PAC does not distinguish between primary and secondary hyperaldosteronism. The highest PAC values occur with adrenocortical tumours, in which baseline aldosterone concentrations are often >1000 pmol/l. However, PAC values vary widely with both primary and secondary hyperaldosteronism, and mean PAC >2000 pmol/l has been reported in cats with chronic renal disease. Furthermore, in early cases of PHA, and particularly in bilateral adrenal hyperplasia cases, PAC can be within the upper end of the reference interval at initial presentation. Therefore, ideally PAC needs to be interpreted together with plasma renin activity (PRA), which would be expected to be elevated in cases of secondary hyperaldosteronism. There are difficulties with measuring PRA (discussed in more detail below) and, as a consequence, demonstration of the presence of adrenocortical neoplasia concurrently with a markedly elevated PAC is considered sufficient to make a diagnosis of aldosterone-secreting adrenocortical tumour in cats, especially in conjunction with persistent hypokalaemia and hypertension. However, it is possible that an incidental non-functional adrenal neoplasm can occur in conjunction with secondary hyperaldosteronism. Histopathological confirmation of the neoplasm, together with resolution of clinical signs and PAC measurements, postoperatively assist in confirming the diagnosis.

Non-tumourous PHA is more difficult to diagnose without assessment of PRA (see later discussion). Potential causes of secondary hyperaldosteronism should be excluded with appropriate investigations, including those for renal, liver and cardiac disease. This is, however, particularly problematic in the case of concurrent azotaemia, given that non-tumourous PHA can cause progressive renal disease, in addition to renal disease being a cause of secondary hyperaldosteronism.

The physical appearance of some cats with PHA is so characteristic that clinicians may initially suspect a differential diagnosis of hyperadrenocorticism. Cats with PHA typically exhibit normal cortisol suppression after dexamethasone administration. Cortisol responses to ACTH response tests are variable. In reports to date, cats with hyperaldosteronism and hyperprogesteronism related to an adrenocortical tumour have normal to low baseline concentrations of cortisol with subnormal responses to ACTH stimulation. It is not known whether this subgroup of cats has normal, low or elevated concentrations of endogenous ACTH. If endogenous ACTH concentration is low, there is need for a more comprehensive survey of adrenocortical steroids to identify whether there is a steroid other than progesterone that may be exerting glucocorticoid effects.

Plasma renin activity

Reliably distinguishing primary from secondary hyperaldosteronism requires assessment of activity of the renin–angiotensin system. The most commonly employed analysis has been PRA. This can be problematic, as the assay is not widely commercially available (in the UK, offered by Cambridge Specialist Laboratory Services) and plasma samples must be processed quickly and kept frozen until assay to minimize degradation of renin prior to assay. Furthermore, PRA may also be influenced by certain drugs (e.g. angiotensin-converting enzyme inhibitors and beta-blockers) and dietary salt intake.

Plasma renin activity results have been reported in six cases of feline PHA due to adrenal neoplasia. Results were low in two cases, within reference interval in three cases and normal and then low when measured on 2 consecutive days in one further case. A reference interval PRA value does not, therefore, exclude the possibility that the hyperaldosteronism is caused by an adrenal tumour.

In humans, the ratio of PAC to PRA, known as the aldosterone:renin ratio (ARR) is regarded as the most reliable screening test, with a high ARR being indicative of PHA. Use of the ARR has been described in cats, where it assisted in the diagnosis of PHA in the eleven reported cases of non-tumourous PHA. These cats had high-normal to slightly increased PAC and low-normal or decreased PRA at presentation. Elevation of the ARR was the evidence used for diagnosing inappropriate excess of aldosterone secretion.

Mineralocorticoid function tests

In humans, there may be false positive results with the ARR, and mineralocorticoid function tests (MFTs) are used as confirmatory tests for PHA (Funder et al., 2008). The MFTs used in humans assess the response to treatments designed to suppress the RAAS and thus decrease circulating concentrations of aldosterone. Examples of MFTs include oral sodium loading, saline infusion, fludrocortisone administration with sodium supplementation, and the captopril challenge test.

Mineralocorticoid function tests are now being investigated for use in cats. A recent report assessed changes of the urinary aldosterone:creatinine ratio in healthy cats in response to increased dietary salt or administration of fludrocortisone acetate (Djajadiningrat-Laanen et al., 2008). In the reported study, healthy cats exhibited the most consistent decrease of the urinary aldosterone: creatinine ratio with administration of fludrocortisone acetate compared with dietary salt supplementation. One cat with an aldosterone-secreting adrenal carcinoma had an elevated ratio with no suppression in response to fludrocortisone acetate. Another recent study showed that twice-daily administration of enalapril (0.5 mg/kg) for 5 days did not suppress baseline serum aldosterone or decrease systolic blood pressure in healthy cats (Gal et al., 2009).

Due to the current difficulty of measuring PRA and lack of a defined mineralocorticoid suppression test in cats, two different diagnostic algorithms are suggested. Both are based initially on identification of appropriate clinical signs and documentation of an elevated PAC. One is further based on the ideal situation where PRA and/or MFTs are available (Figure 19.12). The other is an alternative algorithm which can be used when there is no available PRA and/or MFTs (Figure 19.13). A related algorithm based on

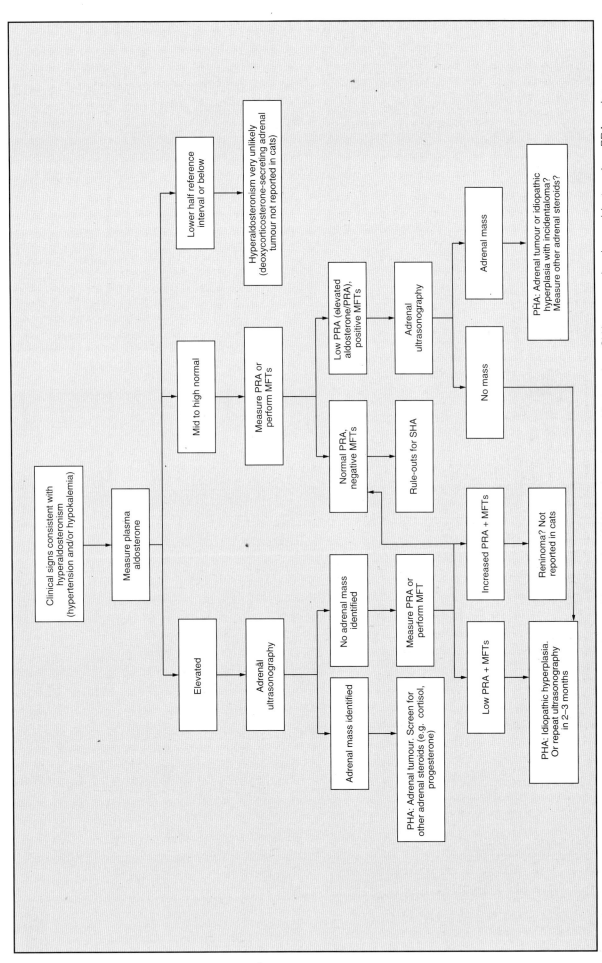

19.12 Algorithm demonstrating the diagnostic pathway of hyperaldosteronism. PHA = primary hyperaldosteronism; PRA = plasma renin activity; MFTs = mineralocorticoid function tests.(Reproduced and adapted from Refsal and Harvey (2010) with the permission of Saunders Elsevier)

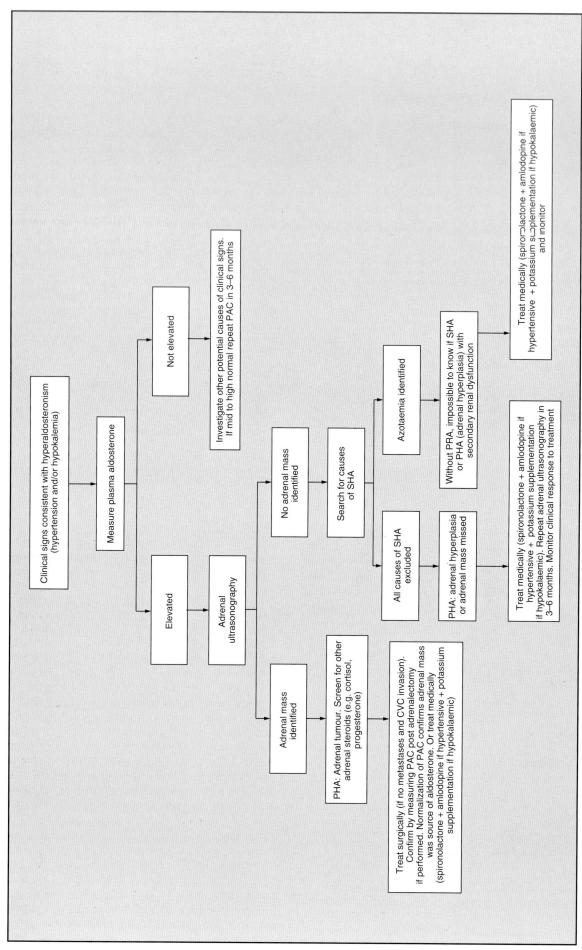

19.13 Algorithm demonstrating the diagnostic pathway of hyperaldosteronism when PRA/MFTs not available. PHA = primary hyperaldosteronism; SHA = secondary hyperaldosteronism; PRA = plasma renin activity; MFTs = mineralocorticoid function tests. (Reproduced and adapted from Refsal and Harvey (2010) with the permission of Saunders Elsevier)

initial identification of an adrenal mass has also been previously suggested (Shiel and Mooney, 2007).

Treatment

Initial treatment of PHA is directed at controlling hypokalaemia and/or hypertension. Potassium supplementation using potassium gluconate at 2–6 mmol orally q12h is recommended. However, intravenous potassium chloride may be required in more severely hypokalaemic cases. Amlodipine besylate (0.625–1.25 mg/cat orally q24h) is the initial treatment of choice for hypertension. Most hypertensive cats become normotensive with amlodipine treatment, but higher doses are sometimes required. Hypertension can become refractory to treatment in time.

Spironolactone, a competitive aldosterone receptor antagonist, is also recommended (2–4 mg/kg orally q24h) and assists in the control of both hypokalaemia and hypertension. Severe facial dermatitis has been reported recently in Maine Coon cats receiving spironolactone for management of hypertrophic cardiomyopathy (MacDonald et al., 2008), but has not been encountered elsewhere. Spironolactone has lesser but significant affinity for progesterone and androgen receptors, and other adverse reactions of spironolactone in human patients include gynaecomastia and menstrual irregularities. Eplerenone has been developed as an alternative aldosterone receptor antagonist that has more selective affinity for mineralocorticoid receptors but there are no reports yet of its use in cats. Although medical treatment alone is unlikely to normalize circulating potassium concentrations, control of clinical signs associated with myopathy is usually achieved.

Adrenalectomy (Figure 19.14) is a potentially curative treatment for unilateral adrenal masses. However, the procedure has been associated with high perioperative mortality: approximately 33% of

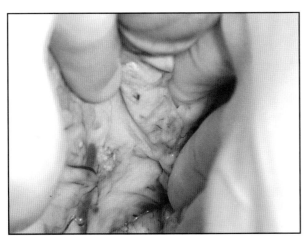

19.14 Intraoperative view of an aldosterone-secreting adrenal adenoma. Note the white cauliflower-like appearance of the adrenal tumour. Adrenalectomy was successful in this patient with no surgical complications. The cat was clinically well with no medical management 12 months postoperatively. (Courtesy of Laura Owen, University of Cambridge)

reported cases died intraoperatively or postoperatively, most commonly as a result of severe acute haemorrhage from the caudal vena cava. Patients should be stabilized medically prior to surgery and meticulous preoperative planning is required. A detailed description of perioperative and intraoperative management of an aldosterone-secreting adrenocortical carcinoma with attached caval thrombus has been reported (Rose et al., 2007). Although clinicians must be vigilant, complications of postoperative adrenal insufficiency have not been associated with excision of aldosterone-secreting tumours in cats. Approximately 5% of human patients develop postoperative hyperkalaemia, requiring transient administration of fludrocortisone, and the authors are aware of similar occurrences in cats.

Cats with concurrent hyperprogesteronism or hypercortisolaemia pose additional surgical risks, including wound dehiscence, sepsis and thromboembolic disease. Effective medical management necessitates suppression of progestin, glucocorticoid and mineralocorticoid production, with the possibility of the additive effect of spironolactone. To date, a protocol for such treatment has not been defined. Trilostane has been used in one of the authors' cases with concurrent hyperaldosteronism and hyperprogesteronism. Treatment was only attempted for a short period of time when the clinical signs were quite advanced, and was not successful in suppressing progesterone concentrations. Use of aminoglutethimide also has been reported for preoperative stabilization in one case but was of questionable benefit.

Prognosis

When medical management with combinations of potassium supplementation, amlodipine and spironolactone is the chosen course of treatment, reported survival times in four of five treated cats ranged from 7 to 32 months, with cats succumbing most commonly to chronic kidney or thromboembolic disease. The survival time in one cat receiving medical treatment alone was limited to 50 days, attributed to non-compliance of the owners. In some cases, hypertension becomes refractory to medical management. For patients who undergo adrenalectomy and survive the immediate perioperative and postoperative periods, the prognosis is good: 8 of 17 adrenalectomized cats survived for at least 1 year, and 2 were alive 3.5 and 5 years postoperatively. However, given the high perioperative mortality rate, the decision to perform surgery should not be taken lightly. Interestingly, the presence of an adrenal carcinoma does not appear to be associated with a poorer prognosis. Only 1 of 3 cats euthanased as a result of perioperative haemorrhage associated with surgery had an adrenal carcinoma. One cat with a carcinoma survived 1045 days following adrenalectomy.

The prognosis for the non-tumourous PHA cases is less well documented to date. Successful management of non-tumourous PHA is possible with potassium supplementation, amlodipine besylate and spironolactone. However, currently there is a lack of histopathological results and long-term follow-up available to be able to give further advice on prognosis in these cases.

References and further reading

Ash RA, Harvey AM and Tasker S (2005) Primary hyperaldosteronism in the cat: a series of 13 cases. *Journal of Feline Medicine and Surgery* **7**, 173–182

Briscoe K, Barrs VR, Foster DF and Beatty JA (2009) Hyperaldosteronism and hyperprogesteronism in a cat. *Journal of Feline Medicine and Surgery* **11**(9), 758–762

De Clue AE, Breshears LA, Pardo ID *et al.* (2005) Hyperaldosteronism and hyperprogesteronism in a cat with an adrenal cortical carcinoma. *Journal of Veterinary Internal Medicine* **19**, 355–358

Djajadiningrat-Laanen SC, Galac S, Cammelbeeck SE, *et al.* (2008) Urinary aldosterone to creatinine ratio in cats before and after suppression with salt or fludrocortisone acetate. *Journal of Veterinary Internal Medicine* **22**, 1283–1288

Eger CE, Robinson WF and Huxtable CR (1983) Primary aldosteronism (Conn's syndrome) in a cat; a case report and review of comparative aspects. *Journal of Small Animal Practice* **24**, 293–307

Funder JW, Carey RM, Fardella C *et al.* (2008) Case detection, diagnosis, and treatment of patients with primary hyperaldosteronism: an Endocrine Society practice guideline. *Journal of Clinical Endocrinology and Metabolism* **93**, 3266–3281

Gal A, Ridge T and Graves TK (2009) Effects of twice daily enalapril on serum aldosterone and systolic blood pressure in cats. *Journal of Veterinary Emergency and Critical Care* **19**, A3 [abstract]

Javadi S, Djajadiningrat-Laanen SC, Kooistra HS *et al.* (2005) Primary hyperaldosteronism, a mediator of progressive renal disease in cats. *Domestic Animal Endocrinology* **28**, 85–104

MacDonald KA, Kittelson MD and Kass PH (2008) Effect of spironolactone on diastolic function and left ventricular mass in Maine coon cats with familial hypertrophic cardiomyopathy. *Journal of Veterinary Internal Medicine* **22**, 335–341

Mackey AD, Holt PE and Sparkes AH (1999) Successful surgical treatment of a cat with primary aldosteronism. *Journal of Feline Medicine and Surgery* **1**, 117–122

Quante S, Sieber-Ruckstuhl N, Wilhelm S *et al.* (2009) Hyperprogesteronism due to bilateral adrenal carcinomas in a cat with diabetes mellitus. *Schweizer Archiv für Tierheilkunde* **151**, 437–442

Refsal KR and Harvey AM (2010) Primary hyperaldosteronism. In: *Consultations in Feline Internal Medicine, Vol.6,* ed. JR August, pp. 254–267. Saunders Elsevier, St Louis

Refsal KR and Mazaki-Tovi M (2009) Baseline concentrations of progesterone, cortisol and corticosterone in a laboratory survey of feline sera submitted for assay of aldosterone. In: *Proceedings, 19th ECVIM-CA Congress, Porto*, pp.270–271 [abstract]

Reimer SB, Pelosi A, Frank JD *et al.* (2005) Multiple endocrine neoplasia type 1 in a cat. *Journal of American Veterinary Medical Association* **227**, 101–104

Rose SA, Kyles AE, Labella P *et al.* (2007) Adrenalectomy and caval thrombectomy in a cat with primary hyperaldosteronism. *Journal of the American Animal Hospital Association* **43**, 209–214

Shiel R and Mooney C (2007) Diagnosis and management of primary hyperaldosteronism in cats. *In Practice* **29**, 194–201

20

Investigation of polyuria and polydipsia

Rhett Nichols and Mark E. Peterson

Introduction

Polydipsia is defined as a fluid intake of >90–100 ml/kg/day in dogs and >45 ml/kg/day in cats. Polyuria is defined in both dogs and cats as a urine output of >50 ml/kg/day (Hardy, 1982; Feldman and Nelson, 2004; DiBartola, 2006). A healthy dog or cat drinks approximately 20–90 ml/kg/day, depending on the moisture content of its diet, and normal urine output varies between 20 and 45 ml/kg/day (Breitschwerdt, 1981; Barsanti *et al.*, 2000; DiBartola, 2006). Thirst and the renal control of salt and water excretion are the two main mechanisms for balancing water intake with water loss.

There are many potential causes of polyuria and polydipsia (PU/PD). Primary disorders of water balance (i.e. central diabetes insipidus, primary nephrogenic diabetes insipidus and primary polydipsia), although uncommon, should always be considered in the differential diagnoses of polyuria and polydipsia. In general, animals with these disorders have only one laboratory abnormality: a low urine specific gravity (SG) or osmolality. In most instances, the more common causes of PU/PD (e.g. hyperadrenocorticism, chronic renal failure, pyelonephritis and pyometra) have other specific and obvious abnormalities on screening laboratory tests (complete blood cell count, serum biochemical profile and urinalysis). In some cases, however, a low urine SG is the only abnormality found in animals with these latter disorders. The work-up for PU/PD can be tedious, time-consuming, expensive, confusing and not without significant patient morbidity, especially in those dogs and cats with normal or near-normal screening test results. This chapter focuses on the diagnostic approach, especially the problems associated with testing, and the treatment of dogs and cats with disorders of water balance.

Physiology of water balance

Urine concentration is under the controlling influence of arginine vasopressin (AVP), also known as antidiuretic hormone (ADH). This hormone is produced in the hypothalamus and stored in the posterior lobe of the pituitary. The most important stimulus for its release under physiological conditions is plasma osmolality. Once released, it binds to specific V2 receptors on the serosal surfaces of renal tubular cells, where it acts to increase water permeability and resorption from the tubular lumen. The thirst mechanism also plays a role but is stimulated at a higher threshold than AVP production. The physiology of water balance is described in greater detail in Chapter 3.

Conditions for maximal urine concentration

In order for an animal to concentrate its urine, the following three conditions must be met:

- As described above, there must be an adequate secretion of AVP and the kidneys must be able to respond normally to its action
- At least a third of the nephrons in both kidneys must be functional; if more than two-thirds of the nephron mass is lost, the kidneys lose their ability to concentrate urine, no matter what the circulating AVP concentration. It is also important to remember that in animals with early renal failure, azotaemia does not develop until three-quarters of the nephrons have become non-functional
- Inasmuch as increased medullary hypertonicity is the driving force for passive water reabsorption in the distal tubule and collecting duct in the presence of AVP, a reduction in medullary solute concentration (medullary washout) will also result in dilute urine and excessive water loss, even in the presence of excessive AVP secretion. The tonicity of the renal medullary interstitium is decreased to some degree with all polyuric disorders (DiBartola, 2006).

Differential diagnosis

The causes of PU/PD can be divided into those that cause primary polydipsia (with secondary polyuria) and those that cause primary polyuria (with compensatory polydipsia). The major cause of primary polydipsia in dogs is thought to be psychogenic. In contrast, the causes of primary polyuria are much more numerous and can be sub-divided into: central diabetes insipidus; primary nephrogenic diabetes insipidus; secondary nephrogenic diabetes insipidus; and osmotic diuresis (Figure 20.1).

Primary polydipsia
• Psychogenic polydipsia (compulsive water drinking) • Dipsogenic diabetes insipidus (thirst centre abnormality) • Metabolic disorders (e.g. hyperthyroidism, hepatic failure)
Primary polyuria

• Central diabetes insipidus (neurogenic, cranial, AVP-responsive):
  – Idiopathic
  – Trauma-induced
  – Neoplastic
  – Post-hypophysectomy
• Primary nephrogenic diabetes insipidus (congenital or familial)
• Secondary nephrogenic diabetes insipidus (acquired)
  – Acromegaly
  – Chronic renal disease
  – Drug administration
  – Liver disease
  – Hyperadrenocorticism
  – Hypercalcaemia
  – Hyperthyroidism
  – Hypoadrenocorticism
  – Hypokalaemia
  – Atypical leptospirosis
  – Pyelonephritis
  – Pyometra
  – Renal failure
• Osmotic diuresis (increased renal tubular solute load)
  – Diabetes mellitus
  – Primary renal glucosuria (e.g. Fanconi syndrome)
  – Post-obstructive diuresis

20.1 Differential diagnoses for polyuria and polydipsia in dogs and cats.

Primary polydipsia

Psychogenic polydipsia, or compulsive water drinking, is usually the manifestation of a behavioural problem triggered by an environmental or emotional stimulus (Barsanti *et al.*, 2000; Feldman and Nelson, 2004). Affected animals are typically hyperactive dogs kept in an exercise-restrictive environment. Although psychogenic polydipsia develops most commonly in dogs, it does appear to develop occasionally in cats as a behavioural manifestation of hyperthyroidism (Peterson *et al.*, 1983).

Primary polydipsia could also result from a defect in the thirst mechanism, leading to excessive thirst. The cause of this dipsogenic diabetes insipidus is usually idiopathic but may result from a variety of infectious, neoplastic or traumatic brain injuries. All of these causes of primary polydipsia are associated with suppression of AVP secretion secondary to excessive thirst. Abnormal AVP release has also been reported in dogs with suspected primary polydipsia, suggesting a primary disturbance in the regulation of AVP secretion in some cases (Van Vonderen *et al.*, 1999; Van Vonderen *et al.*, 2004).

Primary polyuria

Central diabetes insipidus (CDI) (also called pituitary, neurogenic, cranial or AVP-responsive diabetes insipidus) is a rare condition caused by a complete or partial deficiency of AVP. Deficiency of AVP varies in severity. In most animals it is probably caused by loss or destruction of the majority of the AVP-producing neurons. In most dogs and cats, CDI is idiopathic, although the disorder may be familial in some cases. Less commonly, CDI develops as a sequel to head trauma, neoplasia (i.e. invasive pituitary tumour or tumour metastasis to the pituitary gland or hypothalamus) or hypophysectomy for treatment of hyperadrenocorticism (Harb *et al.*, 1996; Meij 2001; Feldman and Nelson, 2004).

In the broadest sense, the term 'nephrogenic diabetes insipidus' (NDI) may be used to describe a diverse group of disorders in which structural or functional abnormalities interfere with the ability of the kidneys to concentrate urine. In animals with NDI, the renal tubules are insensitive to the antidiuretic effects of AVP, despite appropriate AVP release from the pituitary gland.

Primary NDI is due to an extremely rare congenital structural or functional defect of the kidneys. Secondary or acquired NDI, in contrast, is the most common cause of PU/PD in dogs and cats and may be a consequence of a number of renal, endocrine and metabolic disorders. These disorders include:

- Renal failure
- Pyelonephritis
- Hyperadrenocorticism
- Hypokalaemia
- Hypercalcaemia
- Liver disease
- Pyometra.

Many of the acquired forms of NDI are potentially reversible with correction of the underlying illness or disorder. Again, renal medullary washout can contribute to polyuria in animals with any of these disorders because increased tubular flow and volume decreases the reabsorption of sodium and urea, and reduces the medullary interstitial hypertonicity of the kidneys.

Osmotic diuresis

Osmotic diuresis occurs when the concentration of an osmotic solute (e.g. urea, glucose) present in the glomerular filtrate exceeds the proximal tubular capacity for reabsorption. This impairs the passive reabsorption of water and results in increased obligatory water loss. Conditions in which solute or osmotic diuresis contributes to polyuria include diabetes mellitus, primary renal glucosuria and chronic renal failure, as well as the diuresis that follows relief of a postrenal obstruction (post-obstructive diuresis).

Diagnostic approach

Differentiating between the causes of PU/PD is relatively easy when the different disorders are manifested in their classic forms. For example, polyuria that develops after a known head trauma, which continues after water restriction and decreases after AVP administration does not require additional tests to justify the diagnosis of CDI. A diagnosis of congenital

NDI is equally clear if polyuria occurs in a young animal with similarly affected littermates that have normal screening laboratory tests (including renal function), negative urine cultures and whose polyuria fails to respond to fluid restriction or administration of AVP analogues (e.g. desmopressin). Often, however, the clinical setting is of minimal help in making a diagnosis and it is then necessary to perform more detailed diagnostic tests. The initial information gathered should allow the inclusion or exclusion of the many common medical disorders associated with PU/PD before a diagnostic work-up for the less common disorders of CDI, primary NDI or psychogenic polydipsia is embarked upon (Figure 20.2).

History

An accurate history is invaluable when initially investigating an animal with PU/PD, and may help to rule out some of the more common differential diagnoses. When an owner complains of an animal's excessive urination, it is important first to determine whether PU/PD truly exists as opposed to dysuria, pollakiuria, stranguria or incontinence. Consideration must also be given to the animal's overall health, diet and recent drug administration, as well as environmental factors.

Signalment

Some disorders that cause PU/PD develop more frequently in certain age groups or breeds of dogs or cats. For example, hyperadrenocorticism (one of the most common causes of PU/PD in dogs) typically develops in middle-aged to older dogs of smaller breeds such as the Miniature Poodle (Peterson, 1984). Most of the other common causes of PU/PD (e.g. diabetes mellitus, renal disease and pyometra) are also found in older animals, whereas primary polydipsia occurs most frequently in young, hyperexcitable, large-breed dogs (Feldman and Nelson, 2004; Van Vonderen et al., 2004). Renal failure, diabetes mellitus and hyperthyroidism – the three most common causes of PU/PD in cats – all typically develop in older cats.

The reproductive history may also provide helpful clues as to the cause of PU/PD, especially in dogs. For example, pyometra is typically a disorder of middle-aged intact bitches, with clinical signs of PU/PD developing during or immediately after the dioestrus phase of the oestrous cycle (Dunn, 1998). With hyperadrenocorticism, intact bitches may show prolonged anoestrus, whereas males may develop testicular atrophy or have a decreased libido (Peterson, 1984).

Overall health

The presence of non-specific clinical signs (e.g. anorexia, polyphagia, lethargy, weight loss or gain) may be helpful in determining the cause of PU/PD. For example, lethargy and gastrointestinal signs could suggest hepatic disease, renal failure or hypoadrenocorticism. Polyphagia could suggest hyperadrenocorticism or diabetes mellitus in dogs, or hyperthyroidism or diabetes in cats. Weight gain is common in animals with hyperadrenocorticism, whereas weight loss is one of the most common signs in hyperthyroid cats.

Diet

When evaluating an animal with PU/PD, the nature and composition of the diet should always be taken into account (Dunn, 1998). This is especially true if PU/PD develops around the time of a dietary change. Food is an important source of water, and dogs or cats fed primarily on dry food invariably drink more water than those fed on moist canned food. Feeding a low-protein diet can result in renal medullary washout and polyuria (Dunn, 1998).

Recent drug administration

In all animals with PU/PD, any current or recent administration of drugs should be ruled out. Medications that frequently cause PU/PD include glucocorticoids, phenobarbital, primidone and diuretics (Feldman and Nelson, 2004). Chronic administration

Signalment and history
• Age, breed and sex • Reproductive history (intact female?) • Changes in diet or environment? • Overall general health (weight loss or gain, lethargy, vomiting or diarrhoea?) • Appetite normal, increased or decreased? • Drug administration (glucocorticoids, anticonvulsants, diuretics?)
Physical examination
• Kidneys small or misshapen? (chronic renal disease) • Kidneys large? (pyelonephritis, lymphosarcoma) • Hepatomegaly? (hyperadrenocorticism, diabetes mellitus) • Peripheral lymphadenopathy? (lymphosarcoma with hypercalcaemia) • Perianal mass? (anal sac adenocarcinoma with hypercalcaemia) • Vaginal discharge? (pyometra) • Alopecia? Pot belly? (hyperadrenocorticism) • Thyroid mass? (hyperthyroidism)
Complete blood count (CBC), serum biochemical profile and electrolytes, serum thyroxine
• High urea or creatinine? (renal failure) • Hyperglycaemia? (diabetes mellitus) • High alkaline phosphatase activity (hyperadrenocorticism) • Hypercholesterolaemia? (hyperadrenocorticism) • Hypercalcaemia? • Hypokalaemia? • High thyroxine? (hyperthyroidism)
Complete urinalysis and urine culture
• Low urine specific gravity (confirms and defines polyuria) • Proteinuria? (hyperadrenocorticism, pyometra, pyelonephritis, glomerulonephritis) • Glucosuria ± ketonuria? (diabetes mellitus) • Active urine sediment? (infection, pyelonephritis) • Positive bacterial culture? (infection, pyelonephritis)
Abdominal radiography or ultrasonography
• Small kidneys with ill-defined renal or irregular border (renal failure) • Increased cortical echogenicity, indistinct corticomedullary junction (renal failure) • Dilated renal pelvis (pyelonephritis)

20.2 Initial work-up for polyuria and polydipsia in dogs and cats.

of progestogens to intact bitches for oestrous suppression can lead to acromegaly (growth hormone excess), which causes secondary diabetes mellitus (and PU/PD) in many dogs (see Chapter 5).

Environmental factors

In dogs with primary polydipsia it may be possible to identify a stressful lifestyle change that preceded the onset of polydipsia and polyuria. Common examples include the arrival of a new baby, or moving to a new house or apartment. In contrast, polyuria that develops after head trauma could suggest damage to the AVP-secreting neurons or disruption of the pituitary stalk resulting in CDI.

Physical examination

Many common disorders associated with PU/PD can be ruled out by performing a careful and complete physical examination.

- The animal's abdomen must be palpated with special care to evaluate kidney and liver size.
- In intact bitches external genitalia should be examined for vaginal discharge suggestive of pyometra.
- Lymph nodes should be palpated, as generalized enlargement could suggest lymphoma with secondary hypercalcaemia.
- The perianal area should also be palpated carefully, particularly in bitches, for anal sac adenocarcinoma, which can cause hypercalcaemia.
- Findings suggestive of hyperadrenocorticism include pot belly, bilaterally symmetrical hair loss and hepatomegaly.
- In animals with pyelonephritis, fever or perirenal pain may be present.
- The presence of cataracts in dogs, or hindlimb neuropathy in cats, suggests diabetes mellitus.
- In cats, the cervical area should always be palpated to look for a thyroid nodule, because hyperthyroidism is a relatively common cause of PU/PD (Peterson et al., 1983).

In contrast, dogs and cats with diabetes insipidus or primary (psychogenic) polydipsia are typically alert and active and seldom show any abnormalities on physical examination. Dehydration is rarely detected on physical examination, as this would develop only if the animal's access to water had been restricted by the owner.

Measurement of water consumption

The first step in any suspected case of PU/PD is to establish that the problem truly exists, preferably by a combination of history, random urine SG determinations and, if necessary, home measurement of water consumption over several days.

If the daily water intake is found to be normal, or if a random urine SG determination is >1.030 (dogs) or >1.035 (cats), additional history should be obtained to rule out other urinary tract disorders (such as urinary incontinence or dysuria) that are commonly confused with polyuria.

If, however, random urine SG measurements are consistently <1.030 in dogs and <1.035 in cats, and daily water intake is >100 ml/kg for dogs and 45 ml/kg for cats, PU/PD is indeed present and a diagnostic work-up to determine the cause is warranted.

Minimum clinicopathological data

Once a problem of water balance has been confirmed, a practical diagnostic approach is first to rule out the more common causes of PU/PD in dogs and cats, listed in Figure 20.3 in order of most to least common. Recommended initial diagnostic tests include:

- Complete blood cell count (CBC)
- Serum biochemical profile with electrolytes
- Serum total thyroxine (T_4) determination in middle-aged to older cats.

Dogs
<ul><li>Hyperadrenocorticism</li><li>Diabetes mellitus</li><li>Chronic renal failure</li><li>Pyelonephritis</li><li>Pyometra</li><li>Hypercalcaemia</li><li>Atypical leptospirosis</li><li>Psychogenic polydipsia</li><li>Diabetes insipidus</li><li>Liver disease</li><li>Hypoadrenocorticism</li><li>Acromegaly</li></ul>

Cats
<ul><li>Chronic renal failure</li><li>Diabetes mellitus</li><li>Hyperthyroidism</li><li>Hypercalcaemia</li><li>Pyelonephritis</li><li>Hypokalaemia</li><li>Acromegaly</li><li>Post-obstructive diuresis</li><li>Hyperadrenocorticism</li><li>Hypoadrenocorticism</li><li>Diabetes insipidus</li></ul>

20.3 Differential rule outs for polyuria and polydipsia in dogs and cats, listed from most to least common.

A careful evaluation of this initial database, together with the history and results of physical examination, usually provides the diagnosis immediately (e.g. overt renal failure, hyperthyroidism or diabetes mellitus) or offers clues as to the underlying cause of the PU/PD (see Figure 20.2). For example, dogs with hyperadrenocorticism commonly have a stress leucogram (i.e. neutrophilia, lymphopenia and eosinopenia). Over 90% of dogs with hyperadrenocorticism also have high alkaline phosphatase (ALP) activity, whereas over 50% have hypercholesterolaemia (Peterson, 1984).

In contrast, physical examination findings and routine blood work are generally unremarkable in animals with less common causes of polyuria and polydipsia, such as central diabetes insipidus, primary nephrogenic diabetes insipidus and psychogenic polydipsia. When abnormalities are present, they are usually secondary to dehydration caused by water restriction by the owner. Such abnormalities may include a slightly increased packed cell volume (PCV) or hypernatraemia.

Complete urinalysis

Urinalysis is a major key in determining the presence of a water balance problem and the disorder causing the PU/PD (see Figure 20.2). The most important features of urinalysis are: the SG or osmolality; the presence or absence of glucose, protein or bacteria; and the cellularity of the sample.

A urine SG <1.030 in dogs and <1.035 in cats suggests a concentrating defect and supports the complaint of polyuria (Behrend, 2002; Feldman and Nelson, 2004). Persistent glucosuria is diagnostic for primary renal glucosuria or, more commonly, diabetes mellitus. Significant proteinuria in the presence of an inactive urinary sediment and dilute urine can be associated with hyperadrenocorticism, pyelonephritis, pyometra, glomerulonephritis or other glomerulopathy.

An active urine sediment (pyuria, haematuria or bacteriuria) in a sample obtained by catheterization or cystocentesis supports urinary tract infection and possible pyelonephritis. Because urine sediment examination may be misleading in an extremely dilute urine sample, a urine culture should always be done to rule out pyelonephritis, regardless of sediment examination findings.

If the results of the above tests are unhelpful, the direction of further diagnostic work-up can often be based on the urine SG (Figure 20.4). For example, dogs and cats with an SG >1.030–1.035 without glucosuria, are probably not polyuric and need no further work-up, at least for PU/PD.

Urine SG 1.001–1.007

- Atypical hyperadrenocorticism (most common; always rule out first!)
- Atypical leptospirosis
- Psychogenic polydipsia
- Diabetes insipidus (complete)

Urine SG 1.008–1.029

- Atypical hyperadrenocorticism (most common)
- Atypical leptospirosis
- Early renal disease
- Typical and occult pyelonephritis
- Hyperthyroidism (cats)
- Psychogenic polydipsia
- Diabetes insipidus (partial)

Urine SG >1.030 (dogs) and >1.035 (cats) without glucosuria

- Probably not polyuric
- No further work-up for PU/PD needed

20.4 Differential diagnosis based on urine specific gravity (SG) determination in animals with normal results on initial tests (CBC, serum biochemical profile and urinalysis).

Urine SG <1.008

A urine SG consistently <1.008 in a middle-aged to older dog is usually associated with diabetes insipidus, psychogenic polydipsia, atypical hyperadrenocorticism or atypical leptospirosis.

In those dogs with atypical hyperadrenocorticism, PU/PD is a major clinical sign but other characteristic clinical signs are mild or absent (Barsanti *et al.*, 2000; Nichols, 2001). In addition, those dogs with atypical disease may lack the serum biochemistry abnormalities commonly associated with hyperadrenocorticism (i.e. elevated serum alkaline phosphatase activity and hypercholesterolaemia). Results of adrenal function tests in these dogs are usually consistent with mild hyperadrenocorticism.

More recently, an atypical form of leptospirosis has been recognized. These dogs present with an acute onset polyuria and polydipsia, hyposthenuria or isosthenuria, but no other laboratory abnormalities. The urine concentration defect is thought to be an acquired form of nephrogenic DI. Azotaemia does not develop. In dogs not previously vaccinated for leptospirosis, *Leptospira* infection can be confirmed by positive leptospirosis serology or use of molecular detection of leptospiral DNA by PCR testing of urine samples. In dogs previously vaccinated for leptospirosis, a 4-fold rise in convalescent titres is often diagnostic of the atypical form of this disease. Treatment is achieved using antibiotics such as penicillins or doxycycline.

In general, when considering polyuric dogs with a urine SG <1.008, hyperadrenocorticism and atypical leptospirosis should be ruled out first before testing for CDI and primary polydipsia. There are several reasons for making this recommendation: the latter two disorders of water metabolism are much less common than is hyperadrenocorticism (see Figure 20.3); the diagnostic tests of choice to differentiate these disorders – the water deprivation test or a therapeutic trial with the AVP-analogue desmopressin – are time-consuming and expensive (Nichols, 2001; Feldman and Nelson, 2004). Also, dogs with hyperadrenocorticism may respond to these tests in a manner similar to dogs with CDI, resulting in a misdiagnosis (Mulnix *et al.*, 1976; Hardy, 1982). Moreover, water deprivation testing a dog with leptospirosis would be a major contraindication because of the possibility of causing significant patient morbidity.

In cats, a urine SG consistently <1.008 is associated with either diabetes insipidus or hyperthyroidism. Hyperthyroidism should be ruled out first before initiating testing procedures for diabetes insipidus.

It is also important to realize that the finding of a urine SG <1.008 in a cat or dog excludes mild (occult) renal disease, so precautions associated with the water deprivation test are not necessary.

Urine SG between 1.008 and 1.029

A urine SG of >1.008 but <1.030 can be associated with hyperadrenocorticism (dogs), hyperthyroidism (cats), or stage 1 renal insufficiency (including atypical leptospirosis) or pyelonephritis, as well as psychogenic polydipsia and partial forms of diabetes insipidus.

Hyperadrenocorticism and hyperthyroidism should be ruled out first. Pyelonephritis and early renal insufficiency should be ruled out next before evaluating the animal for psychogenic polydipsia and diabetes insipidus with a water deprivation test. Performing a water deprivation test as a diagnostic tool in the face of unsuspected renal insufficiency or pyelonephritis could induce overt renal failure or urosepsis (Barsanti *et al.*, 2000; Nichols, 2001; Feldman and Nelson, 2004; DiBartola, 2006). To avoid this complication, a sensible approach is to do the following.

1. Perform a urine culture to help exclude pyelonephritis and associated urinary tract infection.
2. Consider leptospirosis serology and urine PCR testing.
3. Evaluate renal size and architecture by abdominal radiography or, preferably, renal ultrasonography. The ultrasonographic appearance of renal parenchymal disease (chronic renal failure) includes increased cortical echogenicity and loss of a distinct corticomedullary junction (Konde, 1985). The kidneys may appear smaller than normal and have an ill-defined or irregular border. Similar sonographic findings, in addition to a dilated renal pelvis, are characteristic of pyelonephritis.

If urine culture results are negative, leptospirosis serology and urine PCR testing are negative, and radiographic or ultrasonographic findings are equivocal, a creatinine or iohexol clearance test (Brown *et al.*, 1996; DiBartola, 2006) or renal biopsy may be indicated. In rare cases, the urine culture may be negative even if pyelonephritis is present. If clinical or ultrasonographic findings suggest occult pyelonephritis, a therapeutic trial with an appropriate antibiotic (e.g. enrofloxacin) should be instituted.

Specific tests to differentiate diabetes insipidus from primary polydipsia

Several different diagnostic approaches can be used to confirm CDI, NDI or primary (psychogenic) polydipsia. The water deprivation test is generally considered by most authorities to be the best diagnostic test for differentiating between these disorders. However, it is labour-intensive, difficult to perform correctly, unpleasant for the animal, relies heavily on repeated emptying of the bladder, and can lead to untoward complications and misdiagnosis in some animals. Another common diagnostic approach is to consider a therapeutic trial with the AVP analogue desmopressin (Nichols and Hohenhaus 1994; Nichols, 2000). See Chapter 3 for more information.

References and further reading

Barsanti JA, DiBartola SP and Finco DR (2000) Diagnostic approach to polyuria and polydipsia. In: *Kirk's Current Veterinary Therapy. XIII. Small Animal Practice*, ed. JD Bonagura, pp. 831–835. WB Saunders, Philadelphia

Behrend EN (2002) Managing diabetes insipidus and other causes of polyuria and polydipsia. *Veterinary Medicine* **97**, 753–761

Breitschwerdt EB (1981) Clinical abnormalities of urine concentration and dilution. *Compendium on Continuing Education for the Practicing Veterinarian* **3**, 412–414

Brown SA, Finco DR, Boudinot FD, Wright J, Taver SL and Cooper T (1996) Evaluation of a single injection method, using iohexol, for estimating glomerular filtration rate in cats and dogs. *American Journal of Veterinary Research* **57**, 105–110

Cohen M and Post GS (2002) Water transport in the kidney and nephrogenic diabetes insipidus. *Journal of Veterinary Internal Medicine* **16**, 510–517

DiBartola SP (2006) Disorders of sodium and water: hypernatremia and hyponatremia. In: *Fluid Therapy in Small Animal Practice, 3rd edn*, ed. SP DiBartola, pp. 47–79. Elsevier, Philadelphia

Dunn JK (1998) The dog with polydipsia and polyuria. In: *BSAVA Manual of Small Animal Endocrinology, 2nd edn*, ed. AG Torrance and CT Mooney, pp. 3–9. BSAVA, Cheltenham

Feldman EC and Nelson RW (2004) Water metabolism and diabetes insipidus. In: *Canine and Feline Endocrinology and Reproduction, 3rd edn*, ed. EC Feldman and RW Nelson, pp. 2–44. WB Saunders, Philadelphia

Greene CE, Sykes JE, Brown CA and Hartmann K (2006) Leptospirosis. In: *Infectious Diseases of the Dog and Cat, 3rd edn*, ed. CE Greene, pp. 402–417. Elsevier, Philadelphia

Harb MF, Nelson RW, Feldman EC, Scott-Moncrieff JC and Griffey SM (1996) Central diabetes insipidus in dogs: 20 cases (1986–1995). *Journal of the American Veterinary Medical Association* **209**, 1884–1888

Hardy RM (1982) Disorders of water metabolism. *Veterinary Clinics of North America: Small Animal Practice* **12**, 353–373

Harkin KR, Roshto YM and Sullivan JT (2003) Clinical application of a polymerase chain reaction assay for diagnosis of leptospirosis in dogs. *Journal of the American Veterinary Medical Association* **222**, 1224–1229

Konde LJ (1985) Sonography of the kidney. *Veterinary Clinics of North America: Small Animal Practice* **15**, 1149–1158

Meij B P (2001) Hypophysectomy as a treatment for canine and feline Cushing's disease. *Veterinary Clinics of North America: Small Animal Practice* **31**, 1015–1041

Mulnix JA, Rijnberk A and Hendriks HJ (1976) Evaluation of a modified water-deprivation test for diagnosis of polyuric disorders in dogs. *Journal of the American Veterinary Medical Association* **169**, 1327–1330

Nichols R (2000) Clinical use of the vasopressin analogue DDAVP for the diagnosis and treatment of diabetes insipidus. In: *Kirk's Current Veterinary Therapy. XIII. Small Animal Practice*, ed. JD Bonagura, pp. 325–326. WB Saunders, Philadelphia

Nichols R (2001) Polyuria and polydipsia. Diagnostic approach and problems associated with patient evaluation. *Veterinary Clinics of North America: Small Animal Practice* **31**, 833–844

Nichols R and Hohenhaus AE (1994) Use of the vasopressin analogue desmopressin for polyuria and bleeding disorders. *Journal of the American Veterinary Medical Association* **205**, 168–173

Peterson ME (1984) Hyperadrenocorticism. *Veterinary Clinics of North America: Small Animal Practice* **14**, 731–749

Peterson ME, Kintzer PP, Cavanagh PG et al. (1983) Feline hyperthyroidism: pretreatment clinical and laboratory evaluation of 131 cases. *Journal of the American Veterinary Medical Association* **183**, 103–110

Van De Maele I, Claus A, Haesebrouck F and Daminet S (2008) Leptospirosis in dogs: a review with emphasis on clinical aspects. *Veterinary Record* **163**, 409–413

Van Vonderen IK, Kooistra HS, Sprang EP and Rijnberk A (1999) Disturbed vasopressin release in 4 dogs with so-called primary polydipsia. *Journal of Veterinary Internal Medicine* **13**, 419–425

Van Vonderen IK, Kooistra HS, Timmermans-Sprang EP, Meij BP and Rijnberk A (2004) Vasopressin response to osmotic stimulation in 18 young dogs with polyuria and polydipsia. *Journal of Veterinary Internal Medicine* **18**, 800–806

21

Investigation of hypercalcaemia and hypocalcaemia

Patricia A. Schenck and Dennis J. Chew

Introduction

Calcium in serum or plasma exists in three fractions: ionized, complexed and protein-bound. In healthy dogs, protein-bound, complexed and ionized calcium accounts for 34%, 10% and 56% of total serum concentration, respectively. There is a similar distribution in cats (40%, 8% and 52%, respectively).

Ionized calcium (iCa) is the biologically active fraction of calcium and is important for many physiological functions. It is required for: enzymatic reactions; membrane transport and stability; blood coagulation; nerve conduction; neuromuscular transmission; muscle contraction; vascular smooth muscle tone; hormone secretion; bone formation and resorption; control of hepatic glycogen metabolism; and cell growth and division. Calcium ions directly bind to iCa-specific cell membrane receptors, and the iCa concentration is maintained within a narrow range by interactions between iCa, phosphorus, parathyroid hormone (PTH, parathormone), vitamin D metabolites, and calcitonin. These mechanisms must be disrupted for hypercalcaemia or hypocalcaemia to develop.

The intestine, kidney, and bone are the major target organs involved in calcium regulation. PTH is secreted by the parathyroid glands in response to a decrease in iCa concentration. The actions of PTH are to increase:

- Tubular reabsorption of calcium (with decreased loss of calcium in the urine)
- Bone resorption
- Formation of 1,25-dihydroxycholecalciferol (1,25(OH)$_2$-vitamin D; calcitriol) by the kidney.

The net effects of increased PTH are to increase iCa and decrease serum phosphate concentration. Calcitonin is secreted from the thyroid gland in response to hypercalcaemia, but its role in calcium homeostasis is relatively minor (Schenck et al., 2006).

1,25(OH)$_2$-vitamin D is the active metabolite of vitamin D, and increases serum iCa and phosphorus concentrations by stimulating the resorption of bone, increasing calcium, phosphate, and magnesium absorption in the intestine, and increasing renal tubular resorption of calcium and phosphate by the kidney. As dogs and cats produce little vitamin D in the skin, they are dependent on an adequate dietary intake of vitamin D. Hydroxylation of vitamin D occurs in the liver to produce 25-hydroxycholecalciferol (25(OH)-vitamin D; calcidiol), which is then hydroxylated to 1,25(OH)$_2$-vitamin D in the proximal tubules of the kidney. This process is upregulated by serum PTH concentration and downregulated by serum phosphate and calcitriol concentrations.

Measurement of calcium

Total calcium

Serum or heparinized plasma samples are suitable for analysis; oxalate, citrate, and EDTA anticoagulants should not be used as calcium is bound by these and is therefore unavailable for analysis. Fasting samples are recommended to prevent problems associated with hyperlipidaemia.

Mean serum total calcium concentrations in healthy mature dogs and cats are approximately 2.5 mmol/l (reference interval 2.3–2.8 mmol/l) and 2.25 mmol/l (reference interval 2.1–2.8 mmol/l), respectively. Dogs <3 months old have slightly higher serum total calcium concentrations (mean of approximately 2.75 mmol/l) than dogs >1 year old, most likely because of increased bone turnover in the younger animals.

Interpretation of abnormal serum calcium concentrations in dogs and cats is frequently required. The magnitude of altered serum calcium concentration often does not suggest a specific diagnosis or the extent of disease. Furthermore, a normal serum total calcium concentration does not eliminate a disorder of calcium homeostasis. The calcium status of animals is usually initially based on serum total calcium concentration, despite the fact that the iCa fraction is the only physiologically active portion. The reliance on measurement of serum total calcium is based on the assumption that it is directly proportional to iCa concentration, which can lead to erroneous interpretation in clinical conditions.

In dogs, serum total calcium concentration fails to predict ionized calcium status just over 25% of the time, and in cats, approximately 40% of the time. In dogs, total calcium measurement overestimates normocalcaemia and underestimates hypocalcaemia (Schenck and Chew, 2005b). In cats, both hypercalcaemia and normocalcaemia are underestimated, and hypocalcaemia is overestimated when using serum total calcium to predict iCa status (Schenck and Chew, 2010). The use of serum total calcium to predict ionized calcium status can therefore lead to errors in treatment, due to misclassification of true calcium status.

It has been suggested that canine serum total calcium concentrations should be 'adjusted' relative to the serum total protein or albumin concentration, in order to improve diagnostic interpretation or more accurately reflect actual calcium status. Adjustment formulas, however, were developed without verification by iCa measurements. In canine samples, the use of an adjustment formula to predict iCa status showed a higher diagnostic disagreement (38%) than did measurement of serum total calcium alone (27%). In dogs with chronic renal failure (CRF), diagnostic disagreement between adjusted total calcium and iCa measurement increased to 53%, indicating the poor performance of the adjustment formulas in the prediction of iCa status, particularly in certain disease states. Adjustment formulas perform poorly because they only take into account the protein-bound fraction of calcium and ignore the complexed fraction. Complexed calcium is not constant, especially in canine chronic renal failure patients where it can range from 6 to 39% of the total calcium measured. Serum total or adjusted calcium measurements are unacceptable predictors of iCa status due to the high level of discordance, especially in CRF patients. Changes in serum protein concentration, individual protein-binding capacity and affinity, and alterations in the complexed concentration can all change total calcium independently of iCa. The use of adjustment formulas to predict iCa status is not recommended, as it increases diagnostic errors in prediction of true ionized calcium status.

Direct measurement of iCa

For accurate measurement of calcium status, iCa must be measured directly. Analysers utilizing an ion-selective electrode allow easy and accurate measurement of iCa. Serum iCa concentration in healthy dogs and adult cats is approximately 1.2–1.4 mmol/l. Young dogs and cats have serum iCa concentrations that are 0.025–0.1 mmol/l higher than those in older animals. Accurate determination of iCa concentration requires that samples be collected and processed correctly. The protein binding of calcium is influenced by pH; an alkaline pH that occurs with the loss of CO_2 favours calcium binding to protein, decreasing the amount of iCa. If serum samples are collected anaerobically, iCa is stable in samples stored for 72 hours at 23°C or 4°C, and for 7 days at 4°C (Schenck et al., 1995). Exposure of serum to air results in an increased pH with decreased iCa concentration. Anaerobic collection of serum is technically difficult; therefore accurate aerobic methods for iCa measurement have been developed. Species-specific correction formulae can be developed to correct the measured iCa concentration of aerobically handled samples to a pH of 7.4, with excellent correlation to iCa measured in anaerobically handled samples.

One study has shown that iCa measurement in aerobically handled serum is stable for up to 48 hours at 4°C; however, in this study samples were allowed to sit and had minimal mixing with air (Brennan et al., 2006). However, in the authors' experience, during shipment to a laboratory serum mixes considerably with air, causing a significant decrease in iCa (with an increase in pH). Thus, the authors do not recommend the measurement of iCa in shipped aerobically handled samples without adjustment to a standard pH of 7.4. Typically, serum is used for iCa measurement, although heparinized plasma or whole blood can also be used. The amount and type of heparin used can impact iCa measurement; therefore, when using analysers that utilize heparinized whole blood, a rigid protocol for collection should be established. Results using heparinized whole blood cannot be directly compared to serum results, as iCa concentrations are typically lower in heparinized whole blood (Schenck and Chew, 2008a).

Hypercalcaemia

Clinical features

Polydipsia, polyuria, anorexia, lethargy and weakness are the most common clinical signs in dogs with hypercalcaemia. The severity of clinical signs depend on the magnitude of hypercalcaemia and on its rate of development and duration. Clinical signs are most severe when hypercalcaemia develops rapidly, as occurs with vitamin D intoxication. Dogs with similar magnitudes of hypercalcaemia may display minimal clinical signs when hypercalcaemia has developed gradually. Clinical signs become more severe as the magnitude of hypercalcaemia increases. Serum total calcium concentrations of approximately 3.0–3.5 mmol/l may not be associated with severe clinical signs, but most animals with concentrations >3.7 mmol/l show systemic signs. Dogs with serum calcium concentrations >4.5 mmol/l are often severely ill, and concentrations >5.0 mmol/l may constitute a life-threatening crisis. Some dogs, however, are severely affected by mild hypercalcaemia, whereas others are relatively unaffected by severe hypercalcaemia. Clinical signs are more likely to develop the longer hypercalcaemia has been present, regardless of its magnitude. Progressive hypercalcaemia may contribute to the severity of clinical signs, as occurs in animals with malignant neoplasia or hypervitaminosis D related to rat bait ingestion.

Differential diagnosis

Characterization of the hypercalcaemia as transient or persistent, pathological or non-pathological, mild or severe, progressive or static, and acute or chronic is helpful in determining its cause (Figure 21.1). Persistent, pathological hypercalcaemia occurs most often in association with malignancy. Most studies in dogs attribute hypercalcaemia to malignancy in >50% of cases. In the majority of cats, hypercalcaemia is reported to be due to chronic kidney

Non-pathological causes
• Non-fasting (minimal increase) • Physiological growth of the young • Laboratory error • Spurious (lipaemia)

Transient or inconsequential causes
• Haemoconcentration • Hyperproteinaemia • Severe environmental hypothermia (rare)

Pathological or consequential to persistent causes

• Parathyroid-dependent – primary hyperparathyroidism
• Parathyroid-independent
  – Malignancy-associated (most common cause in dogs)
    o Humoral hypercalcaemia of malignancy
    o Lymphoma (common)
    o Anal sac apocrine gland adenocarcinoma (common)
    o Carcinoma (sporadic): lung, pancreas, skin, nasal cavity, thyroid, mammary gland, adrenal medulla
    o Thymoma (rare)
    o Haematological malignancies (local osteolytic hypercalcaemia)
      ▪ Lymphoma
      ▪ Multiple myeloma
      ▪ Myeloproliferative disease (rare)
      ▪ Leukaemia (rare)
    o Metastatic or primary bone neoplasia (very uncommon)
  – Idiopathic hypercalcaemia (most common association in cats)
  – Chronic renal failure (± ionized hypercalcaemia)
  – Hypoadrenocorticism
  – Hypervitaminosis D
    o Iatrogenic
    o Plants (calcitriol glycosides)
    o Rodenticide (cholecalciferol)
    o Anti-psoriasis creams (calcipotriol or calcipotriene)
  – Granulomatous disease
    o Blastomycosis
    o Dermatitis
    o Panniculitis
    o Injection reaction
  – Acute renal failure (diuretic phase)
  – Skeletal lesions (non-malignant) (uncommon)
    o Osteomyelitis (bacterial or mycotic)
    o Hypertrophic osteodystrophy
    o Disuse osteoporosis (immobilization)
  – Excessive calcium-containing intestinal phosphate binders
  – Excessive calcium supplementation (calcium carbonate)
  – Hypervitaminosis A
  – Raisin/grape toxicity

21.1   Differential diagnosis of hypercalcaemia.

disease followed by malignancy. Though not reported recently, it appears that the most common type of ionized hypercalcaemia in cats is idiopathic, followed by chronic kidney disease and then malignancy-associated. Hypoadrenocorticism, primary hyperparathyroidism, hypervitaminosis D and inflammatory disorders sporadically account for hypercalcaemia. Hypercalcaemic cats have parathyroid-independent hypercalcaemia more commonly than dogs. It is often difficult to determine the cause of hypercalcaemia in animals with mild or transient hypercalcaemia (Schenck and Chew, 2008b). Approximately 30% of dogs with ionized hypercalcaemia in a recent study had no confirmed diagnosis (Messinger *et al.*, 2009).

Diagnostic approach
It is important to ensure that the hypercalcaemia initially detected is repeatable (Figure 21.2). Measurement of serum iCa is important to determine whether the increase is clinically significant. The likely cause of hypercalcaemia may be obvious from findings in the history or from physical examination (Schenck and Chew, 2006).

Assessment of calciotropic hormones
Serum iCa should be measured in association with PTH to assess the appropriateness of PTH response to serum iCa concentration. The first step is to determine whether the hypercalcaemia is parathyroid-dependent (disease of the parathyroid

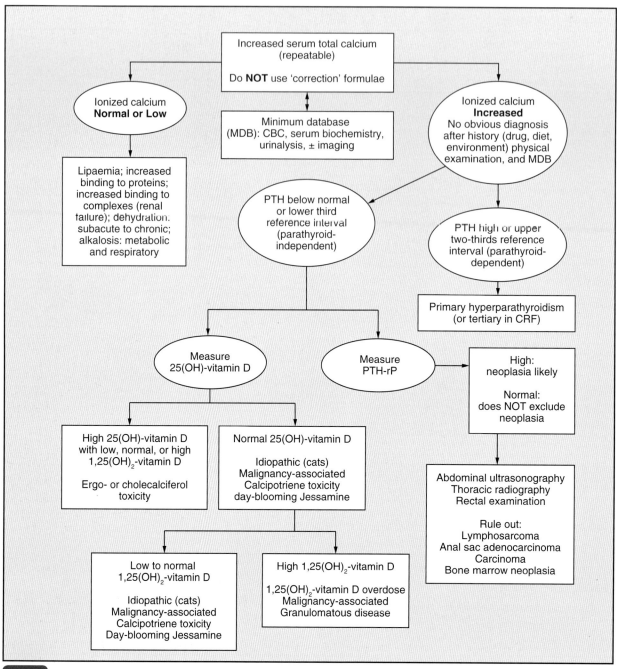

21.2 An approach to the diagnosis of hypercalcaemic disorders.

glands causing hypercalcaemia) or parathyroid-independent (normal parathyroid glands with appropriately suppressed PTH secretion in response to hypercalcaemia).

Measurement of PTHrP is helpful if malignancy is suspected, but PTHrP concentrations are not always increased in malignancy. Measurement of 25(OH)-vitamin D is useful in cases of potential cholecalciferol or ergocalciferol ingestion. Measurement of $1,25(OH)_2$-vitamin D is occasionally useful if excess calcitriol is the cause of hypercalcaemia. The anticipated changes in calcium hormones and serum biochemistry in disorders causing hypercalcaemia are presented in Figure 21.3.

Different types of PTH assays are available. Some assays that measure intact PTH have been

used successfully in animal species. These assays bind at the carboxy terminus and the amino-terminal antibody binds in the region of the 7th–10th amino acid. Depending on the exact site of binding, some assays perform well and others do not, because of species differences at the binding site. The intact PTH assay is capable of measuring PTH 7–84 fragments that may be increased, resulting in a falsely elevated PTH concentration. Intact PTH assays are being discontinued in favour of whole PTH assays. Whole PTH assays measure PTH (1–84) in its entirety, and thus do not measure the 7–84 fragment. At this time there are limited data on the use of whole PTH assays in animal species; however, these assays may provide more accurate assessment of PTH concentration.

Condition/causes	Parameter							
	tCa	*iCa*	*Albumin*	*Phosphate*	*PTH*	*PTH-rP*	*25(OH)-vitamin D*	*1,25(OH)₂-vitamin D*
Primary hyperparathyroidism	↑	↑	N	↓ or N	↑ or N	N	N	N or ↑
Secondary hyperparathyroidism – nutritional	N or ↓	N or ↓	N	N or ↑	↑	N	↓ or N	N or ↓
Secondary hyperparathyroidism – renal	N or ↓ or ↑	N or ↓	N	↑ or N	↑	N	N or ↓	N or ↓
Tertiary hyperparathyroidism	↑	↑	N	↑	↑	N	N or ↓	↓ or N
Malignancy-associated:								
Humoral hypercalcaemia	↑	↑	N or ↓	↓ or N	↓ or N	↑ or N	N	↓ or N or ↑
Local osteolytic	↑	↑	N or ↓	N or ↑	↓ or N	N or ↑	N	N
Hypervitaminosis D:								
Cholecalciferol-associated	↑	↑	N	↑ or N	↓	N	↑	N or ↑
1,5(OH)₂-vitamin D-associated	↑	↑	N	N or ↑	↓	N	N	↑
Calcipotriene-associated	↑	↑	N	↑ or N	↓	N	N	↓ or N
Hypoadrenocorticism	↑	↑	N or ↓	↑ or N	↓ or N	N	N	↓ or N
Hypervitaminosis A	↑	↑	N	N	↓	N	N	N or ↓
Idiopathic (cat)	↑	↑	N	N or ↑	↓ or N	N	N	N or ↓ or ↑
Dehydration	↑	N or ↑	↑ or N	N or ↑	N or ↓	N	N	N
Aluminium exposure (renal failure)	↑	↑	N	↑ or N	↓ or N	N	N	N or ↓
Raisin/grape toxicity (dog)	↑	–	N	N or ↑	–	–	–	–

21.3 Anticipated biochemical and hormonal changes associated with disorders of hypercalcaemia. iCa = ionized calcium; PTH = parathyroid hormone; PTHrP = parathyroid hormone-related protein; tCa =total calcium; N = normal; ↑ = increased; ↓ = decreased; – = no data.

Cervical ultrasonography

High-frequency ultrasonography of the cervical region can be performed to help determine whether the hypercalcaemia is parathyroid-dependent or parathyroid-independent. A single enlarged parathyroid gland is found in most cases of parathyroid-dependent hypercalcaemia, though multiple gland enlargement can be encountered occasionally. In parathyroid-independent hypercalcaemia, parathyroid glands are not enlarged or may not be identified; some may be atrophic if ionized hypercalcaemia of malignancy or hypervitaminosis D has been of long standing.

Other diagnostic tests

When the cause is not immediately apparent, thoracic and abdominal radiography and abdominal ultrasonography are recommended. Patients with evidence of cytopenias should undergo bone marrow evaluation if the diagnosis has not yet been established. Radiography of all bones is sometimes useful in finding lesions, even in those without demonstrable bone pain (multiple myeloma). Bone scintigraphy may be considered in those for which a diagnosis is lacking.

Treatment

The approach to treatment depends on the severity of clinical signs, the underlying cause of hypercalcaemia and the magnitude of hypercalcaemia. How quickly hypercalcaemia develops (acute *versus* chronic), trend for continued increase in calcium level, presence of hyperphosphataemia, presence of severe acid–base disturbances and status of renal and brain function all have an impact on the decision-making process as to how aggressive treatment should be. Rapidly rising levels of hypercalcaemia justify more aggressive intervention.

There is no single treatment protocol consistently effective for all causes of hypercalcaemia (Figure 21.4). Removal of the underlying cause is the definitive treatment for hypercalcaemia, but this is not always immediately possible. The goal of supportive treatment is to enhance urinary excretion of calcium and to prevent calcium resorption from bone.

Parenteral fluids and furosemide provide the first tier of treatment. The goal of fluid therapy is to induce diuresis and also to correct dehydration, because haemoconcentration contributes to increased serum iCa concentration. Furosemide is given following rehydration and fluid volume expansion for treatment

Treatment	Dose	Indications	Comments
Volume expansion			
Subcutaneous saline (0.9%)	75–100 ml/kg q24h	Mild hypercalcaemia	Contraindicated if peripheral oedema is present
Intravenous saline (0.9%)	5 ml//kg/h	Moderate to severe hypercalcaemia	Care in congestive heart failure and hypertension
Diuretics			
Furosemide	2 mg/kg i.v., s.c., orally, q8–12h	Moderate to severe hypercalcaemia	Volume expansion is necessary prior to use of this drug
Glucocorticoids			
Prednisolone	1 mg/kg i.v., s.c., orally, q12–24h	Moderate to severe hypercalcaemia	Use of these drugs prior to identification of aetiology may make definitive diagnosis difficult
Dexamethasone	0.1–0.22 mg/kg i.v., s.c., q12h		
Inhibition of bone resorption			
Calcitonin [a]	Initial 4 IU/kg i.v. infusion followed by 4–8 IU/kg s.c. q12–24h	Hypervitaminosis D toxicity	Response may be short lived. Vomiting and anorexia may occur
Bisphosphonates			
EHDP-etidronate [a]	5–15 mg/kg q12–24h	Moderate to severe chronic hypercalcaemia	Expensive
Clodronate [a]	20–25 mg/kg in a 4-hour i.v. infusion	Moderate to severe chronic hypercalcaemia	Expensive
Pamidronate [a]	1.3–2.0 mg/kg in 150 ml 0.9% saline in a 2-hour i.v. infusion; can repeat after 1–3 weeks	Moderate to severe hypercalcaemia. Well studied in hypervitaminosis D in dogs	Expensive
Alendronate [a]	5–20 mg orally once weekly after overnight fast. Must ensure animal swallows drug appropriately by administration of water or other substance that stimulates swallowing	Idiopathic hypercalcaemia–cats	Safety and efficacy yet to be reported; pilot study at Ohio State University suggests safe and effective

21.4 Treatment of hypercalcaemia. [a] Not authorized for use in dogs in the UK.

of persistent and severe hypercalcaemia to increase calcium excretion into urine (Schenck and Chew, 2008b). Thiazide diuretics should be avoided as they can promote renal tubular calcium reabsorption.

Glucocorticoids provide a second tier of treatment for hypercalcaemia that does not respond adequately to intravenous fluids and furosemide. Glucocorticoids can reduce the magnitude of persistent hypercalcaemia in patients with lymphosarcoma (cytolysis), multiple myeloma, hypoadrenocorticism, hypervitaminosis D, or granulomatous disease, but they have minimal effect on other causes of hypercalcaemia. Steroids exert their effect mainly by reducing bone resorption, decreasing intestinal calcium absorption, and increasing renal calcium excretion. However, glucocorticoids should be withheld if a definitive diagnosis has not yet been established. Chronic steroid administration may be needed to control hypercalcaemia in cats with idiopathic hypercalcaemia in which dietary alterations are not effective.

The third tier is to add a bisphosphonate for the more chronic control of hypercalcaemia. Bisphosphonates assist in lowering serum calcium by reducing the number and action of osteoclasts. Higher-fibre or alkalinizing diets may be helpful for management of chronic idiopathic hypercalcaemia in some cats.

Malignancy-associated hypercalcaemia

Hypercalcaemia in dogs is most commonly associated with cancer (Messinger et al., 2009). Neoplasia can cause hypercalcaemia through humoral hypercalcaemia of malignancy (HHM), or local osteolytic mechanisms (local osteolytic hypercalcaemia, LOH). LOH may develop following metastasis to bone, or from haematological malignancies in bone marrow and local production of bone-resorbing factors.

Clinical findings in HHM include hypercalcaemia, hypophosphataemia, hypercalciuria, increased fractional excretion of phosphate, and increased osteoclastic bone resorption. Increased osteoclastic bone resorption is a consistent finding and increases calcium release from bone. Excessive secretion of biologically active PTHrP plays a central role in the pathogenesis of hypercalcaemia in HHM, but cytokines such as interleukin 1, TNF-α

and transforming growth factor (TGF)-β and −γ, or calcitriol may have synergistic actions with PTHrP.

Malignancies commonly associated with HHM in dogs include T cell lymphoma and adenocarcinomas derived from the apocrine glands of the anal sac. In a recent study, lymphoma accounted for >58% of the cases with ionized hypercalcaemia overall. Of those with cancer and ionized hypercalcaemia, lymphoma was the diagnosis in 78% of the cases (Messinger *et al.*, 2009). Most dogs with lymphoma and hypercalcaemia have HHM because increased osteoclastic resorption is present in bones without evidence of tumour metastasis. Tumours in the apocrine glands of the anal sac appear primarily in middle-aged dogs. Clinical signs are referable to hypercalcaemia (polyuria, polydipsia, anorexia, and weakness), a mass in the perineum (tenesmus, ribbon-like stools, increased odour, and protruding mass), a mass in the sublumbar region, or more distant metastases.

Cases of HHM also occur in dogs with thymoma, myeloma, melanoma, or carcinomas originating in the lungs, pancreas, thyroid gland, skin, mammary gland, nasal cavity or adrenal medulla. Concentrations of PTHrP are highest in dogs with apocrine adenocarcinomas of the anal sac and carcinomas associated with HHM.

Lymphoma and squamous cell carcinoma are the two most common causes of hypercalcaemia in cats. Lymphoma comprises approximately one-third of the cases, with cancer and hypercalcaemia occurring considerably less frequently in the cat than in the dog; carcinomas comprise about one-third of the tumours in cats associated with hypercalcaemia (Savary *et al.*, 2000). Tumours also associated with hypercalcaemia in cats include: multiple myeloma; bronchogenic carcinoma/adenocarcinoma; osteosarcoma; fibrosarcoma; undifferentiated sarcoma; undifferentiated renal carcinoma; anaplastic carcinoma of the lung and diaphragm; and thyroid carcinoma.

Solid tumours that metastasize to bone can produce hypercalcaemia through the induction of local bone resorption associated with tumour growth. Carcinomas of the mammary gland, prostate, liver, and lung are most frequently reported to metastasize to bone in dogs, and the humerus, femur, and vertebrae are the most common sites of metastasis. Primary bone tumours are not often associated with hypercalcaemia in dogs or cats. Some types of haematological malignancies present in the bone marrow produce hypercalcaemia by inducing bone resorption locally. This effect occurs most commonly in multiple myeloma and lymphoma.

Chronic renal failure

Many dogs and cats with CRF have reference interval serum total calcium concentrations. Total hypercalcaemia occurs sporadically in dogs and cats with CRF, and CRF is usually listed as second or third in frequency of causes of hypercalcaemia (Savary *et al.*, 2000). The finding of hypercalcaemia and primary renal azotaemia poses a special diagnostic problem because hypercalcaemia can cause renal failure or develop as a consequence of CRF. Elevated total calcium occurs in up to 14% of dogs and 38% of cats with CRF. The prevalence of hypercalcaemia increases with severity of azotaemia, and in dogs the increase is most commonly due to an increase in the complexed calcium fraction (Schenck and Chew, 2003).

Deleterious effects of hypercalcaemia occur only if there is increased serum iCa concentration. Measurement of serum iCa concentration to assess calcium status in CRF patients is critical.

Fewer than 10% of all dogs with CRF have increased serum iCa concentrations. Cats with CRF appear to have a higher prevalence of ionized hypercalcaemia as compared with dogs, occurring in approximately 29% of cases. Increases in serum iCa do not show a strong association with the degree of azotaemia. Serum PTH concentration is often increased in patients with hypercalcaemia related to renal failure, and these animals must be differentiated from those with primary hyperparathyroidism (see Chapter 6). Serum iCa concentration is increased in primary hyperparathyroidism but is usually normal or low in patients with CRF. Rarely, tertiary hyperparathyroidism occurs, where there is an increased serum iCa concentration with an increase in PTH. Tertiary hyperparathyroidism occurs in those with long-standing secondary hyperparathyroidism and is most likely due to an alteration in the setpoint for circulating iCa.

Idiopathic hypercalcaemia in cats

Within the past 20 years, IHC has been recognized in cats and is considered the most common type of hypercalcaemia in cats. Although some suggest that IHC is a geographically local phenomenon, it is widespread across the United States and is also found in other parts of the world. Cats with IHC range in age from 0.5 to 20 years, and longhaired cats are over-represented (Midkiff *et al.*, 2000; Schenck and Chew, 2005a). Many cats (approximately 50%) have no obvious clinical signs. In the remaining cats, history and clinical signs can include mild weight loss, diarrhoea, chronic constipation, vomiting and anorexia. Uroliths are observed in approximately 15% of cases, with calcium oxalate stones noted in 10%. Serum iCa concentration is increased and PTH concentration is below or within the reference interval. PTHrP is not elevated and both serum magnesium and 25(OH)-vitamin D concentrations are normal. Serum $1,25(OH)_2$-vitamin D is usually suppressed.

Specific treatment for IHC is impossible because the pathogenesis remains unknown. The feeding of increased dietary fibre decreases serum calcium in some cats but not in others. Higher-fibre diets may decrease intestinal absorption of calcium, but the effects of fibre are complex and depend on the types and amounts of fibre present. The feeding of veterinary renal diets may result in normocalcaemia in some cats with IHC. These diets are generally low in calcium and phosphorus and are considered alkalinizing or at least less acidifying than maintenance diets. Some cats that show an initial decrease in serum calcium concentration following any type of dietary change will return to hypercalcaemia over time.

In those cats that do not respond to a change in diet, prednisolone therapy (5–20 mg q24h) may result in a long-term decrease in iCa. Hypercalcaemia returns in some cats despite maximal doses of prednisolone. When dietary modification and treatment with prednisolone have been unsuccessful, treatment with oral bisphosphonates such as alendronate can be considered. Intravenous treatment with bisphosphonates is almost never needed in IHC, since the hypercalcaemia is chronic and the cats are usually not in an acute crisis. A pilot study on the use of oral alendronate at the Ohio State University shows promise for its chronic use in cats with IHC. No adverse effects were seen in the 12 cats of this pilot study that were given an average dose of 10 mg orally per week. It is important to ensure that the medication does not stick in the oesophagus, which could cause oesophagitis: to minimize the risk, 6 ml of water is administered orally to enhance drug passage to the stomach. Ionized calcium decreased in all cats, many into the reference interval, in the 6-month period reported. The medication should be administered after a 12-hour fast, as food significantly reduces bisphosphonate absorption. It appears that this treatment is safe and effective, but further studies are needed (Hardie B *et al.*, unpublished observations, The Ohio State University). Oral bisphosphonates will likely replace prednisolone as the second choice for treatment of IHC in cats.

Hypoadrenocorticism

Hypoadrenocorticism is the second most common cause of hypercalcaemia in dogs, but is rarely recognized in cats. A correlation between the degree of hyperkalaemia and hypercalcaemia is detected when the serum potassium concentration is >6.0–6.5 mmol/l. Increases in serum iCa may or may not develop in hypoadrenocorticism. Serum total calcium concentration rapidly returns to normal after 1–2 days of glucocorticoid replacement therapy in dogs, and intravenous volume expansion can return serum calcium concentration to reference interval within a few hours. Hypoadrenocorticism should always be included in the differential diagnosis of hypercalcaemia because clinical signs of hypoadrenocorticism and hypercalcaemia are similar.

Hypervitaminosis D

Hypervitaminosis D refers to toxicity resulting from excess cholecalciferol (vitamin D) or ergocalciferol (vitamin D2). Vitamin D metabolites can also exert toxicity, and the term hypervitaminosis D has been extended to include toxicity from 25(OH)-vitamin D, $1,25(OH)_2$-vitamin D, as well as newer analogues of $1,25(OH)_2$-vitamin D. Hypercalcaemia may result from excessive dietary supplementation, or may be caused iatrogenically during treatment. Accurate dosing with cholecalciferol and ergocalciferol is difficult because they have a slow onset and prolonged duration of action. Ingestion of toxic plants that contain glycosides of calcitriol (e.g. *Cestrum diurnum*, *Solanum malacoxylon* and *Trisetum flavescens*) is a potential cause of hypercalcaemia in small animals. *Cestrum diurnum* (day-blooming jessamine) has achieved increasing popularity as a house plant and should not be confused with jasmine, which is an indoor climbing plant without active vitamin D metabolites.

A diagnosis of hypervitaminosis D in dogs and cats increased with the introduction of cholecalciferol-containing rodenticides in 1985, but this source of intoxication is less common today. Cholecalciferol bait pellets are palatable and are very toxic when ingested.

Hypercalcaemia usually develops within 24 hours of ingestion, and hypercalcaemia is often severe unless serum samples were obtained within 24 hours of ingestion. Mild hyperphosphataemia is often noted. Azotaemia is initially absent but can develop subsequently and can be marked. It may take as long as 72 hours for azotaemia to develop as a result of renal lesions caused by hypercalcaemia. Measurement of serum 25(OH)-vitamin D concentration can provide evidence for hypervitaminosis D after exposure to cholecalciferol or ergocalciferol.

Topical ointments containing vitamin D analogues (calcipotriene) for treatment of human psoriasis can result in hypercalcaemia when toxic quantities are ingested by dogs or cats (Hare *et al.*, 2000). The minimal toxic dose is 10 µg/kg, minimal lethal dose is 65 µg/kg and the oral LD_{50} is between 100 and 150 µg/kg in dogs. Serum phosphate, total calcium, and iCa are elevated with calcipotriene toxicity and most develop acute renal failure. Hypercalcaemia decreases after several days rather than being prolonged for weeks to months as seen in cholecalciferol toxicity.

Raisin/grape toxicity

The ingestion of grapes or raisins may result in hypercalcaemia in dogs. Over 90% of dogs with renal failure associated with grape or raisin ingestion had increased serum total calcium and increased serum phosphate concentrations 24 hours to several days following ingestion. Vomiting following ingestion of a trivial quantity of raisins or grapes in some dogs leads to the development of acute renal failure within 48 hours. In four dogs, ingestion was estimated to be from 0.41–1.1 ounces (11.6–31.2 g) of grapes or raisins per kilogram of bodyweight. Not all dogs that consume grapes or raisins develop clinical signs or acute renal failure. Of 132 dogs reported with raisin or grape ingestion, 33 developed no clinical signs or azotaemia, 14 developed clinical signs but no azotaemia and 43 developed clinical signs and acute renal failure. The pathogenesis of nephrotoxicity associated with raisins and grapes remains unknown as does the origin of the hypercalcaemia (Eubig *et al.*, 2005; Gwaltney-Brant *et al.*, 2001; Morrow *et al.*, 2005). Serum or plasma ionized calcium concentrations were not reported.

Approximately 58% of dogs with acute renal failure from grape/raisin ingestion survive, but several weeks of hospitalization with intensive fluid treatment is often needed. Initial and peak serum total calcium concentration and initial and peak calcium x phosphorus product are significantly higher in those that do not survive as compared with those that do survive. Approximately 50% of affected dogs can be expected to develop oliguria or anuria. Aggressive treatment is recommended for any dogs suspected of having ingested large, or even small, quantities of grapes or raisins, including induction of emesis, gastric lavage, and administration of activated charcoal, followed by intravenous fluid therapy for a minimum of 48 hours. Serum total calcium concentration returns to the reference interval in approximately 11 days. However, some dogs may consume relatively large quantities of grapes or raisins without development of ill effects.

Primary hyperparathyroidism

Primary hyperparathyroidism is an uncommon cause of hypercalcaemia in dogs and is even less common in cats. Excessive and inappropriate secretion of PTH by the parathyroid glands relative to the serum iCa concentration characterizes this condition. Further details are presented in Chapter 6.

Hypocalcaemia

Hypocalcaemia based on serum total calcium is relatively common and is observed in approximately 13% of sick dogs (Chew and Meuten, 1982). Hypocalcaemia is usually defined as a total calcium concentration <2.0 mmmol/l in dogs and <1.75 mmol/l in cats. When serum iCa concentration is used, hypocalcaemia is generally defined as a concentration <1.25 mmol/l in dogs and <1.1 mmol/l in cats. However, clinically significant hypocalcaemia is generally not apparent until the total and ionized calcium decrease to <1.5 and <0.8 mmol/l, respectively. Samples will usually be submitted when patients have persistent moderate to severe hypocalcaemia for which a known cause cannot be determined. Most samples will be submitted with suspicion of primary hypoparathyroidism (Schenck and Chew, 2008c).

Unexplained differences between iCa and total calcium concentrations have been found in hypocalcaemic conditions, and is not predictable. In sick dogs, approximately 27% have low total calcium concentration, and 31% have low iCa concentration (Schenck and Chew, 2005b). In sick cats, approximately 50% have low serum total calcium concentration, with only 27% having low iCa concentration (Schenck and Chew, 2010). Thus, in dogs total calcium measurement underestimates ionized hypocalcaemia, and in cats hypocalcaemia was overestimated when using serum total calcium concentration to predict iCa status.

Differential diagnosis

Hypocalcaemia develops when bone mobilization of calcium is reduced, skeletal calcium accretion is enhanced, urinary losses of calcium are increased, gastrointestinal absorption of calcium is reduced,

calcium is translocated intracellularly, or as a result of a combination of these mechanisms. The conditions associated with hypocalcaemia in dogs and cats are listed in Figure 21.5. The anticipated changes in calcium hormones and serum biochemistry in disorders causing hypocalcaemia are presented in Figure 21.6.

Common causes
• Hypoalbuminaemia
• Chronic renal failure
• Puerperal tetany (eclampsia)
• Acute renal failure
• Acute pancreatitis
• Undefined (mild hypocalcaemia)

Occasional causes
• Soft tissue trauma or rhabdomyolysis
• Hypoparathyroidism
• Ethylene glycol intoxication
• Phosphate enema
• After $NaHCO_3$ administration

Uncommon causes
• Laboratory error
• Improper anticoagulant (EDTA)
• Infarction of parathyroid gland adenoma
• Rapid i.v. infusion of phosphates
• Intestinal malabsorption or severe starvation
• Hypovitaminosis D
• Blood transfusion (citrated anticoagulant)
• Hypomagnesaemia
• Nutritional secondary hyperparathyroidism
• Tumour lysis syndrome

21.5 Differential diagnosis of hypocalcaemia.

Diagnostic approach

Much like the initial approach to hypercalcaemia, it is helpful to make the initial distinction as to whether hypocalcaemia is parathyroid-dependent or parathyroid-independent (Figure 21.7). Ionized calcium concentration must be evaluated in conjunction with serum PTH to determine whether PTH production is appropriate. Patients with low iCa and low PTH concentrations have absolute hypoparathyroidism (parathyroid-dependent). A reference interval PTH when iCa is low is inappropriate because normal parathyroid glands should respond with increased PTH. Hypocalcaemic patients with increased PTH are classified as having parathyroid-independent hypocalcaemia. In cases of parathyroid-independent hypocalcaemia, hypocalcaemia exists from redistribution of calcium into other body spaces, excess phosphate effects, or from deficiencies of vitamin D or dietary calcium (Schenck and Chew, 2008c).

Patients with persistent moderate to severe hypocalcaemia based on serum total calcium should be evaluated for iCa and PTH concentrations; measurement of 25(OH)-vitamin D and serum phosphate is also helpful, and in rare circumstances measurement of $1,25(OH)_2$-vitamin D may help provide a definitive diagnosis.

Condition	Parameter							
	tCa	iCa	Albumin	Phosphate	PTH	PTHrP	25(OH)-vitamin D	1,25(OH)$_2$-vitamin D
Primary hypoparathyroidism	↓	↓	N	↑ or N	↓ or N	N	N	N or ↓
Pseudohypoparathyroidism	↓	N or ↓	N	↑ or N	↑	N	N	N or ↑
Sepsis/critical care	↓ or N	↓	N	N or ↑	↑ or N	N	N	N
Ethylene glycol toxicity	↓	↓	N	↑ or N	↑	N	N	↓ or N
Phosphate enema toxicity	↓	↓	N	↑	↑	N	N	N or ↓ or ↑
Eclampsia	↓	↓	N	↓	Mildly ↑ or N	N	N	N or ↓
Hypoalbuminaemia	↓	↓ or N	↓	N	N or ↑	N	N	N or ↑

21.6 Anticipated biochemical and hormonal changes associated with disorders of hypocalcaemia. iCa = ionized calcium; PTH = parathyroid hormone; PTHrP = parathyroid hormone-related protein; tCa = total calcium; N = normal; ↑ = increased; ↓ = decreased.

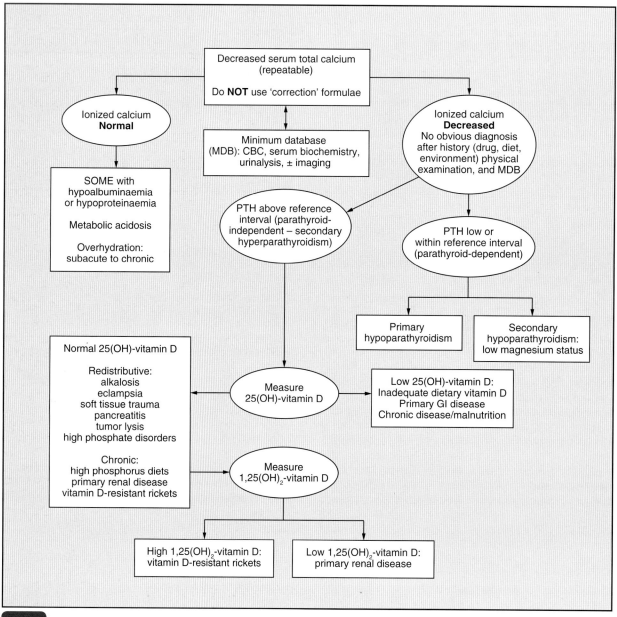

21.7 An approach to the diagnosis of hypocalcaemic disorders.

Treatment

General treatments for hypocalcaemia are listed in Figure 21.8.

Hypoalbuminaemia

Hypoalbuminaemia is the most common disorder associated with decreased total calcium concentration, but it is the least important clinically. Nearly 50% of dogs with low total calcium also have hypoalbuminaemia. The decrease in serum total calcium associated with hypoalbuminaemia is usually mild, and no signs referable to hypocalcaemia are observed. Application of calcium correction formulae to serum total calcium concentrations in dogs or cats with hypoproteinaemia or hypoalbuminaemia has been advocated in the past. However, these correction formulae do not improve the prediction of actual iCa concentration and in many cases increase the level of diagnostic discordance. Use of correction formulae to adjust serum total calcium concentration to serum total protein or albumin concentration is not recommended.

Renal failure

Renal failure is the second most common disorder associated with hypocalcaemia in dogs. Decreased $1,25(OH)_2$-vitamin D synthesis by diseased kidneys, and mass law interactions of calcium with markedly increased serum phosphate concentrations contribute to the development of hypocalcaemia. Low serum total calcium concentration is detected in approximately 10% of dogs with CRF, whereas low serum iCa concentration is found in approximately 30% of cases (Schenck and Chew, 2010). In cats with CRF, hypocalcaemia is found more commonly with higher magnitudes of azotaemia. With moderate CRF, approximately 14% of cats have low serum iCa, and with advanced CRF over 50% have low

Drug	Preparation	Calcium content	Dose	Comment
Parenteral calcium [a, b]				
Calcium gluconate	10% solution	9.3 mg of Ca/ml	0.5–1.5 ml/kg slow i.v. to effect	Stop if bradycardia or shortened QT interval occurs
			6.5–10 ml/kg i.v. q24h	Infusion to maintain normal calcium
Calcium chloride	10% solution	27.2 mg of Ca/ml	0.16–0.5 ml/kg i.v.	Only given i.v., as extremely caustic perivascularly
Calcium borogluconate	20% solution	15 mg of Ca/ml	0.3-0.9 ml/kg i.v.	
Oral calcium [c]				
Calcium carbonate	Many sizes	1 mg of Ca/2.5 mg tablet	25–50 mg/kg q24h	Most common calcium supplement
Calcium lactate	Many sizes (325, 650 mg tablets, etc.)	1 mg of Ca/7.7 mg tablet		
Calcium gluconate	Many sizes	1 mg of Ca/11.2 mg tablet		
Oral vitamin D				
Vitamin D2 (ergocalciferol)			Initial: 4000–6000 IU/kg q24h; Maintenance: 1000–2000 IU/kg once daily to once weekly	Time for maximal effect to occur: 5–21 days Time for toxicity effect to resolve: 1–18 weeks
1,25-dihydroxycholecalciferol ($1,25(OH)_2$-vitamin D; calcitriol)			Initial: 20–30 ng/kg q24h for 3–4 days Maintenance: 5–15 ng/kg q24h	Time for maximum effect to occur: 1–4 days Time for toxicity effect to resolve: 2–7 days
Alfacalcidol			0.01–0.03 µg/kg q24h	
Dihydrotachysterol			Initial: 0.02–0.03 mg/kg q24h. Can be reduced for longer-term management to 0.01–0.02 mg/kg q24–48h or as required	Onset of action within 24 hours; peak activity within 7 days.

21.8 Treatment of hypocalcaemia. [a] Subcutaneous calcium salts can cause severe skin necrosis or mineralization, even when diluted. It is best not to give any calcium salts s.c. [b] Do not mix calcium solution with bicarbonate-containing fluids as precipitation may occur. [c] Calculate dose on elemental calcium content.

serum iCa concentrations (Barber and Elliott, 1998). Hypocalcaemia was underappreciated when based on results of total calcium measurement, especially with advancing azotaemia. Clinical signs of hypocalcaemia are uncommon in renal failure.

Critical illness
Ionized hypocalcaemia is common in the critically ill, and is more common in septic patients (Lind *et al.,* 2000). The magnitude of hypocalcaemia is correlated with the severity of illness. The causes of hypocalcaemia in critical illness appear to be multifactorial; sepsis, systemic inflammatory response syndrome, hypomagnesaemia, blood transfusions and renal failure have all been associated with the condition. The presence of proinflammatory cytokines during sepsis is related to the development of hypocalcaemia in septic patients. PTH is commonly elevated, even when normocalcaemia exists. The impact of hypocalcaemia on survival has not been determined; hypocalcaemia and higher concentrations of PTH may be more frequently associated with fatality. Ionized hypocalcaemia was recently described in 16% of critically ill dogs, and was associated with longer ICU and hospital stays but not with decreased survival. Septic dogs with positive blood culture results were more likely to have ionized hypocalcaemia (Holowaychuk *et al.,* 2009). Ionized hypocalcaemia was reported in 75% of cats with urethral obstruction; hypocalcaemia was considered to be mild in 37.5%, moderate in 25% and severe in 12.5% of affected cats (Drobatz and Hughes, 1997).

Puerperal tetany (eclampsia)
Puerperal tetany typically occurs between 1 and 3 weeks postpartum in the dog, and is attributed to loss of calcium into milk during lactation. Bitches of small breeds and with large litters are most commonly affected. Proposed mechanisms for hypocalcaemia include: a poor dietary source of calcium; major loss of calcium during lactation; fetal skeletal ossification; and abnormal parathyroid gland function, including parathyroid gland atrophy. Hypophosphataemia may accompany the hypocalcaemia, and clinical signs rarely occur before whelping. Clinical signs most often include seizures, trembling, twitching, shaking and stiffness. Non-typical signs include panting, behavioural changes, collapse, and whining; vomiting, diarrhoea, and choking are rare. Rectal temperature is usually elevated, attributable to increased muscle activity. After treatment with intravenous calcium gluconate, serum iCa concentration normalizes within 25 minutes in most dogs (Drobatz and Casey, 2000).

Puerperal tetany is rare in cats, and usually occurs 3–17 days before parturition. Signs of depression, weakness, tachypnoea and mild muscle tremors are most common; vomiting and anorexia are less common, and prolapse of the third eyelid occurs in some cats. Hypothermia, instead of hyperthermia as seen in dogs, is observed (Fascetti and Hickman, 1999).

Pancreatitis
Acute pancreatitis may be associated with hypocalcaemia. In cats with acute pancreatitis, 61% have low serum iCa concentration (Kimmel *et al.,* 2001). In pancreatitis, hypocalcaemia may be due to:

- Sequestration of calcium into peripancreatic fat (saponification)
- Increased free fatty acids
- Increased calcitonin secondary to increased glucagon
- PTH resistance or deficit resulting from the effects of hypomagnesaemia.

Nutritional secondary hyperparathyroidism
Vitamin D deficiency and nutritional secondary hyperparathyroidism (NSHP) associated with low calcium and/or high phosphorus concentrations in the diet result in low to normal serum iCa and normal to high serum phosphate concentrations, with an increase in PTH secretion. NSHP also occurs when severe gastrointestinal disease is present, which limits the absorption of calcium and vitamin D. The occurrence of NSHP has decreased dramatically since the advent of feeding commercially available, nutritionally complete and balanced pet foods. Renal secondary hyperparathyroidism preferentially affects the bones of the face (fibrous osteodystrophy), whereas NSHP tends to cause osteopenia of the long bones and vertebrae. Both lesions are more likely to be seen in young, growing animals. With the feeding of unbalanced homemade diets, the occurrence of NSHP is more likely (DeLay and Laing, 2002). Clinical signs of hypocalcaemia are uncommon.

Tumour lysis syndrome
Tumour lysis syndrome occurs when there is rapid destruction of sensitive tumour cells following chemotherapy. Release of intracellular products can result in hyperkalaemia, hyperphosphataemia and hyperuricaemia. Hypocalcaemia develops as calcium phosphate salts are deposited into soft tissues, and acute renal failure may result. Tumour lysis syndrome with clinical signs of hypocalcaemia occurs uncommonly.

Ethylene glycol toxicity
Metabolites of ethylene glycol can chelate calcium and become deposited in soft tissues, resulting in hypocalcaemia. Both dogs and cats exhibit hypocalcaemia after ethylene glycol ingestion. Seizures have been observed in dogs within hours of ingestion; renal function is often normal at this time. Hypocalcaemia often develops later, when renal function is severely reduced from acute renal failure and when hyperphosphataemia is severe.

Hypoparathyroidism
Hypoparathyroidism is a condition characterized by absolute or relative deficiency of PTH secretion that can be permanent or transient. Hypocalcaemia and clinical signs referable to low iCa concentration are

the hallmarks of this condition. Hypoparathyroidism in dogs is most commonly idiopathic, whereas surgical removal of or injury to the parathyroid gland during thyroidectomy to correct hyperthyroidism is the most common cause in cats. Further details are presented in Chapter 7.

References and further reading

Barber PJ and Elliott J (1998) Feline chronic renal failure: calcium homeostasis in 80 cases diagnosed between 1992 and 1995. *Journal of Small Animal Practice* **39**, 108–116

Brennan SF, O'Donovan J and Mooney CT (2006) Changes in canine ionized calcium under three storage conditions. *Journal of Small Animal Practice* **47**, 383–386

Chew DJ and Meuten DJ (1982) Disorders of calcium and phosphorus metabolism. *Veterinary Clinics of North America: Small Animal Practice* **12**, 411–438

DeLay J and Laing J (2002) Nutritional osteodystrophy in puppies fed a BARF diet, *AHL Newsletter* **6**, 23

Drobatz KJ and Casey KK (2000) Eclampsia in dogs: 31 cases (1995–1998). *Journal of the American Veterinary Medical Association* **217**, 216–219

Drobatz KJ and Hughes D (1997) Concentration of ionized calcium in plasma from cats with urethral obstruction. *Journal of the American Veterinary Medical Association* **211**, 1392–1395

Eubig PA, Brady MS, Gwaltney-Brant SM *et al.* (2005) Acute renal failure in dogs after the ingestion of grapes or raisins: a retrospective evaluation of 43 dogs (1992–2002). *Journal of Veterinary Internal Medicine* **19**, 663–674

Fascetti AJ and Hickman MA (1999) Preparturient hypocalcemia in four cats. *Journal of the American Veterinary Medical Association* **215**, 1127–1129

Gwaltney-Brant S, Holding JK, Donaldson CW *et al.* (2001) Renal failure associated with ingestion of grapes or raisins in dogs. *Journal of the American Veterinary Medical Association* **218**, 1555–1556

Hare WR, Dobbs CE, Slayman KA *et al.* (2000) Calcipotriene poisoning in dogs. *Veterinary Medicine* **95**, 770–778

Holowaychuk MK, Hansen BD, DeFrancesco TC and Marks SL (2009) Ionized hypocalcemia in critically ill dogs. *Journal of Veterinary Internal Medicine* **23**, 509–513

Kimmel SE, Washabau RJ and Drobatz KJ (2001) Incidence and prognostic value of low plasma ionized calcium concentration in cats with acute pancreatitis: 46 cases (1996–1998). *Journal of the American Veterinary Medical Association* **219**, 1105–1109

Lind L, Carlstedt F, Rastad J *et al.* (2000) Hypocalcemia and parathyroid hormone secretion in critically ill patients. *Critical Care Medicine* **28**, 93–99

Messinger JS, Windham WR and Ward CR (2009) Ionized hypercalcemia in dogs: a retrospective study of 109 cases (1998–2003). *Journal of Veterinary Internal Medicine* **23**, 514–519

Midkiff AM, Chew DJ, Randolph JF, Center SA and DiBartola SP (2000) Idiopathic hypercalcemia in cats. *Journal of Veterinary Internal Medicine* **14**, 619–626

Morrow CMK, Valli VE, Volmer PA *et al.* (2005) Canine renal pathology associated with grape or raisin ingestion: 10 cases. *Journal of Veterinary Diagnostic Investigation* **17**, 223–231

Savary KC, Price GS and Vaden SL (2000) Hypercalcemia in cats: a retrospective study of 71 cases (1991–1997). *Journal of Veterinary Internal Medicine* **14**,184–189

Schenck PA and Chew DJ (2003) Calcium fractionation in dogs with chronic renal failure. *American Journal of Veterinary Research* **64**, 1181–1184

Schenck PA and Chew DJ (2005a) Idiopathic hypercalcemia in cats. *Waltham Focus* **15**(3), 20–24

Schenck PA and Chew DJ (2005b) Prediction of serum ionized calcium concentration by use of serum total calcium concentration in dogs. *American Journal of Veterinary Research* **66**(8), 1330–1336

Schenck, PA and Chew DJ (2006) Diseases of the parathyroid gland and calcium metabolism. In: *Manual of Small Animal Practice*, 3rd Edition, ed. SJ Birchard and RG Sherding, pp. 343–356. Elsevier, St. Louis

Schenck PA and Chew DJ (2008a) Calcium: Total or ionized? *Veterinary Clinics of North America: Small Animal Practice* **38**(3), 497–502

Schenck PA and Chew DJ (2008b) Hypercalcemia: a quick reference. *Veterinary Clinics of North America: Small Animal Practice* **38**(3), 449–454

Schenck PA and Chew DJ (2008c) Hypocalcemia: a quick reference. *Veterinary Clinics of North America: Small Animal Practice* **38**(3): 455–458

Schenck PA and Chew DJ (2010) Prediction of serum ionized calcium concentration by serum total calcium measurement in cats. *Canadian Journal of Veterinary Research* **74**, 209–213

Schenck PA, Chew DJ and Brooks CL (1995) Effects of storage on serum ionized calcium and pH values in clinically normal dogs. *American Journal of Veterinary Research* **56**, 304–307

Schenck PA, Chew DJ, Nagode LA and Rosol TJ (2006) Disorders of calcium: hypercalcemia and hypocalcemia. In: *Fluid Therapy in Small Animal Practice*, 3rd edition, ed. S. Dibartola, pp. 122–194. Elsevier, St. Louis

22

Investigation of unstable canine diabetes mellitus

Lucy J. Davison

Introduction

Diabetes mellitus is caused by a relative or absolute lack of insulin, and by the time it is diagnosed in most dogs, irreversible pancreatic damage has usually occurred. Currently there is no universally accepted veterinary classification for canine diabetes; however, with few exceptions, patients can be considered insulin-dependent. It is increasingly clear that despite the similar clinical signs, the process by which a dog becomes diabetic may be different in each individual (Rand *et al.*, 2004; Catchpole *et al.*, 2005). Superimposed on a background of genetic susceptibility (often breed-associated), several factors are capable of 'triggering' diabetes. These include hormonal antagonism (e.g. steroid treatment, hyperadrenocorticism, dioestrus), pancreatitis and autoimmunity (see Chapter 12).

Identifying the cause of diabetes mellitus

Where possible, it is vital to establish the underlying cause of diabetes in a patient, as this can impact significantly on the glycaemic control that might be reasonably expected. Not only is this useful for the veterinary surgeon in charge of the case, but it can also act as a prognostic guide for owners as they embark on the journey of diabetic stabilization and management. For example, a dog whose diabetes is the result of ongoing waxing and waning episodes of pancreatitis might exhibit more 'brittle' glycaemic control than a patient whose diabetes became clinically apparent during dioestrus and who was subsequently neutered. Patients who present for the first time in ketoacidosis rather than as 'well' newly diagnosed patients might also be more prone to episodes of instability in the future. This topic is discussed in depth in Chapter 12.

Management of diabetes mellitus

In the management of human type 1 diabetes, patients assess their blood glucose concentration several times each day and often use a combination of insulins to achieve tight glycaemic control. Human diabetic patients face many decades of treatment and such tight control is required to minimize complications, such as vascular and renal disease, which develop over a number of years. This degree of glycaemic control is impractical for canine diabetes in most cases and potentially less necessary, as dogs are often >7 years old at diagnosis, hence management is likely to be required for no longer than a few years. As with many examples of human medical treatment being applied to veterinary patients, a degree of compromise is required, since the main aim is to preserve the patient's quality of life. Using a 'human' diabetic stabilization protocol, involving multiple daily blood glucose tests and several daily insulin injections, would arguably have a significant negative impact on the dog's quality of life, hence a more simple approach can usually be adopted, with one or two daily injections. It is important for owner and veterinary surgeon to recognize this compromise and to be aware that perfect glycaemic control cannot always be obtained with one or two insulin injections a day. Despite this, good control with an excellent quality of life for several years is certainly achievable in the majority of patients, with careful control of food, exercise and insulin.

Aims of therapy
The aims of therapy include:

- Resolution of clinical signs such as polyuria/polydipsia
- Maintenance of a good appetite and stable bodyweight
- Owner perception that the patient has a good quality of life and is able to undertake a reasonable amount of daily exercise
- Minimal complications, such as ketosis, hypoglycaemia, infections and cataracts.

It is important to note that most of these aims are subjective and can be achieved in some animals despite small elevations in fructosamine and intermittent mild glucosuria. As discussed in Chapter 12, fructosamine measurements are best used to compare a patient with itself over a period of time, as they can be misleading if interpreted without reference to the clinical outcomes discussed here.

Recognition of instability

The definition of an *unstable* diabetic patient includes those dogs that show one or more of the clinical signs listed in Figure 22.1.

- Ongoing polyuria and polydipsia
- Weight loss
- Inconsistent appetite
- Hypoglycaemic episodes
- Ketotic or ketoacidotic episodes
- Increasing sequential serum fructosamine concentrations (rather than a single fructosamine concentration being above the laboratory reference range)
- No apparent change in blood glucose in response to injected insulin
- Cataracts (although even dogs with acceptable glycaemic control may develop cataracts)

22.1 Clinical signs of unstable diabetes mellitus.

It is clear that the best way to manage instability in diabetic patients is to recognize and correct deterioration in glycaemic control as early as possible. This relies on conscientious record-keeping and monitoring by both owner and veterinary surgeon or veterinary nurse, as discussed in Chapter 12. Unstable diabetic patients tend to fall into two general categories:

- Patients that have never been well controlled
- Patients that have been previously well controlled but whose glycaemic control deteriorates to the point that clinical signs become unacceptable or a 'crisis' point such as hypoglycaemia or diabetic ketoacidosis is reached.

The number of patients falling into the first category can be reduced by following strict guidelines during the stabilization period, discussed in Chapter 12. These include the use of twice-daily insulin where possible, careful attention to dietary management factors, the use of small incremental insulin doses with an equilibration time between each dose, regular monitoring, and awareness of concurrent diseases such as pancreatitis.

Investigation of instability

Investigation of diabetic instability is a very challenging and time-consuming process, requiring a lot of patience and very good client communication skills. An outline of a suitable approach to the unstable diabetic patient is discussed below and summarized in Figure 22.2.

History
One of the most important parts of the investigation is establishing a thorough history of the patient's general health and diabetes control. It is preferable to set aside a specific period of time when neither the veterinary surgeon nor the owner feels time-restricted. In these circumstances, owners might reveal important information that they had previously thought insignificant, as well as giving the veterinary surgeon a chance to assess the whole time course of decision-making in the case. It is vital to revisit the factors that were used to decide changes in

HISTORY – Factors relating to treatment and management
- Insulin type, doses, injection technique, feeding, diet, exercise, monitoring
- Check entire females have been spayed
- Look for evidence of concurrent disease – e.g. vomiting, urinary signs, abdominal pain and check whether any other treatment is being given

CLINICAL EXAMINATION
- Full physical examination including lymph node palpation, rectal examination (prostate, anal sacs), dental, ophthalmological and neurological examinations

PROBLEM LIST and DIFFERENTIAL DIAGNOSES
- Including all abnormalities discovered during history and clinical examination.
- Consider and investigate any differential diagnoses that might not be related to diabetes mellitus (e.g. renal disease, malignancy)

EVALUATION OF POTENTIAL UNDERLYING CAUSES OF POOR GLYCAEMIC CONTROL
- **Baseline information** – blood glucose curve, urinalysis (including culture), routine haematology, serum biochemistry

CATEGORIZATION OF POSSIBLE MECHANISM OF INSTABILITY
With special testing ONLY if appropriate clinical signs
1. Rule out management factors (history).

If patient is receiving a high insulin dose:
2. Rule out Somogyi overswing (history ± blood glucose curve).
3. Rule out infection or inflammation – particularly pancreatitis, urinary tract infection, dental disease (history, clinical examination, blood glucose curve, urine culture, cPLI, TLI, diagnostic imaging – radiography and ultrasonography).
4. Rule out hormonal antagonism e.g. progesterone, hypo- or hyperadrenocorticism, hypothyroidism (reproductive and clinical history, ACTH simulation test, T4 and cTSH concentrations), exogenous steroids or progestogens.

If patient is showing erratic response to insulin:
5. Poor insulin activity – test response to intramuscular dose of soluble insulin. If poor response, re-check for infection, inflammation, hormonal antagonism. If good, consider change of insulin preparation or route of delivery.

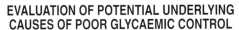
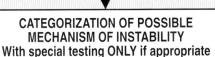

22.2 A summarized approach to the unstable diabetic dog.

management regime, such as insulin dose and diet, and whether these changes led to clinical improvement or deterioration.

Factors contributing to instability might also come to light during this consultation, e.g. the use of a new type of syringe, a change in the person giving the insulin injection or the site of injection, the use of new dietary supplements or factors affecting the storage of insulin. All of these changes can have a profound impact on glycaemic control, yet none of them would be revealed by clinical examination, diagnostic imaging or biochemical testing. The use of both 'open' and 'closed' questions is recommended and a non-exhaustive list of examples is given in Figure 22.3.

Clinical history relating to the time of diagnosis of diabetes

- Was there concurrent ketoacidosis?
- Were there clinical signs of pancreatitis?
- Was there a hormonal trigger, e.g. exogenous steroids, dioestrus?
- How long were clinical signs present before diagnosis?
- Was glycaemic control ever achieved and how long did this take?
- Are there any factors that the owner feels have contributed to the clinical deterioration?

Clinical history relating to the daily/weekly diabetic routine

- Food – type, amount, timing with respect to insulin and any changes in routine
- Scavenging behaviour
- Insulin – type, amount, dose, route, frequency and site of injection
- Insulin storage, mixing and administration practices
- Exercise
- Monitoring at home and diary keeping
- Other treatments – oral or topical, supplements, preventive healthcare measures

Clinical history relating to the investigation and management of instability

- Clinical signs of instability and whether they are progressing
- Other clinical signs that might or might not be related to poor glycaemic control (e.g. vomiting, diarrhoea, hair loss, dysuria)
- How glycaemic control has been monitored since diagnosis
- Serial weight measurements and serial fructosamine measurements (if available)
- Historical blood glucose curve results and diagnostic imaging results (if available)
- Historical changes in insulin dose, frequency and preparation along with rationale for each change, exact dates and whether it led to improvement or deterioration
- Discussion of who has been deciding about the daily insulin dose and changes to that dose
- Other treatments that have been administered (e.g. antibiotics, topical treatments, NSAIDs), reasons for this and clinical effects
- Other investigations that have been performed so far and their results
- The historical points at which the owner feels the patient has been least stable and most stable (subjective assessment of quality of life)

22.3 Examples of questions to ask, and factors to consider, when taking a history from the owner of an unstable diabetic dog.

Physical examination

Once a comprehensive history has been taken, the focus should be on a complete and thorough clinical examination, including neurological and ophthalmological assessment, lymph node palpation, blood pressure measurement and rectal palpation. Poor glycaemic control can often be secondary to other diseases, e.g. pyelonephritis, pancreatitis, dental abscess. Alternatively, clinical signs that suggest unstable diabetes (e.g. polyuria/polydipsia) might equally be the result of a completely unrelated disease process (e.g. hypercalcaemia of malignancy).

Establishing a problem list

Once the complete history has been recorded and a clinical examination performed, a problem list should be established for the patient. This list will include abnormalities detected during the history taking (e.g. episodes of abdominal pain, polydipsia, hypoglycaemia), abnormalities detected during previous investigations (e.g. elevated fructosamine) and those recorded during clinical examination (e.g. patchy hair coat, dental disease, heart murmur).

Differential diagnosis

Using the problem-oriented approach to medicine cases, the problem list is then expanded by the construction of a differential diagnosis list for each problem. Although 'unstable diabetes' could be considered a 'problem' in its own right, when investigating an unstable diabetic patient it is often helpful in complex cases to make a more detailed list of specific clinical abnormalities, e.g. polydipsia, weight loss, recurrent infections. For many of these problems, unstable diabetes is only one of the potential differential diagnoses and this approach reminds the clinician to consider diseases other than diabetes mellitus as the possible cause of the patient's problems, e.g. renal failure, hyperadrenocorticism, urinary tract infection, malignancy. This process can be time-consuming, as many unstable diabetic dogs have several concurrent problems, but it is a very worthwhile investment of time. Potential differential diagnoses should be investigated with further tests, such as diagnostic imaging, specialized biochemical or endocrine testing and urinalysis where appropriate.

Once concurrent disease has been ruled out, the outstanding differential diagnosis for each problem on the list will remain as 'unstable diabetes mellitus'. When this point is reached, it is advisable to continue with a very methodical approach, dividing the possible causes of instability into broad categories (Figure 22.4), each to be worked through in turn. Available tools at this stage include fructosamine measurement, blood glucose curve, urinalysis, diagnostic imaging, endocrine function tests, routine haematology, serum biochemistry and measurement of pancreatic inflammatory markers.

Generally, routine haematology, serum biochemistry and urinalysis (including culture and sensitivity testing), if not already performed, and blood glucose curves represent a good starting point. It must be remembered, however, that blood glucose curves are time-consuming and are not a substitute for a problem-oriented approach. There is considerable day-to-day variability in serial glucose curves, even in stable patients (Fleeman and Rand, 2003) and so they should be interpreted with caution. More details

---

- Management and practical factors
- Insulin-induced hyperglycaemia
- Infection or inflammation
- Hormonal antagonism
- Inadequate insulin activity

22.4 Possible causes of poor glycaemic control in a diabetic patient.

of blood glucose curve analysis, continuous glucose monitoring (Davison *et al.,* 2003b) and home glucose monitoring (Casella *et al.,* 2003) are discussed in Chapter 12.

Causes of instability

Management factors

The contribution of management factors to the instability of a diabetic dog can only be established by very careful history taking. As detailed in Chapter 12, problems with injection technique, insulin storage, diet or exercise can only be discovered by discussion with the owner. Examples of cases where management factors have been the cause of instability include:

- An owner who does not exercise their dog during the week but takes it on long walks at weekends
- An owner who thinks it is a good idea to re-use syringes, but independently decides to rinse them out in ethanol between injections, inactivating all but the first dose of insulin given with each syringe
- A dog who lives next door to a fruit farm and becomes unstable every autumn after eating windfall apples
- A dog who becomes increasingly unstable towards the end of each bottle of insulin in the summer, as the insulin bottle was not always kept in the fridge when the owner visited their caravan
- A friend who cares for the dog shaking the bottle of insulin aggressively before giving the injection, resulting in a loss of insulin activity.

Short duration of insulin action

Most intermediate-acting (lente) insulins have a duration of activity significantly shorter than 24 hours and this is often a problem in those treated with once-daily insulin injections. An inadequate duration of action will be avoided by switching once-daily treated patients to twice-daily insulin if they appear to be unstable. Patients that would benefit from such a change can usually be identified by their history of instability on once-daily insulin, frequent morning hyperglycaemia and glucosuria, and history of overnight polyuria and polydipsia. If necessary, and particularly if the owner is reluctant to use twice-daily insulin, it should be possible to demonstrate inadequate duration of insulin activity using a blood glucose curve, in which glucose concentration will start to rise within 8–16 hours of the first injection. An inadequate duration of activity cannot be compensated for by increasing the insulin dose, although occasionally an alternative preparation with a longer duration of activity (e.g. protamine zinc insulin, although this is not currently widely available) can result in successful glycaemic control with once-daily treatment. Generally, however, in difficult diabetic patients, better glycaemic control is more likely to be achieved with twice-daily treatment (Hess *et al.,* 2000; Fleeman and Rand, 2001).

When changing a patient from once-daily to twice-daily insulin of the same preparation, the new dose used will depend on many factors. If the effect of the insulin has clearly stopped by 12 hours after the morning injection, then the same dose that was used once daily can be given twice daily. If the patient is receiving a particularly high insulin dose, or if there is any suggestion of a Somogyi overswing (see below) or evidence of some residual insulin effect at 12 hours, then 0.5 IU/kg q12h can be a useful guide to a starting dose, with small adjustments made every 4–5 days, depending on progress.

Insulin-induced hyperglycaemia (Somogyi overswing)

The administration of a high dose of insulin (usually >1.5 IU/kg) once daily can lead to the phenomenon of a paradoxical insulin-induced hyperglycaemia. This occurs because of the initial rapid drop in blood glucose caused by the high insulin dose. The body's natural response to low blood glucose (usually <3.5 mmol/l), particularly if it has occurred rapidly, is to counteract this by the secretion of a combination of hormones to antagonize the hypoglycaemic effect of insulin, often raising blood glucose to very high concentrations (>20 mmol/l), as illustrated in Figure 22.5. These hormones include glucagon, cortisol and adrenaline (which can also result in an accompanying hypertension). It is important to note that in a non-diabetic patient that experiences hypoglycaemia, compensatory overswing is less of a problem, as it can be counteracted by endogenous insulin secretion.

Although the Somogyi overswing is theoretically simple to detect using a blood glucose curve, it is not always straightforward: the period of hypoglycaemia can be very short, and is easily missed, even with hourly blood samples; and the effect of the antagonistic hormones can persist for >24 hours after the hypoglycaemic event, limiting the development of hypoglycaemia in response to the same insulin dose on the subsequent day(s).

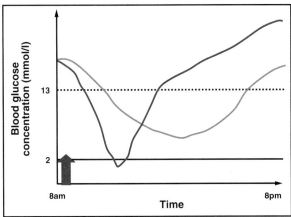

22.5 Insulin-induced hyperglycaemia (Somogyi overswing) caused by an excessive once-daily dose of insulin. Blue line: blood glucose concentration after an acceptable twice-daily insulin dose. Pink line: blood glucose concentration after a high once-daily insulin dose (given at 8 am); there is rebound hyperglycaemia.

As this 'overswing' effect is not always apparent on blood glucose curves, other factors must be used to determine whether this is the cause of instability in a patient. A comprehensive history will already have established the current dose of insulin and how changes in insulin doses were undertaken. The Somogyi overswing effect is more likely in a patient whose history includes two or more of the factors listed in Figure 22.6. Should a Somogyi overswing be detected (or strongly suspected), and other causes of insulin resistance have been ruled out, it is often helpful to switch the patient to twice-daily insulin at a lower dose (e.g. 0.5 IU/kg) with close monitoring. The blood glucose curve can then be repeated after 4–5 days and the insulin dose adjusted accordingly (see Chapter 12).

- Patient is receiving once-daily lente insulin treatment
- Home urine monitoring has been used to adjust insulin
- Blood glucose is often very high, whatever time of day it is measured
- Insulin dose adjustments have been in large (>2 IU) increments
- Insulin dose adjustments have been made very frequently, without adequate time to equilibrate between dose changes (at least 2–3 days)
- Insulin dose is approaching or above 2 IU/kg per injection
- Patient displays more marked polyuria/polydipsia overnight (if receiving once daily treatment)
- There was an initial clinical improvement at the time of diagnosis when insulin treatment was started, but this has not been sustained as insulin dose has risen

22.6 Factors increasing the risk of insulin-induced hyperglycaemia.

Infection or inflammation

Any focus of infection or inflammation can result in insulin resistance in a diabetic patient. As hyperglycaemia is a risk factor in the establishment of bacterial and fungal disease, infections are very common in diabetic dogs and hence should always be carefully considered in the unstable patient (Hess *et al.*, 2000). Signs of infection or inflammation in a diabetic dog can be very obvious (e.g. purulent nasal discharge, severe dental disease) or they can be more subtle (e.g. prostatic infection, respiratory infection, urinary tract disease, pancreatitis).

Screening for infection or inflammation can include routine haematology, urinalysis and diagnostic imaging (e.g. thoracic radiography, abdominal ultrasonography), as well as other more specific tests if indicated by history and clinical signs (e.g. blood culture, joint aspirates, pancreatic enzyme measurement, echocardiography, rhinoscopy). Any bacterial infection should ideally be treated on the basis of a positive culture and sensitivity result, and often a protracted course of antibiotics is required to control infection completely and prevent recurrence. Fungal infections in diabetic patients can be even more tenacious, and antifungal therapy is often required for a minimum of 6–8 weeks. Where possible, contributory factors to infection should also be addressed (e.g. periodontal disease, prostatic disease, urethral sphincter mechanism incompetence).

Urinary tract infection

As urinary tract infection is common in unstable diabetic dogs, urinalysis (including culture and sensitivity testing) of a sample obtained by cystocentesis should always be performed (in addition to clinical examination). Long-standing infections can also result in the formation of crystals or cystic calculi, which can perpetuate the problem, even if there was previously a temporary improvement on an empirical course of antibiotics. For this reason, diagnostic imaging of the urinary tract is also recommended. Urinary tract infections are a particularly important complication, as their clinical signs (such as frequent urination and polydipsia) can easily be dismissed as simply a result of diabetic polyuria. Whilst urinary tract infections are a common cause of instability, it must also be remembered that they can arise as a secondary complication of poor glycaemic control which has arisen by another mechanism. Treatment of such infections is therefore paramount for the restoration of glycaemic control, but is not always the only factor that needs to be addressed.

Pancreatitis

As discussed in Chapter 12, canine diabetes can be a consequence of pancreatitis, and stabilization can be very challenging in such patients. A recent survey of post-mortem findings in the non-diabetic canine population detected a prevalence of pancreatic inflammation of 34% (Watson *et al.*, 2007) in patients with no obvious clinical signs of pancreatic disease, suggesting that the disease may be clinically underdiagnosed. This is because clinical signs of chronic pancreatitis are variable and there is no *ante mortem* 'gold standard' test that can easily be applied to clinical cases. Although classic signs of acute pancreatitis (abdominal pain, inappetence, colitis signs and/or vomiting) can be present at diagnosis of diabetes or intermittently during the disease course, often chronic pancreatitis signs are restricted to glycaemic instability along with intermittent and unpredictable bouts of depression, anorexia or signs of colitis. During the history taking, should there be any suggestion that the patient has 'off days' or has experienced any signs of abdominal pain, consideration should be given to assessment for pancreatitis.

There are several ways in which pancreatic inflammation can be assessed (see *BSAVA Manual of Canine and Feline Gastroenterology*). Diagnostic tests for chronic pancreatitis will be most sensitive if performed when the patient is in an 'unwell' phase. Classical elevations in serum amylase and lipase can be helpful in acute pancreatic inflammation but false negative results are common in chronic disease (Mansfield *et al.*, 2003). A newer pancreas-specific lipase assay, canine pancreatic lipase immunoreactivity (cPLI), promises improved specificity and sensitivity, and can be helpful in patients showing appropriate clinical signs (Steiner *et al.*, 2008). In addition to biochemical testing, ultrasonography can be used to assess the pancreas for signs of oedema, tumour, cystic or abscess-related changes. Although this technique can be helpful, it is very operator-and machine-dependent and changes seen on pancreatic ultra-sonography are often regarded as non-specific.

Management of pancreatitis and diabetes:
Management of acute pancreatic inflammation in the diabetic patient uses the same principles as treatment for the non-diabetic patient:

- Careful monitoring of fluid balance, including intravenous fluid and electrolyte therapy if necessary
- Appropriate initial and ongoing analgesia
- Anti-emetic therapy if required
- Low fat food (assuming the patient is not vomiting).

Insulin therapy in such patients is more of a challenge as it must be matched to food eaten, with an awareness that the pancreatic inflammation will result in a variable degree of insulin resistance. Small doses (0.2 IU/kg) of soluble (neutral) insulin every 2–4 hours, depending on blood glucose concentration and food eaten, are often more appropriate than attempting to control blood glucose with a longer- acting insulin preparation in an acute pancreatitis patient (see Chapter 12 for discussion regarding current availability of soluble insulin for veterinary use). In the long term, patients should be managed on a low fat diet and not allowed to become overweight.

Sometimes it can be just as challenging to treat the acute pancreatitis patient as to manage the diabetic patient on a day where signs of chronic pancreatitis 'flare up', particularly if this leads to a change in appetite. Such patients are often not unwell enough to warrant overnight hospitalization or intravenous fluid therapy, but nonetheless can benefit from appropriate analgesia, anti-emetic therapy and, if there is any suggestion of small intestinal bacterial overgrowth, a short course of antibiotic treatment (e.g. metronidazole). It is also easier to manage these patients if they are receiving twice-daily insulin, so that following a 'missed' injection as the result of inappetence, therapy can easily be re-started within 12 rather than 24 hours.

Exocrine pancreatic insufficiency
Whilst awareness of pancreatitis at diagnosis can imply a more difficult stabilization period, it also reminds the clinician that the exocrine pancreatic tissue might become functionally compromised in future. An important consequence of chronic pancreatitis in some dogs is damage to the exocrine tissue as well as the beta cells (Watson, 2003; Watson *et al.*, 2007). This can result in exocrine pancreatic insufficiency (EPI), which is another cause of glycaemic instability and weight loss in diabetic patients. Documentation of a low serum trypsin-like immunoreactivity (TLI) will confirm a diagnosis of EPI but, as TLI can be elevated (into or above the reference interval) with acute pancreatic inflammation, it is theoretically preferable to collect a blood sample for EPI diagnosis when the patient is in a 'well' phase. Should a diagnosis of EPI be

confirmed, treatment with pancreatic enzyme supplementation should be instigated. This will result in an improvement in digestion and absorption of food, so is likely to necessitate some adjustment in insulin dose.

Hormonal antagonism
Many hormones can antagonize the effect of insulin, including corticosteroids, growth hormone and progestogens (Hess *et al.*, 2003). Hypothyroid dogs can also suffer from insulin resistance.

Unstable diabetes mellitus caused by hormonal antagonism can be naturally occurring or iatrogenic, with even topical preparations being enough to destabilize diabetes in some dogs. It is therefore very important to check that diabetic dogs have not been receiving eye, ear or skin preparations containing steroids with or without the clinician's knowledge. It must also be remembered that when insulin sensitivity is restored following withdrawal of such a therapy or treatment of an underlying condition, a lower insulin dose will be required, otherwise the patient is at risk of hypoglycaemia.

Insulin resistance is usually defined in a patient where an insulin dose of >2.2 IU/kg/injection is not enough to control clinical signs and a Somogyi overswing (see above) has been ruled out. Hormonal antagonism is a common underlying cause for profound insulin resistance, although chronic undiagnosed infection and inflammation can result in tolerance of similarly high doses of insulin. Despite the fact that animals suffering from hormonal antagonism are often receiving high insulin doses, hypoglycaemic episodes are rare because of the high level of one or more hormones antagonistic to insulin, tending to raise the blood glucose.

Hormonal antagonism can be a contributory factor to the initial presentation of the diabetic patient, e.g. treatment with high doses of prednisolone can precipitate diabetes in a susceptible individual. Alternatively, it can arise later in the disease course, turning a previously stable patient into a challenging case of insulin resistance (e.g. dioestrus in an intact bitch).

Reproductive hormones
It is vital that entire females are neutered as soon as possible after the diagnosis of diabetes. This is because the predominance of progestogens in the dioestrus phase antagonizes insulin and causes dramatic insulin resistance in many cases, sometimes precipitating ketoacidosis. This is exacerbated by a unique feature of the bitch, in which the mammary glands produce growth hormone, which is also diabetogenic, during this progesterone-dominated phase. Together, the two hormones can cause very sudden and severe instability, which will recur and may increase in severity with each subsequent oestrous cycle (Eigenmann *et al.*, 1983).

Although it is best to neuter a diabetic bitch before she has a chance to come into oestrus and, subsequently, dioestrus, this is not always possible. Sometimes the diagnosis is made during the dioestrus phase and the patient is already acutely unwell; occasionally, presentation is complicated further by the presence of a pyometra. Theoretically, there is a chance of reversal of diabetes by neutering such cases immediately, but this carries an increased anaesthetic risk (particularly in the presence of ketosis or ketoacidosis) and early intervention very rarely prevents the dog from becoming insulin-dependent in the long term. These cases are best managed on an individual basis; it is often helpful to treat the ketoacidosis (see Chapter 24) and stabilize the patient as far as possible before embarking on surgery. On occasion, however, for example in the case of progesterone-secreting tumours or pyometra, patients may become increasingly unwell despite intensive insulin therapy, and immediate ovariohysterectomy can be life-saving in restoring some level of insulin sensitivity. Careful monitoring of blood glucose after surgery is necessary, as much lower insulin doses will be required once the source of insulin resistance has been removed.

Hyperadrenocorticism

Canine hyperadrenocorticism (see Chapter 16) can occur concurrently with diabetes mellitus. Disease should be suspected where there are consistent clinical signs (e.g. hair loss, pot belly, skin thinning) as well as evidence of insulin resistance. Such patients are also at risk of concurrent infections (another contributory factor to their insulin resistance), hypertension and thromboembolic disease.

Pituitary-dependent disease accounts for approximately 80% of hyperadrenocorticism cases, resulting in bilateral adrenal enlargement. The remaining 20% of cases are the result of an adrenal tumour, usually leading to atrophy of the contralateral adrenal gland. These changes are usually detectable by ultrasonography, although the stress of chronic illness can also result in adrenal enlargement, so this is not a specific test. The diagnosis of hyperadrenocorticism in an unstable diabetic patient is challenging, as many of the clinical, biochemical and haematological abnormalities seen in hyperadrenocorticism (e.g. hepatomegaly, polyuria, polydipsia, elevated liver enzymes, stress leucogram) are nonspecific and are also detectable in unstable diabetes. In particular, the ACTH stimulation test and low dose dexamethasone suppression tests can give false positive results in a chronically stressed animal. As well as convincing insulin resistance and clinical signs, at least one positive screening test result must be obtained before treatment for hyperadrenocorticism is instigated.

If hyperadrenocorticism and diabetes mellitus are suspected concurrently, it is often more straightforward to attempt to stabilize the diabetes and limit the development of ketoacidosis as a priority, before embarking on any concurrent investigation or treatment of the hyperadrenocorticism. It is imperative too that the patient is assessed and, if necessary, treated for any urinary tract infection, as this will compromise attempts at stabilization if left untreated. Such patients will often need larger doses of insulin to control clinical signs until therapy for hyperadrenocorticism is instigated.

The authorized medication for canine pituitary-dependent hyperadrenocorticism in the UK is trilostane, a reversible inhibitor of 3β-hydroxysteroid dehydrogenase (see Chapter 16). It is important to be aware that trilostane can have an effect on serum cortisol concentrations within hours, and its effect will last 12–24 hours in most canine patients. This means that insulin resistance can improve dramatically and quickly with treatment, so patients must be monitored carefully for hypoglycaemia as soon as therapy with trilostane is started. As a guide, it is prudent to reduce insulin dose by approximately 50% when treatment for hyperadrenocorticism is instigated, and to monitor glucose every 1–3 hours initially. The prognosis for diabetes with concurrent hyperadrenocorticism is poorer than for diabetes alone. In one study the median survival of diabetic patients was 3 years, whereas for diabetic dogs with hyperadrenocorticism it was 1 year, although this might have been related to the difference in age at diagnosis of the two groups (Graham and Nash, 2005).

Other endocrinopathies

It is not unusual for more than one endocrinopathy to occur in a patient, particularly if the diabetes mellitus is considered to be immune-mediated, as such animals can be predisposed to immune-mediated destruction of other endocrine glands. Concurrent endocrinopathies can be a cause of instability and hence initiation of treatment often necessitates a change in insulin dose or frequency.

Hypothyroid patients in particular can be insulin-resistant, requiring careful dose reduction once levothyroxine supplementation is started. Thyroxine has insulin antagonistic properties, but the mechanism of insulin resistance in hypothyroid dogs is unclear. Care should be taken with a diagnosis of hypothyroidism, as suppression of T4 can be seen in dogs with unstable diabetes due to sick euthyroid syndrome (see Chapter 8). Thyroid testing should be restricted to those patients showing appropriate clinical signs (bradycardia, lethargy, hypercholesterolaemia, hair loss, heat-seeking behaviour), and thyroid-stimulating hormone (TSH, thyrotropin) should also be measured to improve diagnostic specificity.

Dogs with hypoadrenocorticism (see Chapter 15) represent a further challenge, as their treatment can require the intermittent use of physiological doses of corticosteroids, which can result in insulin resistance and instability. Even a patient who only requires mineralocorticoid therapy may still need insulin adjustments, as fludrocortisone, the most commonly used mineralocorticoid preparation in UK veterinary practice, has a small amount of glucocorticoid activity and hence can have an effect on glycaemic control.

Acromegaly, as a result of increased growth hormone production, is exceptionally rare in the dog, although its incidence associated with diabetic instability in cats appears to be increasing. Unlike cats, dogs do not appear to have any predisposition to growth hormone-secreting pituitary macroadenomas.

In canine patients, acromegaly is more likely to result from excess growth hormone from the mammary glands, under the influence of progesterone, as previously mentioned. Such cases of long-term growth hormone excess may develop thickened facial features and extremities, widened interdental spaces, insulin resistance and hypertension (Eigenmann *et al.* 1983). Excess growth hormone has also recently been associated with hypothyroidism and is a potential but reversible explanation for insulin resistance in such a state (Chapter 8). Even more rarely, glucagonoma and phaeochromocytoma have been associated with insulin-resistant diabetes in canine patients.

Inadequate insulin activity

The final category of instability in the canine diabetic patient is the least specific and often the most challenging to investigate and treat. If other causes of insulin resistance (infection, inflammation, hormonal antagonism) and management factors have been ruled out, as discussed above, it is possible that the insulin is being antagonized by some other mechanism in the periphery or that the insulin is being poorly absorbed, although very few practical tests exist to confirm this.

The patient that is still unstable on twice-daily insulin at an appropriate dose, with management factors and concurrent diseases ruled out, represents a great challenge and unfortunately it is not always possible to determine the exact cause of the instability. It is possible, however, to make some changes in management, even in these patients, that can improve glycaemic control.

Poor absorption

One reason for poor insulin absorption is scar tissue or excess fatty tissue at injection sites. Sometimes this is easy to palpate but occasionally there are no detectable physical changes at the injection site. A useful technique in these circumstances is to assess the glycaemic response (every 30 minutes for 2–3 hours) to a test dose of neutral (soluble) insulin given by the intramuscular route. A dose of 0.2 IU/kg should be enough to bring about a reduction in blood glucose concentration in patients with normal insulin sensitivity. Should no reduction in blood glucose concentration occur, this implies insulin resistance and further attention should be paid to assessment for infection, inflammation or hormonal antagonism. If a convincing reduction in blood glucose is seen then insulin sensitivity is confirmed and a change of injection site and/or preparation should be considered. Some poorly-controlled diabetic patients respond well to (unauthorized) soluble insulin given by the intramuscular route at mealtimes, and many owners can be taught to administer the insulin by this route as a long-term solution if necessary.

Anti-insulin antibodies

Anti-insulin antibodies, induced by the injected insulin being from a 'foreign' species, are often quoted as a cause of insulin resistance. In practice, however, recent research has shown that although anti-insulin antibodies are present in the majority of dogs who have received heterologous bovine insulin therapy, they do not appear to be generally associated with instability or deleterious side effects (Davison *et al.*, 2003a, 2008). In fact, it is also theoretically possible that anti-insulin antibodies act to prolong the activity of insulin, so some practitioners believe that they might even be beneficial. Anti-insulin antibodies are less likely to be induced by homologous preparations, such as porcine insulin, so swapping the species of preparation might help if antibodies are a concern. As there is variability in the pharmacokinetics and pharmacodynamics of different insulin preparations, so that one insulin preparation might suit a particular animal more than another, a change of preparation might be appropriate in an unstable diabetic patient regardless of anti-insulin antibody status. If antibodies are a concern, it is important to remember that anti-insulin antibodies are not species-specific and so are likely to cross-react with the new insulin, and it could take several months for their concentration to decline.

Conclusion

Unstable diabetic patients are a challenge for the whole practice, as not all diabetic cases behave in a predictable fashion: some are straightforward and rarely need any intervention, whereas others may be complicated and very frustrating. Successful stabilization will be achieved more easily with small dose changes at infrequent intervals of usually no more than every 3 days, hence patience is certainly required by both the owner and veterinary surgeon. When investigating instability, it is also important not to change more than one thing at a time if possible; otherwise it becomes difficult to assess the effects of that change. Good client communication and regular contact with even apparently 'stable' patients are the keys to successful management of diabetes and prevention of instability.

References and further reading

Casella M, Wess G, Hassig M *et al.* (2003) Home monitoring of blood glucose concentration by owners of diabetic dogs. *Journal of Small Animal Practice* **44**, 298–305

Catchpole B, Kennedy LJ, Davison LJ *et al.* (2008) Canine diabetes mellitus: from phenotype to genotype. *Journal of Small Animal Practice* **49**, 4–10

Catchpole B, Ristic JM, Fleeman LM *et al.* (2005) Canine diabetes mellitus: can old dogs teach us new tricks? *Diabetologia* **48**, 1948–1956

Davison LJ, Ristic JM, Herrtage ME *et al.* (2003a) Anti-insulin antibodies in dogs with naturally occurring diabetes mellitus. *Veterinary Immunology and Immunopathology* **91**, 53–60

Davison LJ, Slater LA, Herrtage ME *et al.* (2003b) Evaluation of a continuous glucose monitoring system in diabetic dogs. *Journal of Small Animal Practice* **44**, 435–442

Davison LJ, Walding B, Herrtage ME *et al.* (2008) Anti-insulin antibodies in diabetic dogs before and after treatment with different insulin preparations. *Journal of Veterinary Internal Medicine* **22**, 1317–1325

Eigenmann JE, Eigenmann, RY, Rijnberk A *et al.* (1983) Progesterone-controlled growth hormone overproduction and naturally occurring canine diabetes and acromegaly. *Acta Endocrinologica (Copenhagen)* **104**, 167–176

Fall T, Hamlin HH, Hedhammar A *et al.* (2007) Diabetes mellitus in a population of 180,000 insured dogs: incidence, survival, and breed distribution. *Journal of Veterinary Internal Medicine* **21**, 1209–1216

Fleeman LM and Rand JS (2001) Management of canine diabetes. *Veterinary Clinics of North America: Small Animal Practice* **31**, 855–880

Fleeman LM and Rand JS (2003) Evaluation of day-to-day variability of serial blood glucose concentration curves in diabetic dogs. *Journal of the American Veterinary Medical Association* **222**, 317–321

Graham PA and Nash AS (2005) How long will my diabetic dog live? *BSAVA Congress 2005 Scientific Proceedings: Veterinary stream* p. 217

Hess RS, Kass PH and Van Winkle TJ (2003) Association between diabetes mellitus, hypothyroidism or hyperadrenocorticism, and atherosclerosis in dogs. *Journal of Veterinary Internal Medicine* **17**, 489–494

Hess RS, Saunders HM, Van Winkle TJ *et al.* (2000) Concurrent disorders in dogs with diabetes mellitus: 221 cases (1993–1998). *Journal of the American Veterinary Medical Association* **217**, 1166–1173

Hess RS and Ward CR (2000) Effect of insulin dosage on glycemic response in dogs with diabetes mellitus: 221 cases (1993–1998).

Journal of the American Veterinary Medical Association **216**, 217–221

Jensen AL (1995) Glycated blood proteins in canine diabetes mellitus. *Veterinary Record* **137**, 401–405

Mansfield CS, Jones BR and Spillman T (2003) Assessing the severity of canine pancreatitis. *Research in Veterinary Science* **74**, 137–144

Rand JS, Fleeman LM, Farrow HA *et al.* (2004) Canine and feline diabetes mellitus: nature or nurture? *Journal of Nutrition* **134**, 2072–2080

Steiner JM, Newman S, Xenoulis P *et al.* (2008) Sensitivity of serum markers for pancreatitis in dogs with macroscopic evidence of pancreatitis. *Veterinary Therapy* **9**, 263–273

Watson PJ (2003) Exocrine pancreatic insufficiency as an end stage of pancreatitis in four dogs. *Journal of Small Animal Practice* **44**, 306–312

Watson PJ, Roulois AJ, Scase T *et al.* (2007) Prevalence and breed distribution of chronic pancreatitis at post-mortem examination in first-opinion dogs. *Journal of Small Animal Practice* **48**, 609–618

23

Investigation of unstable feline diabetes mellitus

Danièlle Gunn-Moore and Nicki Reed

Introduction

Diabetes mellitus is defined as a disorder caused by a relative or absolute lack of insulin. It is a common endocrine disease of cats (see Chapter 13). Despite being likened to type 2 diabetes mellitus of humans, the majority of cats require insulin therapy together with dietary management to control hyperglycaemia and increase the chance of diabetic remission. Although adequate glycaemic control is attained in many cats, a variety of factors can result in diabetic instability (Figure 23.1). These can generally be categorized into:

- Management issues
- Inappropriate type and dose of insulin
- Misinterpretation of blood glucose curves
- Fluctuating insulin requirements
- Insulin resistance.

- Failure to adhere to consistent regime
  - Variable timing of injections
  - Variable timing of feeding
- Variable diet
  - Switching types of diet
  - Excess food intake
  - Too little food
  - Changes in caloric requirements not considered
- Inactive insulin
  - Out of date
  - Incompletely mixed
  - Vigorously shaken
  - Incorrectly stored
- Poor injection technique
  - Inappropriate syringe type
  - Variable doses of insulin drawn up
  - Dilution of insulin
  - Consistent injection in same site
- Poor subcutaneous absorption
- Inappropriate insulin dose
  - Underdosing
  - Overdosing resulting in Somogyi overswing
- Fluctuating insulin requirements
- Short duration of insulin activity
- Insulin antibodies
- Poor owner monitoring
- Stress hyperglycaemia
- Concurrent disease
- Diabetogenic medications, e.g. corticosteroids

23.1 Potential reasons for apparent diabetic instability in cats.

Management issues

Management issues include such things as changes in diet or exercise, poor owner compliance, and inappropriate monitoring. It is most common for these problems to arise in the early stages of stabilization. They may be fairly easy to identify and correct after detailed communication with the owner.

Incorrect storage and handling of insulin and poor injection technique

Insulin may be ineffective if it is out of date, incompletely mixed, damaged from vigorous shaking or poorly stored. Although it is not strictly necessary to refrigerate insulin, this does avoid inactivation caused by increases in ambient temperature or direct sunlight. In addition, insulin will bind to the rubber stopper of the dispensing bottle if it is stored upside down or on its side, thereby resulting in decreased insulin activity within the injection.

It is important to use the correct syringe for the insulin concentration (40 or 100 IU/ml). Incorrect doses can be administered through mismatching; it is possible to recalculate the volume of insulin to be administered when using mismatched syringes, but such a step adds an unnecessary complication, increasing the risk of inappropriate dosing.

Some owners may be unable to draw up the correct insulin dose accurately because they have arthritic hands or poor vision. In such cases, the dose administered may frequently change, resulting in significant under- or overdosing at each injection time. Overdosing can lead to insulin-induced hyperglycaemia (Somogyi overswing) (see below). Even for those adept at injecting, accurate drawing up of the small doses of insulin usually required to treat cats can be difficult to achieve consistently. Diluting insulin in order to achieve more accurate dosing may have been recommended, but such dilution can itself be associated with unpredictable results.

Although subcutaneous injections are relatively simple, poor injection technique may be a complicating factor in diabetic instability. This may be particularly important in longhaired cats or those with very dense coats. In such cases, owners may initially benefit from injecting into an area that has been clipped so that they can visualize the technique until greater experience is gained.

Adherence to a consistent daily regime is of vital importance in maximizing the chances of good glycaemic control. Problems can arise if, for example, insulin is given at different times each day. There may then be prolonged periods when insulin activity has waned (injection interval too long) or where insulin doses are piggybacked on to each other (injection interval too short).

Other management changes

Consistency in the feeding regimen is also important and problems may arise if variable quantities or types of food are being offered. Some owners may persist in giving extra food at weekends, switching between wet food on some days and dry on others, giving *ad libitum* meals on some days and set meals on others, or feeding treats that contain large amounts of soluble sugars. Careful questioning is often required to elucidate the problem as it is more typically children, or occasionally neighbours, that offer the additional food.

There may, however, be occasions when significant changes in energy requirements arise. These include changes in environmental temperature and/or exercise regime. Owners of diabetic cats that previously hunted and exercised outside may find it easier to keep their cat indoors. Equally, the introduction of a new kitten may entice a diabetic cat to play. In such cases, a change in energy intake may be required, as significant changes in bodyweight (either weight gain or weight loss) can result in significant changes to insulin requirements.

Poor owner monitoring

Good owner observation is important in determining the degree of glycaemic control in a diabetic cat. Ideally, owners should regularly monitor their diabetic cat for changes in demeanour, appetite, thirst, urination, bodyweight, body condition score and muscle tone, coat condition, mobility and ability to jump. This is easier for some owners than for others. Adequate information may not be available if a number of different people are involved in the cat's care or if the cat spends a great deal of time away from the house or urinates outside. Where significant changes have occurred and the owner has not noticed them, the cat may be presented to the veterinary practice with severely unstable diabetes mellitus, with a greater risk of the development of diabetic ketoacidosis.

Recognition of hypoglycaemia is one of the most important owner considerations. Hypoglycaemic cats rarely exhibit polyphagia but may show a sudden desire to hide, be excessively quiet, weak or lethargic, tremble, become ataxic, collapse or even lose consciousness. Unfortunately, in most affected cats these signs are often subtle and can easily be missed.

Type and dose of insulin

Cats can be unpredictable in their response to insulin and no single type of insulin or dosing regime is suitable for all cats. Individual responses to exogenous insulin vary not only from cat to cat but also from day to day in the same cat. Therefore, the recommended doses and dosing frequencies are merely guidelines and must be adjusted appropriately based on response.

In cats, lente insulin's time to peak activity can vary from 2 to 10 hours and duration of action can vary from 6 to 16 hours. However, it is usually considered as having a duration of activity close to, though often less than, 12 hours. This compares to protamine zinc insulin (PZI), which has a time to peak activity of 3–12 hours and a duration of activity that varies from 6 to 24 hours. Glargine insulin has a peak effect at approximately 14 hours and duration of action of approximately 24 hours, but often considerably less. Detemir insulin appears to have a similar activity profile to glargine insulin.

Therefore, twice-daily dosing with lente insulin is usually required for adequate glycaemic control, and unstable diabetes mellitus often results from once-daily dosing. If once-daily insulin injections are desired then PZI may be used, although there are currently problems with availability of authorized veterinary preparations. Additionally, some cats cannot absorb PZI effectively and its use may be associated with poor glycaemic control.

Selecting too high an initial dose of insulin can be problematic. Some authors recommend a starting dose of 0.5 IU insulin/kg per injection, but this is inappropriately high if the blood glucose concentration is <20 mmol/l. A more appropriate starting dose in such cases is 0.25 IU insulin/kg per injection.

Frequent dose changes, particularly if of high magnitude, can also result in wide swings in glycaemic control. It takes approximately 3 days for glucose homeostasis to adjust after starting or altering insulin doses and, as a consequence, insulin doses should only be increased in small steps (e.g. by a total of 0.5–1.0 IU per injection) followed by a period of at least 3–5 days before reassessing the cat to monitor changes in glycaemic control.

Insulin may be of porcine or bovine origin, recombinant human insulin or synthetic. Of all the insulins available, none is identical to cat insulin. However, although antibody formation to the administered insulin is a theoretical risk, it has not been shown to be of clinical significance in cats.

Interpreting blood glucose curves

Blood glucose curves are frequently made for the assessment of unstable diabetic cats. The various different types of blood glucose curves typically found are outlined in Figure 23.2. Blood glucose curves can provide important information on the absolute nadir blood glucose concentration, the precise time of the nadir, the duration of effect of insulin, the presence of a Somogyi overswing and the degree by which there is a glucose-lowering effect or not.

Unfortunately, the use of blood glucose curves can be limited in cats for a number of reasons. These include the stress of hospitalization that can itself result in significant hyperglycaemia, the day-to-day variability of blood glucose curves even within the

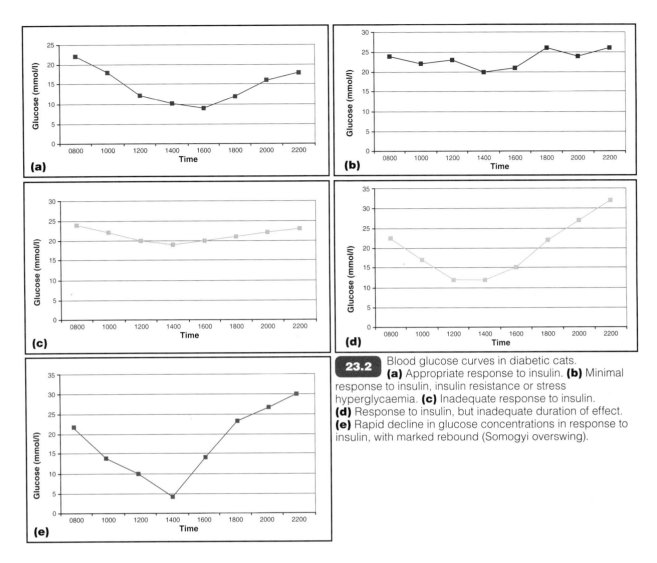

23.2 Blood glucose curves in diabetic cats.
(a) Appropriate response to insulin. **(b)** Minimal response to insulin, insulin resistance or stress hyperglycaemia. **(c)** Inadequate response to insulin. **(d)** Response to insulin, but inadequate duration of effect. **(e)** Rapid decline in glucose concentrations in response to insulin, with marked rebound (Somogyi overswing).

same cat, the possible short duration of hypoglycaemia and the often prolonged duration of any resultant Somogyi overswing.

The effect of stress

It is meaningless to obtain a blood glucose curve from a cat with stress hyperglycaemia. Unfortunately, stress may not be visibly apparent and can be present even in cats that do not struggle or vocalize. In addition, although stress rarely results in blood glucose concentrations of >16 mmol/l, this is still sufficient to confuse the interpretation of a blood glucose curve. A stressed cat can be hospitalized, allowed to calm down in its kennel and then reassessed. Other measures to minimize stress include using peripheral ear or paw pad veins (see Chapter 13). Alas, some cats exhibit stress hyperglycaemia every time they are hospitalized. For these cats it may be preferable to train their owners to measure blood glucose concentrations in the home environment. Alternatively, an implanted subcutaneous glucose device and monitor could be used.

Blood glucose measurement

It is important to ensure that the same type of glucometer is used throughout data collection for each blood glucose curve and for every subsequent blood glucose curve in an individual cat. Human glucometers tend to read feline glucose concentrations lower than the actual value but may variably under- or overestimate values at very high or low concentrations depending on the individual glucometer used. Glucometers validated for feline blood (e.g. Abbott AlphaTRAK) are more likely to give values similar to those from a standard reference laboratory.

Variability

Whilst blood glucose curves can provide useful information, they can also vary widely from day to day in individual cats. It is therefore important that major changes to treatment are not based on the results from a single blood glucose curve. A blood glucose curve should instead be interpreted in conjunction with the cat's clinical status, fructosamine concentration and the environment in which the curve was obtained. The most important thing to consider is the *trend* of change, so comparing the current curve with previous blood glucose curves is important.

Somogyi overswing

The Somogyi overswing describes a normal physiological response to hypoglycaemia induced by excessive insulin administration. This commonly occurs when insulin doses are increased too quickly with inadequate monitoring, or if the cat has fluctuating insulin requirements. When blood glucose concentrations reduce to <3.5 mmol/l or when they fall precipitously (>10 mmol/l in 1 hour), counter-regulatory hormones such as cortisol, glucagon and adrenaline are secreted, resulting in a rebound hyperglycaemia within a few hours. This hyperglycaemia persists for at least 24 hours in most cases, but can last for up to 72 hours, and occasionally even longer. Clinical signs of hypoglycaemia are rarely seen.

A diagnosis of Somogyi overswing is achieved by demonstrating hypoglycaemia or a rapid fall in blood glucose concentration followed by hyperglycaemia. Unfortunately, the hypoglycaemia can be missed if blood samples are taken less frequently then every hour at peak insulin activity and the subsequent rebound hyperglycaemia and insulin resistance can last for considerably more than 24 hours. A cyclic history of 1–2 days of good glycaemic control followed by several days of poor control should raise particular suspicion for the Somogyi overswing. If considered a possibility, the insulin dose should be reduced by 0.5–1.0 IU or 25–30% and the cat monitored for the next few days. If originally overdosed, the cat should become more stable; if not, it is likely to become more polydipsic and polyuric.

Fluctuating insulin requirements

It is not unusual for some cats to have fluctuating insulin requirements, with apparently uncontrolled diabetes mellitus at one time and hypoglycaemia or hyperglycaemia the next. The most common reasons for this are:

- Transient diabetes mellitus (see Chapter 13)
- The development of a concurrent disease that causes variable insulin resistance and later resolves spontaneously, or waxes and wanes.

Insulin resistance

The majority of diabetic cats can be controlled with insulin doses of approximately 0.4–0.6 IU/kg administered twice daily. Poor glycaemic control and/or insulin resistance are generally defined by an insulin requirement of >1.5–2.0 IU/kg. This can be associated with a wide variety of different problems and conditions (Figure 23.3) and can be complex to investigate.

As diabetic cats tend to be older, it is not surprising that there is a risk of concurrent disorders that may affect diabetic stability. The presence of any concurrent disease, especially those involving an inflammatory response or infectious focus, can cause marked insulin resistance. One study found concurrent disease in 22% of diabetic cats (Crenshaw and Peterson, 1996). Those commonly diagnosed include chronic kidney disease, hyperthyroidism, pancreatitis, urinary tract infection (UTI), acromegaly and hyperadrenocorticism (Goossens *et al.*, 1998; Feldman and Nelson, 2004). While

- Recent weight gain (common)
- Infection, e.g. urinary tract infection (12–14%) or gingivitis
- Pancreatitis or other forms of pancreatic pathology (acute or chronic pancreatitis 6–50%; pancreatic adenocarcinoma 19%; exocrine pancreatic insufficiency 4%)
- Administration of diabetogenic drugs (9%), e.g. corticosteroids, progestogens
- Hyperthyroidism (9–29%)
- Acromegaly (14–19%)
- Hyperadrenocorticism (14–17%)
- Kidney disease (15–33%)
- Liver disease (2–10%)
- Inflammatory bowel disease (3%)
- Neoplasia (2–9%)
- Congestive heart failure (up to 15%)
- Eosinophilic granuloma complex (3%)
- Asthma (2%)
- Immune-mediated disease (2%)
- FIV-positive (2%)

23.3 Concurrent disease that may potentially result in insulin resistance in diabetic cats. The percentages refer to the frequency of occurrence in cats with diabetes mellitus (data from Goossen *et al.*,1998; Feldman and Nelson, 2004).

these different diseases may occur concurrently, some occur together more frequently and are potentially related to the development of diabetes mellitus or its consequences (pancreatitis, acromegaly). For some of the disorders highlighted in Figure 23.3 (eosinophilic granuloma complex, asthma, neoplasia, immune-mediated disease) the administration of systemic corticosteroids for their management can result in unstable diabetes mellitus rather than the presence of the condition itself.

Obesity
Any increase in bodyweight is likely to cause significant insulin resistance. Recent weight gain despite poor diabetic control is most commonly due to acromegaly, although it can occasionally be seen with hyperadrenocorticism or excessive feeding.

Infection
In diabetic cats, infection is most likely to affect the mouth (gingivostomatitis and/or periodontal disease), urinary tract, or skin. Diabetic animals are predisposed to infection because of systemic immunosuppression resulting from decreased peripheral blood supply, impaired humoral immunity and antibody production, abnormal neutrophil chemotaxis and defects in phagocytosis and intracellular processing of infectious agents (Joshi *et al.*, 1999).

Pancreatitis
Pancreatitis and other forms of pancreatic pathology often result in variable insulin requirements. Pancreatitis may be more common than previously thought, as >50% of diabetic cats have evidence of past or current pancreatitis at necropsy. Pancreatitis can occur together with inflammatory bowel disease (IBD) and cholangitis ('triaditis'). Where this occurs, the presence of these conditions can further complicate diabetic stability, particularly if they remain undiagnosed. Chronic pancreatitis can eventually

lead to significant loss of pancreatic function with possible development of exocrine pancreatic insufficiency (EPI). Unfortunately, pancreatitis can be difficult to diagnose and affected cats may show few or non-specific clinical signs, such as anorexia and lethargy. Measurement of feline pancreatic lipase immunoreactivity (fPLI) is the most sensitive diagnostic test available, but a reference interval fPLI does not exclude pancreatitis. Abdominal ultrasonography and pancreatic biopsy can be useful tools for the diagnosis of pancreatitis. Achieving a diagnosis of pancreatitis is unlikely to alter the treatment regimen for the diabetes mellitus but provides some explanation as to why a cat may have extremely variable insulin requirements.

Hyperthyroidism

Hyperthyroidism complicates the diagnosis and treatment of diabetes mellitus. The duration of action of exogenous insulin may be shorter than expected in cats with concurrent hyperthyroidism, and any endogenous insulin secretion may be reduced. Unfortunately, the possibility of concurrent hyperthyroidism may be missed in cats with diabetes mellitus as the clinical signs can be similar. In addition, a diagnosis of hyperthyroidism is complicated by the suppressive effect of diabetes mellitus on total thyroxine (T4) concentrations. Circulating fructosamine concentration may also be lowered by hyperthyroidism, suggesting better glycaemic control than is actually present. Evaluation of free T4 concentration may help in the diagnosis of hyperthyroidism.

Acromegaly

Acromegaly (Chapter 5) is an uncommonly reported, but probably underdiagnosed, condition in cats. It results from overproduction of growth hormone (GH) from a pituitary tumour, typically an adenoma of the pars distalis. In addition to diabetes mellitus, cats with acromegaly usually exhibit enlargement of the head, paws and abdomen and inferior prognathism. Some cats may also develop neurological signs, osteoarthritis, and cardiac and kidney disease. Definitive diagnosis of acromegaly requires demonstration of elevated concentrations of GH or insulin-like growth factor-1 (IGF-1) together with a pituitary mass, by either computed tomography (CT) or magnetic resonance imaging (MRI). As growth hormone assays and advanced imaging techniques are poorly available, an elevated IGF-1 concentration (especially if >131 nmol/l), together with clinical signs consistent with acromegaly, are usually considered adequate for a diagnosis. The possibility of underlying acromegaly should be considered in any unstable diabetic cat. A particularly high index of suspicion should be present in any older, large, male diabetic cat that is gaining weight despite the presence of unstable diabetes mellitus.

Hyperadrenocorticism

Hyperadrenocorticism is a rare but also possibly underdiagnosed disease in cats (see Chapter 17). In approximately 80% of cases it is caused by adrenocorticotropic hormone (ACTH)-secreting pituitary tumours, most of which are adenomas. In a few cases, hyperadrenocorticism is caused by a functional adrenal tumour, which can be either adenomatous (approximately 50% of cases) or carcinomatous.

Hyperadrenocorticism is typically seen in middle-aged to older cats (range 4–16 years) with no apparent sex or breed predisposition. The history and clinical signs often include polyuria, polydipsia, polyphagia, weight loss, generalized muscle loss and lethargy, and may include a history of recurrent infections and/or abscesses. Affected cats often have a coat that is in poor condition, with spontaneous alopecia, and fragile thin inelastic skin that bruises easily (fragile skin syndrome). Occasionally, they develop seborrhoea and/or bacterial dermatitis and a pot-bellied appearance that results from weakened abdominal muscles, obesity and, in some cases, hepatomegaly. As cortisol antagonizes insulin, the majority of cases develop diabetes mellitus and are frequently insulin resistant.

In cats, screening tests include the urine cortisol: creatinine ratio (UCCR), low-dose dexamethasone suppression test (LDDST) and the ACTH response test, while differentiation of pituitary from adrenal dependency may involve measurement of endogenous ACTH concentration or diagnostic imaging modalities (adrenal glands by ultrasonography, or CT/MRI assessment of pituitary gland). Some cases that mimic hyperadrenocorticism actually have progestogen-secreting adrenal tumours.

Kidney disease

Kidney disease is commonly seen in cats with diabetes mellitus and in one study was found in approximately one-third of cases (Goossens et al., 1998). Kidney disease is not uncommon in older cats but might also be caused or exacerbated by ascending bacterial infections, diabetic nephropathy or significant hypotension in those cases with diabetic ketoacidosis or severe pancreatitis. As renal function deteriorates, significant insulin resistance may develop. However, the anorexia associated with kidney disease potentially increases the risk of hypoglycaemia, resulting in fluctuating insulin requirements in affected cats. Monitoring of diabetic control becomes more difficult, as the degree of polyuria and polydipsia is obviously affected by renal function.

Liver disease

Liver disease may occur in diabetic cats. Hepatic lipidosis may develop in unstable or newly diagnosed cats, while cholangitis often occurs concurrently with IBD and/or pancreatitis.

Neoplasia

Neoplasia anywhere in the body can lead to inflammation and insulin resistance. The tumours seen most commonly in unstable diabetic cats are pancreatic adenocarcinoma, lymphoma and mast cell tumours (Ogilvie et al., 1997).

Administration of diabetogenic drugs

Diabetogenic drugs include corticosteroids (dexamethasone is more diabetogenic than equipotent doses of prednisolone) or progestogens such as megestrol, particularly when given at high doses and/or for long courses. Corticosteroids do not require systemic administration to influence diabetic control, as topical eye and ear preparations can be absorbed sufficiently to affect insulin requirements.

Other problems

A failure of insulin absorption mimics the insulin resistance seen with concurrent disorders. It may be a result of injecting the insulin at the same site every day or injecting the insulin into fat depots. It can also be a feature of long-acting insulin administration. In dogs, insulin antibodies potentially result in insulin resistance. However, such antibodies appear to be rare in cats.

Investigation of instability

Investigation of diabetic instability can be challenging, time-consuming and expensive. Each category of instability should be considered by obtaining an appropriate history, completing a thorough physical examination and pursuing additional diagnostic tests as considered necessary. A step-by-step approach is outlined in Figure 23.4.

History

The first important step when investigating problems of diabetic stabilization is to ask the owner detailed questions about their cat's daily management regime, particularly any recent changes. Many problems with stabilization result from poor owner compliance, which in turn often results from poor direction, support and communication from the veterinary team. When investigating an unstable diabetic cat it is necessary to ensure that clients understand the importance of adhering to a consistent regime of insulin administration, diet and exercise. Careful questioning will usually reveal if such problems are possible, but if they are not identified at this point it may be necessary to ask the owner to demonstrate how they mix and inject the insulin, in order to check that this is being done correctly. Any such problems can be easily rectified without the need for further protracted investigations.

If problems of management or insulin administration are eliminated then further questioning may be necessary. Owners need to be asked about changes in their cat's health and behaviour, including ascertaining information on demeanour, appetite, thirst, urination, bodyweight, muscle tone, coat condition, mobility and ability to jump. Questions should focus on those concurrent diseases that can significantly complicate the treatment of diabetes. Cats with unstable diabetes resulting from chronic pancreatitis may have a history that includes episodes of depression, anorexia, vomiting, diarrhoea and/or abdominal

pain, and if most of the pancreas has been destroyed these clinical signs may also be accompanied by signs of EPI (i.e. a voracious appetite and large quantities of voluminous fatty faeces). Cats with acromegaly may present with weight gain despite diabetic instability, while those with hyperthyroidism may lose weight despite significant polyphagia.

Physical examination

Each cat should have a full physical examination, including assessment of bodyweight, calculation of percentage bodyweight change since the previous visit, body condition score, retinal examination and systemic blood pressure measurement.

It is important to differentiate signs of diabetic instability from signs of another underlying or concurrent illness. Signs of diabetic instability include an unkempt coat, hepatomegaly and a plantigrade stance. Cats with UTI may additionally exhibit signs of cystitis such as bladder and/or kidney discomfort, dehydration. The mouth should be carefully checked as severe periodontal disease is a possible reason for insulin resistance. Concurrent pancreatitis may result in dehydration, abdominal discomfort and, in severe cases, jaundice. The neck should be carefully palpated for goitre.

Blood glucose curve

The next step in the investigation depends on the abnormalities detected from the history and on physical examination. Where significant concomitant disease is suspected, further investigations should include routine clinicopathological analyses (see below). However, where this is not the case and a problem with insulin dose or dosing frequency is suspected, it is more appropriate to obtain a blood glucose curve (see above and Chapter 13). Such curves may provide information on short duration of activity or the possibility of a Somogyi overswing (see Figure 23.2). If either of these problems is identified then the frequency of dosing should be increased or the dose decreased, respectively. If insulin resistance is noted, then other causes should be considered.

Routine clinicopathological analyses

Each cat should have a full haematology, serum biochemistry (including electrolytes, total T4 concentration and fructosamine concentration), plus full urine analysis with sediment assessment and bacterial culture.

Haematology

Haematological changes may result from associated systemic infections or severe stress. The most typical changes are a mild non-regenerative anaemia, lymphopenia and either neutropenia or neutrophilia. Acute pancreatitis may present with severe red cell fragility and haemolytic anaemia, and/or sequestration of neutrophils resulting in a degenerate left shift. Severe cases may develop haematological changes consistent with disseminated intravascular coagulation.

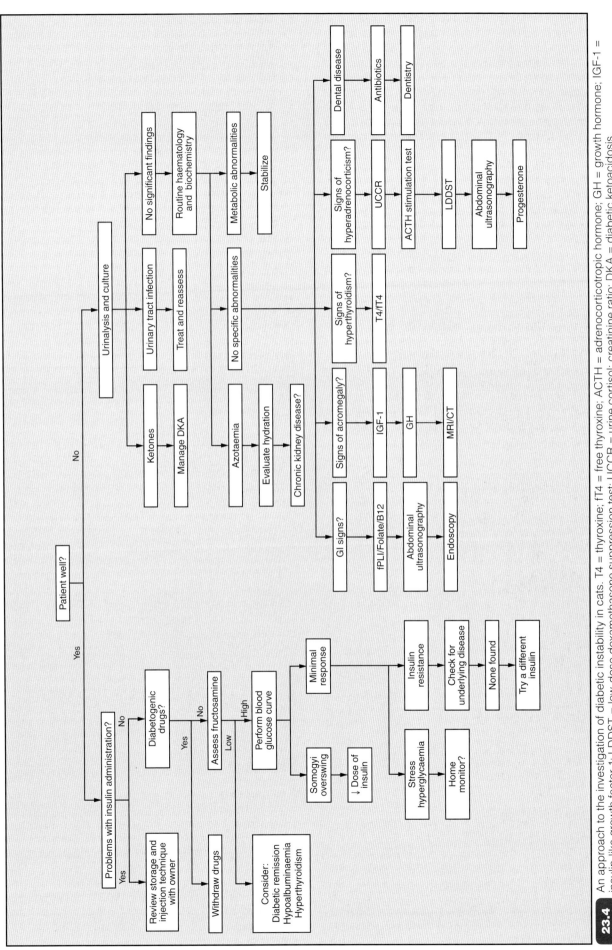

23.4 An approach to the investigation of diabetic instability in cats. T4 = thyroxine; fT4 = free thyroxine; ACTH = adrenocorticotropic hormone; GH = growth hormone; IGF-1 = insulin-like growth factor 1; LDDST = low-dose dexamethasone suppression test; UCCR = urine cortisol: creatinine ratio; DKA = diabetic ketoacidosis.

Serum biochemistry

Serum biochemistry can be helpful in detecting concurrent and complicating disease but changes associated with unstable diabetes mellitus need to be considered. Many cats with diabetes mellitus have mild to moderate increases in serum concentrations of cholesterol and liver enzymes. More severe changes including hyperbilirubinaemia and azotaemia usually indicate the presence of a complicating disorder.

Fructosamine concentration

Assessing serum fructosamine concentration can be useful, as it gives an indication of how elevated the blood glucose concentration has been for the preceding 1–2 weeks. High concentrations (>500 µmol/l) indicate poor glycaemic control. However, such high values may occur both in insulin resistant states and with insulin overdose if it results in Somogyi overswing. Care is also required as fructosamine can be raised where there has been prolonged stress hyperglycaemia. Additionally, it may not be raised in the initial stages of diabetic instability and can be falsely lowered in some conditions such as hyperthyroidism that increase protein turnover.

Total thyroxine concentration

Circulating total T4 concentration should be assessed to rule out the presence of concurrent hyperthyroidism. Care should be taken in its interpretation as the presence of diabetes mellitus can result in suppression of a previously mildly elevated total T4 concentration into the reference interval. In the absence of hyperthyroidism, total T4 concentrations would be expected in the lower half of the reference interval in diabetic cats.

Urine analysis

Urinalysis is essential to assess the presence of ketones and glucosuria as indicators of diabetic instability. However, caution is advised as stress hyperglycaemia can result in glucosuria. The urine specific gravity should be noted and interpreted appropriately, as the presence of 2% or 4+ glucosuria will increase the specific gravity by 0.008–0.010, which may complicate the diagnosis of concurrent kidney disease. Sediment examination will help in the diagnosis of UTIs but some of these cats have a non-active urinary sediment. It is therefore essential to collect a sample by cystocentesis and perform urine culture regardless of the sediment findings.

Further investigation

Depending on other findings this may involve additional testing as follows:

- GH and/or IGF-1 and assessment of pituitary size when investigating acromegaly
- UCCR, LDDST, endogenous ACTH concentration, and assessment of adrenal and pituitary size by ultrasonography, CT or MRI when investigating hyperadrenocorticism
- Serum fPLI, fTLI, cobalamin and folate concentrations when investigating pancreatic and/or intestinal pathology
- Survey radiographs of thorax and abdomen for cardiac, respiratory disease or evidence of neoplasia
- Abdominal ultrasonography (paying particular attention to the pancreas, liver, kidneys and adrenal glands)
- Gastrointestinal endoscopy and biopsy for diagnosing IBD
- Hepatic biopsy and/or bile culture to diagnose cholangitis.

More detailed information on the diagnosis and treatment of other endocrine disorders is presented in relevant chapters.

References

Crenshaw KL and Peterson ME (1996) Pretreatment clinical and laboratory evaluation of cats with diabetes mellitus: 104 cases (1992–1994). *Journal of the American Veterinary Medical Association* **209**, 943–949

Crenshaw KL, Peterson ME, Heeb LA, Moroff SD and Nichols R (1996) Serum fructosamine concentration as an index of glycemia in cats with diabetes mellitus and stress hyperglycemia. *Journal of Veterinary Internal Medicine* **10**, 360–364

Elliott DA, Feldman EC, Koblik PD, Samii VF and Nelson RW (2000) Prevalence of pituitary tumors among diabetic cats with insulin resistance. *Journal of the American Veterinary Medical Association* **216**, 1765–1768

Feldman EC and Nelson RW (2004) Canine diabetes mellitus; Feline diabetes mellitus In: *Canine and Feline Endocrinology and Reproduction, 3rd edn*, ed. EC Feldman and RW Nelson, pp. 486–538; 539–579. WB Saunders, Philadelphia

Forcada Y, German AJ, Noble PJM *et al.* (2008) Determination of serum fPLI concentrations in cats with diabetes mellitus. *Journal of Feline Medicine and Surgery* **10**, 480–487

Goossens MMC, Nelson RW, Feldman EC and Griffey SM (1998) Response to insulin treatment and survival in 104 cats with diabetes mellitus (1985–1995). *Journal of Veterinary Internal Medicine* **12**, 1–6

Joshi N, Caputo GM, Weitekamp MR and Karchmer AW (1999) Infections in patients with diabetes mellitus. *New England Journal of Medicine* **341**, 1906–1912

Koenig A, Drobatz KJ, Beale AB and King LG (2004) Hyperglycemic, hyperosmolar syndrome in feline diabetics: 17 cases (1995–2001). *Journal of Veterinary Emerging and Critical Care* **14**, 30–40

Kraus MS, Calvert CA, Jacobs GJ and Brown J (1997) Feline diabetes mellitus: a retrospective mortality study of 55 cats (1982-1994). *Journal of the American Animal Hospital Association* **33**, 107–111

Little CJL and Gettinby G (2008) Heart failure is common in diabetic cats: findings from a retrospective case-controlled study in first-opinion practice. *Journal of Small Animal Practice* **49**, 17–25

Niessen S (2010) Feline acromegaly: an essential differential diagnosis for the difficult diabetic. *Journal of Feline Medicine and Surgery* **12**, 15–23

Ogilvie GK, Walters L, Salman MD *et al.* (1997) Alterations in carbohydrate metabolism in dogs with nonhematopoietic malignancies. *American Journal of Veterinary Research* **58**, 277–281

Rand JS (2002) Understanding feline diabetes. *Compendium on Continuing Education for the Practicing Veterinarian* **24(5)**, Supplement B, 2–6

Reusch CE, Kley S, Casella M *et al.* (2006) Measurements of growth hormone and insulin-like growth factor 1 in cats with diabetes mellitus. *Veterinary Record* **158**, 195–200

24

Ketoacidosis

Amanda K. Boag

Introduction

Ketoacidosis occurs when there is excessive production and accumulation of ketoacids, notably β-hydroxybutyrate and acetoacetate, within the circulation. Although low concentrations of these acids may be found in healthy patients, when excessive amounts accumulate they overwhelm the buffering capacity of the body and a metabolic acidosis and acidaemia develop. Large concentrations of ketoacids may be produced in a few selected pathophysiological scenarios, but in small animal patients significant ketoacidosis is almost invariably associated with diabetes mellitus.

Aetiology

Ketoacidosis is a severe and potentially life-threatening complication of diabetes mellitus (DM), and may occur in both cats and dogs. It may be present at the time of initial diagnosis of DM but it can also develop in a previously diagnosed diabetic patient that is already undergoing treatment.

DM occurs when there is an absolute or relative deficiency of insulin (see Chapters 12 and 13). Insulin is required for the metabolism of ketones and there may be a low rate of ketone production in untreated uncomplicated DM. However, this is typically insufficient to cause acidaemia. The development of ketoacidosis generally requires a concurrent relative excess of glucagon or, less commonly, other 'counter-regulatory' hormones (cortisol, growth hormone and adrenaline). This most commonly occurs when there is a second triggering condition or stressor that is superimposed on the underlying DM. Commonly identified triggering conditions are depicted in Figure 24.1, although it should be noted that *any* concurrent disease could act as a trigger.

Hormonally, the distinction between uncomplicated DM and diabetic ketoacidosis (DKA) is that there is an excess of glucagon, concurrent with subnormal concentrations of endogenous insulin, and hence an increase in the glucagon:insulin ratio. High concentrations of glucagon tend to promote metabolism of free fatty acids and ketone production. Coupled with the subnormal concentrations of insulin, this leads to rapid ketogenesis. The low concentrations of insulin inhibit ketone metabolism and the rate of ketone production thus quickly overwhelms

Bacterial infections

• Any significant bacterial infection but especially consider:
  – Urinary tract infection [b]
  – Pneumonia
  – Pyometra
  – Pyoderma
  – Prostatitis

Inflammatory disease
• Pancreatitis [a][b]
Endocrinopathy
• Hyperadrenocorticism [a] • Hypothyroidism (dog) • Hyperthyroidism (cat) • Acromegaly
Physiological endocrine change
• Dioestrus phase of oestrous cycle
Miscellaneous
• Chronic renal failure [b] • Neoplasia [b]
Iatrogenic
• Administration of corticosteroids (including topical)

24.1 Conditions that may trigger diabetic ketoacidosis. [a] Conditions identified as the most common concurrent diagnoses in a population of dogs presenting with diabetic ketoacidosis (Hume *et al.*, 2006). [b] Conditions identified as the most common concurrent diagnoses in a population of cats presenting with diabetic ketoacidosis (Bruskiewicz *et al.*, 1997).

the body's excretory ability, with consequent accumulation of ketoacids and development of ketoacidosis and acidaemia.

Acidaemia has many negative physiological effects (Figure 24.2), including vomiting and anorexia. As diabetic ketoacidosis develops, the patients therefore tend to reduce water intake and also to undergo increased fluid and electrolyte loss through the gastrointestinal tract. This occurs in the face of the obligatory polyuria seen in all diabetics, due to the osmotic diuresis caused by glucosuria and exacerbated by the presence of ketones in the urine. This leads to a rapid decline in intravascular volume status (development of shock) and mental deterioration.

Cardiovascular
• Reduction in cardiac output • Reduction in cardiac contractility • Reduced inotropic response to catecholamines • Predisposition to arrhythmia • Arterial vasodilation and reduction in arterial blood pressure
Respiratory
• Tachypnoea and hyperpnoea as compensatory mechanisms (Kussmaul breathing in human patients)
Neurological
• Depression • Coma
Miscellaneous
• Insulin resistance • Anorexia • Nausea • Muscle weakness

24.2 Negative physiological effects of metabolic acidosis.

Clinical features

Patients with DKA typically present in a collapsed state with a relatively short (hours to several days) history of vomiting, inappetence and progressive lethargy (Figure 24.3). They may have previously been diagnosed with DM and already be undergoing insulin treatment, or they may not have had a prior diagnosis. In the former scenario, owners should be carefully questioned about any recent changes in insulin administration and patient stability. In the latter case the owners are likely to report a more chronic history of polyuria and polydipsia (PU/PD), polyphagia and weight loss that may have been present for many months.

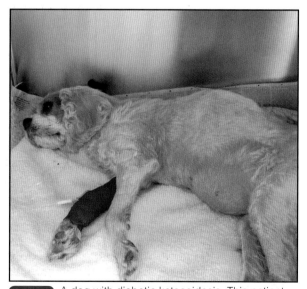

24.3 A dog with diabetic ketoacidosis. This patient was subsequently diagnosed as suffering from concurrent hyperadrenocorticism.

History and physical examination

In consideration of the importance of triggering conditions in the aetiology of DKA, a thorough history should always be taken, with the aim of identifying any possible concurrent disorders or at least prioritizing the differential diagnosis list.

The initial physical examination should focus on the major body systems (cardiovascular, respiratory and neurological). Examination of the cardiovascular system usually reveals evidence of hypovolaemic shock, which may range from mild to severe. Dependent on the severity of the shock, patients exhibit varying degrees of tachycardia, with concomitant changes in pulse quality, mucous membrane colour and capillary refill time. These patients frequently also have an increased skin tent and dry mucous membranes, suggestive of concurrent dehydration. They are usually tachypnoeic without being dyspnoeic, as the respiratory system acts to compensate for the metabolic acidosis. Auscultation of the lungs is typically unremarkable although it should be carried out carefully, as aspiration pneumonia is possible either as a consequence of the vomiting in a depressed animal or as the triggering condition. Animals are usually depressed but without specific neurological deficits. In many cases, the depression merely reflects the presence of shock, but occasionally severe disturbances in electrolytes and osmolality may contribute to the mental depression. Other commonly identified findings on initial physical examination include being overweight or underweight, cranial organomegaly and abdominal pain. Icterus is also commonly noted in cats as a consequence of concurrent disease (Bruskiewicz *et al.*, 1997).

DKA and its treatment are associated with a number of potential life-threatening complications, including acute renal failure, significant electrolyte disturbances and development of anaemia. It is important that the owner is questioned on when the animal was last noted to urinate; an animal that has not been observed to urinate for several hours, especially if previously polydipsic and polyuric, should be carefully monitored for production of urine, with placement of a urinary catheter if possible.

Diagnosis

DKA should be considered in any patient presenting with collapse and vomiting and with a history of PU/PD, regardless of whether there is a pre-existing diagnosis of DM. On initial examination, the presence of a 'pear-drop' ketone smell on the patient's breath is highly suggestive of ketoacidosis, although not everyone is able to detect this. The index of suspicion is increased if initial in-house blood work reveals moderate to significant hyperglycaemia. Identification of a metabolic acidosis on a venous blood gas and electrolyte panel further suggests DKA, and necessitates assessment for ketones. Metabolic acidosis is identified when measured pH is low or just within the lower end of the reference interval and there is a negative base excess (< −4) or low bicarbonate concentration. The pCO_2 is often also low, reflecting respiratory compensation. An anion gap should also be calculated, using the formula:

$$\text{anion gap} = (Na^+ + K^+) - (HCO_3^- + Cl^-)$$

DKA is typically associated with a high anion gap metabolic acidosis. The differential diagnosis of metabolic acidosis is shown in Figure 24.4.

High anion gap (normochloraemic)
• Diabetic ketoacidosis [a]
• Lactic acidosis [a]
• Uraemic acidosis [a]
• Toxins (e.g. ethylene glycol, salicylates)

Normal anion gap (hyperchloraemic)
• Diarrhoea [a]
• Renal tubular acidosis
• Drugs (e.g. carbonic anhydrase inhibitors)
• Dilutional acidosis

24.4 Differential diagnosis of metabolic acidosis. [a] Diagnoses encountered most frequently in clinical practice.

DKA is confirmed when high concentrations of ketones are identified. In-house diagnostic tests utilize either multi-purpose or specifically designed urine dipsticks, with an appropriate colour change on the stick confirming the presence of ketones. Historically, urinalysis was used as the principal means of confirming the diagnosis. However, recent publications have highlighted the use of serum or plasma with urine dipstick and other methodologies when evaluating for the presence of ketones (Brady *et al.*, 2003; DiTommaso *et al.*, 2009). This can be particularly useful in patients that do not have palpable bladders on presentation but where an urgent diagnosis is required. The serum obtained from a spun-down packed cell volume (PCV) tube can be placed on the ketone square of a urine dipstick with the same colour change expected as for urine confirming the presence of ketonaemia. Serum could also be sent to external laboratories for more accurate assessment and characterization of ketone concentrations although this is rarely necessary.

It is important to note that the dipstick methodology utilizes the nitroprusside reaction, which detects acetone and acetoacetate but does **not** detect β-hydroxybutyrate. In clinical patients, the ketone bodies formed are a mixture of β-hydroxybutyrate and acetoacetate, with the relative proportion produced dependent upon the redox state of the liver mitochondria. In states of hypoperfusion and shock this tends to mean that β-hydroxybutyrate is produced in larger quantities than acetoacetate. It is thus theoretically possible to have a patient with DKA that is negative for ketones on serum or urine dipstick. Practically, this seems to occur rarely; a more common scenario is for the ketonuria or ketonaemia apparently to become more

pronounced during the first few hours or days of treatment, as β-hydroxybutyrate is metabolized to acetoacetate prior to its oxidation to acetyl co-A.

Although diagnosis of DKA is confirmed by the identification of hyperglycaemia with metabolic acidosis and ketonaemia or ketonuria, it is also strongly recommended that a number of other diagnostic tests are performed. These act either as an aid to identifying the concurrent triggering condition or as a baseline to aid stabilization and early treatment. DKA may be associated with a large number of potential metabolic disturbances, and success in the early phase of treatment depends as much (if not more) on consideration of these as on the primary underlying insulin abnormality. Recommended diagnostic tests are summarized in Figure 24.5 and described below.

• Blood gas and electrolyte panel
• Haematology
• Biochemistry, including phosphate
• Urinalysis, including culture
• Thoracic radiography
• Abdominal ultrasonography
• cPLI/fPLI

24.5 Diagnostic tests that should be considered when evaluating a patient with diabetic ketoacidosis. Further endocrine testing (ACTH stimulation test, thyroid function tests) should generally be delayed until the patient is stable.

Electrolytes

DKA is associated with several concurrent electrolyte disturbances, some or all of which may need addressing during the initial treatment phase.

Sodium concentration

On presentation, the serum sodium concentration may be less than, within or above the reference interval, reflecting the balance of free water *versus* electrolyte loss in the individual patient. When hyponatraemia is identified, and before any specific treatment is instituted, the question of whether it could represent artefactual or spurious hyponatraemia or whether it is a 'real' hyponatraemia should be considered. Artefactual hyponatraemia may occur when serum sodium is measured by a flame photometry methodology (used by most commercial laboratories) in patients with concurrent hyperlipidaemia or hyperproteinaemia. In this situation the true serum sodium is likely to be within the reference interval. Spurious hyponatraemia may occur due to the presence of large numbers of other osmotically active particles, notably glucose. The elevated serum glucose concentration has a significant osmotic effect and draws water into the vasculature leading to dilution of serum sodium. It is expected that for every 1 mmol/l increase in glucose concentration, the serum sodium concentration is reduced by approximately 0.3–0.4 mmol/l. The hyponatraemia may thus correct with correction of the hyperglycaemia itself. Measurement of serum sodium concentration is strongly recommended as, if abnormal, it may contribute to mental depression. Also, knowledge of baseline sodium is important as it is vital the serum sodium concentration is not changed too rapidly during treatment by the use of inappropriate fluid therapy (see Treatment, below).

Potassium concentration

On presentation, the serum potassium concentration may be less than, within or above the reference interval. Hyperkalaemia may occur secondary to a shift of intracellular potassium to an extracellular location secondary to the acidosis, lack of insulin and plasma hyperosmolarity. It may also reflect reduced urine output secondary to oliguric or anuric renal failure. Hypokalaemia is, however, more common and may be dramatic, especially once treatment is instituted. Regardless of initial measured serum values, most patients are whole body potassium-depleted, reflecting the chronic increased renal loss of potassium that occurs with marked PU/PD, coupled with increased loss through the gastrointestinal tract (if the patient is vomiting) and inadequate intake (if the patient has been inappetent). Most patients will develop worsening hypokalaemia with treatment, as insulin administration causes potassium to move from the extracellular to the intracellular space. Potassium concentration should be closely monitored.

Chloride concentration

Serum chloride concentration typically changes in the same way as sodium and does not need specific treatment.

Azotaemia

Patients with DKA are often azotaemic on presentation. Most commonly, this simply reflects a prerenal azotaemia in the face of hypovolaemia with an obligatory diuresis. Differential diagnoses, however, include both acute (oliguric or anuric) and chronic renal failure. As mentioned above, it is vital to ascertain when the animal last urinated; if it has not been observed to urinate for several hours this must be monitored very closely. Blood urea and creatinine concentrations should also be closely monitored during early treatment to ensure resolution of azotaemia is occurring as expected. If urea and creatinine fail to normalize with appropriate fluid therapy, diagnostic tests to rule out other differentials should be considered.

Phosphate concentration

Many patients with DKA have had chronic increased phosphate loss secondary to the muscle catabolism that occurs with DM. Serum phosphate concentration may drop further with treatment as translocation from the extracellular to the intracellular space occurs.

Liver enzymes

Both alanine aminotransferase (ALT) and alkaline phosphatase (ALP) are typically increased. This may be attributable to the triggering condition (e.g. hypercortisolaemia). However, it may also occur secondary to the direct effects of either the DM (hepatic lipidosis) or the hypoperfusion that commonly accompanies DKA.

Haematology

The haematocrit may be less than, within or above the reference interval on presentation. As it is likely to change as treatment progresses, close monitoring is warranted. Many DKA patients have a leucocytosis secondary to a mature neutrophilia on presentation. Identification of a high proportion of band cells or toxic change within the neutrophils should increase the index of suspicion for an infectious or severe inflammatory triggering condition and prompt thorough evaluation to identify any potential focus.

Urinalysis

Urinalysis should include: measurement of specific gravity (SG), dipstick evaluation, and sediment examination. Considering the high frequency of urinary tract infection in diabetic patients, it is strongly recommended that a urine culture is submitted; this should be considered mandatory if the sediment examination suggests infection.

In the presence of azotaemia, urine SG is typically used to evaluate whether the azotaemia is renal or prerenal in origin. In patients with DKA, however, this process is complicated by several factors.

- Regardless of intrinsic renal function, DM leads to an osmotic diuresis that is enhanced by the presence of ketones in the urine; this would tend to create a hypo- or isosthenuric urine
- The presence of large amounts of glucose and ketones in the urine means that the linear relationship between SG and urine osmolality is no longer valid and SG can no longer be taken to be a reflection of urine osmolality
- Isosthenuria is typically considered to be 1.008– 1.012, but this is in the face of a normal serum osmolality. Patients with DKA may have significantly increased serum osmolality and hence, in the absence of other factors, isosthenuria may actually be reflected by a higher SG.

Measured SG must be interpreted in the light of these considerations; it is not possible to be precise, but it is not uncommon for a patient with DKA to have a prerenal azotaemia with a urine SG of 1.020 and 4+ glucose.

Sediment examination and evaluation of whether a urinary tract infection is present is particularly important, as such infections are a common trigger for the development of ketoacidosis. If infection is suspected, a sample should be taken via cystocentesis and submitted for culture ideally prior to institution of antimicrobial therapy.

Tests for triggering disease

The list of potential triggering conditions for DKA is long (see Figure 24.1). Diagnostic tests should be tailored to the individual patient and based on prioritization of the differential list by signalment, history and physical examination findings. Imaging of both the thorax and abdomen should be strongly considered, as should additional diagnostic laboratory tests such as cPLI/fPLI in appropriate cases. If infection is suspected, the site should be sampled and cultured.

Treatment

Fluid therapy and correction of electrolyte disturbances are the two most important components of initial therapy and can be started prior to a definitive diagnosis. Once a diagnosis is made, informed owner consent for ongoing treatment is vital. Ketoacidotic patients can be very rewarding to treat, with approximately 70% of treated dogs and cats being discharged from the hospital (Bruskiewicz *et al.*, 1997; Hume *et al.*, 2006). However, the owners must be made aware at an early stage that treatment of the initial episode is likely to involve a moderate to prolonged period of hospitalization (average of 5–6 days), with concurrent financial and emotional impact. Furthermore, the primary underlying disease (DM) is chronic and requires lifelong treatment in all dogs and many cats. The owners must be prepared and willing to undertake this commitment.

Fluid therapy, electrolytes and acid–base balance

Disturbances in intravascular volume status, hydration and electrolytes are a key cause of morbidity in DKA patients and should be addressed as a priority. With appropriate use of fluid boluses, it should be possible to address hypovolaemia within 1–2 hours of admission. Insulin therapy should only be started once the patient's intravascular volume status is being addressed and is thought to be close to normal. Starting insulin therapy prior to addressing intravascular volume depletion increases the risk of rapid changes in glucose and electrolytes and the development of metabolic complications.

Treatment for hypovolaemia

Stabilization can start prior to a confirmed diagnosis and involves administration of one or more fluid boluses. The size and speed of administration of the bolus is dependent on the animal's clinical signs; suggested bolus doses for dogs are shown in Figure 24.6. In cats it is harder to judge the severity of hypoperfusion on physical examination and high rates of fluids are less well tolerated; a more stepwise approach is recommended, with administration of incremental boluses of 5–10 ml/kg of isotonic crystalloid. The aim of the bolus dose is to normalize perfusion and its associated physical examination parameters. For this initial stage of fluid resuscitation, it is recommended that an isotonic replacement crystalloid solution (e.g. 0.9% NaCl, Hartmann's solution) is used. The fluid chosen should be one with a sodium concentration close to the animal's serum sodium, to avoid inducing rapid changes in the patient's serum sodium concentration.

Ongoing fluid therapy

Once any hypovolaemia is resolved, an ongoing fluid rate should be chosen for the patient. This should include consideration of:

- Maintenance requirements – considered to be approximately 2.5 ml/kg/h
- Replacement of estimated hydration losses – the animal's fluid deficit should be calculated based on the estimated percentage dehydration. This estimated fluid deficit should be replaced over the first 12–24 hours of treatment
- Ongoing losses – this should include consideration of any ongoing gastrointestinal losses (vomiting, diarrhoea) as well as the extra renal losses caused by the ongoing osmotic diuresis. This can be difficult to estimate; placement of a urinary catheter with accurate measurement of urine production is appropriate in some patients.

All three of the above components are estimates and hence the final fluid rate decided upon represents a judgement rather than a precise calculation. Monitoring of the patient is therefore vitally important to ensure that the fluid rate is optimized for the patient as the disease and treatment progress.

Sodium supplementation

Measured serum sodium is variable in DKA patients at the time of diagnosis and will change as treatment progresses. The key challenge is to ensure that it does not change too rapidly. The maximum rate of change of sodium in either direction should not exceed 0.5 mmol/l/h. Rates of change greater than this put the patient at risk of either cerebral

Clinical parameter	Mild hypovolaemia	Moderate hypovolaemia	Severe hypovolaemia
Heart rate	130–150	150–170	170–220
Mucous membrane colour	Normal to pinker than normal	Pale pink	Grey, white or muddy
Capillary refill time	Rapid (<1 second)	Approximately normal (1–2 seconds)	Prolonged (>2 seconds) or absent
Pulse amplitude	Increased	Mild to moderately decreased	Severely decreased
Pulse duration	Mildly reduced	Moderately reduced	Severely reduced
Metatarsal pulse	Easily palpable	Just palpable	Absent
Suggested initial bolus dose of replacement isotonic crystalloid	10–20 ml/kg over 30 min to 1 hour	20–40 ml/kg over 30 min to 1 hour	40–60 ml/kg over 15 min to 1 hour

24.6 Suggested initial bolus doses of isotonic replacement crystalloid to be used in dogs with varying degrees of hypoperfusion.

oedema (if patient's sodium decreases too rapidly) or cerebral dehydration (if patient's sodium increases too rapidly). Osmotic demyelinization has also been suspected in a small number of patients where hyponatraemia has undergone rapid correction. As discussed above, initial fluid resuscitation for hypovolaemia should use a crystalloid fluid with a sodium concentration similar to the animal's serum sodium concentration. Following this initial resuscitation, serum sodium concentration should be measured regularly and ongoing fluids chosen dependent on this monitoring. It is not uncommon for patients being treated for DKA to become hypernatraemic over the first few days of treatment. This occurs as ongoing fluid losses (notably large volumes of urine secondary to osmotic diuresis) contain more water than sodium. In this scenario, a hypotonic fluid (e.g. 0.45% NaCl) may be used as a component of the overall fluid therapy plan.

Potassium supplementation

Patients with DKA may be hypokalaemic on presentation and invariably become hypokalaemic once insulin treatment commences. Hypokalaemia may be severe enough to cause signs of muscular weakness and hypoventilation if unrecognized or untreated. Hypokalaemia should be treated by supplementation of parenteral fluids with an appropriate amount of potassium chloride (Figure 24.7) and/or potassium phosphate. Infusion rates should not exceed 0.5 mmol/l/h except in exceptional circumstances. In a patient that requires high rates of potassium supplementation, the author recommends that a separate bag of parenteral fluids is made containing this high level of supplementation. This should be administered through a separate intravenous line at the desired rate; this approach minimizes the risk of alterations in the patient's ongoing fluid therapy plan leading to changes in the rate of potassium delivery. It should be noted that even when maximal supplementation rates are used, patients may remain hypokalaemic for the first few days of treatment.

Acid–base balance

The use of sodium bicarbonate in the treatment of DKA is controversial. Generally, if appropriate fluid and insulin therapy is used, the acidosis will resolve

Serum potassium (mmol/l)	mmol KCl to add to 1 litre of fluids	Maximum recommended infusion rate for supplemented fluids (ml/kg/h)
3.5–5.0	20	25
3.0–3.5	30	18
2.5–3.0	40	12
2.0–2.5	60	8
<2.0	80	6

24.7 Guidelines for supplementation of intravenous fluids with potassium chloride for the treatment of hypokalaemia.

and does not need specific treatment. The use of bicarbonate may also be associated with the development of complications, such as paradoxical cerebrospinal fluid acidosis and hypernatraemia. However, there are many negative effects of severe acidaemia (see Figure 24.2). Generally, use of sodium bicarbonate is not recommended unless pH is <7.1 and does not show an upward trend within the first few hours of treatment. In addition, it should not be used unless the patient's acid–base and electrolyte status can be monitored frequently. When bicarbonate is used, the dose can be calculated as:

$$NaHCO_3^- \text{ (mmol/l/h)} = \text{base deficit} \times 0.3 \times \text{bodyweight (kg)}$$

One-third to one-half of this dose is administered by slow intravenous infusion over 15–30 minutes and the acid–base status is reassessed. The remainder can be added to the patient's intravenous fluids and delivered over a period of hours if necessary.

Insulin treatment

Insulin administration is an important part of the management of the DKA patient. Neutral (soluble) insulin **must** be used in the early stages of treatment. It has several advantages over the more familiar medium- and long-acting formulations, notably its rapid onset and short duration of action and, importantly, the fact it can be administered by numerous routes, including intravenously and intramuscularly.

Subcutaneous administration of insulin is not recommended during initial treatment of the ketotic patient as absorption is unpredictable, especially if the patient is dehydrated. Use of neutral insulin by both intravenous and intramuscular routes allows the clinician to titrate the delivery of insulin to the patient's needs. Both intravenous and intramuscular protocols can be used successfully and an example of each technique is described in Figure 24.8.

It is preferable to use the intravenous constant rate infusion (CRI) technique if suitable facilities are available, since this avoids the need for multiple intramuscular injections, which is of benefit from both a patient welfare and a staff time management perspective. The disadvantage of the CRI technique is the need for a suitable infusion pump or syringe driver.

Regardless of which protocol is used, it is likely that blood glucose will fall towards the reference interval long before the ketoacidosis resolves. Hypoglycaemia must be avoided; therefore, it may be necessary to supplement the ongoing intravenous crystalloid fluids with 2.5% or 5% dextrose. This allows continued delivery of insulin required for ketone metabolism, whilst avoiding hypoglycaemia. Glucose supplementation should start once blood glucose falls to <15 mmol/l. It is recommended that the fluids are supplemented initially with 2.5% dextrose if glucose is between 10 and 15 mmol/l, and with 5% dextrose if glucose is <10 mmol/l. This dextrose-supplemented fluid should then be delivered at maintenance rates alongside whatever other fluid is required to manage the patient's overall fluid and

Intravenous constant rate infusion protocol

1. Make up insulin infusion solution in 0.9% NaCl to a concentration of 0.05 IU/ml by adding 25 IU neutral insulin to a 500 ml bag or 2.5 IU to a 50 ml syringe.
2. Infuse at 1 ml/kg/h until the blood glucose is <15 mmol/l. With normal insulin sensitivity, blood glucose typically falls at 1–3 mmol/l/h.
3. Once blood glucose is <15 mmol/l, reduce insulin infusion rate to 0.5 ml/kg/h and add glucose supplementation of 2.5% or 5% to ongoing fluid therapy.

NB: As insulin adsorbs to plastic, 50–100 ml of the insulin infusion fluid should be run through the infusion line prior to starting the infusion. The insulin infusion should be freshly made up on a daily basis.

Intramuscular protocol

1. Begin treatment with an intramuscular injection of neutral insulin at 0.2 IU/kg.
2. Blood glucose should be measured on an hourly basis, with repeat injections of 0.1 IU/kg as necessary until blood glucose is in the 10–15 mmol/l range.
3. If blood glucose is in the 10–15 mmol/l range but ketoacidosis persists, intravenous fluids should be supplemented with 2.5% or 5% dextrose and neutral insulin intramuscular injections continued at 0.1 IU/kg q1–4h.

24.8 Examples of soluble insulin protocols to be used in the treatment of patients with diabetic ketoacidosis. Other intravenous protocols have been described (Macintire, 1993).

electrolyte balance. The percentage glucose supplementation should be adjusted in light of further glucose measurements such that serum glucose is held in the 10–15 mmol/l range. Insulin administration may need to be temporarily discontinued if blood glucose falls to <8 mmol/l.

Other considerations

Hypophosphataemia/haemolytic anaemia
Hypophosphataemia is a common complication of DKA therapy and is often most marked 1–2 days following initiation of insulin therapy as phosphorus translocates into an intracellular location. Severe hypophosphataemia may lead to haemolysis and can contribute to development of anaemia. It is recommended that both PCV and serum phosphate concentration are monitored every 6–12 hours during the first 48–72 hours of treatment. Phosphate supplementation is recommended if the serum phosphate concentration drops below 0.35 mmol/l. The recommended phosphate supplementation rate is 0.01–0.03 mmol/kg/h for 6 hours, although on occasion this is found to be insufficient, and doses up to 0.12 mmol/kg/h for 12–48 hours may be required. Regular monitoring of phosphate (every 4–12 hours) is necessary, especially if higher dose rates are used. The phosphate supplementation rate should be adjusted dependent on the patient's response. Iatrogenic hyperphosphataemia and consequent hypocalcaemia should be avoided. As phosphate is generally supplied as potassium phosphate, the additional potassium supplementation should be taken into account when calculating the dose of potassium chloride supplementation required.

Hypomagnesaemia
Hypomagnesaemia is a recognized complication of DKA in human patients and is associated with clinical signs including refractory hypokalaemia, cardiac conduction disturbances and increased neuromuscular excitability. It has not been identified as a significant problem in dogs with DM (Fincham et al., 2004); however, normalization of serum magnesium levels is recommended if serum magnesium is low and one or more compatible clinical signs is present.

Antiemetics
Patients with DKA frequently exhibit profuse vomiting. Antiemetic medication with maropitant or metoclopramide should be considered.

Nutrition
Patients with DKA are frequently inappetent on presentation. Appetite usually returns as the ketoacidosis is controlled. If appetite is poor for a prolonged period of time, alternative methods of nutritional supplementation, such as use of feeding tubes, should be considered.

Treatment of triggering disease
As discussed above, DKA is frequently associated with a concurrent triggering disease process. Specific treatment for this disease may also be required. Dependent on the diagnosis, specific treatment may form part of the initial treatment plan (e.g. antibiosis for an infectious trigger) or may be delayed until the initial DKA crisis is resolved and stabilization of the DM has started (e.g. trilostane treatment for hyperadrenocorticism).

Monitoring
DKA patients are frequently critically ill on presentation, with the potential for the development of complications during treatment. Frequent monitoring of both physical examination and clinicopathological parameters, with early intervention if complications develop, is a vital part of a successful outcome. The monitoring should be tailored to the individual patient and should change with time. Suggested parameters to monitor are shown in Figure 24.9.

As regular repeat bloodwork and multiple intravenous infusions may be required, consideration should be given to placement of a central venous catheter at an early stage. These catheters have several advantages over peripheral catheters, notably: blood sampling can be performed in an easy and patient welfare-friendly way; multiple infusions can be given via the same catheter; the catheter can remain in place for 7–10 days; and the catheters are generally well tolerated and easy to maintain.

Transition to chronic therapy
The initial goal of treatment of DKA patients should be to manage the ketoacidotic crisis and any subsequent complications until the patient is ready for transition to a chronic management phase of their DM, using medium- or long-acting insulin (see Chapters 12 and 13). Subcutaneous insulin can be introduced once the patient is well hydrated

Physical examination
• Perfusion parameters (heart rate, mucous membrane colour, CRT, pulse quality) initially every 1–2 hours, reducing to every 4–8 hours
• Respiratory rate and effort with thoracic auscultation every 4–8 hours
• Neurological status initially every 1–2 hours, reducing to every 4–8 hours
• Body temperature every 4–8 hours
• Bodyweight every 8–12 hours

Clinicopathological parameters
• Blood glucose initially every hour, reducing to every 2–4 hours
• PCV/total solids initially every 2 hours, reducing to every 4–8 hours
• Venous blood gas and electrolyte panel initially every 2 hours, reducing to every 4–8 hours
• Urine or serum ketone dipstick evaluation every 12 hours

Other parameters
• Urine output: initially assess every 2–4 hours; if urinary catheter in place measure urine output and adjust fluids accordingly every 4 hours

24.9 Suggested parameters to be monitored in patients with diabetic ketoacidosis.

and eating and drinking without vomiting. The patient should have negative or trace ketones on urine dipsticks. Dependent on the blood glucose concentration, the neutral insulin should be discontinued. Subcutaneous insulin can be started within a few hours of that discontinuation, with the dose chosen dependent on the severity of the hyperglycaemia at that time. Care should be taken to avoid hypoglycaemia.

Hyperglycaemic hyperosmolar syndrome

A second much less common, but similarly severe, complication of DM is the development of hyperglycaemic hyperosmolar syndrome. This syndrome is characterized by severe hyperglycaemia (>33 mmol/l) and a serum osmolality >350 mOsm/kg coupled with minimal or absent ketones. As with DKA, patients typically also have a concurrent disease process; the precise detail of how the pathogenesis of DKA differs from hyperosmolar syndrome is unknown. However, it is thought that it is associated with one of the following:

- The presence of small amounts of insulin and hepatic glucagon resistance, which together lead to an inhibition of lipolysis and ketogenesis
- A reduction in glomerular filtration rate, allowing the development of severe hyperglycaemia.

History and physical examination features are generally similar to those for DKA, except for the recent onset of neurological signs, although it appears coma is uncommon in veterinary patients.

Diagnosis is based on fulfilling the criteria mentioned above. Osmolality can rarely be measured in clinical veterinary medicine but may be calculated using the following formula (with all measurements in mmol/l):

$$\text{Serum osmolality}_{(calc)} = 2(Na^+ + K^+) + BUN + glucose$$

Treatment revolves around meticulous fluid, electrolyte and insulin therapy to resolve the hyperosmolarity and gain control of the underlying DM. Identification and treatment of any concurrent disease process is also important. Great care must be taken during the initial treatment period to ensure that hyperosmolarity does not resolve too quickly, as exacerbation of neurological signs may then occur. During hyperosmolarity the brain generates substances known as idiogenic osmoles, which protect it from dehydration. As hyperosmolarity resolves, these idiogenic osmoles will be slowly eliminated; however, if the hyperosmolar state resolves quickly, these idiogenic osmoles act to pull water into the brain, leading to cerebral oedema.

Prognosis is guarded. In one study of feline clinical patients, long-term (>2 month) survival was only 12% (Koenig et al., 2004).

Summary

DKA represents a severe and potentially life-threatening complication of a common endocrine disease. Patients presenting with DKA require intensive 24-hour care in the initial stages of their management. The development of additional metabolic complications during the early part of treatment is common, and diligent monitoring is required to maximize the chance of a successful outcome.

References and further reading

Brady MA, Dennis JS and Wagner-Mann C (2003) Evaluating the use of plasma hematocrit samples to detect ketones utilizing urine dipstick colorimetric methodology in diabetic dogs and cats. *Journal of Veterinary Emergency and Critical Care* **13**, 1–6

Bruskiewicz KA, Nelson RW, Feldman EC *et al.* (1997) Diabetic ketosis and ketoacidosis in cats: 42 cases (1980–1995). *Journal of the American Veterinary Medical Association* **211**, 188–192

DiTommaso M, Aste G, Rocconi F *et al.* (2009) Evaluation of a portable meter to measure ketonaemia and comparison with ketonuria for diagnosis of canine diabetic ketoacidosis. *Journal of Veterinary Internal Medicine* **23**, 466–471

Fincham SC, Drobatz KJ, Gillespie TN and Hess RS (2004) Evaluation of plasma ionized magnesium concentration in 122 dogs with diabetes mellitus; a retrospective study. *Journal of Veterinary Internal Medicine* **18**, 612–617

Hess RS (2009) Diabetic ketoacidosis. In: *Small Animal Critical Care Medicine*, ed. DC Silverstein DC and K Hopper, pp. 288–291. Elsevier Saunders, St Louis

Hume DZ, Drobatz KJ and Hess RS (2006) Outcome of dogs with ketoacidosis: 127 dogs (1993–2003). *Journal of Veterinary Internal Medicine* **20**, 547–55

Koenig A, Drobatz KJ, Beale AB and King LG (2004) Hyperglycaemic hyperosmolar syndrome in feline diabetics 17 cases (1995–2001). *Journal of Veterinary Emergency and Critical Care* **14**, 30–40

Macintire DK (1993) Treatment of diabetic ketoacidosis in dogs by continuous low-dose intravenous infusion of insulin. *Journal of the American Veterinary Medical Association* **202**, 1266–1272

25

Investigation of hypoglycaemia

Johan P. Schoeman

Introduction

Hypoglycaemia is defined as a blood glucose concentration of <3.5 mmol/l. It is a common complication in the treatment of insulin-dependent diabetes mellitus and a frequent, but poorly recognized, cause of weakness and collapse. In the critically ill or sedated patient hypoglycaemia is a clinically silent, yet life-threatening, disorder that necessitates swift and decisive treatment to prevent lasting neuronal damage.

The most frequent clinical manifestations of hypoglycaemia include weakness, trembling, altered state of consciousness, collapse and seizures. Hypoglycaemia is typically a consequence of:

- Decreased glucose production, which may be caused by:
  - Inadequate dietary intake of glucose or other gluconeogenic substrates (e.g. anorexia in neonates or toy breeds)
  - Impaired hepatic gluconeogenesis (e.g. portosystemic shunt)
  - Deficiency of glucose counter-regulatory hormones (e.g. cortisol, glucagon)
- Excessive glucose utilization, which may be caused by:
  - Increased endogenous insulin production (insulinoma)
  - Overzealous insulin administration
- A combination of the above mechanisms (e.g. in sepsis).

Many causes of hypoglycaemia span the above mechanisms and the list of differential diagnoses are therefore given according to the DAMNIT system (Figure 25.1). The cause is frequently evident after reviewing the history, signalment, physical examination and minimum clinicopathological database (complete blood count, serum biochemistry profile and urinalysis), but a small proportion of cases need advanced diagnostic testing. This chapter presents an overview of the basic pathophysiology of hypoglycaemia and describes a rational, problem-oriented approach to the diagnosis of the potential underlying causes.

More detailed information on insulinoma, a potential cause of hypoglycaemia, and its treatment can be found in Chapter 14.

Developmental

- Hepatic vascular anomalies [a]
- Hepatic enzyme deficiency [a]
  - Von Gierke's disease (type 1 glycogen storage disease)
  - Cori's disease (type 3 glycogen storage disease)

Artefactual

- Prolonged sample storage [b]
- Delayed serum separation [b]
- Laboratory error [d]
- Uncalibrated handheld glucometers [d]

Miscellaneous

- Severe polycythaemia [b]
- Prolonged starvation or malnutrition [a]
- Extreme exertion [b]

Metabolic

- Hepatic insufficiency [a]
  - Acute liver failure
  - Acquired portosystemic shunts
  - Chronic liver fibrosis/cirrhosis
- Hypoadrenocorticism [a]
- Panhypopituitarism [a]
- Renal failure [c]

Neoplastic

- Pancreatic beta cell tumours (insulinoma) [b]
- Extra-pancreatic neoplasia [b]
  - Hepatocellular carcinoma
  - Hepatoma
  - Haemangiosarcoma
  - Leiomyoma/sarcoma

Idiopathic hypoglycaemia

- Hunting dog hypoglycaemia [b]
- Neonatal hypoglycaemia [c]
- Juvenile hypoglycaemia (especially toy breeds) [c]

Iatrogenic

- Excess insulin therapy [b]
- Sulphonylurea therapy [b]
- Therapy with other oral hypoglycaemic drugs, acarbose [a], metformin [b]
- Propranolol therapy [a]

25.1 Causes of hypoglycaemia according to the DAMNIT classification system. Causes are denoted as follows: [a] decreased glucose production; [b] increased glucose utilization; [c] combination of decreased glucose production and increased glucose utilization; [d] analytical errors. (continues)

Infectious

• Canine babesiosis [c]
• Canine parvovirus infection [c]
• Sepsis [c]
  – Endocarditis
  – Chemotherapy-associated neutropenia
  – Severe pneumonia
  – Peritonitis, etc.

Toxic
• Ethanol poisoning [a] • Ethylene glycol poisoning [a] • Xylitol poisoning [b]

25.1 (continued) Causes of hypoglycaemia according to the DAMNIT classification system. Causes are denoted as follows: [a] decreased glucose production; [b] increased glucose utilization; [c] combination of decreased glucose production and increased glucose utilization; [d] analytical errors.

Pathophysiology

Glucose represents the major source of energy for mammalian cells. It is obtained directly from the diet when carbohydrates are catabolized to glucose for absorption and transport to the liver and other organs. In addition, the liver produces glucose from substrates such as amino acids via gluconeogenesis and glycogen via glycogenolysis. Glucose is stored in the liver and muscles as glycogen. Blood glucose concentrations are regulated by dietary intake, hormones (e.g. insulin, glucagon, catecholamines, cortisol, growth hormone), and tissue utilization.

Brain cells and red blood cells are heavily dependent on glucose as an energy source. Indeed, although the brain only constitutes 2% of the total body mass, it utilizes 25% of the total body glucose (Peters *et al.*, 2004). The brain relies on a large and sustained supply of glucose; this is because it has three times the metabolic rate of peripheral tissues yet contains 10–30% less glucose (Levin *et al.*, 2004). Mammalian cells, especially those of the blood–brain barrier (BBB), are generally impermeable to polar molecules; the transport of glucose across cell membranes therefore requires specific transport proteins. The endothelium of the BBB appears to have the highest concentration of glucose transporters of all mammalian tissue. Two classes of glucose transport protein have been described: the sodium-dependent glucose co-transporter, expressed in the kidney and small intestines; and the facilitative glucose transporter (GLUT), expressed by most other cells. Different isoforms of GLUT exist, the most clinically relevant of which is GLUT 4, since this isoform is responsible for the transport of glucose into muscle and adipose tissue under the influence of insulin (Zhao and Keating, 2007).

When blood glucose concentrations decline, glucosensors are stimulated. These initiate neurohormonal compensatory mechanisms that increase plasma glucose concentrations, increase glucose

delivery to and uptake by the brain, and alter glucose metabolic pathways. This compensatory response involves the following.

• A decrease in insulin secretion, with a resultant increase in glucagon concentration that induces hepatic glycogenolysis and gluconeogenesis.
• Adrenaline and noradrenaline are released at the onset of hypoglycaemia. Like glucagon, adrenaline release promotes hepatic glycogenolysis and gluconeogenesis, but will also stimulate muscle glycogenolysis, lipolysis and ketogenesis; it also mobilizes gluconeogenic precursors (lactate, alanine and glycerol) and inhibits glucose utilization by insulin-sensitive tissues.
• If hypoglycaemia persists for longer, a third mechanism, namely the secretion of cortisol and growth hormone, is initiated (Cryer, 1997). This robust cortisol response to hypoglycaemia has also been shown in natural canine infection (Schoeman and Herrtage, 2007).

In certain circumstances, these physiologic safeguards fail and hypoglycaemia develops.

Methods of measurement

A diagnosis of hypoglycaemia is made by documenting a subnormal blood glucose concentration. Misrepresentation of the patient's true glycaemic status due to a laboratory or processing error is a common occurrence in practice. The clinician should be aware of artefactual causes of hypoglycaemia, such as a poorly calibrated handheld glucometer, polycythaemia, prolonged storage of blood or lack of plasma/serum separation from blood cells. Blood glucose concentrations obtained with most portable glucometers read lower than the reference hexokinase method. This difference is typically exacerbated as the true blood glucose concentrations decrease (Wess and Reusch, 2000). However, the recently licensed AlphaTRAK meter showed higher concentrations than the reference method in 43% of measurements. Portable glucometers misclassified blood glucose concentrations in terms of hypo-, eu-, or hyperglycaemia 2.1–38.7% of the time (Cohen *et al.*, 2009).

It is therefore always good practice to re-sample the patient in order to verify hypoglycaemia, using a reference laboratory method, before embarking on an extensive diagnostic work-up. Blood should ideally be collected in fluoride oxalate tubes (grey or yellow top); serum (red top) or heparinized tubes (green top) can be used, but have to be centrifuged and the serum/plasma separated within 30 minutes of sample collection.

• Normal plasma glucose concentrations range from approximately 3.5 to 6.5 mmol/l in dogs and from 3.5 to 7.0 mmol/l in cats, with small variations depending on the laboratory and methodology used.

- When plasma glucose concentrations are reduced to below approximately 3.5 mmol/l, clinical signs indicative of sympathetic nervous system activation, such as nervousness, tremors and tachycardia, are observed in a range of species, including dogs and cats.
- When plasma glucose concentrations fall to <1 mmol/l, seizure activity, severe brain damage, coma and death can occur as a result of marked neuronal dysfunction and cell death.

Differential diagnosis

Decreased glucose production

This can be the result of substrate, hormone or enzyme deficiencies. Substrate deficiencies are most commonly caused by malnutrition, inadequate food intake or liver disease. Insufficient functional hepatic mass (<75%), as a result of either portosystemic shunt or acute and chronic liver failure, is a common cause of hypoglycaemia. These hepatic disorders also result in impaired insulin catabolism that further exacerbates the hypoglycaemia.

Inadequate production or release of insulin-antagonizing hormones, such as cortisol and growth hormone, can result in hypoglycaemia. The blood glucose concentrations in these disorders are usually only slightly below normal and other clinical and biochemical findings, such as dwarfism in panhypopituitarism and electrolyte abnormalities in classic hypoadrenocorticism, often predominate. Isolated glucocorticoid deficiency in 'atypical hypoadrenocorticism' presents a diagnostic challenge, unless the clinician retains a high index of suspicion for this disorder (see Chapter 15).

Enzyme deficiencies are the least common cause of decreased glucose production. Dogs with glycogen storage diseases due to specific glycogenolytic enzyme deficiencies are unable to release glucose from the liver, with resultant glycogen accumulation, hepatomegaly and organ dysfunction.

Increased glucose utilization

A common cause of excessive glucose utilization is in cases of insulinoma, where there is increased insulin production by malignant pancreatic islet beta cells (see Chapter 14). Recently, a pancreatic beta cell tumour has been described that caused hypoglycaemia in a dog, not by oversecretion of insulin, but by oversecretion of insulin-like growth factor type II (Finotello et al., 2009).

Severe malarial infection in humans results in hypoglycaemia, due to the overproduction of insulin by the parasites, and some evidence of elevated insulin concentrations exist in hypoglycaemic cases of canine babesiosis (Rees and Schoeman, 2008).

Overzealous administration of exogenous insulin to diabetic patients, in the form of overdosing, double-dosing or persistent dosing in the face of anorexia, are common iatrogenic causes of hypoglycaemia, resulting in excessive glucose utilization. Previously well regulated diabetic cats can suddenly experience bouts of hypoglycaemia due to dramatically reduced insulin requirements. This is due to a reversal of 'glucose toxicity', whereby weeks to months of insulin treatment can lead to a restoration in beta cell insulin secretory ability, rendering further exogenous insulin administration redundant and potentially dangerous.

The concomitant administration of sulphonylurea drugs, such as glipizide and other oral hypoglycaemics, to type 2 diabetic patients can also lead to excessive glucose utilization and resultant hypoglycaemia. Xylitol, a sweetener that is increasingly found in sugar-free products such as gums and baked goods, is a recently described cause of excessive insulin secretion and hepatic necrosis in dogs, with resultant profound hypoglycaemia (Dunayer, 2004).

Hyperinsulinaemia drives glucose out of the plasma and into the cells, whilst simultaneously inhibiting the mobilization of energy stored as amino acids, triglycerides or glycogen in muscle, fat and liver, respectively. This dual effect of increased utilization and decreased mobilization can lead to profound hypoglycaemia.

Hypoglycaemia insensitivity in diabetic patients

Hypoglycaemia insensitivity is a condition in human diabetic patients caused by impaired compensatory responses to hypoglycaemia. These patients develop decreased glucagon release and decreased hepatic responsiveness to adrenaline. Lower plasma glucose levels are thus endured without stimulation of normal compensatory mechanisms, and these patients become more prone to hypoglycaemic episodes (Korytkowski et al., 1998; Ovalle et al., 1998). The author has also encountered this in some canine diabetics; practitioners should maintain an awareness for these patients.

Diagnostic approach

The most important step in solving this problem is the recognition of hypoglycaemia as the cause of the clinical signs. If hypoglycaemia is strongly suspected, yet not documented on the first occasion, the clinician is advised to repeat 2-hourly blood glucose concentration measurements over a 12-hour period of fasting. This fasting period might have to be prolonged to 24–72 hours. When hypoglycaemia (plasma glucose <3.5 mmol/l) is confirmed, the sequence of diagnostic tests is mainly governed by results obtained after a thorough review of the history, signalment, clinical examination and minimum clinicopathological data findings. Additional diagnostics such as serum insulin concentration, ACTH response test, hepatic function tests, radiography, ultrasonography, blood culture and, occasionally, organ biopsy are then rationally employed on the basis of these initial findings (Figure 25.2).

Signalment

Young animals are more prone to developing hypoglycaemia due to starvation, neonatal or juvenile

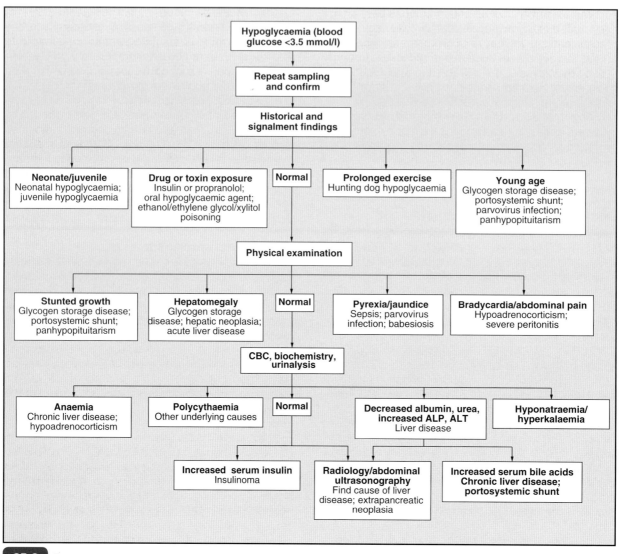

25.2 Flowchart for use as an aid in identifying the underlying causes of hypoglycaemia.

hypoglycaemia, portosystemic shunt, parvovirus infection, babesiosis or glycogen storage disease. Middle-aged to older animals are more likely to be affected by insulinoma, other neoplastic conditions, acquired hepatic disease and hypoadrenocorticism. Bearded Collies and West Highland White Terriers may be predisposed to hypoadrenocorticism, whereas Yorkshire, Cairn and Maltese Terriers as well as Irish Wolfhounds are more likely to have portosystemic shunt, and Boxers and Irish Setters are more likely to develop insulinoma.

Historical features

Animals with hypoadrenocorticism and insulinoma usually have a more prolonged history (spanning a few months) of intermittent weakness and collapse and even peripheral neuropathy in the case of insulinoma. Hunting dog hypoglycaemia cases have an obvious history of activity-associated clinical signs in lean individuals, whereas parvovirus-infected dogs have a classic history of vomiting or diarrhoea immediately (a few hours to days) preceding the weakness and collapsed state. Tick exposure and a short history of weakness,

associated with marked anaemia, characterizes hypoglycaemia associated with virulent canine babesiosis (Keller *et al.*, 2004). Sepsis should be suspected in patients that have received chemotherapy or are splenectomized, those with parvovirus infection and those with abnormal hepatic function or endocarditis. A history of exposure to hypoglycaemic drugs, such as propranolol or insulin, or toxins such as ethanol, ethylene glycol, and especially the ingestion of chewing gum containing xylitol, should be borne in mind in dogs with acute onset weakness and collapse (Dunayer, 2004). Other appropriate areas of questioning include: age of onset and whether siblings are affected (glycogen storage diseases); temporal relationship to meals (insulinoma, portosystemic shunt); vaccination history (parvovirus infection); and quality of the diet (malnutrition/starvation) or the presence of persistent diarrhoea (severe malassimilation).

Physical examination

Affected patients may show a variety of focal and generalized neurological signs. The most common clinical signs are intermittent, brief episodes (a few seconds to minutes) of altered or clouded consciousness (depression, coma), weakness, ataxia, collapse and seizures. The exact clinical signs are dependent on the rapidity of the fall in blood glucose, the duration of hypoglycaemia and the absolute blood glucose concentration reached – some animals can tolerate quite low glucose concentrations without showing clinical signs. With a rapid fall in glucose, additional signs such as muscle fasciculation, tachycardia and vomiting are observed, which are mainly attributable to sympathetic system activation.

Clinical signs unrelated to the hypoglycaemia, such as pyrexia, jaundice or bradycardia, are helpful in localizing the cause of hypoglycaemia.

Patients suffering from insulinoma may show signs of lower motor neuron dysfunction, such as decreased spinal reflexes related to the presence of peripheral neuropathy. They are generally in very good body condition due to the anabolic effects of insulin, whereas patients with advanced renal failure or prolonged starvation are clearly emaciated. Failure to identify abnormalities on physical examination in an older, large-breed dog is an important clue to the potential presence of an insulin-secreting tumour.

Patients with portosystemic shunt may have small stature and poor growth. Acquired or end-stage chronic liver disease patients are also generally in poor body condition with concomitant jaundice and ascites. Patients with other extrapancreatic neoplastic conditions are usually presented for clinical signs referable to these, such as hepatomegaly and other abdominal masses with or without ascites. Polycythaemic patients might present with brick-red mucous membranes and seizures. Lactating bitches with eclampsia (hypocalcaemia) could have concurrent hypoglycaemia. Hypoglycaemia should always be suspected in any dog presenting in status epilepticus, either as an inciting cause or as a complicating factor.

The cardiovascular and neurological systems should be thoroughly evaluated during the physical examination, because abnormalities in these are important differentials for weakness, collapse, syncope and seizures.

Minimum clinicopathological data

A complete haematological and biochemical profile will enable the confirmation of hypoglycaemia and help to rule out other causes of weakness and collapse such as hypo- or hypercalcaemia. Abnormalities that provide very useful pointers as to which test might have to be employed next include:

- Polycythaemia
- Non-regenerative anaemia in the case of chronic kidney disease
- Neoplastic diseases
- Acute haemolytic anaemia in the case of babesiosis
- Marked neutropenia in the case of parvovirus infection
- A degenerative left shift neutrophilia that might indicate sepsis.

Full serum biochemistry will elucidate potential liver involvement if liver enzyme activities and bile acid concentrations are elevated, whilst electrolyte disorders such as hyperkalaemia, hyponatraemia, hypercalcaemia (with or without eosinophilia) and lymphocytosis might point to hypoadrenocorticism. Elevated urea and creatinine concentrations in the face of unconcentrated urine are consistent with chronic kidney disease or hypoadrenocorticism. Hypoglycaemic states caused by excessive insulin administration will often show hypokalaemia and hypophosphataemia, which is also present in cases of xylitol poisoning, but with additional profound elevations in hepatic enzymes (Dunayer and Gwaltney-Brant, 2006).

Hepatic function tests

The bile acid stimulation test is the most practical and reliable way to assess liver function in practice. It involves taking a serum sample, giving the patient a fatty meal and then re-sampling 2 hours later. Hypoalbuminaemia, low serum urea, hyperbilirubinaemia and prolonged bleeding times are additional indications of hepatic dysfunction. Serum cholesterol concentrations in hepatobiliary disease are variable; hypercholesterolaemia is seen in cholestatic disease, whereas hypocholesterolaemia is observed in end-stage liver disease.

Insulin concentration

Blood insulin concentrations should lie below the reference interval in hypoglycaemic patients. When the blood insulin concentration of hypoglycaemic patients falls within or above the upper reference interval, this is abnormal and a diagnosis of insulinoma is very likely. The guidelines for the interpretation of fasting insulin concentrations are detailed in Chapter 14.

ACTH response test

This test is employed to assess adrenal reserve. Normal dogs should stimulate to serum cortisol values of >200 nmol/l one hour after injection of exogenous ACTH, depending on background lifestyle stress and resultant adrenal size. Dogs with hypoadrenocorticism will typically have cortisol concentrations of <30 nmol/l both pre- and post-ACTH.

Diagnostic imaging

Abdominal radiography is generally of limited value in detecting insulinomas. It is, however, used to identify potential neoplastic conditions denoted by hepatomegaly, or to detect metastatic disease that might present as decreased serosal detail or a radiological mass-effect. Thoracic radiography may indicate pulmonary metastatic disease.

Abdominal ultrasonography is probably the most useful test to use in hypoglycaemic dogs where the underlying cause is not immediately apparent after reviewing the preceding findings. It will reveal changes to the liver parenchyma in diseases such as chronic cirrhosis or may reveal anomalous blood vessels consistent with portosystemic shunting. Ultrasonography is also useful for the detection of extrapancreatic neoplasms such as renal adenocarcinoma, which can be associated with hypoglycaemia (Battaglia *et al.,* 2005).

Most insulinomas are quite small (<4 cm) and are isoechoic when compared with surrounding pancreatic parenchyma. The ultrasonographic detection of insulinomas is difficult, even in experienced hands; a negative ultrasonographic examination does not therefore rule the condition out. Changes to the hepatic parenchyma and enlargement of the regional lymph nodes can be detected and are the most common potential metastatic sites for insulinoma. Intraoperative ultrasonography enables more accurate detection of primary pancreatic tumours.

Scintigraphic studies with radiolabelled somatostatin analogues can detect insulinomas that express these somatostatin receptors and are helpful in a subgroup of cases with negative ultrasonographic findings (Robben *et al.,* 1997; Robben *et al.,* 2005). Low serum fructosamine can also be helpful in the diagnosis of insulinoma (Mellanby and Herrtage, 2002).

Blood culture

Positive blood cultures are consistent with sepsis, but this is not a very sensitive test. Sensitivities can be increased by taking at least three cultures over a 12-hour period and ensuring that blood samples are taken before the onset of antibiotic therapy.

Organ biopsy

The method of biopsy is influenced by organ size and degree of ascites, the suspected diagnosis and the clinical condition/haemorrhage risk of the patient. Ultrasound-guided biopsy can be a high-yielding procedure in diffuse disorders, such as liver cirrhosis or focal conditions in which suspicious lesions can be targeted. Fine-needle aspirates are preferred in patients with bleeding disorders, large cavitatory lesions or abscesses, and may yield diagnostic samples and even reveal infectious agents that can be missed on histopathology. However, in patients that can tolerate the procedure, hepatic wedge biopsy upon exploratory laparotomy gives the most reliable results and is often the only procedure resulting in a definitive diagnosis in diseases with subtle lesions or uneven distribution.

References and further reading

Battaglia L, Petterino C, Zappulli V and Castagnaro M (2005) Hypoglycaemia as a paraneoplastic syndrome associated with renal adenocarcinoma in a dog. *Veterinary Research Communications* **29**, 671–675

Cohen TA, Nelson RW, Kass PH, Christopher MM and Feldman EC (2009) Evaluation of six portable blood glucose meters for measuring blood glucose concentration in dogs. *Journal of the American Veterinary Medical Association* **235**, 276–280

Cryer PE (1997) Hierarchy of physiological responses to hypoglycemia: relevance to clinical hypoglycemia in type I (insulin dependent) diabetes mellitus. *Hormone and Metabolic Research* **29**, 92–96

Dunayer EK (2004) Hypoglycemia following canine ingestion of xylitol-containing gum. *Veterinay and Human Toxicology* **46**, 87–88

Dunayer EK and Gwaltney-Brant SM (2006) Acute hepatic failure and coagulopathy associated with xylitol ingestion in eight dogs. *Journal of the American Veterinary Medical Association* **229**, 1113–1117

Finotello R, Marchetti V, Nesi G *et al.* (2009) Pancreatic islet cell tumor secreting insulin-like growth factor type-II in a dog. *Journal of Veterinay Internal Medicine* **23**, 1289–1292

Keller N, Jacobson LS, Nel M *et al.* (2004) Prevalence and risk factors of hypoglycemia in virulent canine babesiosis. *Journal of Veterinary Internal Medicine* **18**, 265–270

Korytkowski MT, Mokan M, Veneman TF et al. (1998) Reduced beta-adrenergic sensitivity in patients with type 1 diabetes and hypoglycemia unawareness. *Diabetes Care* **21**, 1939–1943

Levin BE, Routh VH, Kang L, Sanders NM and Dunn-Meynell AA (2004) Neuronal glucosensing: what do we know after 50 years? *Diabetes* **53**, 2521–2528

Mellanby RJ and Herrtage ME (2002) Insulinoma in a normoglycaemic dog with low serum fructosamine. *Journal of Small Animal Practice* **43**, 506–508

Ovalle F, Fanelli CG, Paramore DS *et al.* (1998) Brief twice-weekly episodes of hypoglycemia reduce detection of clinical hypoglycemia in type 1 diabetes mellitus. *Diabetes* **47**, 1472–1479

Peters A, Schweiger U, Pellerin L *et al.* (2004) The selfish brain: competition for energy resources. *Neuroscience and Behavioural Reviews* **28**, 143–180

Rees P and Schoeman JP (2008) Plasma insulin concentrations in hypoglycaemic dogs with *Babesia canis rossi* infection. *Veterinary Parasitology* **152**, 60–66

Robben JH, Pollak YW, Kirpensteijn J *et al.* (2005) Comparison of ultrasonography, computed tomography, and single-photon emission computed tomography for the detection and localization of canine insulinoma. *Journal of Veterinary Internal Medicine* **19**, 15–22

Robben JH, Visser-Wisselaar HA, Rutteman GR *et al.* (1997) In vitro and in vivo detection of functional somatostatin receptors in canine insulinomas. *Journal of Nuclear Medicine* **38**, 1036–1042

Schoeman JP and Herrtage ME (2007) The response of the pituitary-adrenal and pituitary-thyroidal axes to the plasma glucose perturbations in *Babesia canis rossi* babesiosis. *Journal of the South African Veterinary Association* **78**, 215–220

Wess G and Reusch C (2000) Evaluation of five portable blood glucose meters for use in dogs. *Journal of the American Veterinary Medical Association* **61**, 1587–1592

Zhao FQ and Keating AF (2007) Functional properties and genomics of glucose transporters. *Current Genomics* **8**, 113–128

26

Investigation of symmetrical alopecia in dogs

Rosario Cerundolo

Introduction

Hair loss in dogs is usually a major cause of concern for both owners and breeders. This is especially true when the dog has been bred for its coat characteristics or for showing purposes. Conscientious owners and breeders easily recognize subtle changes in coat density, which may or may not lead to eventual alopecia, and often seek veterinary advice early on. In some cases the alopecia may be purely cosmetic, yet may still cause distress to owners.

As a cosmetic problem, changes in haircoat density represent no risk to the patient. However, such changes may be indicative of cutaneous or internal disease, with potentially serious consequences. A methodical approach and an accurate diagnosis are therefore essential for the successful management of these cases.

Disorders causing *symmetrical* alopecia are usually acquired during a dog's lifetime and include:

* Severe folliculitis (e.g. demodicosis, dermatophytosis, superficial pyoderma)
* Abnormalities of hair follicle anatomy or cycling (e.g. follicular dysplasias, endocrinopathies, alopecia X)
* Self-trauma, often caused by pruritic conditions (e.g. allergies).

In some cases the hair may be so short that it can simulate a classic form of alopecia. Initially, hair loss may be localized; however, the affected areas may expand if there is an underlying cause that is not properly addressed, and the alopecia may become symmetrical or generalized. The purpose of this chapter is to provide a diagnostic approach to symmetrical alopecia that should help veterinary surgeons better manage these cases. Further details on alopecia and on dermatological testing may be found in the *BSAVA Manual of Canine and Feline Dermatology*.

Diagnostic approach

The diagnostic approach to follow when presented with a case of symmetrical alopecia is summarized in Figure 26.1. This includes: identifying breed predisposition; looking into sex status; taking a detailed history of the patient; completing a physical and dermatological examination; and, finally, exploring the most appropriate diagnostic tests.

1. Breed predisposition.
2. Sexual status.
3. History:
   – Age of onset
   – Presence of pruritus
   – Signs of internal/systemic disease
   – Initial location of alopecia and progression
   – Response to previous therapy.
4. Physical and dermatological examination.
5. Routine dermatological tests (skin scrapings, trichogram, cytology).
6. Routine haematology and biochemistry tests.
7. Hormonal tests:
   – Thyroid function evaluation: thyroxine (T4) and free T4; thyroid-stimulating hormone (TSH); anti-thyroglobulin autoantibodies
   – Pituitary–adrenal gland axis function evaluation: ACTH response and low-dose dexamethasone suppression tests
   – Sex hormone measurements in intact dogs.
8. Skin biopsy.

26.1 Step-by-step diagnostic approach to follow when presented with a case of symmetrical alopecia. ACTH = adrenocorticotropic hormone.

Signalment

Breed predisposition

Certain types of alopecia are observed most commonly in particular breeds. It is therefore crucial to consider breed-specific diseases when dealing with alopecic patients. Hereditary forms of alopecia have been reported anecdotally in various dog breeds, although genetic proof is lacking. Certain forms of hereditary alopecia may only appear later in life.

Some conditions are linked to coat colour (Figure 26.2). Breeds or coat colours allegedly affected by hereditary forms of alopecia include: Rottweilers (follicular lipidosis); dogs with black coats (black hair follicular dysplasia) (Figure 26.3); dogs with a dilute coat colour, such as blue coat Dobermanns (Figure 26.4); and Dachshunds and Yorkshire Terriers (colour dilution alopecia).

Other breed-specific forms of canine alopecia that are not linked to coat colour have been described in Irish Water Spaniels (Figure 26.5a), Portuguese Water Dogs, Nordic breeds, Keeshonds (Figure 26.5b), Pomeranians (Figure 26.5c), Greyhounds, Curly Coated Retrievers and Chesapeake Bay Retrievers (Figure 26.5d).

Coat colour-linked

- Follicular lipidosis
- Black hair follicular dysplasia
- Colour-dilution alopecia

Non-coat colour-linked

- Infectious/parasitic diseases
- Alopecia X (see Figure 26.11)
- Hypothyroidism
- Hyperadrenocorticism
- Sex hormone imbalance (see Figure 26.11)
- Pattern alopecia
- Canine recurrent flank alopecia (see Figure 26.11)
- Follicular dysplasia

26.2 Coat colour-linked and non-coat colour-linked forms of alopecia.

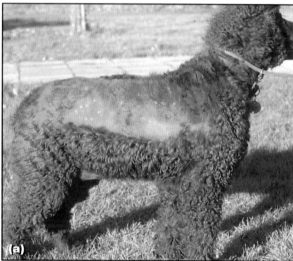

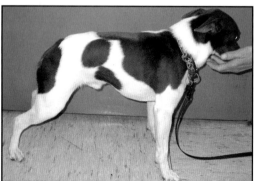

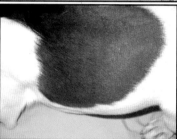

26.3 Hair loss affecting the black areas of the coat in a 2-year-old Rat Terrier. The close-up view shows the left side of the dog's chest.

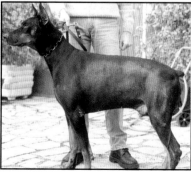

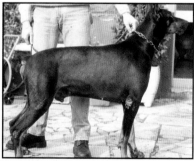

26.4 Bilateral and symmetrical alopecia of a Dobermann with colour-dilution alopecia.

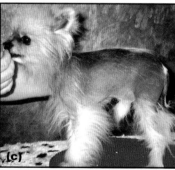

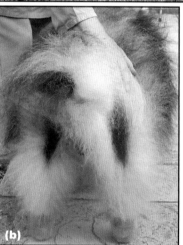

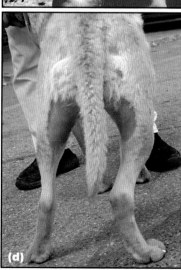

26.5 Alopecia linked to breed but not to coat colour.
(a) Alopecia of the side of the trunk spreading over the dorsum of an Irish Water Spaniel with follicular dysplasia.
(b) Bilateral symmetrical alopecia of the thighs of a Keeshond with alopecia X.
(c) Alopecia and cutaneous hyperpigmentation in a Pomeranian with alopecia X.
(d) Bilaterally symmetrical alopecia of the thighs of a Chesapeake Bay Retriever with follicular dysplasia.

Hyperadrenocorticism is the most common endocrinopathy of small breeds such as Miniature Poodles, Dachshunds and terriers, while hypothyroidism is more common in various large-breed dogs. Pattern alopecia is more common in Manchester and Yorkshire Terriers (Figure 26.6), Miniature Pinschers, Dachshunds, Whippets, Italian Greyhounds, Greyhounds and Boston Terriers, whereas cyclic recurrent flank alopecia is more often seen in Dobermanns, Boxers, Airedale Terriers, English Bulldogs and also in cross-breeds (Figure 26.7).

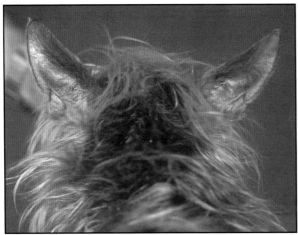

26.6 Bilateral symmetrical alopecia of the pinnae of a Yorkshire Terrier with pattern baldness.

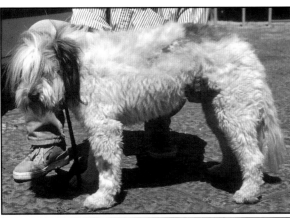

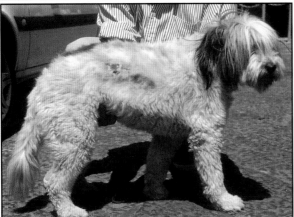

26.7 Bilateral symmetrical alopecia of a crossbred dog with canine recurrent flank alopecia.

Conditions that bring about an inflammatory form of alopecia occur more commonly in particular breeds; for example demodicosis is more prevalent in short-coated dog breeds (e.g. Pugs, Boxers, Dobermanns and terriers) whereas sebaceous adenitis is more prevalent in Akitas, Vizslas, Hovawarts and Poodles.

Sex status

Intact dogs may develop tumours of the gonads. This may lead to feminization in male dogs with oestrogen-producing testicular tumours, while bitches may develop ovarian disorders and subsequent hyperoestrogenism. Hyperoestrogenism, as well as Sertoli cell tumours in male dogs, may cause alopecia.

History

Taking a detailed history of the patient before physical examination is a vital step in the diagnostic work-up. It is important to consider asking the questions listed in Figure 26.8.

- What type of environment is the patient exposed to?
- Are other animals or humans that live in the same environment exhibiting any skin/coat lesions?
- Is the patient showing any systemic clinical signs or has it been affected by other illnesses?
- Has the patient undergone any recent surgical interventions, blood loss, pregnancy or stressful events?
- How long has the disease been present and how did it progress?
- Is the dog pruritic: any scratching, licking, chewing, or rubbing at the alopecic area?
- At what age did the hair loss start?
- Are siblings or parents affected?
- Has the alopecia been waxing and waning?
- On which part of the body did the problem start?
- Has the alopecia slowly progressed and spread to other parts of the body?
- Is the alopecia related to the season of the year or to the oestrous cycle?
- Has the patient shown any response to previous or current therapy for their alopecia?
- Is the patient currently undergoing treatment for a different illness, or has it received any such treatment in recent months?

26.8 Questions to consider asking the owner in order to obtain a detailed history of the patient.

Age of onset

The age at which alopecia first occurred can be helpful in narrowing the differential diagnoses. Non-inflammatory alopecia during the first year of life is suggestive of ectodermal or follicular dysplasia or dysplasia of the hair follicle pigmentary unit. Late-onset alopecia is common in some forms of follicular dysplasia or endocrinopathies. In contrast, inflammatory alopecia with or without pruritus can occur at any age.

Pruritus

The presence of pruritus should be clearly evaluated, as it may suggest a traumatic aetiology. However, diseases that are normally non-inflammatory, such as endocrinopathies, may become pruritic if complicated by a secondary bacterial/yeast infection; hair regrowth may not be complete unless these infections are properly controlled. Re-evaluation of these cases after an appropriate course of therapy may be helpful.

Progression of alopecia

Abrupt hair loss may occur in dogs following certain drug therapies (see below). Sudden profuse hair loss (telogen effluvium) that lasts for a few weeks may be a transient disorder of excess hair shedding, resulting from a synchronous cessation of hair growth. It usually follows pregnancy, lactation, severe illness or a stressful event that occurred 1–3 months previously. Seasonal or cyclic episodes of non-inflammatory symmetrical truncal alopecia, usually followed by spontaneous hair regrowth, are typical of canine recurrent flank alopecia. Spontaneous regrowth can also be seen in the follicular dysplasia of the Portuguese Water Dog. Most endocrinopathies and inflammatory disorders tend to be progressive and generalized without intermittent remission. Burns or scalds can be followed by scarring alopecia that develops several days after the injury.

Underlying disease

Dogs with alopecia that is associated with an underlying endocrine disorder may also exhibit other signs, such as polyuria, polydipsia and polyphagia in hyperadrenocorticism, and lethargy and weight gain in hypothyroidism.

Additionally, a dog's response to previous therapy for alopecia, or the lack of response, is helpful in the diagnostic process; for example failure of hair regrowth after 3–5 months of appropriate thyroid hormone supplementation suggests that hypothyroidism is an unlikely cause of alopecia.

Drug administration

Long-term glucocorticoid therapy may cause iatrogenic hyperadrenocorticism and hair cycle arrest in dogs. Oestrogens may also interfere with the hair cycle. Dogs receiving chemotherapy (doxorubicin and cyclophosphamide) may develop hair follicle dystrophy resulting in hair loss; this is especially seen in Miniature Poodles, Labradors and Golden Retrievers.

Physical examination

A general physical examination should be undertaken before dermatological examination; this should rule out concurrent diseases or systemic conditions that may affect the skin and coat. For example, the presence of a pendulous abdomen and/or panting should raise suspicion of hyperadrenocorticism, whilst the presence of lethargy, hypothermia and bradycardia may suggest hypothyroidism. Gynaecomastia, pendulous prepuce and atrophic testicles may indicate a Sertoli cell tumour.

Dermatological examination

Examining coat condition

The coat condition should be carefully examined. It is important to consider the factors outlined in Figure 26.9. Discoloration of the coat (leucotrichia) is not uncommon in dogs with hyperadrenocorticism; a change in coat colour to brown (salivary staining) is a hallmark of licking, especially in white dogs. The severity of hair loss should be recorded to allow documentation of progression or resolution of the disease.

- Is the hair missing or merely broken?
- Is the coat around the alopecic area normal?
- Is the hair easily epilated?
- Is the hair easily broken by touching the coat?
- Is the coat normal or does it look dry/greasy, matted/dirty?
- Are the primary and/or secondary hairs missing?
- Is the hair thinner than normal in some areas of the body?
- Has the hair density changed?
- Has the coat colour changed?
- Has the skin colour changed?
- Is the skin dry and scaly?
- Are there any other primary or secondary lesions in addition to the alopecia?

 26.9 Factors to consider when examining the coat condition and the skin.

In most cases of symmetrical alopecia, hairs are in telogen and there is hair follicle arrest. Consequently, the areas of the body that are subject to continuous friction (e.g. the lateral neck, thighs and tail) may undergo fracture of the hairs, with subsequent hair loss. Interestingly, the head and distal extremities of dogs with symmetrical alopecia are largely unaffected, or less severely affected, than other parts of the body; this most likely reflects the differences in hair genetics at different body locations.

Examining the skin

After evaluating and recording the degree of alopecia, the skin should be carefully examined (Figure 26.9) for the presence of other primary or secondary lesions. Occasionally, certain forms of alopecia that are initially non-pruritic may become pruritic because of secondary/concurrent infections or infestations.

The dermatological examination should first concentrate on signs of follicular inflammation and infection, differentiating them from non-inflammatory diseases. However, there may be cases of follicular dysplasia or endocrinopathies with secondary bacterial infections that need to be carefully evaluated.

In addition, signs that are specific for some dermatoses should be carefully evaluated:

- Erythema, papules, pustules, thickening of the skin or lichenification, self-trauma (recognized by broken hairs), excoriations, erosions, and ulcerations are all suggestive of an inflammatory process with pruritus
- Thinning of the skin, with prominent subcutaneous vessels or calcium deposits along dermal collagen fibres (calcinosis cutis), is pathognomonic for hyperadrenocorticism
- Hypothyroidism is often accompanied by thickened and hyperpigmented skin without inflammation
- In canine recurrent flank alopecia, the affected area of the skin is well demarcated, hyperpigmented and feels cold.
- Hyperpigmentation of the alopecic areas is common in dogs with alopecia X
- Hyperpigmentation and lichenification are also seen in response to chronic inflammation.

Careful examination should distinguish inflammatory from non-inflammatory hyperpigmentation. Depigmentation will occur with scarring.

Location and progression
Symmetrical alopecia on the head or thighs suggests a genetic type of hair loss, such as pattern baldness or follicular dysplasia. Bilateral alopecia of the trunk or flanks suggests follicular dysplasia or canine recurrent flank alopecia. If presented with alopecia that started as symmetrical or bilateral and then progressed to generalized, endocrine disease, alopecia X or follicular dysplasia should be suspected. Alopecia cases that start as focal or multifocal and then progress to generalized should be investigated for ectoparasites and infections.

Diagnostic tests
Routine dermatological investigations (Figure 26.10) carried out at the time of the initial visit should rule out the presence of ectoparasites, fungi or infections.

Trichogram
The trichogram is one of the most important tests in alopecic patients. Under physiological conditions, a trichogram will reveal hair shafts in anagen (growing) and in telogen (resting) stage. Telogen hairs are easily epilated and anagen hairs can be pulled out by applying some traction. Some dog breeds will show very high numbers of hair follicles in the telogen stage.

Examining the hair tips of plucked hairs with a microscope may help to differentiate broken hair shafts or split ends from the fine-peaked ends of normal hairs. This is often the best way to diagnose alopecia caused by self-trauma. Furthermore, the hair shaft can reveal clumped melanin and thus will draw attention towards colour-dilution alopecia or black hair follicular dysplasia. Microscopic examination of plucked hairs mounted on a glass slide with mineral oil can be used to search for ectoparasites and arthrospores or dermatophytes within or along the hair shaft. Abnormal cycling of hair follicles can be detected by an altered ratio of anagen to telogen hairs. Hair shafts may be covered by keratinosebaceous material (follicular casts), suggesting abnormalities within the hair follicle and the sebum production.

Clinicopathological investigations
Specific laboratory tests, such as routine haematology, biochemistry and hormone tests, are often required for a definitive diagnosis in most cases of symmetrical alopecia. These will not be discussed in detail, as they are covered in other relevant chapters on specific endocrine disorders. A summary of the important diagnostic points in the investigation of alopecia X, sex hormone imbalance and recurrent flank alopecia is given in Figure 26.11.

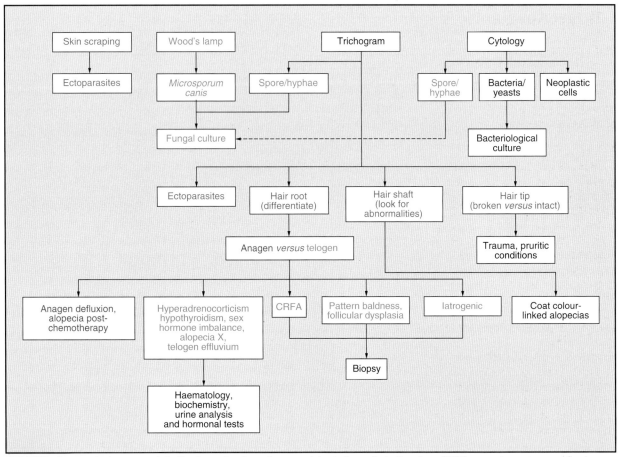

26.10 Suggested approach to the investigation of symmetrical alopecia in the dog. CRFA = canine recurrent flank alopecia.

Characteristic	Alopecia X	Sex hormone imbalance	Canine recurrent flank alopecia
Breed predisposition	Pomeranian, Miniature Poodle, Nordic breeds	None – can occur in any breed	Many breeds, including the Airedale Terrier, Boxer, Dobermann, Giant Schnauzer and English Bulldog
Age of onset	2–6 years	Adult to old	8 months to 11 years
Clinical pattern of alopecia	Truncal progressive hair loss and/or woolly coat quality; with or without cutaneous hyperpigmentation	Truncal progressive hair loss which may also affect neck, tail and thighs; with or without cutaneous hyperpigmentation, ceruminous otitis	Thoracolumbar progressive, ultimately well demarcated hair loss (November to March) with cutaneous hyperpigmentation. Spontaneous hair regrowth within 3–8 months followed by hair loss at the same time the following year. Some dogs may develop permanent alopecia
Systemic clinical signs	Absent	Male: pendulous prepuce, gynaecomastia, enlarged testicle in the scrotum or abdomen. Female: enlarged vulva, prolonged oestrous cycle, nymphomania	Absent
Haematology and biochemistry	Normal	Aplastic anaemia and normal biochemical findings	Normal
Thyroid function	Normal	Normal	Normal
Pituitary–adrenal axis function	See UCCR, below	Normal	Normal
Steroidogenesis	Abnormal steroidogenesis: increased concentration of 17-hydroxyprogesterone pre- and/or post-ACTH stimulation	See Oestradiol, below	Normal
Urine cortisol: creatinine ratio (UCCR)	Increased in most urine samples collected over a 10-day period. Mild or moderate suppression of UCCR by the (blood or oral) low-dose dexamethasone suppression test	Normal	Normal
Oestradiol concentration	Often increased in the Keeshond	Increased	Normal
Diagnostic imaging tests	Ultrasonography	Ultrasonography and radiography	Not applicable
Histological findings	Tricholemmal keratinization of the hair follicles	Skin: non-specific findings Gonads: cystic or neoplastic ovary or testicular tumour	Follicles with marked infundibular orthokeratotic hyperkeratosis extending to secondary follicles ('witch's feet' or 'octopus-like' hair follicles)
Therapy	Cosmetic disease. Dogs are otherwise healthy and treatment is not necessary. Castration may lead to temporary hair regrowth. Melatonin is safe, cheap and may induce hair regrowth. Trilostane effective though costly: bewware side effects	Castration or ovariohysterectomy	Cosmetic disease. Dogs are otherwise healthy and treatment is not necessary. Melatonin may speed up the hair regrowth or, if given early enough during the autumn, may prevent hair loss

26.11 A comparative summary of the history, clinical features, diagnostics and treatment of canine alopecia X, sex hormone imbalance and canine recurrent flank alopecia.

Skin biopsy

Skin biopsy is indicated in cases where the diagnosis cannot be readily confirmed by any other means. It is useful to confirm or rule out alopecia linked to coat colour, recurrent flank alopecia and follicular dysplasias. As a general rule, multiple biopsy specimens should be collected from alopecic areas.

Skin biopsy is impractical for the diagnosis of endocrine diseases, since these conditions bring about similar changes in the skin and hair follicles, which are hard to differentiate. Nevertheless, skin biopsy is a valuable test, as it can be used to rule out the so-called 'endocrine impersonators'. Occasionally, the histopathological changes observed in skin biopsy specimens are subtle and only experienced dermatopathologists are capable of evaluating them clearly.

Treatment

On the whole, alopecia caused by endocrinopathies are easily treated using a relevant therapy (see relevant chapters in this Manual).

Alopecia in dogs with follicular dysplasia is usually permanent, since no specific therapy is available. Hormonal supplementation without a specific indication should not be prescribed. Trial hormonal therapies in dogs with follicular dysplasia should be avoided. Palliative therapy is normally used in these cases to control secondary bacterial infections, and topical therapy is used to control dryness and scaliness.

Conclusion

The diagnostic approach to alopecia is complex. Symmetrical or generalized alopecia are often signs of hormonal, metabolic congenital/genetic or neoplastic disease. Skin biopsy for histopathology is often needed for definitive diagnosis. Clients should be discouraged from using home remedies and human hair-loss medications, as these are ineffective and can be toxic. For example, the vasodilator medication minoxidil can cause cardiac disease, weakness, lethargy and collapse in dogs. Thyroid supplementation trials should also be avoided unless hypothyroidism is confirmed. Breeding of dogs with genetic causes of alopecia should be avoided.

References and further reading

Cerundolo R, Lloyd DH, Persechino A, Evans H and Cauvin A (2004) Treatment of canine alopecia X with trilostane. *Veterinary Dermatology* **15**, 285–293

Linek M (2009) How to approach alopecic diseases – clinical aspects. In: *Hair Loss Disorders in Domestic Animals*, ed. L Meckelenburg *et al.*, pp. 65–76. Wiley-Blackwell, Ames, Iowa

27

Investigation of adrenal masses

Carlos Melian

Introduction

Dogs and cats with adrenal tumours present in a variety of ways, from those with severe clinical signs to those that are apparently asymptomatic. The tumours may be benign or malignant, functional or non-functional. When functional, either one or several hormones may be secreted. Based on these considerations, the finding of an adrenal mass represents a significant diagnostic and therapeutic challenge.

An adrenal mass can be found in dogs or cats with suspected adrenal disease (hyperadrenocorticism, hyperaldosteronism, phaeochromocytoma). Alternatively, it may be an incidental finding in patients undergoing diagnostic imaging tests for reasons other than adrenal disease, or during necropsy. The increasing expertise and availability of ultrasonography has improved detection of such unsuspected adrenal masses, the so-called 'adrenal incidentalomas'.

Adrenal incidentalomas are common findings in human patients undergoing abdominal ultrasonography and computed tomography (CT) or magnetic resonance imaging (MRI) scans. Prevalence approaches 3% in middle age and increases to as much as 10% in the elderly (Mansmann *et al.,* 2004). Most humans with an adrenal incidentaloma have a benign, non-functional adrenal mass. Adrenocortical carcinoma and hormone hypersecretion are reported in <10% and 20% of affected patients, respectively. After a 30-month follow-up period in 229 human patients with benign non-functional masses, the mass increased significantly in size (>5 mm) in only 7% of these patients. No patients developed malignancy in this period (Bülow *et al.,* 2006).

Canine and feline adrenal tumours may be large or small, primary or metastatic, and benign or malignant. They may appear similar to adrenal cysts, granulomas, nodular hyperplasia or haematomas. Although adrenal incidentalomas have recently been diagnosed with increased frequency in small animals, there are no prospective studies with a large number of cases.

Adrenal-dependent hyperadrenocorticism is the most common consequence of adrenal tumours in dogs and cats. However, other adrenal masses, including aldosteronoma, sex hormone-secreting neoplasms, non-functional adrenal masses or phaeochromocytoma, should also be considered (Figure 27.1).

Adrenal cortex [a]
• Cortisol-secreting tumour (adrenal hyperadrenocorticism)
• Mineralocorticoid-secreting tumour (aldosterone or other mineralocorticoids)
• Sex hormone-secreting tumour
• Non-functional adrenal mass
• Nodular hyperplasia (pituitary-dependent hyperadrenocorticism)

Adrenal medulla
• Phaeochromocytoma
• Ganglioneuroma

Adrenal metastasis
• Carcinomas (mammary gland, pulmonary, prostate, bladder, gastric and pancreatic)
• Lymphoma
• Melanoma
• Haemangiosarcoma

Other adrenal masses
• Myelolipoma
• Granulomatous disease (fungal, feline infectious peritonitis)
• Teratoma
• Cyst
• Haematoma

Extra-adrenal masses
• Extra-adrenal phaeochromocytoma (paraganglioma)
• Masses arising from kidney, pancreas, spleen, lymph nodes and blood vessels

27.1 List of differential diagnoses in a patient with a suspected adrenal mass. [a] Tumours arising from the adrenal cortex may secrete more than one type of hormone (i.e. glucocorticoids and mineralocorticoids, glucocorticoids and sex hormones, or mineralocorticoids and sex hormones).

Diagnostic approach

In clinical practice, it is essential to separate adrenal masses that require intervention (functional or malignant tumours) from those that can safely be left untreated (non-functional and benign incidentalomas). It is important first to ensure that an adrenal mass truly exists. Ultrasonography is the most commonly used tool for visualizing adrenal lesions and for differentiating adrenal hyperplasia from neoplasia. Normal adrenal glands are hypoechoic, flattened, peanut-shaped organs located craniomedial to the kidneys. Maximum thickness on ultrasound evaluation is generally <7.5 mm in healthy dogs and <5.5 mm in healthy cats (Grooters *et al.*, 1996; Zatelli *et al.*, 2007). In dogs and cats with bilateral hyperplasia (e.g. patients with pituitary-dependent hyperadrenocorticism) the adrenal glands appear mildly to moderately enlarged and their shape is maintained. An adrenal mass is suspected if there is significant enlargement (width >15 mm) and a change of shape to a rounded or irregularly rounded mass (Figure 27.2). Adrenal masses may invade or compress adjacent structures. Their echogenicity is variable, ranging from a solid to a mixed-cystic appearance. The adrenal mass should be a reliably repeatable finding on abdominal ultrasonography.

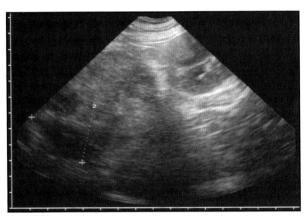

27.2 Left adrenal mass (72 x 74 mm) found incidentally on ultrasound evaluation of a 9-year-old female Siberian Husky.

Once an adrenal mass has been found, ultrasonographic evaluation of the contralateral adrenal gland is important. In dogs with adrenal-dependent hyperadrenocorticism, the adrenal mass may produce excessive amounts of cortisol that is capable of chronically suppressing adrenocorticotropic hormone (ACTH) release, leading to atrophy of the contralateral adrenal gland. In these patients, the contralateral adrenal gland is expected to be thin and more difficult to identify. However, in some dogs with a functional adrenocortical tumour, significant atrophy of the contralateral adrenal gland is not detected. In this instance, the size of the contralateral adrenal gland may be within reference limits (Hoerauf and Reusch, 1999; Gould *et al.*, 2001).

Adrenal ultrasonography has limitations. For example, it may be difficult, if not impossible, to differentiate a cortisol-producing adrenal tumour from other adrenal tumours, such as phaeochromocytoma, aldosteronoma, metastatic or non-functional tumours. In dogs with confirmed hyperadrenocorticism, ultrasonography is helpful in differentiating adrenal (usually unilateral adrenal mass) from pituitary-dependent disease (generally bilaterally symmetric hyperplasia), but in a few cases dogs with pituitary-dependent hyperadrenocorticism present with bilateral nodular hyperplasia that can be difficult to differentiate from bilateral adrenal tumours.

Other imaging studies, including CT and MRI, may be helpful in determining the extent of disease. CT is effective in lesion location and in assessment for local invasion and metastases. MRI is considered highly sensitive for the detection of phaeochromocytoma in humans (Gilson *et al.*, 1994; McNiel and Husbands, 2005) but it has not yet been well evaluated in dogs.

Once an adrenal mass has been confirmed, the diagnostic and therapeutic approach is based on clinical presentation (age, clinical signs, laboratory findings, blood pressure measurement) and the characteristics of the adrenal mass (size, likelihood of hormonal activity, presence of metastasis and invasion of other structures). A detailed history and physical examination is of immense value in determining the diagnostic plan, as some clinical signs may have gone largely unnoticed or their significance may have been misinterpreted (Figure 27.3).

Measurement of blood pressure is important for the diagnostic investigation and treatment plan. Demonstrating increased blood pressure increases the likelihood of a functional adrenal mass, as hyperadrenocorticism, hyperaldosteronism and phaeochromocytoma are all known to cause hypertension.

Condition	History	Physical examination	Expected results in diagnostic tests
Adrenal-dependent hyperadrenocorticism	Polyuria/polydipsia, polyphagia, panting, lethargy, weakness, abdominal distension	Hepatomegaly, alopecia	Hypertension. Increased ALP, ALT and cholesterol. No suppression on low- or high-dose dexamethasone suppression tests. ACTH stimulation test high only in 50% patients. Serum concentration of sex hormones or mineralocorticoids may also be elevated
Aldosteronoma	Polymyopathy (cervical ventroflexion (cats), weakness and pain), polyuria/polydipsia	Extreme weakness	Hypertension. Hypokalaemia. High plasma aldosterone concentration
Sex hormone excess	Asymptomatic or clinical signs similar to those of hyperadrenocorticism, or behavioural signs (i.e. aggression)	Asymptomatic or clinical signs similar to those of hyperadrenocorticism	Normal results on low-dose dexamethasone suppression tests. Normal or subnormal ACTH test results. Elevated pre- and/or post-ACTH concentrations of sex hormones
Phaeochromocytoma	Asymptomatic or lethargy, weight loss, panting, anorexia or polyuria/polydipsia	Tachypnoea, tachycardia	Hypertension. High concentrations of urine catecholamines and their metabolites

27.3 Classical clinical presentation and expected results of diagnostic tests in dogs and cats with an adrenal mass.

Adrenal-dependent hyperadrenocorticism

A cortisol-producing adrenal mass causing clinical signs of hyperadrenocorticism is the most common adrenal neoplasm in dogs and cats. If a patient with an adrenal mass is showing appropriate clinical signs (see Figure 27.3), adrenal function tests should be performed to confirm or rule out hyperadrenocorticism. The ACTH response test is commonly used to diagnose hyperadrenocorticism in dogs. However, the sensitivity of this test is much lower in dogs with adrenal-dependent hyperadrenocorticism (approximately 50%) compared to dogs with pituitary-dependent hyperadrenocorticism (approximately 85%). In a dog with clinical signs of hyperadrenocorticism and a confirmed adrenal mass, a reference interval ACTH response test result does not rule out a cortisol-producing adrenal tumour.

Dogs and cats with adrenal-dependent hyperadrenocorticism have high circulating cortisol concentrations secreted autonomously by the adrenal mass. This leads to chronic suppression of ACTH release. As ACTH concentration is therefore already suppressed, the use of other ACTH suppressants (such us dexamethasone at low or high doses) has minimal effect on ACTH and cortisol concentrations. Such a lack of suppression supports a diagnosis of hyperadrenocorticism. In dogs with adrenal-dependent hyperadrenocorticism, the sensitivity of the low-dose dexamethasone suppression (LDDS) test for the diagnosis of hyperadrenocorticism is high, at virtually 100% (Hoerauf and Reusch, 1999); however, this should be interpreted carefully as test specificity is low, and results consistent with hyperadrenocorticism can occur in dogs with other diseases, inclu ding phaeochromocytoma (Melian and Peterson, 2000; Kook et al., 2007). The clinical, diagnostic and therapeutic aspects of adrenal-dependent hyperadrenocorticism are further discussed in Chapters 16 and 17.

Although most cases of adrenal-dependent hyperadrenocorticism are caused by a unilateral adrenal mass, bilateral adrenocortical neoplasia is not uncommon, occurring in up to 20% of cases. Phaeochromocytoma may also occur concurrently in dogs with a cortisol-producing adrenocortical mass.

Hyperaldosteronism

Hyperaldosteronism should be suspected in any dog or cat with weakness, hypokalaemia and hypertension of unknown origin. Hyperaldosteronism is considered uncommon in dogs but appears to be more common in cats. Generally, primary hyperaldosteronism is caused by high circulating aldosterone concentrations produced by a functional tumour, arising from the outer layer of the adrenal cortex (zona glomerulosa). Such tumours are also called aldosteronomas and their presence is the defining symptom of the disorder Conn's syndrome (Ash et al., 2005).

Idiopathic primary hyperaldosteronism has also been described in humans and in cats. In these patients, primary hyperaldosteronism is confirmed by demonstration of increased plasma concentrations of aldosterone and low plasma renin activity, but in the absence of an adrenal tumour (Javadi et al., 2005). Diagnostic imaging reveals no, or only minimal, changes in the adrenal glands compatible with nodular hyperplasia. Adrenal gland histopathology in cats with idiopathic primary hyperaldosteronism demonstrates extensive micronodular hyperplasia extending from the zona glomerulosa into the zona fasciculata and zona reticularis.

Cats with an adrenocortical tumour causing hyperaldosteronism can present with concurrent hyperprogesteronism. In addition to the clinical signs of hyperaldosteronism, these patients may present with a pot-bellied appearance, muscle wasting, marked thinning and fragility of the skin and/or bilaterally symmetrical alopecia (Briscoe et al., 2009).

Although most cases of recognized mineralocorticoid excess are caused by an adrenal tumour that secretes aldosterone, its effects can also be mimicked by high concentrations of an aldosterone precursor, such us deoxycorticosterone (Reine et al., 1999). Plasma deoxycorticosterone concentration should be evaluated in dogs or cats with a suspected aldosteronoma that have reference interval or low plasma aldosterone concentrations. The diagnosis and management of feline hyperaldosteronism is described in Chapter 19.

Sex hormone-secreting adrenal neoplasia

Adrenocortical tumours can potentially produce and secrete excessive amounts of several sex hormones, including progestogens, oestrogens and androgens. In humans, adrenal carcinomas are usually inefficient in conversion of cholesterol to cortisol. This might result from aberrant biosynthetic pathways or enzyme deficiencies, and can give rise to high circulating concentrations of hormone precursors. By contrast, adrenal adenomas exhibit more efficient steroidogenesis, and production of precursors may be low or normal in relation to cortisol production. Similarly, in dogs and cats, when the main secretory product is a steroid other than cortisol then the adrenal tumour is usually a carcinoma.

Dogs and cats with adrenocortical carcinomas and clinical signs consistent with hyperadrenocorticism may have reference interval ACTH response and LDDS test results. In such cases, the clinical signs may be related to sex hormones rather than to hypercortisolaemia. Hormone concentrations that may be increased in different combinations include 17α-hydroxyprogesterone, progesterone, oestradiol, testosterone and androstenedione. Evaluation of pre- and post-ACTH concentration of these hormones is recommended in dogs and cats with obvious clinical signs of hyperadrenocorticism but without the expected abnormalities on ACTH response and LDDS testing.

Progesterone has direct glucocorticoid effects, and high concentrations of progesterone may also result in clinical signs of hypercortisolaemia by displacing cortisol from cortisol-binding proteins (Syme *et al.,* 2001). This results in high concentrations of free cortisol, even if total serum cortisol concentration is decreased. As the unbound cortisol is the active portion, it is able to exert its effects on a variety of tissues and clinical signs of cortisol excess may develop.

Clinical signs

Clinical signs described in cats with unilateral or bilateral carcinoma producing high concentrations of progesterone include polyuria, polydipsia, polyphagia, abdominal distension and alopecia. Hyperglycaemia and glucosuria can also occur (Boord and Griffin, 1999; Quante *et al.,* 2009). A similar presentation has been described in dogs. Two dogs with clinical signs consistent with hyperadrenocorticism (polyuria, polydipsia, polyphagia) showed a subnormal ACTH test result and low concentrations of endogenous ACTH. Several sex hormones, including progesterone and 17α-hydroxyprogesterone, were elevated before and after ACTH administration, and the clinical signs were attributed, at least in part, to high concentration of these hormones (Syme *et al.,* 2001). Pre- and/or post-ACTH concentration of sex hormones, including progesterone, 17α-hydroxyprogesterone and dihydroepiadrostenedione, are also commonly increased in dogs with pituitary-dependent hyperadrenocorticism; therefore hyperadrenocorticism should always be ruled out before testing for sex hormone excess (Frank *et al.,* 2001).

Patients with an excess of sex hormones from an adrenal neoplasia may present differently. Spraying urine and behavioural changes including aggressiveness can be the presenting complaints of cats with high concentrations of androgens. One castrated cat presented with these signs and on physical examination spines were detected on the penis, despite being castrated. Abdominal ultrasonography revealed a mass in the region of the right adrenal gland, and the results of adrenal hormonal analyses demonstrate considerable increases in serum concentrations of androstenedione and testosterone (Millard *et al.,* 2009).

Phaeochromocytoma

A phaeochromocytoma is a catecholamine-producing tumour of chromaffin cells of the adrenal medulla or sympathetic paraganglia (Barthez *et al.,* 1997). It is an uncommon ante-mortem diagnosis in dogs and is rare in cats. These tumours are considered APUDomas, since they comprise cells characterized by amine precursor uptake and decarboxylation (APUD). The term APUD describes the common biochemical feature of the cells, which involves the synthesis and secretion of biologically active amines.

Phaeochromocytomas are generally unilateral, although they can involve both adrenal glands. In humans, several multiple endocrine neoplasia (MEN) syndromes are well described, and characterized by hypersecretion of more than one endocrine organ. MEN type 2 syndrome consists of

medullary thyroid carcinoma, phaeochromocytoma, and primary hyperparathyroidism (Raue and Frank-Raue, 2007). Dogs with phaeochromocytoma may also present with another endocrine disorder, particularly adrenocortical or corticotropic tumours (von Dehn *et al.,* 1995). Whether these truly represent MEN-type syndromes is unclear.

Phaeochromocytomas are benign or malignant. These tumours commonly compress or invade the vena cava and phrenicoabdominal vein, although they can also involve the aorta, renal vessels, adrenal vessels, hepatic veins or the kidneys. Metastasis to lung, regional lymph nodes, spleen, liver, heart, bone, pancreas and central nervous system can occur.

Clinical signs

Dogs with phaeochromocytoma have a median age at presentation of 11 years. There is no apparent sex predisposition. Any breed can be affected, although certain breeds are at increased risk (McNiel and Husbands, 2005). Approximately half of dogs with phaeochromocytoma remain apparently asymptomatic; in these patients, the diagnosis occurs incidentally when they are evaluated for other problems or at necropsy (Figure 27.4). Clinical manifestations may develop as a result of an excessive secretion of catecholamine and its effect on blood pressure and cardiac function or, less commonly, as a result of the space-occupying nature of the tumour and its metastasis (Gilson *et al.,* 1994; Barthez *et al.,* 1997).

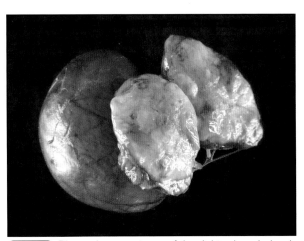

27.4 Phaeochromocytoma of the right adrenal gland found unexpectedly on necropsy of a 16-year-old female Yorkshire Terrier. The cause of death was attributed to advanced congestive heart failure. (Courtesy of the Pathology Department, Veterinary Faculty, University of Las Palmas de Gran Canaria)

Catecholamine secretion in patients with phaeochromocytoma is sporadic and unpredictable. Clinical signs suggestive of catecholamine excess include weakness, episodic collapse, tachypnoea and polyuria/polydipsia (Figure 27.5). The finding of systemic hypertension is variable (25–86%) and non-pathognomonic. Severe hypertension may cause nasal, gingival or ocular haemorrhage. Tachycardia is common amongst dogs with phaeochromocytoma, but as it is frequently cyclic it may

Clinical signs	Number of dogs	Percentage among symptomatic dogs (%)
Asymptomatic	59	
Symptomatic	52	
History		
Weakness/lethargy	26	50
Weight loss	16	31
Anorexia/decreased appetite	13	25
Polyuria/polydipsia	10	19
Collapse	10	19
Vomiting	5	10
Cough	5	10
Convulsive episodes	4	8
Paraparesis	2	4
Physical examination		
Tachypnoea	13	25
Tachyarrhythmia	9	17
Dyspnoea	6	12
Pale mucous membranes	6	12
Abdominal distension	6	12
Palpable abdominal mass	2	4
Fever	2	4

27.5 Clinical signs in 111 dogs with phaeochromocytoma. (Data adapted from Barthez *et al.*, 1997 and Gibson *et al.*, 1994)

not be detected on clinical evaluation and the diagnosis of phaeochromocytoma cannot be ruled out based on its absence. In addition, dogs with phaeochromocytoma may present with collapsing episodes, due to a bradyarrhythmia associated with brief periods of high-grade second-degree AV block. The cause of the AV block might be attributed to a high vagal tone occurring as a reflex response to systemic hypertension (Brown *et al.*, 2007).

The size of the mass may correlate with the presence or absence, and the severity, of clinical signs. Large masses that compress or invade surrounding structures commonly cause clinical signs, increasing the likelihood of ante-mortem diagnosis. The growth of these tumours is unpredictable and can be very rapid. In approximately one-third of dogs with phaeochromocytoma, a thrombus can be detected within the caudal vena cava. Local invasion can also involve the renal vein and the kidney. Non-traumatic rupture can occur in dogs, resulting in life-threatening blood loss into the peritoneal cavity or retroperitoneal space (Whittemore *et al.*, 2001).

Diagnosis

The findings of complete blood count, biochemical profiles and urinalysis in dogs and cats with phaeochromocytoma are non-specific. However, these routine tests are necessary to rule out other diseases. Anaemia is relatively common in dogs with phaeochromocytoma, occurring in 15–60% of these patients. Anaemia could result from chronic illness or from haemorrhage. Catecholamines cause neutrophil demargination, which could explain the leucocytosis found in 25–40% of dogs. Leucocytosis could also be connected to tumour-related necrosis or inflammation, or to concurrent diseases.

Plasma or urine catecholamine concentration can be useful for confirming the diagnosis in dogs and cats with suspected phaeochromocytoma. These determinations, however, have been infrequently performed in suspected phaeochromocytoma cases because of limited availability of techniques, problems in obtaining a reliable sample (24-hour urine sample), expense or a lack of established reference intervals for dogs and cats. Plasma catecholamine measurements are rarely used, mainly because of their limited availability and efficacy. The mean half-life of these hormones is short, leading to significant fluctuation in plasma concentration. Plasma catecholamines may be normal in patients with phaeochromocytoma and can be high in sick or stressed patients without phaeochromocytoma.

The concentrations of urine catecholamine and its metabolites (metanephrine, normetanephrine and vanillylmandelic acid) exhibit a lesser degree of fluctuation and constitute the traditional approach to the biochemical diagnosis of phaeochromocytoma in human medicine. Collecting a 24-hour urine sample minimizes the influence of stress.

Urine catecholamine- and metanephrine-to-creatinine ratios have been evaluated in healthy dogs and dogs with phaeochromocytoma using a single morning urine sample. Stress associated with a hospital visit may increase urinary catecholamine and metanephrine excretion in healthy dogs. For this reason, the urine sample should ideally be collected at home or after an adaptation to the sampling process (Kook *et al.*, 2007). A recent study has shown that urine normetanephrine:creatinine ratio may be useful in the diagnosis of canine phaeochromocytoma, even when samples are collected during initial evaluation and when differentiating phaeochromocytoma from hyperadrenocorticism (Kook *et al.*, 2010; Quante *et al.*, 2010).

Scintigraphy has been used to identify phaeochromocytomas in dogs and might be useful to evaluate tumour extension and metastasis. Meta-iodobenzylguanidine (MIBG) is a guanethidine-derived analogue that shares the same cellular uptake mechanism as noradrenaline at the sympathetic nerve terminal (Berry *et al.*, 2002). In most dogs with phaeochromocytoma, however, the diagnosis currently relies on histopathology following surgical adrenalectomy or a biopsy procedure.

Non-functional adrenal mass

Adrenal tumours can produce normal or excessive amounts of one or several hormones or hormone precursors, but equally may be hormonally inactive. It is difficult to confirm a non-functional adrenal mass because of the problems in completely evaluating and precluding all other possible functional tumours.

A non-functional adrenal mass should be suspected in those dogs and cats that remain apparently asymptomatic, normotensive and maintain reference interval routine clinicopathological laboratory results. In addition, patients with non-functional masses should have normal pituitary–adrenal function when evaluated for hyperadrenocorticism, hyperaldosteronism and sex hormone hypersecretion.

In patients with a small adrenal mass that is likely non-functional, a conservative approach is recommended. In these asymptomatic animals, tumour growth should be assessed by repeating an ultrasound study after 4–6 weeks. If the mass has changed little in appearance at that time, the patient should be rechecked in another 3 months. If the adrenal mass does not change in size, the time between ultrasound evaluations can be increased to every 4–6 months. However, if the adrenal mass is increasing in size, adrenalectomy should be considered.

References and further reading

Ash RA, Harvey AM and Tasker S (2005) Primary hyperaldosteronism in the cat: a series of 13 cases. *Journal of Feline Medicine and Surgery* **7**, 173–182

Barthez PY, Marks SL, Woo J, Feldman EC and Matteucci M (1997) Pheochromocytoma in dogs: 61 cases (1984–1995) *Journal of Veterinary Internal Medicine* **11**, 272–278

Berry CR, DeGrado TR, Nutter F *et al.* (2002) Imaging of pheochromocytoma in 2 dogs using p-[18F] fluorobenzylguanidine. *Veterinary Radiology and Ultrasound* **43**, 183–186

Boord M and Griffin C (1999) Progesterone-secreting adrenal mass in a cat with clinical signs of hyperadrenocorticism. *Journal of the American Veterinary Medical Association* **214**, 666–669

Briscoe K, Barrs VR, Foster DF and Beatty JA (2009) Hyperaldosteronism and hyperprogesteronism in a cat. *Journal of Feline Medicine and Surgery* **11**, 758–762

Brown AJ, Alwood AJ and Cole SG (2007) Malignant pheochromocytoma presenting as a bradyarrhythmia in a dog. *Journal of Veterinary Emergency and Critical Care* **17**, 164–169

Bülow B, Jansson S, Juhlin C *et al.* (2006) Adrenal incidentaloma – follow-up results from a Swedish prospective study. *European Journal of Endocrinology* **154**, 419–423

Frank LA, Schmeitzel LP and Oliver JW (2001) Steroidogenic response of adrenal tissues after administration of ACTH to dogs with hypercortisolemia. *Journal of the American Veterinary Medical Association* **218**, 214–216

Gilson SD, Withrow SJ, Wheeler SL and Twedt DC (1994) Pheochromocytoma in 50 dogs. *Journal of Veterinary Internal Medicine*, **8**, 228–232

Gould SM, Baines EA, Mannion PA, Evans H and Herrtage ME (2001). Use of endogenous ACTH concentration and adrenal ultrasonography to distinguish the cause of canine hyperadrenocorticism. *Journal of Small Animal Practice* **42**, 113–121

Grooters AM, Biller DS, Theisen SK and Miyabayashi T (1996) Ultrasonographic characteristics of the adrenal glands in dogs with pituitary dependent hyperadrenocorticism: comparison with normal dogs. *Journal of Veterinary Internal Medicine* **10**, 110–115

Hoerauf A and Reusch C (1999) Ultrasonographic characteristics of both adrenal glands in 15 dogs with functional adrenocortical tumors. *Journal of the American Animal Hospital Association* **35**, 193–199

Javadi S, Kooistra HS, Mol JA *et al.* (2003) Plasma aldosterone concentrations and plasma renin activity in healthy dogs and dogs with hyperadrenocorticism. *Veterinary Record* **153**, 521–525

Javadi S, Djajadiningrat-Laanen SC, Kooistra HS *et al.* (2005) Primary hyperaldosteronism, a mediator of progressive renal disease in cats. *Domestic Animal Endocrinology* **28**, 85–104

Kook PH, Boretti FS, Hersberger M, Glaus TM and Reusch CE (2007) Urinary catecholamine and metanephrine to creatinine ratios in healthy dogs at home and in a hospital environment and in 2 dogs with pheochromocytoma. *Journal of Veterinary Internal Medicine* **21**, 388–393

Kook PH, Grest P, Quante S, Boretti FS and Reusch CE (2010) Urinary catecholamine and metadrenaline to creatinine ratios in dogs with a phaeochromocytoma. *Veterinary Record* **166**,169–174

Mansmann G, Lau J, Balk E *et al.* (2004) The clinically inapparent adrenal mass: update in diagnosis and management. *Endocrine Reviews* **25**, 309–340

McNiel E and Husbands BD (2005) Pheochromocytoma. In: *Textbook of Veterinary Internal Medicine, 6th edn,* ed. SJ Ettinger and EC Feldman, pp. 1632–1638. Elsevier Saunders, Missouri

Melian C and Peterson ME (2000) Management of incidentally discovered adrenal masses. In: *Kirk's Current Veterinary Therapy. XIII. Small Animal Practice,* ed. JD Bonagura, pp. 368–372. WB Saunders, Philadelphia

Millard RP, Pickens EH and Wells KL (2009) Excessive production of sex hormones in a cat with an adrenocortical tumor. *Journal of the American Veterinary Medical Association* **234**, 505–508

Peterson ME, Randolph JF, Zaki FA and Heath H III (1982) Multiple endocrine neoplasia in a dog. *Journal of the American Veterinary Medical Association* **180**, 1476–1478

Quante S, Boretti FS, Kook PH *et al.* (2010) Urinary catecholamine and metanephrine to creatinine ratios in dogs with hyperadrenocorticism or pheochromocytoma, and in healthy dogs. *Journal of Veterinary Internal Medicine* **24**, 1093–1097

Quante S, Sieber-Ruckstuhl N, Wilhelm S *et al.* (2009) Hyperprogesteronism due to bilateral adrenal carcinomas in a cat with diabetes mellitus. *Schweizer Archiv für Tierheilkunde* **151**, 437–442

Raue F and Frank-Raue K (2007) Multiple endocrine neoplasia type 2: 2007 update. *Hormone Research.* **68**, 101–104

Reine NJ, Hohenhaus AE, Peterson ME and Patnaik AK (1999) Deoxycorticosterone-secreting adrenocortical carcinoma in a dog. *Journal of Veterinary Internal Medicine* **13**, 386–390

Syme HM, Scott-Moncrieff C, Treadwell NC *et al.* (2001) Hyperadrenocorticism associated with excessive sex hormone production by an adrenocortical tumor in two dogs. *Journal of the American Veterinary Medical Association* **219**, 1725–1728

von Dehn BJ, Nelson RW, Feldman EC and Griffey SM (1995) Pheochromocytoma and hyperadrenocorticism in dogs: six cases (1982–1992). *Journal of the American Veterinary Medical Association* **207**, 322–324

Whittemore JC, Preston CA, Kyles AE, Hardie EM and Feldman EC (2001) Nontraumatic rupture of an adrenal gland tumor causing intra-abdominal or retroperitoneal hemorrhage in four dogs. *Journal of the American Veterinary Medical Association* **219**, 329–333

Zatelli A, D'Ippolito P, Fiore I and Zini E (2007) Ultrasonographic evaluation of the size of the adrenal glands of 24 diseased cats without endocrinopathies. *Veterinary Record* **160**, 658–660

28

Investigation of hyperlipidaemia

Steve Dodkin and Kostas Papasouliotis

Introduction

Hyperlipidaemia (hyperlipaemia) is the term used to describe an increased concentration of lipids in the blood. These lipids include: free cholesterol; cholesterol esters; phospholipids; triacylglycerols (traditionally known as triglycerides); and free fatty acids. All except free fatty acids exhibit low solubility in water and are consequently transported in the plasma in association with a specific group of proteins, the apolipoproteins (Figure 28.1). The resultant large lipid–protein particles are called lipoproteins. These are composed of a hydrophobic core of triacylglycerols and cholesterol esters, with a relatively hydrophilic surface of protein, phospholipids and free cholesterol. Free fatty acids are predominantly transported bound to albumin.

Hyperlipoproteinaemia refers to the increased plasma concentration of lipoproteins and should be used only in cases where the concentrations of the actual lipoproteins have been measured. In spite of this, the term hyperlipoproteinaemia is often used interchangeably with hyperlipidaemia.

Lipaemia is a term that refers to the turbid or lactescent appearance of serum or plasma due to increased concentration of triacylglycerols (>2 mmol/l) but not cholesterol. It is worth noting that lipaemia can falsely increase or decrease the results of several other biochemical tests depending on the methodology and analyser used (Duncan, 2005).

Lipoprotein metabolism

The lipoproteins form a heterogeneous group of particles in terms of their size, composition and physical characteristics. As a consequence, the grouping of lipoproteins into distinct classes is inevitably an arbitrary process. For the purpose of this brief overview, lipoproteins have been separated into triacylglycerol-rich lipoproteins (TRLs) and cholesterol-rich high-density lipoproteins (HDLs). The traditionally and frequently used terms very low density lipoproteins (VLDLs) and low density lipoprotein (LDLs) will be avoided, as their relevance and accuracy are questionable in species other than humans. Where possible, the pathways outlined below and in Figure 28.2 are based on published data from studies conducted in the dog and cat. However, where specific information is lacking, research conducted in other species has been used.

Component	Function
Endogenous triacylglycerol-rich lipoprotein (TRL)	Synthesized by the liver; transports free fatty acids to the peripheral tissues; in humans, termed low and very low density lipoprotein (LDL and VLDL)
Chylomicrons	Exogenous TRL; synthesized by the enterocytes; transport dietary lipid (primarily triacylglycerol) from the small intestine to peripheral tissues and liver
Apolipoprotein B (ApoB)	Major structural component of TRL
Lipoprotein lipase (LPL)	Hydrolyses triacylglycerols resulting in the formation of remnants
Apolipoprotein C-II (apoC-II)	Activates LPL
Apolipoprotein A-V (apoA-V)	Brings TRL close to LPL at the endothelial surface
Remnant	A smaller triacylglycerol-depleted TRL particle which is removed by the liver
High density lipoproteins (HDL)	Cholesterol rich lipoproteins; transport excess cholesterol from peripheral cells to the liver
Apolipoprotein A-I (apoA-I)	Major component of HDL; activates lecithin-cholesterol acyltransferase (LCAT)
Lecithin-cholesterol acyltransferase (LCAT)	Causes esterification of free cholesterol in HDL, allowing free cholesterol from tissues to be incorporated into HDL
Apolipoprotein E (apoE)	Binds to hepatic receptors facilitating the removal of TRL and HDL from the circulation

28.1 The function of lipoproteins, apolipoproteins and enzymes in lipid metabolism.

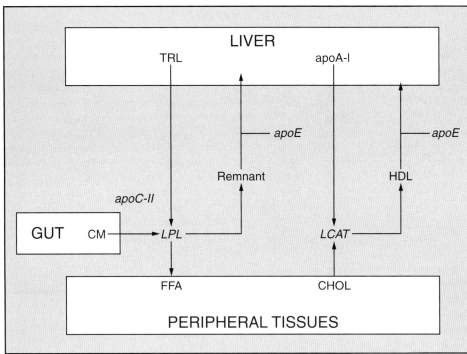

28.2 A schematic representation of lipid metabolism. CHOL = cholesterol; CM = chylomicron; FFA = free fatty acids; HDL = high density lipoprotein; LCAT= lecithin-cholesterol acyltransferase. LPL = lipoprotein lipase; TRL = triacylglycerol-rich lipoprotein.

Triacylglycerol-rich lipoproteins

The principal function of TRLs is to transport free fatty acids to the peripheral tissues, where they serve as an important source of energy. The TRLs are the largest of the lipoproteins and are characterized by the presence of a single molecule of apolipoprotein B (apoB), which has both structural and receptor recognition functions. The TRLs can be divided into those containing lipid of exogenous origin (chylomicrons), synthesized by the enterocyte, and those that contain endogenously produced lipid emanating from the liver (termed, respectively, LDL and VLDL in humans, as outlined above).

Both exogenously derived and endogenously derived TRLs appear to be metabolized through broadly similar pathways, although the rates at which they are metabolized differ. Upon entering the circulation, the TRL particle is rapidly metabolized by the endothelial-associated enzyme lipoprotein lipase (LPL), which catalyses the hydrolysis of triacylglycerols in the core of the lipoprotein particle. The TRL-associated protein apolipoprotein C-II (apoC-II) has long been recognized as an essential cofactor of LPL, but more recently it has become apparent that other proteins also play important roles in the lipolytic process. A crucial role in the process has been demonstrated for apolipoprotein A-V (apoA-V), which appears to function by bringing the TRL particle into close proximity with LPL at the endothelial surface. The action of LPL on TRL results in the formation of a smaller triacylglycerol-depleted remnant particle.

In humans, the TRL remnants of hepatic origin (VLDL remnants) can undergo further processing to give rise to LDL. This transformation involves the transfer of cholesterol esters from HDL to the TRL remnant, a reaction catalysed by cholesterol ester transfer protein (CETP). Only negligible CETP activity is found in canine or feline plasma, and consequently the transformation of remnant particles into LDL is unlikely to be a physiologically significant process in either species. TRL remnant particles are removed by the liver through an apolipoprotein E (apoE)-dependent receptor-mediated process. The identity of the receptor(s) responsible for remnant removal has not been conclusively established in dogs or cats, but the LDL receptor and/or the LDL receptor-related protein 1 (LRP1) are most likely involved.

Cholesterol-rich high density lipoproteins

The particles constituting the HDL fraction are smaller and have a higher protein content than TRL. The major function of HDL is reverse cholesterol transport, in which excess cholesterol is removed from peripheral cells and shuttled to the liver where it is stored, re-exported in newly synthesized TRL particles or secreted into the bile. Other roles that have been ascribed to HDL include involvement in the innate immune response, transport of fat-soluble vitamins, delivery of cholesterol to organs for hormone production, and thyroxine transport in the dog.

The genesis of HDL occurs with the release of apolipoprotein A-I (apoA-I) from the liver (and to a lesser extent from the intestine). ApoA-I acquires free cholesterol from peripheral tissues, through an interaction with the membrane protein ATP-binding cassette A1 (ABCA1), giving rise to discoidal nascent HDL. The free cholesterol in this discoidal particle is then esterified by the enzyme lecithin-cholesterol acyltransferase (LCAT) to produce small spherical HDL, referred to as HDL_2 in the dog. These particles gradually increase in size by acquiring more cholesterol from the periphery, giving rise to large cholesterol-enriched particles referred to as HDL_1 or HDL_c.

HDL particles can be metabolized by the liver through two distinct mechanisms: selective cholesterol uptake, in which cholesterol from the lipoprotein core is transferred to the liver; or complete uptake, in which the whole particle is taken up by endocytosis. It is unclear as yet which of these pathways is predominant in dogs and cats, and whether the relative importance of the two varies in different pathological or physiological states.

Measurement of lipids and lipoproteins

Lipid assays
Measurement of plasma triacylglycerol and total cholesterol concentrations can be performed routinely by enzymatic colorimetric methods, using in-practice or high-volume commercial biochemistry analysers. Hypercholesterolaemia can be associated with an increase in HDL and/or TRL concentrations. Hypertriacylglycerolaemia is mainly associated with an increased concentration of chylomicrons and/or endogenously produced TRLs. Enzymatic colorimetric assays for phospholipids and free cholesterol are also commercially available, but are only offered by a few specialist laboratories.

Chylomicron refrigeration test
The presence of chylomicrons can be identified by leaving a small tube of plasma in the refrigerator (at 4°C) overnight. Due to their low density, chylomicrons will rise to the surface, forming a 'creamy' layer, whilst the presence of other TRLs will result in a uniformly turbid sample (Figure 28.3). However, this test has a poor sensitivity for detecting chylomicrons when compared to ultracentrifugation or lipoprotein electrophoresis.

Ultracentrifugation
Ultracentrifugation is generally considered the method of choice for lipoprotein analysis in human medicine, but is unsuitable for use in species such as the dog, due to comparative differences in the physicochemical properties of the respective lipoprotein particles. In the dog there is a large overlap in the hydrated densities of the TRL and HDL fractions, making it impossible to achieve an adequate separation of the two. Techniques have been developed to overcome this by subjecting ultracentrifugation fractions to a further purification step, using methodologies such as preparative electrophoresis or polyanion precipitation. However, these methodologies are expensive, technically demanding and time-consuming, and are therefore only available in specialist laboratories.

Electrophoresis
Lipoprotein electrophoresis exploits differences in the size and charge of different lipoprotein particles and can typically resolve lipoproteins into up to four fractions (Figure 28.4). The lipoproteins are visualized using specific lipid stains, such as Sudan black B or oil red O. Due to slight differences in the staining characteristics of the major fractions, this technique is not strictly quantitative, but it provides adequate results for establishing lipoprotein phenotypes. This technique is cheaper and more straightforward to perform than ultracentrifugation techniques, and so is generally more readily available.

Polyanion precipitation
Polyanions, such as sodium phosphotungstate and dextran sulphate, used in association with a divalent cation such as magnesium chloride, can cause the precipitation of lipoproteins under low-speed

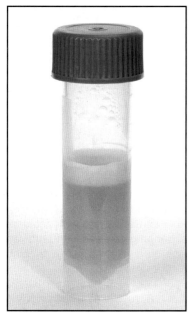

28.3 Canine plasma sample after 12 hours' refrigeration. A 'creamy' layer of chylomicrons has risen to the top. The underlying plasma has a lactescent appearance, indicating the presence of endogenous triacylglycerols.

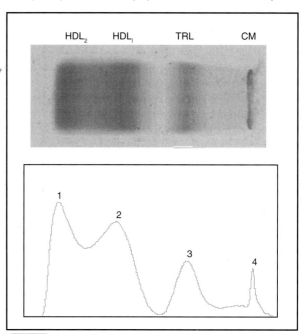

28.4 Lipoprotein electrophoresis of canine plasma. 1, 2, 3, 4 = fractions; HDL = high-density lipoprotein; TRL = triacylglycerol-rich lipoprotein fraction. CM = chylomicrons.

centrifugation. There is a strict relationship between the lipid-to-protein ratio of a lipoprotein particle and the concentration of the precipitant required to affect the precipitation. By careful alteration of the polyanion concentration, it is therefore possible to precipitate discrete lipoprotein fractions selectively. Polyanion precipitation is a quantitative technique that can achieve similar resolution to lipoprotein electrophoresis. However, separation of lipoprotein classes can be problematical when the polyanion technique is applied to samples containing lipoproteins of particularly abnormal composition.

Other tests

Measurements of LPL and LCAT activities can be performed by specialist lipid research laboratories.

Causes of hyperlipidaemia

The three main types of hyperlipidaemia (Figure 28.5) are:

- Physiological (postprandial)
- Secondary to an underlying disease or drug administration
- Primary (familial).

A good history and physical examination, routine clinicopathological data, endocrine testing and imaging modalities are essential in the investigation of hyperlipidaemia.

Physiological (postprandial)

Physiological hyperlipidaemia is caused by the accumulation of chylomicrons in the serum or plasma. In clinically healthy dogs and cats, hyperlipidaemia peaks 6 hours after a meal and is cleared within 12 hours at the latest. Even after consumption of a high-fat meal, blood triacylglycerol concentrations are not expected to exceed 6 mmol/l.

Secondary hyperlipidaemia

In the majority of canine and feline cases, hyperlipidaemia is found to be secondary to an underlying disease. Lipoprotein metabolism is under complex hormonal control and for this reason the most commonly diagnosed diseases are endocrinopathies, in particular hypothyroidism (Dixon *et al.*, 1999; Prieur *et al.*, 2005; Fugier *et al.*, 2006), hyperadrenocorticism (Huang *et al.*, 1999) and diabetes mellitus (Wilson *et al.*, 1986). Although the precise mechanisms involved are still being actively researched, decreased enzyme activity and

Cause	Biochemical abnormalities				
	Cholesterol	**Triacylglycerol**	**Chylomicrons**	**Triacylglycerol-rich lipoproteins**	**High-density lipoproteins**
Physiological	N	↑	↑	N	N
Primary (idiopathic defects)					
Miniature Schnauzer	N or ↑	↑↑	↑	↑	N
Brittany Spaniel	N	↑↑	↑	↑	N
Briard	↑	N	–	N	↑
Dobermann, Rottweiler	↑	N	–	–	–
Rough Collie	↑	N	–	↑	↑
Shetland Sheepdog	↑	N or ↑	–	↑	↑
Beagle	↑	↑	–	↑	↑
Lipoprotein lipase deficiency in cats	N	↑↑	↑	↑ or N	N
Primary hypercholesterolaemia in cats	↑	N	–	↑	N
Secondary					
High dietary fat intake	↑	N or ↑	–	N	↑
Cholestasis	↑	N	–	N	↑
Nephrotic syndrome/protein-losing nephropathy	↑	N or ↑	–	–	–
Hypothyroidism	↑	N or ↑	–	N or ↑	↑
Hyperadrenocorticism	N or ↑	↑	–	↑	N
Diabetes mellitus	↑	↑	–	↑	↑

28.5 Main causes of hyperlipidaemia and associated lipid/lipoprotein abnormalities. N = normal concentration; ↑ = increased concentration; ↑↑ = markedly increased concentration; – = unknown/not reported.

impaired lipoprotein removal from the circulation have been shown to play a role in the development of hyperlipidaemia.

Cholestasis is frequently associated with marked hypercholesterolaemia, due to the appearance in the circulation of an abnormal lipoprotein called Lp-X (Danielsson et al., 1976). Hypercholesterolaemia is also a recognized abnormality of nephrotic syndrome/protein-losing nephropathy, where it occurs as a direct consequence of hypoalbuminaemia. The mechanism(s) behind this is unclear, but may be a part of a more generalized response to reduced oncotic pressure (Marsh, 1996).

Hyperlipidaemia has also been reported following the administration of drugs such as corticosteroids, potassium bromide, phenobarbital, phenytoin and megestrol.

Primary hyperlipidaemia

Compared with humans, there have been relatively few reports of primary hyperlipidaemias in dogs and cats. This is not necessarily a reflection of a significantly lower incidence in these species but is probably, at least in part, a result of a much lower rate of diagnosis. The best characterized primary hyperlipidaemia in the dog is that of the Miniature Schnauzer; this condition has a clearly established familial basis (Rogers et al., 1975a) a remarkably high incidence, and a prevalence that increases with age (Xenoulis et al., 2007; Mori et al., 2010).

There have been some reports of familial conditions in other breeds, although the underlying defect has yet to be determined in any of them. Familial hypercholesterolaemia associated with an increase in HDL concentrations, presumed to be HDL$_c$, has been reported in the Briard (Watson et al., 1993). An increased incidence of hypercholesterolaemia has been reported in Shetland Sheepdogs in Japan, with affected animals showing an increase in HDL$_c$ on electrophoresis (Sato et al., 2000; Mori et al., 2010). Hypercholesterolaemia associated with an increase in HDL$_c$ has also been reported in five related Rough Collies (Jeusette et al., 2004). Familial hypercholesterolaemia with hypertriacylglycerolaemia has been reported in Beagles (Wada et al., 1977).

There are far fewer reports of primary hyperlipidaemia in the cat. Hyperchylomicronaemia as a result of LPL deficiency has been reported in an inbred colony of cats, and the defect has been fully characterized at a molecular level (Jones et al., 1983; Ginzinger et al., 1996). Transient chylomicronaemia has been reported in kittens (Watson et al., 1992; Gunn-Moore et al., 1997). Signs in these animals resolved after weaning and triacylglycerol concentration returned to reference intervals. The exact nature of the defect in these animals is not entirely clear, although there appears to be a clear familial element. A recent study has demonstrated delayed triacylglycerol clearance during an oral fat tolerance test in some Australian Burmese cats, which is suggested to reflect an inborn error of lipid metabolism (Kluger et al., 2009, Kluger et al., 2010).

Clinical manifestations of hyperlipidaemia

In the past, hyperlipidaemias were often considered to be relatively benign conditions in the dog and cat. However, it is apparent that some forms of hyperlipidaemia may predispose the animal to the development of secondary diseases of a potentially more serious nature. Hypertriacylglycerolaemia is a known risk factor for pancreatitis in humans and presumably also in dogs and cats. Both hypercholesterolaemia and hypertriacylglycerolaemia predispose animals to the development of corneal lipidosis (Crispin, 2002; Dodkin, 2009), although other factors also play an important role. Profound hypercholesterolaemia may also cause atherosclerosis in the dog, although this is uncommon as this species appears highly resistant to its development (Mahley et al., 1976). Atherosclerosis has only been convincingly reported in a small number of dogs with hypothyroidism or diabetes mellitus where marked hypercholesterolaemia was also present (Hess et al., 2003). There are some reports of neurological signs associated with hyperlipoproteinaemia, although the evidence for this seems largely anecdotal (Xenoulis and Steiner, 2010).

Management and treatment

Secondary hyperlipidaemias should resolve once the underlying disease has been diagnosed and treated. Dietary or medical treatment of primary or idiopathic hyperlipidaemia may be indicated to decrease the risk of complications. It has been suggested that treatment should aim to maintain circulating triacylglycerol concentration at <5.65 mmol/l (Ford, 1996; Whitney, 1992), and cholesterol concentration at <13 mmol/l (Xenoulis and Steiner, 2010).

Initial treatment of hypertriacylglycerolaemia (hypertriglyceridaemia) typically involves dietary modification, with a low-fat diet containing <20 g fat per 1000 kcal of recommended daily intake (Ford, 1996). Fish oil supplementation (omega-3 fatty acids) has also been shown to reduce triacylglycerol concentrations in healthy dogs, with no major side effects (LeBlanc et al., 2005), but the efficacy of this treatment in hyperlipidaemic animals is unclear.

In instances where dietary modification is ineffective, medical management may be considered. Fibric acid derivatives (gemfibrozil) at a fixed dose of 200 mg/day/dog orally, and niacin at 25–100 mg/day/dog orally have been used in the treatment of canine hypertriaclyglycerolaemia (Bauer, 1995). Fibre supplements (chitin, chitosan), and HMG CoA-reductase inhibitors ('statins') have been developed for the treatment of hypercholesterolaemia in human patients and have been used empirically in dogs. However, canine or feline studies on the efficacy and safety of these lipid-lowering drugs have not yet been published.

References and further reading

Barrie J, Watson TDG, Stear MJ *et al.* (1993) Plasma cholesterol and lipoprotein concentrations in the dog: The effects of age, breed, gender and endocrine disease. *Journal of Small Animal Practice* **34**, 507–512

Bauer JE (1995) Evaluation and dietary considerations in idiopathic hyperlipidemia in dogs. *Journal of the American Veterinary Medical Association* **206**, 1684–1688

Crispin S (2002) Ocular lipid deposits and hyperlipoproteinaemia. *Progress in Retinal and Eye Research* **21**, 169–224

Danielsson B, Ekman R, Johansson BG *et al.* (1976) Abnormal low density plasma lipoproteins occurring in dogs with obstructive jaundice. *FEBS Letters* **63**, 33–36

Dixon RM, Reid SW and Mooney CT (1999) Epidemiological, clinical, haematological and biochemical characteristics of canine hypothyroidism. *Veterinary Record* **145**, 481–487

Dodkin SJ (2009) Ocular lipid deposition in the dog – the use of lipoprotein electrophoresis to identify underlying lipoprotein abnormalities. *BSAVA Congress Scientific Proceedings: Veterinary Programme*, p. 454

Duncan J (2005) Laboratory evaluation of lipid disorders. In: *BSAVA Manual of Canine and Feline Clinical Pathology, 2nd edn*, ed. E. Villiers and L. Blackwood, pp. 241–247. BSAVA Publications, Gloucester

Ford RB (1996) Clinical management of lipemic patients. *Compendium on Continuing Education for the Practicing Veterinarian* **18**, 1053–1060

Fugier C, Tousaint JJ, Prieur X *et al.* (2006) The lipoprotein lipase inhibitor ANGPTL3 is negatively regulated by thyroid hormone. *Journal of Biological Chemistry* **281**, 1153–1159

Ginzinger DG, Lewis MES, Ma Y *et al.* (1996) A mutation in the lipoprotein lipase gene is the molecular basis of chylomicronemia in a colony of domestic cats. *Journal of Clinical Investigation* **97**, 1257–1266

Gunn-Moore DA, Watson TDG, Dodkin SJ *et al.* (1997) Transient hyperlipidaemia and anaemia in kittens. *Veterinary Record* **140**, 355–359

Hess RS, Kass PH and Van Winkle TJ (2003) Association between diabetes mellitus, hypothyroidism, and atherosclerosis in dogs. *Journal of Veterinary Internal Medicine* **17**, 489–494

Huang HP, Yang HL, Liang SL *et al.* (1999) Iatrogenic hyperadrenocorticism in 28 dogs. *Journal of the American Animal Hospital Association* **35**, 200–207

Jeusette I, Grauwels M, Cuvelier C *et al.* (2004) Hypercholesterolaemia in a family of rough collie dogs. *Journal of Small Animal Practice* **45**, 319–324

Jones BR, Wallace A, Harding DR *et al.* (1983) Occurrence of idiopathic, familial hyperchylomicronaemia in a cat. *Veterinary Record* **112**, 543–547

Kluger EK, Caslake M, Baral RM *et al.* (2010) Preliminary post-prandial studies of Burmese cats with elevated triglyceride concentrations and/or presumed lipid aqueous. *Journal of Feline Medicine and Surgery* **12**, 621–630

Kluger EK, Hardman C, Govendir M *et al.* (2009) Triglyceride response following an oral fat tolerance test in Burmese cats, other pedigree cats and domestic crossbred cats. *Journal of Feline Medicine and Surgery* **11**, 82–90

LeBlanc CJ, Bauer JE, Hosgood G *et al.* (2005) Effects of dietary fish oil and vitamin E supplementation on hematologic and serum biochemical analytes and oxidative status in young dogs. *Veterinary Therapeutics* **6**, 325–340

Mahley R, Nelson AW, Ferrans VJ *et al.* (1976) Thrombosis in association with atherosclerosis induced by dietary perturbations in dogs. *Science* **192**, 1139–1141

Marsh JB (1996) Lipoprotein metabolism in experimental nephrosis. *Proceedings of the Society for Experimental Biology and Medicine* **213**, 178–186

Mori N, Lee P, Muranaka S *et al.* (2010) Predisposition for primary hyperlipidaemia in Miniature Schnauzers and Shetland sheepdogs as compared to other canine breeds. *Research in Veterinary Science* **88**, 394–399

Prieur X, Huby T, Coste H *et al.* (2005) Thyroid hormone regulates the hypotriglyceridemic gene APOA5. *Journal of Biological Chemistry* **280**, 27533–27543

Rogers WA, Donovan EF and Kociba GJ (1975a) Idiopathic hyperlipoproteinemia in dogs. *Journal of the American Veterinary Medical Association* **166**, 1087–1091

Rogers WA, Donovan EF and Kociba GJ (1975b) Lipids and lipoproteins in normal dogs and in dogs with secondary hyperlipoproteinemia. *Journal of the American Veterinary Medical Association* **166**, 1092–1100

Sato K, Agoh H, Kaneshige T *et al.* (2000) Hypercholesterolemia in Shetland sheepdogs. *Journal of Veterinary Medical Science* **62**, 1297–1301

Wada M, Minamisono T, Ehrhart LA *et al.* (1977) Familial hyperlipoproteinemia in beagles. *Life Sciences* **20**, 999–1008

Watson P, Simpson KW and Bedford PGC (1993) Hypercholesterolaemia in Briards in the United Kingdom. *Research in Veterinary Science* **54**, 80–85

Watson TDG, Gaffney D, Mooney CT *et al.* (1992) Inherited hyperchylomicronaemia in the cat: Investigations of lipoprotein lipase function and gene structure. *Journal of Small Animal Practice* **33**, 207–212

Whitney MS (1992) Evaluation of hyperlipidemias in dogs and cats. *Seminars in Veterinary Medicine and Surgery (Small Animal)* **7**, 292–300

Wilson DE, Chan IF, Elstad NL *et al.* (1986) Apolipoprotein E-containing lipoproteins and lipoprotein remnants in experimental canine diabetes. *Diabetes* **35**, 933–942

Xenoulis PG and Steiner JM (2010) Lipid metabolism and hyperlipidaemia in dogs. *The Veterinary Journal* **183**, 12–21

Xenoulis PG, Suchodolski JS, Levinski MD *et al.* (2007) Investigation of hypertriglyceridemia in healthy Miniature Schnauzers. *Journal of Veterinary Internal Medicine* **21**, 1224–1230

Index

Page numbers in *italic* refer to figures.

Index

Index

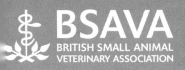

BSAVA Manual of
Canine and Feline
Clinical
Pathology
Second edition

Edited by

Elizabeth Villiers and Laura Blackwood

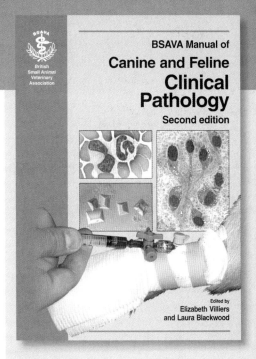

The BSAVA *Manual of Canine and Feline Clinical Pathology* provides a truly useful and accessible resource for clinicians, clinical pathologists and veterinary students. It answers the essential questions:

- which tests to do
- how to do them
- how to get the best samples
- how to interpret the results.

Clinical case examples are included throughout to illustrate how test selection and interpretation are used. Cytology is covered in a large chapter that reviews both sampling and interpretation. Chapters on body cavity effusions, CSF analysis, joint and muscle disease and skin disorders include both biochemical and cytological information. Quick reference appendices provide summaries of the samples required for common tests and list differential diagnoses for many of the abnormalities discussed in detail elsewhere in the book. Colour illustrations throughout enable the reader to identify normal and abnormal blood cells and cytological changes in a range of conditions.

Contributors:
Joy Archer, UK; Laura Blackwood, UK; Sue Dawson, UK; Emma Dewhurst, UK; Joan Duncan, UK; John Dunn, UK; Gary England, UK; Derek Flaherty, UK; Kathleen Freeman, UK; Karen Gerber, UK; Alex German, UK; Peter Graham, UK; Edward Hall, UK; Mike Herrtage, UK; John Innes, UK; Tim Jagger, UK; Clare Knottenbelt, UK; Yvonne McGrotty, UK; Richard Mellanby, UK; Carmel Mooney, Republic of Ireland; Kate Murphy, UK; Tim Nuttall, UK; Natasha Olby, USA; Kostas Papasouliotis, UK; Alan Radford, UK; Ian Ramsey, UK; Marco Russo, Italy; Barbara Skelly, UK; Richard Squires, New Zealand; Tracy Stokol, USA; Kathleen Tennant, UK; Elizabeth Villiers, UK; Penny Watson, UK.

Contents:
Making the most of in-clinic and external laboratory testing; Interpretation of laboratory data; Introduction to haematology; Disorders of erythrocytes; Disorders of leucocytes; Disorders of haemostasis; Disorders of plasma proteins; Electrolyte imbalances; Blood gas analysis and acid-base disorders; Urine analysis; Laboratory evaluation of renal disorders; Laboratory evaluation of hepatic disease; Laboratory evaluation of gastrointestinal disease; Laboratory evaluation of exocrine pancreatic disease; Laboratory evaluation of lipid disorders; Laboratory evaluation of hyperglycaemia and hypoglycaemia; Laboratory evaluation of hypothyroidism and hyperthyroidism; Laboratory diagnosis of adrenal diseases; Laboratory evaluation of the reproductive system; Diagnostic cytology; Body cavity effusions; Laboratory evaluation of joint and muscle diseases; Laboratory evaluation of cerebrospinal fluid; Laboratory evaluation of skin and ear disease; Diagnosis of bacterial, fungal and mycobacterial diseases; Diagnosis of viral infections; Diagnosis of protozoal and arthropod-borne disease; References and further reading; Appendices; Index.

Published 2005
464 pages
ISBN   978 0 905214 79 5

Price to non-members: £89.00

MEMBER PRICE: £50.00

ORDERING DETAILS

British Small Animal Veterinary Association
Woodrow House, 1 Telford Way, Waterwells Business Park, Quedgeley, Gloucester GL2 2AB

Tel: 01452 726700
Fax: 01452 726701
Email: administration@bsava.com
Web: www.bsava.com

BSAVA reserves the right to change these prices at any time

**Order online at
www.bsava.com
to save on P&P**

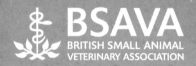

BSAVA Manual of
Canine and Feline
Oncology
Third edition

Edited by
Jane M. Dobson
B. Duncan X. Lascelles

Building on the success of previous editions, the Editors have sought to marry the best of the old with the new. All chapters have been updated or rewritten by international experts to encompass the important advances made over recent years, while keeping the text practical and user-friendly.

The Manual begins by outlining the principles of diagnostics and clinical staging and the main therapeutic modalities. Individual tumour types in the body systems of dogs and cats are then described, using a common approach to aid information retrieval on aetiology and pathogenesis, presentation and clinical signs (including staging/grading of tumours), management and prognosis.

A wealth of new photographs has been included to illustrate the clinical, diagnostic and therapeutic aspects of a range of tumours. The growing importance of ethical considerations and palliative care are also recognized, and exciting developments and treatment possibilities explored.

Contents:

Published January 2011
376 pages
ISBN   978 1 905319 21 3

Price to non-members: £85.00
MEMBER PRICE: £55.00

Order online at
www.bsava.com
to save on P&P

ORDERING DETAILS

British Small Animal Veterinary Association
Woodrow House, 1 Telford Way, Waterwells Business Park, Quedgeley, Gloucester GL2 2AB

Tel: 01452 726700
Fax: 01452 726701
Email: administration@bsava.com
Web: www.bsava.com

BSAVA reserves the right to change these prices at any time